Current Trends in Lifestyle Psychiatry

Current Trends in Lifestyle Psychiatry

Edited by Rachel Hughes

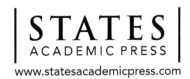

www.statesacademicpress.com

States Academic Press,
109 South 5th Street,
Brooklyn, NY 11249, USA

Visit us on the World Wide Web at:
www.statesacademicpress.com

ISBN: 978-1-63989-762-9

Trademark Notice: Registered trademark of products or corporate names are used only for explanation and identification without intent to infringe.

Cataloging-in-Publication Data

Current trends in lifestyle psychiatry / edited by Rachel Hughes.
p. cm.
Includes bibliographical references and index.
ISBN 978-1-63989-762-9
1. Psychiatry. 2. Mental illness--Treatment. 3. Physical therapy.
4. Diet therapy. 5. Lifestyles. 6. Health behavior. I. Hughes, Rachel.
RC454 .C87 2023
616.89--dc23

Table of Contents

the First Wave of the COVID-19 Pandemic**..203
Yanping Duan, D. L. I. H. K. Peiris, Min Yang, Wei Liang,
Julien Steven Baker, Chun Hu and Borui Shang

Chapter 24   **Experiment *in vivo*: How COVID-19 Lifestyle Modifications
Affect Migraine**..214
Vesselina Grozeva, Ane Mínguez-Olaondo and Marta Vila-Pueyo

Chapter 25   **Mental Disorders, Cognitive Impairment and the Risk of Suicide in
Older Adults**...219
Agnieszka Kułak-Bejda, Grzegorz Bejda and Napoleon Waszkiewicz

              Permissions

              List of Contributors

              Index

Preface

This book aims to highlight the current researches and provides a platform to further the scope of innovations in this area. This book is a product of the combined efforts of many researchers and scientists, after going through thorough studies and analysis from different parts of the world. The objective of this book is to provide the readers with the latest information of the field.

Psychiatry refers to an area of medicine concerned with the diagnosis, prevention and management of behavioral, emotional and mental disorders. There are various types of psychiatric conditions and disorders such as depression, dissociative disorders, neurodevelopmental disorders, anxiety disorders, paraphilic disorders, and bipolar disorder. Maintaining a good lifestyle is critical for the overall physical and mental well-being of any person, which can be achieved through exercise, good nutrition, work-life balance, and getting enough sleep. Lifestyle psychiatry deals with the treatment of psychiatric disorders that are a result of unhealthy lifestyle choices. In order to assist people in managing their psychiatric disorders, it uses an integrated and holistic approach to health, which includes suggestions for sleep, exercise, practicing mindfulness, and nutritious diet. It also entails incorporating techniques such as meditation, yoga, and tai chi, which are known to help prevent and lessen the symptoms of mental illness. This book aims to shed light on some of the unexplored aspects of lifestyle psychiatry and the recent researches in this field. Those in search of information to further their knowledge will be greatly assisted by it.

I would like to express my sincere thanks to the authors for their dedicated efforts in the completion of this book. I acknowledge the efforts of the publisher for providing constant support. Lastly, I would like to thank my family for their support in all academic endeavors.

Editor

Effects of Occupational Fatigue on Cognitive Performance of Staff from a Train Operating Company

Jialin Fan[1,2] and Andrew P. Smith[2]*

[1] School of Psychology, Shenzhen University, Shenzhen, China, [2] Centre for Occupational and Health Psychology, School of Psychology, Cardiff University, Cardiff, United Kingdom

Correspondence:
Andrew P. Smith
SmithAP@Cardiff.ac.uk

Background: Occupational fatigue is a key issue in the rail industry that can endanger staff, passenger, and train safety. There is a need to demonstrate the relationship between workload, fatigue, and performance among rail staff.

Objective: The present study, conducted in the workplace in realistic situations, integrating both subjective and objective measurements, aimed at demonstrating the relationship between workload, fatigue, and cognitive performance with a rail staff sample.

Methods: The "After-Effect" technique was applied in the current study. Online diaries and cognitive performance tasks were used to assess the fatigue, work experiences, and performance of rail staff before and after work on the first and last days of one working week.

Results: Reported fatigue was greater after work on both the first and last day of the working week. There were large individual differences in the change in fatigue and workload ratings. Analysis of covariance with age and the pre-work performance score as covariates and the post-work performance score as the dependent variable showed that high levels of fatigue were associated with impaired performance on both the visual search and logical reasoning tasks. Workload had fewer effects on performance than fatigue.

Conclusion: This field study provided evidence for the relationship between work-related fatigue and performance impairment. The findings show the need for future work on predicting fatigue-related performance decrements, and the necessity of providing interventions and support so that the risk to safety can be reduced.

Keywords: occupational fatigue, rail industry, rail staff, field study, performance

INTRODUCTION

Fatigue is often an indicator of an unhealthy lifestyle. It has found to be associated with higher probability of illness and injury in the workplace (Harma et al., 1998, 2002; Chau et al., 2008). Fatigue is synonymous with a generalized stress response over time. Occupational fatigue may occur during or after work; it may also occur before work when the worker has not fully recovered from previous fatigue through the regular periods of rest before the onset of the next set of demands (Cameron, 1973). It has been found to be associated with impaired cognitive performance, including increased reaction time, decreased vigilance, perceptual and cognitive distortions (reviewed in Krueger, 1989), dropped skill effectiveness (Drew, 1940). Fatigue also leads to impaired memory and information processing (Craig and Cooper, 1992), reductions in concentration, motivation, and activity (Beurskens et al., 2000). In addition, fatigue may impair the sense of agency (i.e., the loss of the sense of being responsible for own's actions; Howard et al., 2016), which increases the safety risks in the workplace. In particular, previous studies show that human agency was reduced by increased out of the loop events which could be associated with fatigue, and decreased control or increased automation in the environment (Berberian et al., 2012; Kumar and Srinivasan, 2012, 2013; Moore, 2016; Di Plinio et al., 2019, 2020). Such effects may also show inter-individual differences (Di Plinio et al., 2019) and also vary with cultural background (Barlas and Obhi, 2014).

In the railway industry, occupational fatigue is a severe problem which jeopardizes not only the staff health but also train and passenger safety, as most jobs are safety-critical. Evidence for fatigue among rail staff has been found in previous studies, in which various methods have been used, including surveys (Cotrim et al., 2017; Fan and Smith, 2017), incident reports (reviewed in Buck and Lamonde, 1993; Ugajin, 1999; Fan and Smith, 2018), simulated driving studies (Dorrian et al., 2007), and interviews (Filtness and Naweed, 2017). In particular, fatigue is considered to be a causal or contributory factor in the majority of train accident and incident investigation reports (British Rail Safety and Standards Board, 2005; British Rail Accident Investigation Branch, 2008, 2010). Fatigue, its impact on task performance, and fatigue-related human errors have been found in previous research in several different transport sectors (e.g., road drivers: Feyer and Williamson, 2001; seafarers: Smith et al., 2006), and has also been suggested as a key issue for train safety (Bowler and Gibbon, 2015). However, the field of rail fatigue research was historically smaller than that of other transport sectors, and the investigation of the effect of fatigue on performance in real time in the workplace is still lacking in this industry.

The causes of occupational fatigue can emanate from either inside or outside the workplace, and mainly include task-related factors and sleep-related factors. Jobs in the rail industry were designed to operate on a 24/7 basis, often with an irregular schedule. A large-scale study (Fan and Smith, 2017) identified the main predictors of fatigue in the rail industry as high job demands (i.e., workload), shift-work, poor job control and support, and noise and vibration in the working environment. Shift work, especially the night and early morning shifts, disrupts the sleep–wake cycle (Ferguson et al., 2008) and deprives workers of sleep (Åkerstedt, 1991). Shift workers have little time to recover when working certain shift hours, which makes them more likely to suffer from cumulative fatigue (Åhsberg et al., 2000). Moreover, Dorrian et al. (2011) indicated that in addition to work hours and sleep length, workload significantly influenced fatigue among train crew. It is notable that mental workload is the major

problem in the modern railway industry rather than traditional physical workload, due to the increasing level of automation in operating systems (Young et al., 2015; Fan and Smith, 2019). The majority of job tasks in this modern industry require more cognitive demands (e.g., selective attention, sustained vigilance), resulting in a heavy mental workload and increased fatigue; meanwhile, fatigue is associated with a deterioration of attention and impaired performance. Failure to maintain such performance at an acceptable level brings danger, especially to those working in safety-critical job roles.

Subjective measurement of fatigue has been validated as a reliable way to distinguish between fatigued and non-fatigued staff (e.g., Chalder et al., 1993; Kim et al., 2010), and this is widely used in different types of job disciplines, both within (Kishida, 1991) and between industries (Kogi et al., 1970; Beurskens et al., 2000). Recently, however, Cheng and Hui-Ning (2019) argued that the ability of rail staff to perceive their own fatigue could be limited, which may due to sleep debt and cumulative sleep loss, particularly following a string of atypical shifts (night or early morning shift). Therefore, it is important to also include objective measurement of fatigue and performance which can be used in the work situation along with subjective measurement to reducing potential subjective biases. However, it can be a challenge to apply certain objective measurements in the railway environment. Railway companies usually have their own rules regarding staff uniforms for consistency and safety, which means that wearing extra instruments for objective measurement, such as Electroencephalography (EEG) or eye-tracking equipment, is not allowed in the workplace, as it may cause distractions and other potential safety risks.

Broadbent (1979) suggested that using the "After-Effect" technique in fatigue measurement could be applicable in realistic situations. This involves measuring performance before and after a specific task or work period, without changing people's normal behaviors during and after the task. The after-effect symptoms of fatigue usually include longer reaction times and reduced accuracy. In the work context, the After-Effect method compares the difference in performance before and after work, and a greater difference reflects a greater effect. This method has already been widely used in workload studies (e.g., Parkes, 1995; Hockey and Earle, 2006). For instance, workload study Parkes's (1995) found that reaction time and accuracy in search tasks and logical reasoning ability showed clear impairments due to the effect of higher workload. It has also been used to assess other factors which contribute to fatigue, such as the common cold (Smith et al., 2000), caffeine (Brice and Smith, 2001; Smith, 2002; Doherty and Smith, 2005), and night work (Åkerstedt, 1988). Recently, Smith and Smith (2017) used the After-Effect method to assess rail engineers' fatigue and performance on the first and last day of the work week and showed that the extent of fatigue could be identified using this methodology.

Online fatigue measures could be a more appropriate tool for detecting fatigue in the workplace due to their convenience and low development cost. Online cognitive tests have been used for the past two decades, and a review of them confirmed their ability to provide realistic simulations of cognitive tasks in daily life, which is the main advantage of computerized cognitive evaluation (see Crook et al., 2009). It is possible for online measures to be used in the workplace and they are often more convenient than offline tests or the use of measures from laboratory experiments. One fatigue study with students, which used a methodology that combined the After-Effect method and online cognitive performance tasks to measure fatigue in a real-life setting (Fan and Smith, 2017), established the relationship between workload, fatigue, and cognitive performance. This study showed that workload increased subjective fatigue after work which then resulted in cognitive performance impairments, including slower reaction time and decreased accuracy, while the effect of time of day on performance was not found significant. However, this study consisted of undergraduate students with risk factors for fatigue due to their study life at university, which are different from fatigue in the actual work life of the railway industry. Thus, a further experiment based on a staff sample is needed.

The present study aimed to use this same methodology to demonstrate the relationship between workload, fatigue, and objective performance with staff from a train operating company. The company was interested in generic fatigue across a range of jobs. Other research has adopted the present approach to study train drivers (Evans, 2019), conductors, guards, and engineers (Smith and Smith, 2017). The methods used in this study consisted of a self-assessment diary, mainly used to record ratings of fatigue and workload, and also objective performance tests. The experimental hypothesis for this study predicted that an increased feeling of fatigue would lead to performance reduction, including delayed reaction time, and lower accuracy rates in both visual search and logical reasoning tests. This methodology was also used to examine whether the effects of fatigue and workload were different.

MATERIALS AND METHODS

Participants

This study recruited participants with different types of jobs from volunteers from a train company in the *United Kingdom* [N = 19, mean (± SD) age = 41.86 ± 9.89 yrs.; 74% male], as all job types may be susceptible to fatigue (Fan and Smith, 2017). The main job types reported were managers, conductors, drivers, station workers, engineers, and administrators. Selection of different job types meant that any obtained results could be generalized across occupations. Participants were fit for work but no other data was collected on health status.

Procedure

This study included four sessions in total, requiring participants to complete the diary and the tests immediately before starting work, and immediately after finishing work on the first and fourth days of a working week. For example, if one participant was off-work on Tuesday and Wednesday, and then worked the following four continuous days, this participants would complete the diary on Thursday (the first day of his or her working week) and on Sunday (the last day of his or her working week). An invitation e-mail with attached information about the study and

an informed consent form was sent to potential participants. Once participants had signed and returned the forms, they were asked to provide the start date of their next work week with four continuous days of working. The links to the four test sections and a familiarization session were then sent to them. The familiarization session included an introduction to the diary and an example of each cognitive task to ensure that the participants were able to complete the tasks correctly before starting the study. On the testing day(s), participants were asked to complete the online diary and cognitive tasks immediately before starting work and immediately after finishing work via a computer or mobile phone.

Participants were free to withdraw from the survey at any point. This study was reviewed and approved by the School of Psychology Research Ethics Committee at Cardiff University and carried out with the informed consent of the volunteers.

Materials

The materials used in this study included a diary and two online cognitive tasks and took about 15 min to complete. These online measures required assessment by mobile phone or computer, and participants responded by touching the screen (if using mobile phone) or clicking on the mouse (if using the computer). All the tasks and data collection were via the Qualtrics online survey platform.

Diary

The diary was used to measure fatigue and the causes of fatigue. It consisted of 15 single-item questions, including six questions to be answered before work and nine questions to be answered after work. **Supplementary Table 1** (in **Supplementary Material**) shows the details of the diary questionnaire. It was designed based on the material used in Smith and Smith's (2017) diary studies, and majority questions were on a 10-point scale. The questions in the pre-work diary covered sleep duration and quality, commute time, fatigue due to the commute, general health status, and alertness before starting work. The questions in the post-work diary recorded workload, effort, fatigue, stress, break duration, work duration, time of work completion, and level of distraction during work. There were extra questions in the post-work diary on the last day, which asked whether the participants had worked at the same time every workday during the working week; if participants answered no, they were asked about their working time for each day.

Online Cognitive Tasks

Two online cognitive tasks were used to assess objective performance in each session: a visual search and a logical reasoning task. These two tests have been widely used in previous workload (e.g., Parkes, 1995) and fatigue studies (e.g., Lamond and Dawson, 1999; Barker and Nussbaum, 2011). The online version of such tests was validated in our previous study with the student sample (Fan and Smith, 2017; Fan, 2019). **Supplementary Figures 1, 2** (in **Supplementary Material**) shows the example of a trial of each task. For both tasks, the inter-trial intervals were 500 ms. The tasks were distributed and the data collection was completed via the Qualtrics online survey platform. Participant would assess the task using either computer or mobile phone, responding by clicking mouse or tapping touch screen.

The visual search task consisted of 12 trials, which randomly appeared from a total of 30 possible trials. In each trial, participants were randomly shown a 60-letter set and one target letter. They were required to find and click the target letter as quickly and accurately as possible on the screen. The response time and accuracy for each trial were recorded.

The logical reasoning task consisted of 24 trials and required the participants to make a decision between two options as quickly and accurately as possible. This test was based on Baddeley's (1968) grammatical reasoning test. The outcome measures were response time and accuracy.

ANALYSIS

Both the diary and the cognitive tasks were presented online using the Qualtrics software package. The diary and performance data were then downloaded into a single SPSS data file. Analysis was carried out using the IBM SPSS 25 package. The main focus of the analysis was on the associations between fatigue and workload and changes in performance over the day. Analyses of covariance with the pre-work measures and age as covariates, and the post-work performance scores as dependent variables were carried out. Fatigue and workload change scores were split into high and low groups (based on the median of scores from these questions in the diary) and these were the between subject factors in the analyses of covariance. Fan and Smith (2017), in a study of university students, found that fatigue reduced visual search accuracy and led to slower logical reasoning speed. Workload had no significant effects. One-tail significance levels were used where the two tailed level was not significant, as it was predicted that high fatigue and high workload would be associated with impaired performance seen in the Fan and Smith (2017) study.

RESULTS

The Sample

Nineteen participants, 14 of whom were male, completed the whole study. The most common job types reported were managers (26.3%), engineers (15.8%), conductors (15.8%), drivers (15.8%), and station workers (15.8%), followed by administrators (10.5%). Most participants did daytime shifts (68.4%), while 31.6% did night shifts (begin between the hours of 7:00 p.m. and 12:00 a.m.) or early morning shifts (begin between the hours of 12:00 a.m. and 6:00 a.m.). Nearly half (43.1%) of the participants worked two or more different shift times during the testing week (4 days).

Fatigue and Workload Ratings

The descriptive statistics for the fatigue ratings and the performance tasks, are shown for pre-work and post work on the first and last day of the working week in **Table 1**.

On the first working day, fatigue ratings showed a large increase over the day (pre-work mean = 2.16; post-work

mean = 6.42). There was considerable variation across individuals with the increase in fatigue having a range from 0 to 800%. A similar profile was seen for the last working day (pre-work mean: 2.47; post-work mean = 7.11), and again there were large individual differences in the change of fatigue over the day (range = −14–900%). Workload ratings were consistent across days (Day 1: mean = 5.79, SD = 2.18; Day 4: mean = 5.42, SD = 2.43) and showed large individual differences (Day 1: range = 1–9; Day 4: range = 1–9).

Changes in fatigue over the day were correlated with age (Day 1: $r = 0.73$, $p < 0.001$). On the last day increased fatigue was associated with greater distraction due to thinking about other things ($r = 0.49$, $p < 0.05$). Workload ratings were associated with ratings of effort ($r = 0.61$, $p < 0.01$), stress ($r = 0.49$, $p < 0.05$), and alertness ($r = −0.49$). These results show that fatigue and workload are different constructs which are only weakly correlated.

Changes in Fatigue, Workload and Performance Changes Over the Day

Analyses of covariance were carried out to examine associations between changes in fatigue, workload and performance after work. Changes of fatigue and workload were divided into high and low groups using a median split. Before work performance measures were covariates for the corresponding after work measure (the dependent variable). Age was also included as a covariate. It was predicted that increases of fatigue and workload would be associated with impaired performance.

On the first day, the high fatigue group had less accurate performance on the visual search task than the low fatigue group ($F = 3.78$, df = 1.13, $p = 0.037$, 1-tail, partial eta squared = 0.225). This result is shown in **Figure 1**.

Also on Day 1, the high workload group had less accurate performance on the logical reasoning task than the low workload group ($F = 5.37$, df = 1,13, $p = 0.037$, partial eta squared = 0.292). This result is shown in **Figure 2**. None of the other effects were significant.

On the last working day, the high fatigue group again had less accurate performance on the visual search task ($F = 5.84$, df = 1,13, $p = -0.031$, partial eta squared = 0.310). This is shown in **Figure 3**.

The high fatigue group were also slower than the low fatigue group on the logical reasoning task on the last day ($F = 3.38$, df = 1,13, $p < 0.045$, 1-tail, partial eta squared = 0.206). This is shown in **Figure 4**.

DISCUSSION

The present research involved a field study using online fatigue tests integrating both subjective and objective measurements, which was validated in a previous fatigue study (Fan and Smith, 2017). The design of the fatigue tests combined online methods and the After-Effect technique. This methodology was suitable and convenient to use in the workplace, especially in the railway industry where wearing

TABLE 1 | Descriptive statistics for fatigue ratings and performance tests (mean [SD]).

	Day 1 Pre-work	Day 1 Post-work	Day 4 Pre-work	Day 4 Post-work
Fatigue ratings (scale of 1–10; high scores = greater fatigue)	2.16 [1.21]	6.42 [2.12]	2.47 [1.61]	7.11 [2.00]
Visual search accuracy (% correct)	97.81 [4.68]	97.81 [4.68]	94.07 [5.77]	90.35 [8.45]
Visual search speed (s)	13.58 [3.15]	14.25 [3.00]	13.93 [3.54]	14.29 [3.06]
Logical reasoning accuracy (% correct)	74.34 [20.00]	77.63 [21.35]	74.78 [22.27]	79.39 [23.63]
Logical reasoning speed (s)	6.28 [1.73]	6.94 [2.39]	5.58 [1.40]	5.66 [1.38]

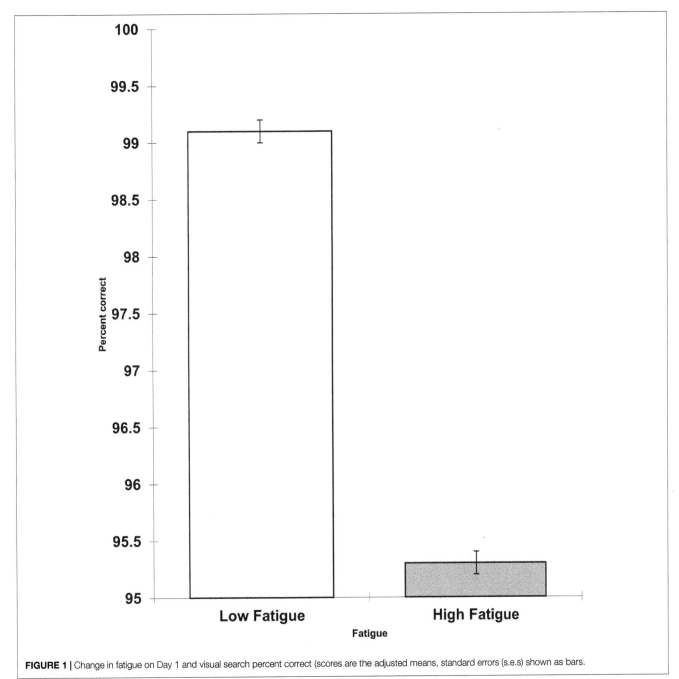

FIGURE 1 | Change in fatigue on Day 1 and visual search percent correct (scores are the adjusted means, standard errors (s.e.s) shown as bars.

extra instruments of objective measurement was not allowed, as this might create distractions and pose other potential safety risks.

Overall, the results of this study with the staff sample were in line with those of previous studies, including our study with a student sample using the same performance tasks

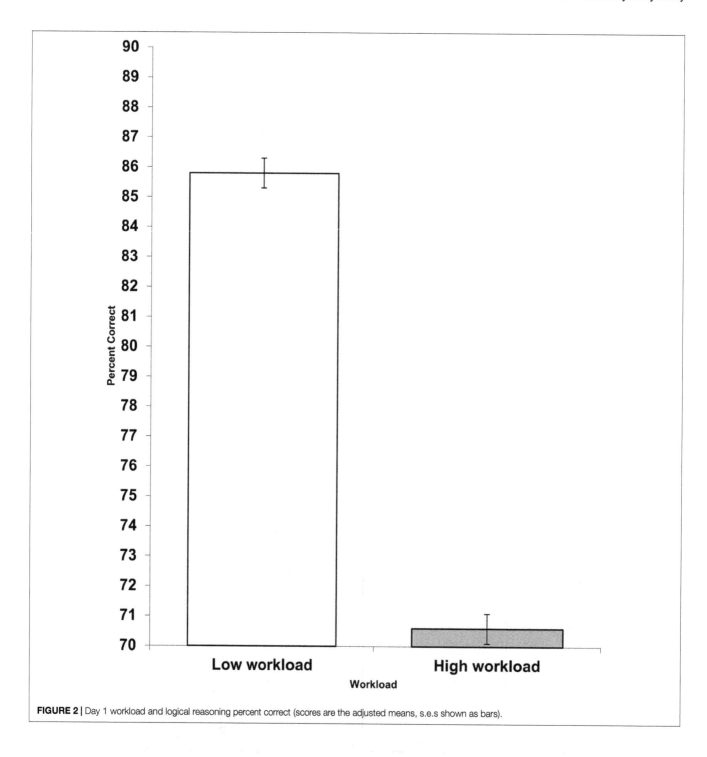

FIGURE 2 | Day 1 workload and logical reasoning percent correct (scores are the adjusted means, s.e.s shown as bars).

(Fan and Smith, 2017) and those carried out in different transport industries (Feyer and Williamson, 2001; Smith et al., 2006; Smith and Smith, 2017) which found that performance was impaired by fatigue. The effects of fatigue on cognitive performance were found with both high and low workloads. However, there was some evidence of independent effects of workload on performance speed, although such effects were less frequent than those of fatigue. In addition, subjective fatigue increased, and general outcomes got worse at the end of the week, suggesting an effect of cumulative work fatigue on outcomes throughout the

working week. This result was very similar to fatigue observed in seafarers, which increased day by day during the tour of duty and continued into leave (Bal et al., 2015).

The main hypothesis of the current study predicted that increased occupational fatigue would lead to performance reduction, including slower RT and lower accuracy rates. Comparable to our student sample study (Fan and Smith, 2017), the results here showed that an increased feeling of fatigue was associated with impaired performance, including decreased accuracy in the visual search task and slower RT in the logical

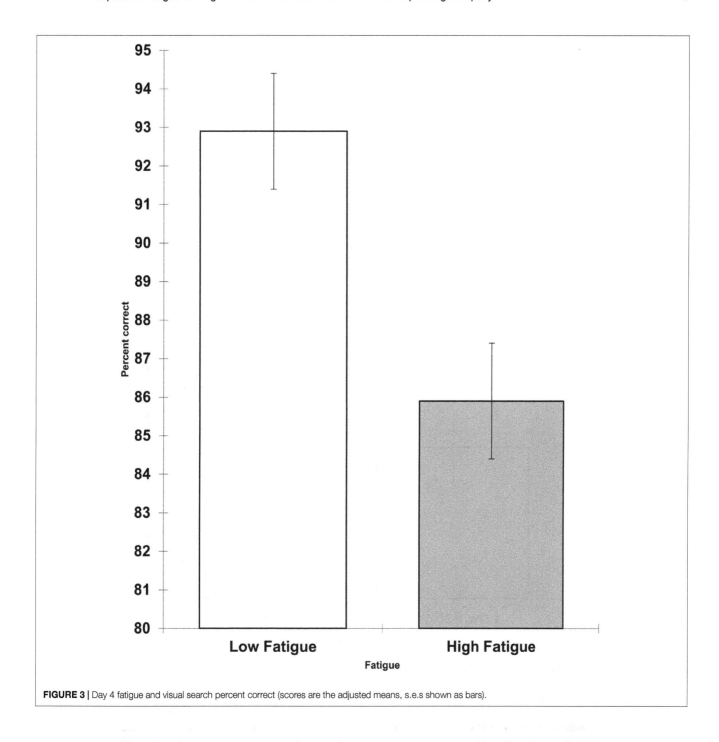

FIGURE 3 | Day 4 fatigue and visual search percent correct (scores are the adjusted means, s.e.s shown as bars).

reasoning task, which supports this hypothesis. The effects of workload were restricted to less accurate performance of the logical reasoning task on the first day.

This study was performed in the United Kingdom and the results were obtained using a United Kingdom sample, and differences in culture (Barlas and Obhi, 2014) were not relevant here. Previous studies have shown that fatigue impaired cognitive performance (e.g., Craig and Cooper, 1992; Beurskens et al., 2000), which was supported by the current study. The results from previous studies also suggest that it could be the increased fatigue, decreased control, and increased automation in the

working environment which resulted in the changed sense of agency (e.g., Berberian et al., 2012; Kumar and Srinivasan, 2012, 2013; Moore, 2016; Howard et al., 2016; Di Plinio et al., 2019, 2020). The modern railway industry has increased the level of automation in operating systems and decreased control by operators (Young et al., 2015; Fan and Smith, 2019), and future studies of fatigue in railway staff samples should focus on changes in the sense of agency.

This study investigated the effect of occupational fatigue on cognitive performance in railway staff, and its results provide insight on current practices regarding fatigue management in

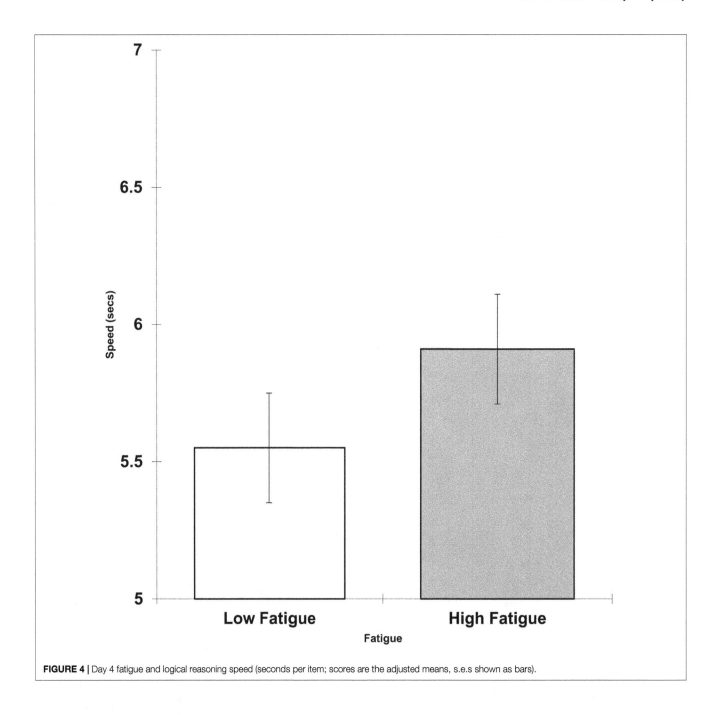

FIGURE 4 | Day 4 fatigue and logical reasoning speed (seconds per item; scores are the adjusted means, s.e.s shown as bars).

the industry. The findings allow us to offer a few suggestions for the railway industry. In general, either organizations or individuals should raise the issue of fatigue and its after-effects, and take action to prevent and manage it and related impaired performance in the workplace. The present research, in line with previous studies (e.g., Dorrian et al., 2011; Fan and Smith, 2017), indicated that workload should be considered as well as fatigue. Considering the nature of jobs in the railway industry, however, it will be not easy to control or reduce the workload, especially with the unpredictability of train problems and unplanned overtime work. Thus, companies and organizations can apply such online fatigue self-assessment and cognitive performance tasks to assess staff fatigue level before and after work. For those with no indication of fatigue, this will not change the normal working behavior of during their duty. For those with fatigue this can be prevented and managed by providing support (e.g., fatigue managing advices or intervention) during times when fatigue is likely to be at a high-risk level. Also, companies may need to improve work patterns and arrange rest times during and after work for recovery from fatigue, which reduces the risk of future fatigue-related performance impairment.

Limitations

The first sets of limitations are common in diary studies. As a method, the online diary study is less controlled than laboratory experiments, although it has the advantage of assessing the effects of fatigue in the context of participants' daily work lives, as well as being able to assess the effect of cumulative fatigue for a longer period of time than in laboratory experiments. One issue is completion of the diary at the correct time. One participant commented that he did not have time to complete the diary immediately after work because he was off very late and caught transport to return home in a hurry. Although this participant completed the post-work diary immediately upon arriving home, his fatigue and performance may have recovered during the commute. Another problem is the completion of the study. Diary studies are also time-consuming, and participants required reminders and encouragement to fully complete the diaries. In this study, it was difficult to recruit participants and have them fully complete all of the four sessions, especially the post-work diary on the last day of the work week. The majority of participants who forgot to fill in the last diary decided to quit the study rather than re-do it. This meant that the major limitation of the present study was the small sample size. The small sample size also meant that it was not possible to consider individual differences, such as job type or the personality of the participants.

Future Research

The current study was an initial trial of studying the effect of fatigue on performance in a real-life setting. There is a plan to conduct more staff experiments to further investigate the effects of fatigue on performance, as well as intervention experiments. Future research requires better control of online diary data collection. While the online diary is an advanced method for assessing fatigue closely in the context of daily work life, reminder texts or e-mails are needed to ensure that participants fill out each diary on time. The diary could be integrated with the HSE Fatigue and Risk Index (a fatigue prediction tool based on shift patterns currently used in the United Kingdom rail industry) in a future study. Although the job demands variable in this index is usually set at a constant level for all staff, it can be measured through the single-item self-assessment in the diary.

CONCLUSION

Occupational fatigue is an important issue in the rail industry and it can endanger passenger, staff and train safety. It is also important in jobs which are not safety critical as it can influence the efficiency of the organization and the health and wellbeing of staff. Our previous research has examined this issue in drivers (Evans, 2019), conductors, guards, and engineers (Smith and Smith, 2017). There is now a need to demonstrate the relationship between workload, fatigue, and performance among a wider range of staff of train operating companies. The present study was carried out in the workplace using an online methodology with both subjective and objective measurements. The aim was to examine the relationship between workload, fatigue, and cognitive performance using staff from a train operating company. The "After-Effect" technique was used with online diaries and cognitive performance tasks assessing the fatigue, work experiences, and performance of staff before and after work on the first and fourth days of one working week.

This field study provided evidence for the relationship between work-related fatigue and performance impairment. The findings show the need for future work on predicting fatigue-related performance decrements, and the necessity of providing interventions and support so that the risk to safety can be reduced. The results demonstrated that the objective performance of staff was impaired due to fatigue, shown as decreased accuracy on a visual search task and the logical reasoning task. These findings were in line with those of previous research in other work contexts. Increased fatigue was associated with higher workload, while fatigue before work was also associated with the quality and duration of sleep. Considering it is not easy to control or reduce the workload due to the nature of the jobs, the rail industry could focus instead on improving the guidelines regarding rest to manage fatigue, which would then reduce the risk of work performance impairment. Future research using an online diary should consider recruiting a larger sample and mitigating the risk of absent or incomplete diary entries.

ETHICS STATEMENT

The studies involving human participants were reviewed and approved by School of Psychology Research Ethics Committee at Cardiff University. The patients/participants provided their written informed consent to participate in this study.

AUTHOR CONTRIBUTIONS

AS formulated the research question, designed the study, and revised the manuscript for important intellectual content. JF conducted the analyses, interpreted the data, and drafted the original manuscript. Both the authors approved the final version for publication and also agreed to be held accountable for all aspects of the work in ensuring that questions related to accuracy and integrity are appropriately investigated and resolved.

ACKNOWLEDGMENTS

The main content of this paper has previously appeared in JF's Ph.D. thesis, available online in Cardiff University's institutional repository. JF would like to thank AS for his supervision and invaluable guidance in her Ph.D. journey.

REFERENCES

Åhsberg, E., Kecklund, G., Åkerstedt, T., and Gamberale, F. (2000). Shiftwork and different dimensions of fatigue. *Int. J. Ind. Ergon.* 26, 457–465. doi: 10.1016/s0169-8141(00)00007-x

Åkerstedt, T. (1988). Sleepiness as a consequence of shift work. *Sleep* 11, 17–34. doi: 10.1093/sleep/11.1.17

Åkerstedt, T. (1991). "Sleepiness at work: Effects of irregular work hours", in *Sleep, Sleepiness and Performance*, ed. T. Monk (Oxford: John Wiley & Sons), 129–152.

Baddeley, A. D. (1968). A 3 min reasoning test based on grammatical transformation. *Psychon. Sci.* 10, 341–342. doi: 10.3758/bf03331551

Bal, E., Arslan, O., and Tavacioglu, L. (2015). Prioritization of the causal factors of fatigue in seafarers and measurement of fatigue with the application of the Lactate Test. *Saf. Sci.* 72, 46–54. doi: 10.1016/j.ssci.2014.08.003

Barker, L. M., and Nussbaum, M. A. (2011). The effects of fatigue on performance in simulated nursing work. *Ergonomics* 54, 815–829. doi: 10.1080/00140139. 2011.597878

Barlas, Z., and Obhi, S. S. (2014). Cultural background influences implicit but not explicit sense of agency for the production of musical tones. *Conscious. Cogn.* 28, 94–103. doi: 10.1016/j.concog.2014.06.013

Berberian, B., Sarrazin, J. C., Le Blaye, P., and Haggard, P. (2012). Automation technology and sense of control: a window on human agency. *PLoS One* 7:e34075. doi: 10.1371/journal.pone.0034075

Beurskens, A. J., Bultmann, U., Kant, I., Vercoulen, J. H., Bleijenberg, G., and Swaen, G. M. (2000). Fatigue among working people: validity of a questionnaire measure. *Occupat. Environ. Med.* 57, 353–357. doi: 10.1136/oem.57. 5.353

Bowler, N., and Gibbon, W. H. (2015). *Fatigue and its Contribution to Railway Incidents.* Derby: British Rail Accident Investigation Branch (RAIB).

Brice, C., and Smith, A. (2001). The effects of caffeine on simulated driving, subjective alertness and sustained attention. *Hum. Psychopharmacol. Clin. Exp.* 16, 523–531. doi: 10.1002/hup.327

British Rail Accident Investigation Branch (2008). *Derailment of Two Locomotives at East Somerset Junction.* Derby: British Rail Accident Investigation Branch.

British Rail Accident Investigation Branch (2010). *Uncontrolled Freight Train Run-Back Between Shap and Tebay, Cumbria.* Derby: British Rail Accident Investigation Branch.

British Rail Safety and Standards Board (2005). *T059 Main Report: Guidelines for the Management and Reduction of Fatigue in Train Drivers.* Derby: British Rail Safety and Standards Board.

Broadbent, D. E. (1979). Is a fatigue test now possible? *Ergonomics* 22, 1277–1290. doi: 10.1080/00140137908924702

Buck, L., and Lamonde, F. (1993). Critical incidents and fatigue among locomotive engineers. *Saf. Sci.* 16, 1–18. doi: 10.1016/0925-7535(93)90003-V

Cameron, C. (1973). A theory of fatigue. *Ergonomics* 16, 633–648. doi: 10.1080/ 00140137308924554

Chalder, T., Berelowitz, G., Pawlikowska, T., Watts, L., Wessely, S., Wright, D., et al. (1993). Development of a fatigue scale. *J. Psychosom. Res.* 37, 147–153. doi: 10.1016/0022-3999(93)90081-p

Chau, N., Bourgkard, E., Bhattacherjee, A., Ravaud, J. F., Choquet, M., Mur, J. M., et al. (2008). Associations of job, living conditions and lifestyle with occupational injury in working population: a population-based study. *Int. Arch. Occupat. Environ. Health* 81, 379–389. doi: 10.1007/s00420-007-0 223-y

Cheng, Y. H., and Hui-Ning, T. (2019). Train drivers' subjective perceptions of their abilities to perceive and control fatigue. *Int. J. Occupat. Saf. Ergon.* 26, 20–36. doi: 10.1080/10803548.2019.1568726

Cotrim, T., Carvalhais, J., Neto, C., Teles, J., Noriega, P., and Rebelo, F. (2017). Determinants of sleepiness at work among railway control workers. *Appl. Ergon.* 58, 293–300. doi: 10.1016/j.apergo.2016.07.006

Craig, A., and Cooper, R. E. (1992). "Symptoms of acute and chronic fatigue," in *Handbook of Human Performance,* Vol. 3, eds A. P. Smith and D. M. Jones (London: Harcourt Brace Jovanovich), 289–339. doi: 10.1016/b978-0-12-650353-1.50017-4

Crook, T. H., Kay, G. G., and Larrabee, G. J. (2009). "Computer-based cognitive testing", in *Neuropsychological Assessment of Neuropsychiatric and Neuromedical Disorders,* eds I. Grant and K. Adams (United States: Oxford University Press), 84–100.

Di Plinio, S., Arnò, S., Perrucci, M. G., and Ebisch, S. J. H. (2019). Environmental control and psychosis-relevant traits modulate the prospective agency in non-clinical individuals. *Conscious. Cogn.* 73:102776. doi: 10.1016/j.concog.2019. 102776

Di Plinio, S., Arnò, S., Perrucci, M. G., and Ebisch, S. J. H. (2020). The evolving sense of agency: context recency and quality modulate the interaction between prospective and retrospective processes. *Conscious. Cogn.* 80:102903. doi: 10. 1016/j.concog.2020.102903

Doherty, M., and Smith, P. M. (2005). Effects of caffeine ingestion on rating of perceived exertion during and after exercise: a meta-analysis. *Scand. J. Med. Sci. Sports* 15, 69–78. doi: 10.1111/j.1600-0838.2005.00445.x

Dorrian, J., Baulk, S. D., and Dawson, D. (2011). Work hours, workload, sleep and fatigue in Australian Rail Industry employees. *Appl. Ergon.* 42, 202–209. doi: 10.1016/j.apergo.2010.06.009

Dorrian, J., Hussey, F., and Dawson, D. (2007). Train driving efficiency and safety:

examining the cost of fatigue. *J. Sleep Res.* 16, 1–11. doi: 10.1111/j.1365-2869. 2007.00563.x

Drew, G. C. (1940). *An Experimental Study of Mental Fatigue. Report No. 227.* Cambridge: Air Ministry, Flying Personnel Research Committee.

Evans, M. S. (2019). *The Development and Validity of an Objective Indicator of Fatigue for Frontline Safety Critical Workers.* PhD Thesis. Cardiff: Cardiff University.

Fan, J. (2019). *An Investigation of Rail Crew Fatigue and Well-Being.* [Doctoral dissertation]. Cardiff: Cardiff University.

Fan, J., and Smith, A. P. (2017). "The impact of workload and fatigue on performance," in *Proceedings of the International Symposium on Human Mental Workload: Models and Applications,* eds L. Longo and M. C. Leva (Cham: Springer), 90–105. doi: 10.1007/978-3-319-61061-0_6

Fan, J., and Smith, A. P. (2018). A preliminary review of fatigue among rail staff. *Front. Psychol.* 9:634. doi: 10.3389/fpsyg.2018.00634

Fan, J., and Smith, A. P. (2019). "Mental workload and other causes of different types of fatigue in rail staff," in *Proceedings of the International Symposium on Human Mental Workload: Models and Applications,* eds L. Longo and M. C. Leva (Cham: Springer), 147–159. doi: 10.1007/978-3-030-14273-5_9

Ferguson, S. A., Lamond, N., Kandelaars, K., Jay, S. M., and Dawson, D. (2008). The impact of short, irregular sleep opportunities at sea on the alertness of marine pilots working extended hours. *Chronobiol. Int.* 25, 399–411. doi: 10. 1080/07420520802106819

Feyer, A. M., and Williamson, A. M. (2001). "Broadening our view of effective solutions to commercial driver fatigue," in *Stress, Workload and Fatigue,* eds P. A. Hancock and P. A. Desmond (New York, NY: Lawrence Erlbaum), 550–565.

Filtness, A. J., and Naweed, A. (2017). Causes, consequences and countermeasures to driver fatigue in the rail industry: the train driver perspective. *Appl. Ergon.* 60, 12–21. doi: 10.1016/j.apergo.2016.10.009

Harma, M., Sallinen, M., Ranta, R., Mutanen, P., and Müller, K. (2002). The effect of an irregular shift system on sleepiness at work in train drivers and railway traffic controllers. *J. Sleep Res.* 11, 141–151. doi: 10.1046/j.1365-2869.2002.00294.x

Harma, M., Suvanto, S., Popkin, S., Pulli, K., Mulder, M., and Hirvonen, K. (1998). A dose–response study of total sleep time and the ability to maintain wakefulness. *J. Sleep Res.* 7, 167–174. doi: 10.1046/j.1365-2869.1998.00115.x

Hockey, G. R. J., and Earle, F. (2006). Control over the scheduling of simulated office work reduces the impact of workload on mental fatigue and task performance. *J. Exp. Psychol. Appl.* 12, 50–65. doi: 10.1037/1076-898x.12.1.50

Howard, E. E., Edwards, S. G., and Bayliss, A. P. (2016). Physical and mental effort disrupts the implicit sense of agency. *Cognition* 157, 114–125. doi: 10.1016/j. cognition.2016.08.018

Kim, E., Lovera, M. J., Schaben, L., Bourdette, D., and Whitham, R. (2010). Novel method for measurement of fatigue in multiple sclerosis: real-time digital fatigue score. *J. Rehabilit. Res. Dev.* 47, 477–484. doi: 10.1682/jrrd.2009.09. 0151

Kishida, K. (1991). "Workload of workers in supermarkets," in *Towards Human Work: Solutions to Problems in Occupational Health and Safety,* eds M. Kmashiro and E. D. Megaw (London: Taylor and Francis), 269–279.

Kogi, K., Saito, Y., and Mitsuhashi, T. (1970). Validity of three components of subjective fatigue feelings. *J. Sci. Lab.* 46, 251–270.

Krueger, G. P. (1989). Sustained work, fatigue, sleep loss and performance: a review of the issues. *Work Stress* 3, 129–141. doi: 10.1080/02678378908 256939

Kumar, D., and Srinivasan, N. (2012). Hierarchical event-control and subjective experience of agency. *Front. Psychol.* 3:410. doi: 10.3389/fpsyg.2012.00410

Kumar, D., and Srinivasan, N. (2013). "Hierarchical control and sense of agency: differential effects of control on implicit and explicit measures of agency," in *Proceedings of the Annual Meeting of the Cognitive Science Society,* Berlin.

Lamond, N., and Dawson, D. (1999). Quantifying the performance impairment associated with fatigue. *J. Sleep Res.* 8, 255–262. doi: 10.1046/j.1365-2869.1999. 00167.x

Moore, J. W. (2016). What is the sense of agency and why does it matter? *Front. Psychol.* 7:1272. doi: 10.3389/fpsyg.2016.01272

Parkes, K. R. (1995). The effects of objective workload on cognitive performance in a field setting: a two-period cross-over trial. *Appl. Cogn. Psychol.* 9, S153–S171. doi: 10.1002/acp.2350090710

Smith, A. (2002). Effects of caffeine on human behavior. *Food Chem. Toxicol.* 40, 1243–1255. doi: 10.1016/s0278-6915(02)00096-0

Smith, A., Thomas, M., and Whitney, H. (2000). Effects of upper respiratory tract illnesses on mood and performance over the working day. *Ergonomics* 43, 752–763. doi: 10.1080/0014013004 04724

Smith, A. P., Allen, P. H., and Wadsworth, E. J. K. (2006). *Seafarer Fatigue: The Cardiff Research Programme*. Cardiff: Centre for Occupational and Health Psychology.

Smith, A. P., and Smith, H. N. (2017). "Workload, fatigue and performance in the rail industry," in *Human Mental Workload: Models and Applications. H-WORKLOAD 2017. Communications in Computer and Information Science*, Vol. 726, eds L. Longo and M. C. Leva (Cham: Springer), 251–263. doi: 10.1007/ 978-3-319-61061-0_17

Ugajin, H. (1999). Human factors approach to railway safety. *Q. Rep. RTRI* 40, 5–8. doi: 10.2219/rtriqr.40.5

Young, M. S., Brookhuis, K. A., Wickens, C. D., and Hancock, P. A. (2015). State of science: mental workload in ergonomics. *Ergonomics* 58, 1–17. doi: 10.1080/ 00140139.2014.956151

2

A Pro-Inflammatory Diet is Associated with an Increased Odds of Depression Symptoms among Iranian Female Adolescents

Nitin Shivappa[1,2], James R. Hebert[1,2], Asal Neshatbini Tehrani[3], Bita Bayzai[3], Farah Naja[4] and Bahram Rashidkhani[3]*

[1] Cancer Prevention and Control Program, University of South Carolina, Columbia, SC, United States, [2] Department of Epidemiology and Biostatistics, Arnold School of Public Health, University of South Carolina, Columbia, SC, United States, [3] Department of Community Nutrition, Faculty of Nutrition Sciences and Food Technology, National Nutrition and Food Technology Research Institute (WHO Collaborating Center), Shahid Beheshti University of Medical Sciences, Tehran, Iran, [4] Nutrition and Food Sciences Department, American University of Beirut, Beirut, Lebanon

*Correspondence:
Bahram Rashidkhani
rashidkhani@yahoo.com;
b_rashidkhani@sbmu.ac.ir*

Background: The relation between dietary inflammation and risk of depression has not been widely explored. We examined the association between the inflammatory effect of the diet and the odds of depression among Iranian female adolescents.

Methods: Using a stratified cluster sampling technique, 300 female adolescents aged 15–18 years were recruited from schools in Tehran between years 2014–2015. Depression was assessed using the Depression, Anxiety and Stress Scale (DASS)- a 21-point scale. The dietary inflammatory index (DII®) was used to evaluate the inflammatory potential of the diet. Dietary intake was assessed using a validated food frequency questionnaire. In addition to descriptive statistics, multivariable linear and logistic regression were used to calculate confounder-adjusted beta estimates and odds ratios.

Results: In total, 88 females (30%) had at least a moderate level of depressive symptoms (DASS > 6). Females with the most pro-inflammatory diet had higher DASS depression score ($\beta = 1.67$; 95% CI = 0.03, 3.31) and were at 3.96 (95% CI = 1.12, 13.97) times higher odds of having at least moderate depressive symptoms, compared to females with the least anti-inflammatory diets.

Conclusion: These data suggest that Iranian adolescent females eating a pro-inflammatory diet, as indicated by higher DII scores, had greater odds of having at least moderate depressive symptoms.

Keywords: dietary inflammatory index, diet, inflammation, depression, Iran

INTRODUCTION

Depression is expected to become the world's second leading disease burden, after cardiovascular disease, by 2020 according the World Health Organization (1). Women are more than twice as likely to be diagnosed with depression compared with men (2). In Iran, major depression is the most prevalent mood disorder, with a prevalence rate of 2.98% among the entire population and 4.38% among women (3). The peak prevalence is between 25 and 44 years of age; however, recent data indicate that depression is occurring at younger ages (4, 5). Several metabolic and inflammatory processes, such as reduced insulin sensitivity, elevations in plasma homocysteine levels and, perhaps more importantly, increased production of pro-inflammatory cytokines and endothelial dysfunction, seem to be the major factors responsible for the depression (3, 4). Proinflammatory cytokines like c-reactive protein and interleukin-6 act by reducing brain monoamine levels, activating neuroendocrine responses, promoting excitotoxicity (increased glutamate levels), and impairing brain plasticity modulate mood behavior which can result in depression (6). Various dietary components have different effects on inflammation (7–9). A prudent dietary pattern high in fish, yogurt, pulses, rice, fruit, vegetables, and pasta has been shown to be associated with lower concentrations of intermediary inflammatory markers (10).

Various studies have been conducted to evaluate dietary exposures in relation to depression (11–15). In general, prospective cohort studies have shown that dietary patterns rich in anti-inflammatory components such as fruits, vegetables, olive oil, and legumes may be protective against depression (16–19). By contrast, increased risk has been observed with "pro-inflammatory" dietary patterns rich in saturated fat, omega 6 fatty acids, and refined carbohydrates (20, 21). A literature-derived, population-based dietary inflammatory index (DII) was developed to assess the inflammatory potential of an individual's diet (22). DII has previously been shown to be associated with various inflammatory markers in different populations (23–28) including among Iranians (29, 30). With respect to health outcomes, DII was significantly associated with different health outcomes ranging from cardiovascular diseases (31–33), cancer (34–37), overall and disease-specific mortality (38–42) to various mental health disorders (43–47). Previously, DII has been shown to be associated with depression in various studies conducted in Western population (48–53) but no study has been conducted in Iran whose dietary habits and culture are very different from Western populations. Our aim was to assess the association between the inflammatory potential of diet of adolescent Iranian females, as indicated by higher DII scores, and dimensions of depression as measured by Depression Anxiety Stress Scale-21 (DASS-21) (54).

METHODS AND MATERIALS

Study Population

This cross-sectional study of 300 adolescents females aged 15–18 years was carried out in Tehran (capital of Iran) from 2014 to 2015. Participants were randomly chosen by stratified cluster sampling. We first stratified the high schools based on socioeconomic status of the districts (low, intermediate, and high). Then we randomly selected 8 high schools from each stratum. Finally, subjects were chosen from a registration list (in each selected high school) by simple random sampling to fulfill the sample size requirement ($n = 300$).We did not include participants who reported major depression and anxiety disorder, using of any anti-depressant or sedative medication and who were pursuing a distinct diet, because there is a high probability that people with these disorders and taking antidepressant or sedative medications would have made lifestyle changes like adopting a healthier diet that may bias the results. The study protocol was approved by the research council of the Research Institute for Nutrition and Food Sciences, Shahid Beheshti University of Medical Sciences. All subjects gave written informed consent in accordance with the Declaration of Helsinki (approval number is 054577).

Assessment of Dietary Intake

Food consumption was based on a reliable and valid Food Frequency Questionnaire (FFQ) consisting of 168 food items with standard serving sizes typically used in Iran (55). FFQs were collected by specifically trained professional interviewers through private face-to-face interviews. Participants reported their daily, weekly, monthly or yearly of intake frequency for each food item. Daily frequencies for each item were computed. Then, by applying the manual for household measures the daily grams of food intake were calculated (56).

Anthropometric Measurement

Body weight was assessed to the nearest 0.1 kilogram by using digital scales (Seca 881® Germany) while participants were in light clothes with bare feet. Height was evaluated by using a stradiometer in the standing position and was recorded to the nearest 0.1 cm. Body Mass Index (BMI) was computed as weight divided by height squared (kg/m^2).

Socio-Demographic Information

Characteristics including age (years), ethnicity (Fars,Tork, Gilak, others), father/mother job (Unemployed, grade 3 (e.g., laborers), grade 2 (e.g., clerks), grade 1 (e.g., managers and higher), father/mother education (<diploma, diploma, university education), marital status of parents (married, unmarried), salary (USD), chronic disease (yes/no) diet supplement (yes, no), and smoking status (never, previous, current) were collected by a general questionnaire for all subjects.

Physical Activity Assessment

Physical activity was assessed using a valid self-reported questionnaire (57) that has been used previously in a sample of Iranian women and demonstrated consistent outcomes (58). Participants were asked to check the activities in which they had participated during the last year. From these reports, the total time spent in particular activities were summed and mean durations were calculated. Total physical activity was expressed as metabolic equivalent-hours per day (Mets/d).

TABLE 1 | Characteristics of participants according to different categories of depressive symptoms, Study of Diet-Inflammation and Depression in Iranian Adolescent Females, 2014 to 2015.

Characteristics[a,b]	Normal symptoms (DASS ≤9) N = 257	At least mild level of depressive symptoms (DASS > 9) N = 43	P-value
Age, (years) (mean ± sd)	16.2 ± 1.0	16.3 ± 1.1	0.69
Physical Activity (METs/d)(mean ± sd)	36.2 ± 5.7	34.7 ± 5.0	0.11
BMI (kg/m2)(mean ± sd)	22.3 ± 4.6	22.3 ± 4.9	0.98
Smoking (%)			0.002
Never	96.9	90.7	
Current/Past	3.1	9.3	
Chronic disease (%)			0.38
Yes	2.3	4.6	
No	97.7	95.4	
Diet supplement use (%)			0.47
Yes	34.0	39.5	
No	66.0	60.5	
Parental marital status (%)			0.20
Yes	95.3	90.7	
No	4.7	8.3	

[a]Significance testing was based on t-test for continuous variables.
[b]Chi-square test was used for categorical variables.

TABLE 2 | Participant characteristics by tertiles of dietary inflammatory index (DII)[c], Study of Diet-Inflammation and Depression in Iranian Adolescent Females, 2014 the 2015.

Characteristics[a,b]	Tertile 1	Tertile 2	Tertile 3	P-value
Age, (years) (mean ± sd)	16.1 ± 1.0	16.3 ± 1.0	16.2 ± 0.9	0.83
Physical activity (METs/d)(mean ± sd)	36.3 ± 5.9	36.2 ± 5.0	35.4 ± 5.9	0.28
BMI (kg/m2)(mean ± sd)	21.4 ± 4.8	22.7 ± 4.4	23.0 ± 4.6	0.02
Smoking (%)				0.39
Never	97.0	97.0	93.0	
Current/Past	3.0	3.0	7.0	
Chronic disease (%)				0.59
Yes	2.0	4.0	2.0	
No	98.0	96.0	98.0	
Diet supplement use (%)				0.17
Yes	42.0	30.3	32.0	
No	58.0	69.0	68.0	
Marital status (%)				0.29
Yes	95.0	97.0	92.0	
No	5.0	3.0	8.0	

[a]Significance testing was based on ANOVA for continuous variables.
[b]Chi-square test was used for categorical variables.
[c]Tertile 3 indicates the group with the most pro-inflammatory diet and tertile 1 indicates the group with most anti-inflammatory diet.

Other Variables

Further information on body image was collected by using 28-items of eating disorder examination questionnaire (EDE-Q-28) (59). The Persian version of EDE-Q-28 which was used in this study (60).

Dietary Inflammatory Index (DII®)

The development and validation of the DII are described in detail elsewhere (22). Briefly, developing the DII involved reviewing and scoring nearly 2,000 scientific articles representing cell culture and laboratory animal experiments, and a variety of human studies on diet and six inflammatory markers (i.e., CRP, interleukin (IL)-1b, IL-4, IL-6, IL-10, tumor necrosis factor (TNF)-α). Developing the DII also entailed creation of a world standard database that involved obtaining 11 data sets from around the world to which individuals' intakes of 45 food parameters (consisting of nutrients, spices and whole foods) on which the DII is based, could then be compared.

FFQ-derived dietary data were used to calculate DII scores for all participants. Dietary data were first linked to the previously described regionally representative world database that provided a robust estimate of a mean and standard deviation for each parameter (22). These then became the multipliers to express an individual's exposure relative to the "standard global mean" as a z-score. This score was computed by subtracting the "standard global mean" from the amount reported and dividing this value by the "global standard deviation" of the world population as represented by the 11 data sets used for comparative purposes. To minimize the effect of "right skewing," this value was then converted to a centered proportion score.

For each individual food parameter, this score was multiplied by the respective food parameter effect score, derived from the literature review, in order to obtain a food parameter-specific DII score (22). All of the food parameter-specific DII scores were then summed to create the overall DII score for each participant in the study, DII = b1*n1+b2*n2...........b31*n31, where b refers to the literature-derived inflammatory effects score for each of the evaluable food parameters and n refers to the food parameter-specific centered percentiles, which were derived from the FFQ-derived dietary data.

For the current study, data on 31 of the 45 DII food parameters could be derived from the FFQ and were thus used for DII calculation. These include: Pro-inflammatory components (energy, carbohydrate, protein, fat, saturated fat, iron, cholesterol, trans-fat, vitamin B12) and anti-inflammatory components (alcohol, fiber, mono-unsaturated fat, poly-unsaturated fat, omega-3, omega-6, niacin, thiamin, riboflavin, magnesium, zinc, vitamin A, vitamin C, vitamin E, vitamin D, vitamin B6, folic acid, beta-carotene, tea, turmeric, garlic, and onions).

Psychological Assessment of Depression, Anxiety and Stress

The Persian version of Depression, Anxiety, Stress Scale-21 (DASS-21) which was introduced by Lovibond and Lovibond (61) has been used to determine the level of depression, anxiety

TABLE 3 | Beta estimates and odds ratios and confidence intervals for the association between DII as tertiles and depressive symptoms, Study of Diet-Inflammation and Depression in Iranian Adolescent Females, 2014 to 2015.

DII[d]	Beta Estimates for depressive symptoms expressed as continuous DASS-21 score				Odds Ratios for at least moderate level of depressive symptoms (DASS-21 > 9)			
	Tertile 1	Tertile 2	Tertile 3	P-trend[c]	Tertile 1	Tertile 2	Tertile 3	P-trend[c]
DASS-21 > 9/DASS ≤ 9					12/88	17/82	14/87	
Model 1[a]	0	1.47 (0.04, 2.89)	1.97 (0.30, 3.64)	0.03	1	2.70 (1.03, 7.12)	3.01 (0.94, 9.59)	0.09
Model 2[b]	0	1.57 (0.19, 2.94)	1.67 (0.04, 3.31)	0.07	1	3.03 (1.11, 8.26)	3.96 (1.12, 13.97)	0.03

[a]Adjusted for age and energy.
[b]Mode 1+physical activity, BMI, smoking, presence of chronic disease, diet supplement use, salary and marital status.
[c]Tests for linear trend were performed by assigning the median value of each category to each participant in that group.
[d]Tertile 3 indicates the group with the most pro-inflammatory diet and tertile 1 indicates the group with most anti-inflammatory diet.

and stress in our sample population. This questionnaire has three subscales and each of them consists of seven items. The score of each subscale is attained by adding the scores of relevant questions. The Persian version of the DASS-21 was found to be a reliable and valid tool to examine the level of depression, anxiety and stress among Iranian adolescents (62).

Statistical Analysis

Study participants' characteristics were described according to two parameters: (1) reporting of at least depressive symptoms and (2) tertiles of the DII. Comparisons were carried out using t-tests and ANOVA for continuous variables and chi-square test for categorical variables. Multiple linear and logistic regression analysis were then used to calculate adjusted beta estimates and odds ratios (ORs) and 95% confidence intervals (CIs) for both DASS-21 as continuous and as categorical variable (DASS-21 > 9) in relation to DII in 2 separate models. Model I adjusted for total energy intake and age, model 2 additionally adjusted for physical activity, marital status, income, smoking, BMI, and presence of chronic disease.

RESULTS

Table 1 describes distribution of characteristics across categories of DASS-21 scores. Females with at least moderate level of depressive symptoms had lower level physical activity and greater dietary supplement use and were either past/current smokers. Table 2 shows distribution of characteristics across tertiles of DII. Females in tertile 3 had higher BMI compared to females in tertile 1. Table 3 describes the results for depression as a continuous score and as a dichotomous outcome where the scores were categorized on having at least a moderate level of depression symptoms (DASS > 9). Significant associations were observed for both types of outcomes for both models. Results are described for the full model, females in the third tertile had significantly higher depression scores (β = 1.67, 95% C.I. 0.04, 3.31); odds of having at least moderate depressive symptoms (DASS-21 > 9) (OR = 3.96, 95% CI 1.12, 13.97) compared to females in tertile 1 (**Table 3**).

DISCUSSION

In this study we report a significant positive association between increasing inflammatory potential of diet and depressive symptoms among adolescent females in Iran. To date, this is the first study to examine this association in adolescent females. A case-control study conducted in Iran showed that a healthy dietary pattern is protective against major depressive disorders, while no such association was observed with the unhealthy dietary patterns. The healthy pattern was characterized by high intakes of fish, poultry, low fat dairy, high fat dairy, coffee, fruits, and nuts, fruit juices, vegetables, legumes, and olives, and low intakes of refined grains, fats, and soft drinks. The unhealthy dietary patterns, on the other hand, were characterized by high intakes of processed meats, red meat, tea, fried potatoes, whole grains, refined grains, snacks, cookies, oils, sugar, and soft drinks (63). Previous reports suggest that men are more likely to have mental health problems than women (64). The current work shows an association between inflammatory potential of diet and depressive symptoms, among the female adolescents. While some of the earlier studies also reported associations between dietary inflammation potential and risk of depression among women; these were female-only cohorts where inflammatory potential of diet was determined by two different methods (inflammatory dietary pattern and DII) (14, 53). Results from the Nurses' Health Study revealed a 30–40% increased risk of depression, among women in the highest quintile compared to women in the lowest quintile of inflammatory dietary pattern (14). Twelve-years' follow-up of middle-aged women in Australia ($n = 6,438$) identified a 20% lower risk of depression among those whose diets were in the highest DII quartile compared to those in the lowest DII quartile (53).

This study is unique because for the first time this association has been examined in a Middle-Eastern population whose dietary habits and culture is very different from the Western population where this relationship has previously been examined (48–53). Traditional Iranian diet consist of food like cooked rice, mixed pilaf, rice, and stew, rice, high protein dishes and stuffed vegetables (65).

In agreement with our findings, the results of the only other study that examined the association between inflammatory potential of diet and depression showed that the hazards ratio for participants in the highest quintile of the DII (strongly pro-inflammatory) was 1.47 (95% confidence interval (CI): 1.17–1.85) compared with those in the bottom quintile, with a significant dose-response relationship (p for trend = 0.01) (66).

The DII, thus far, has been shown to be associated with several inflammatory markers and various chronic inflammation related outcomes. For instance, higher DII scores were positively associated with various inflammatory markers, including C-reactive protein (67, 68), interleukin-6 (69, 70), and homocysteine (69). Additionally, the DII has been shown to be associated with bone mineral density among postmenopausal women in Iran (70), two colorectal cancer case-control studies in Spain and Italy (71, 75) and in a cohort study in women in the USA (37, 71), esophageal cancer (72–74), breast cancer (75), pancreatic cancer (76), prostate cancer (77, 78), cardiovascular diseases (79, 80) and biomarker of aging (81).

The direct association between the DII and the odds of depression observed in this study could be explained by the fact many of the anti-inflammatory components of the index, namely zinc, omega 3 fatty acids, and coffee, have been shown to be negatively associated with the risk of depression (13). On the other hand, pro-inflammatory components of the index, such as energy and carbohydrate, have been linked to a higher risk of depression. For instance, results from a large cohort study conducted in the USA showed that frequent consumption of sweetened beverages, especially diet drinks, increases the risk of depression among older adults, whereas coffee consumption lowered the risk (11). Various studies have been conducted examining the association between dietary pattern and depression. In a systematic review conducted on 21 studies high intakes of fruit, vegetables, fish, and whole grains may be associated with a reduced depression risk (82). There is substantial evidence linking inflammation and depression (83–86).

Despite its strengths, our study had some limitations, which should also be considered in interpreting the results. First, the validity and reliability of FFQ has not been established in the context measuring dimensions of depression measured using DASS-21. Second, we could not directly infer causality due to the cross-sectional nature of the study design. Other limitations include small sample size, and the possibility of recall bias. Fourth, in this study, data were available on 31 of the 45 food parameters; absence of information on the remaining food parameters can be considered as a limitation. Additionally, validity and reliability of FFQ has not been established in the context measuring dimensions of depression measured using DASS-21. Another limitation is the inability to evaluate the history of stressful life events in the last 12 months. Self-reported dietary methods like the FFQ is subjected to bias of under reporting and implausible values for energy intake, the inability to measure this bias and adjust for it in the analyses is a limitation.

In conclusion, female adolescents with a pro-inflammatory diet have greater odds of having at least a moderate level of depressive symptoms. So, promoting diets with a higher concentration of anti-inflammatory foods, such as vegetables and fruits, at younger age may be protective against the development of depression. However, further studies analyzing the link between diet, inflammation and depression are warranted among both men and women to further elucidate the role of diet in the development of depression and other mental disorders.

AUTHOR CONTRIBUTIONS

NS calculated the DII, ran the analyses and also wrote the first draft of the manuscript. Upon receiving comments from the co-authors he also made changes to the manuscript and finalized it. JRH, AN, BB, FN, and BR reviewed and provided important input to the paper.

REFERENCES

World Health Organization. *Mental Health - Disorders Management 2011*, Available online at: from: http://www.who.int/mental_health/management/ depression/ definition/en/. 2011 (Accessed May 07, 2015)

Nolen-Hoeksema S, Girgus JS. The emergence of gender differences in depression during adolescence. *Psychol Bull.* (1994) 115:424–43.

Mohammadi MR, Davidian H, Noorbala AA, Malekafzali H, Naghavi HR, Pouretemad HR, et al. An epidemiological survey of psychiatric disorders in Iran. *Clin Pract Epidemiol Ment Health* (2005) 1:16. doi: 10.1186/1745-0179-1-16

Kessler RC, McGonagle KA, Swartz M, Blazer DG, Nelson CB. Sex and depression in the National Comorbidity Survey. I: lifetime prevalence, chronicity and recurrence. *J Affect Disord.* (1993) 29:85–96.

Zisook S, Rush AJ, Albala A, Alpert J, Balasubramani GK, Fava M, et al. Factors that differentiate early vs. later onset of major depression disorder. *Psychiatry Res.* (2004) 129:127–40. doi: 10.1016/j.psychres.2004.07.004

Bauer ME, Teixeira AL. Inflammation in psychiatric disorders: what comes first? *Ann NY Acad Sci.* (2018) doi: 10.1111/nyas.13712. [Epub ahead of print].

de Mello VD, Schwab U, Kolehmainen M, Koenig W, Siloaho M, Poutanen K, et al. A diet high in fatty fish, bilberries and wholegrain products improves markers of endothelial function and inflammation in individuals with impaired glucose metabolism in a randomised controlled trial: the Sysdimet study. *Diabetologia* (2011) 54:2755–67. doi: 10.1007/s00125-011-2285-3

Khoo J, Piantadosi C, Duncan R, Worthley SG, Jenkins A, Noakes M, et al. Comparing effects of a low-energy diet and a high-protein low- fat diet on sexual and endothelial function, urinary tract symptoms, and inflammation in obese diabetic men. *J Sex Med.* (2011) 8:2868–75. doi: 10.1111/j.1743-6109.2011.02417.x

Luciano M, Mottus R, Starr JM, McNeill G, Jia X, Craig LC, et al. Depressive symptoms and diet: their effects on prospective inflammation levels in the elderly. *Brain Behav Immun.* (2012) 26:717–20. doi: 10.1016/j.bbi.2011. 10.007

Wood AD, Strachan AA, Thies F, Aucott LS, Reid DM, Hardcastle AC, et al. Patterns of dietary intake and serum carotenoid and tocopherol status are associated with biomarkers of chronic low-grade systemic inflammation and cardiovascular risk. *Br J Nutr.* (2014) 112:1341–52. doi: 10.1017/S0007114514001962

Guo XG, Park Y, Freedman ND, Sinha R, Hollenbeck AR, Blair A, et al. Sweetened beverages, coffee, and tea and depression risk among older us adults. *PLoS ONE* (2014) 9:e94715. doi: 10.1371/journal.pone.0094715

Hegarty BD, Parker GB. Marine omega-3 fatty acids and mood disorders–linking the sea and the soul. 'Food for Thought' I. *Acta Psychiatr Scand.* (2011) 124:42–51. doi: 10.1111/j.1600-0447.2011.01703.x

Liperoti R, Landi F, Fusco O, Bernabei R, Onder G. Omega-3 polyunsaturated fatty acids and depression: a review of the evidence. *Curr Pharm Design.* (2009) 15:4165–72. doi: 10.2174/138161209789909683

Lucas M, Chocano-Bedoya P, Shulze MB, Mirzaei F, O'Reilly EJ, Okereke OI, et al. Inflammatory dietary pattern and risk of depression among women. *Brain Behav Immun.* (2014) 36:46–53. doi: 10.1016/j.bbi.2013.09.014

Mihrshahi S, Dobson AJ, Mishra GD. Fruit and vegetable consumption and prevalence and incidence of depressive symptoms in mid-age women: results from the Australian longitudinal study on women's health. *Eur J Clin Nutr.* (2015) 69:585–91. doi: 10.1038/ejcn.2014.222

Jacka FN, Kremer PJ, Berk M, de Silva-Sanigorski AM, Moodie M, Leslie ER, et al. A prospective study of diet quality and mental health in adolescents. *PLoS ONE* (2011) 6:e24805. doi: 10.1371/journal.pone.0024805

Jacka FN, Rothon C, Taylor S, Berk M, Stansfeld SA. Diet quality and mental health problems in adolescents from East London: a prospective study. *Soc Psychiatry Psychiatric Epidemiol.* (2013) 48:1297–306. doi: 10.1007/s00127- 012-0623-5

Rienks J, Dobson AJ, Mishra GD. Mediterranean dietary pattern and prevalence and incidence of depressive symptoms in mid-aged women: results from a large community-based prospective study. *Eur J Clin Nutr.* (2013) 67:75–82. doi: 10.1038/ejcn.2012.193.

Sanchez-Villegas A, Delgado-Rodriguez M, Alonso A, Schlatter J, Lahortiga F, Serra Majem L, et al. Association of the Mediterranean dietary pattern with the incidence of depression: the Seguimiento Universidad de Navarra/ University of Navarra follow-up (SUN) cohort. *Arch General Psychiatry* (2009) 66:1090–8. doi: 10.1001/archgenpsychiatry.2009.129

Akbaraly TN, Brunner EJ, Ferrie JE, Marmot MG, Kivimaki M, Singh-Manoux Dietary pattern and depressive symptoms in middle age. *Br J Psychiatry* (2009) 195:408–13. doi: 10.1192/bjp.bp.108.058925

Le Port A, Gueguen A, Kesse-Guyot E, Melchior M, Lemogne C, Nabi H, et al. Association between dietary patterns and depressive symptoms over time: a 10-year follow-up study of the GAZEL cohort. *PLoS ONE* (2012) 7:e51593. doi: 10.1371/journal.pone.0051593.

Shivappa N, Steck SE, Hurley TG, Hussey JR, Hebert JR. Designinganddeveloping a literature-derived, population-based dietary inflammatory index. *Public Health Nutr.* (2014) 17:1689–96. doi: 10.1017/S1368980013002115

Shivappa N, Wirth MD, Murphy EA, Hurley TG, Hebert JR. Association between the Dietary Inflammatory Index (DII) and urinary enterolignans and C-reactive protein from the National Health and Nutrition Examination Survey-2003-2008. *Eur J Nutr.* (2018) doi: 10.1007/s00394-018-1690-5. [Epub ahead of print].

Shivappa N, Schneider A, Hebert JR, Koenig W, Peters A, Thorand B. Association between dietary inflammatory index, and cause-specific mortality in the MONICA/KORA Augsburg Cohort Study. *Eur J Public Health* (2018) 28:167–72. doi: 10.1093/eurpub/ckx060

Wirth MD, Shivappa N, Davis L, Hurley TG, Ortaglia A, Drayton R, et al. Construct validation of the dietary inflammatory index among African Americans. *J Nutr Health Aging* (2017) 21:487–91. doi: 10.1007/s12603-016-0775-1

Julia C, Assmann KE, Shivappa N, Hebert JR, Wirth MD, Hercberg S, et al. Long-term associations between inflammatory dietary scores in relation to long-term C-reactive protein status measured 12 years later: findings from the Supplementation en Vitamines et Mineraux Antioxydants (SU.VI.MAX) cohort. *Br J Nutr.* (2017) 117:306–14. doi: 10.1017/S00071145170 00034

Shivappa N, Hebert JR, Rietzschel ER, De Buyzere ML, Langlois M, Debruyne E, et al. Associations between dietary inflammatory index and inflammatory markers in the Asklepios Study. *Br J Nutr.* (2015) 113:665–71. doi: 10.1017/ S000711451400395X

Boden S, Wennberg M, Van Guelpen B, Johansson I, Lindahl B, Andersson J, et al. Dietary inflammatory index and risk of first myocardialinfarction; a prospective population-based study. *Nutr J.* (2017) 16:21. doi: 10.1186/ s12937-017-0243-8

Vahid F, Shivappa N, Faghfoori Z, Khodabakhshi A, Zayeri F, Hebert JR, et al. Validation of a Dietary Inflammatory Index (DII) and Association with Risk of Gastric Cancer: a Case-Control Study. *Asian Pac J Cancer Prev.* (2018) 19:1471–7. doi: 10.22034/APJCP.2018.19.6.1471

Vahid F, Shivappa N, Hekmatdoost A, Hebert JR, Davoodi SH, Sadeghi M. Association between Maternal Dietary Inflammatory Index (DII) and abortion in Iranian women and validation of DII with serum concentration of inflammatory factors: case-control study. *Appl Physiol Nutr Metab.* (2017) 42:511–6. doi: 10.1139/apnm-2016-0274

Shivappa N, Godos J, Hebert JR, Wirth MD, Piuri G, Speciani AF, et al. Dietary inflammatory index and cardiovascular risk and mortality-a meta-analysis. *Nutrients* (2018) 10:E200. doi: 10.3390/nu10020200

Hodge AM, Bassett JK, Dugue PA, Shivappa N, Hebert JR, Milne RL, et al. Dietary inflammatory index or Mediterranean diet score as risk factors for total and cardiovascular mortality. *Nutr Metab Cardiovasc Dis.* (2018) 28:461– 9. doi: 10.1016/j.numecd.2018.01.010

O'Neil A, Shivappa N, Jacka FN, Kotowicz MA, Kibbey K, Hebert JR, et al. Pro-inflammatory dietary intake as a risk factor for CVD in men: a 5-year longitudinal study. *Br J Nutr.* (2015) 114:2074–82. doi: 10.1017/ S0007114515003815

Shivappa N, Godos J, Hebert JR, Wirth MD, Piuri G, Speciani AF, et al. Dietary inflammatory index and colorectal cancer risk-a meta-analysis. *Nutrients* (2017) 9:E1043. doi: 10.3390/nu9091043

Niclis C, Pou SA, Shivappa N, Hebert JR, Steck SE, Diaz MDP. Proinflammatory dietary intake is associated with increased risk of colorectal cancer: results of a case-control study in argentina using a multilevel modeling approach. *Nutr Cancer* (2018) 70:61–8. doi: 10.1080/01635581.2018.1397710

Shivappa N, Hebert JR, Steck SE, Hofseth LJ, Shehadah I, Bani-Hani KE, et al. Dietary inflammatory index and odds of colorectal cancer in a case- control study from Jordan. *Appl Physiol Nutr Metab.* (2017) 42:744–9. doi: 10.1139/ apnm-2017-0035

Shivappa N, Prizment AE, Blair CK, Jacobs DR, Jr., Steck SE, Hebert JR. Dietary inflammatory index and risk of colorectal cancer in the Iowa women's health study. *Cancer Epidemiol Biomark Prevent.* (2014) 23:2383–92. doi: 10.1158/1055-9965.EPI-14-0537

Park YM, Choi MK, Lee SS, Shivappa N, Han K, Steck SE, et al. Dietary inflammatory potential and risk of mortality in metabolically healthy and unhealthy phenotypes among overweight and obese adults. *Clin Nutr.* (2018) doi: 10.1016/j.clnu.2018.04.002. [Epub ahead of print].

Bondonno NP, Lewis JR, Blekkenhorst LC, Shivappa N, Woodman RJ, Bondonno CP, et al. Dietary inflammatory index in relation to sub-clinical atherosclerosis and atherosclerotic vascular disease mortality in older women. *Br J Nutr.* (2017) 117:1577–86. doi: 10.1017/S0007114517001520

Shivappa N, Steck SE, Hussey JR, Ma Y, Hebert JR. Inflammatory potential of diet and all-cause, cardiovascular, and cancer mortality in National Health and Nutrition Examination Survey III Study. *Eur J Nutr.* (2017) 56:683–92. doi: 10.1007/s00394-015-1112-x

Shivappa N, Harris H, Wolk A, Hebert JR. Association between inflammatory potential of diet and mortality among women in the Swedish Mammography Cohort. *Eur J Nutr.* (2016) 55:1891–900. doi: 10.1007/s00394-015-1005-z

Shivappa N, Blair CK, Prizment AE, Jacobs DR Jr, Steck SE, Hebert JR. Association between inflammatory potential of diet and mortality in the Iowa Women's Health study. *Eur J Nutr.* (2016) 55:1491–502. doi: 10.1007/ s00394-015-0967-1

Shin D, Kwon SC, Kim MH, Lee KW, Choi SY, Shivappa N, et al. Inflammatory potential of diet is associated with cognitive function in an older adult Korean population. *Nutrition* (2018) 55–6:56–62. doi: 10.1016/j.nut.2018.02.026

Hayden KM, Beavers DP, Steck SE, Hebert JR, Tabung FK, Shivappa N, et al. The association between an inflammatory diet and global cognitive function and incident dementia in older women: the Women's Health Initiative Memory Study. *Alzheimers Dement.* (2017) 13:1187–96. doi: 10.1016/j.jalz.2017.04.004

Kesse-Guyot E, Assmann KE, Andreeva VA, Touvier M, Neufcourt L, Shivappa N, et al. Long-term association between the dietary inflammatory index and cognitive functioning: findings from the SU.VI.MAX study. *Eur J Nutr.* (2017) 56:1647–55. doi: 10.1007/s00394-016-1211-3

Frith E, Shivappa N, Mann JR, Hebert JR, Wirth MD, Loprinzi PD. Dietary inflammatory index and memory function: population-based national sample of elderly Americans. *Br J Nutr.* (2018) 119:552–8. doi: 10.1017/ S0007114517003804

Shivappa N, Hebert JR, Rashidkhani B. Association between inflammatory potential of diet and stress levels in adolescent women in Iran. *Arch Iran Med.* (2017) 20:108–12.

Shivappa N, Hebert JR, Veronese N, Caruso MG, Notarnicola M, Maggi S, et al. The relationship between the dietary inflammatory index (DII((R))) and incident depressive symptoms: a longitudinal cohort study. *J Affect Disord.* (2018) 235:39–44. doi: 10.1016/j.jad.2018. 04.014

Phillips CM, Shivappa N, Hebert JR, Perry IJ. Dietary inflammatory index and mental health: A cross-sectional analysis of the relationship with depressive symptoms, anxiety and well-being in adults. *Clin Nutr.* (2017) doi: 10.1016/j. clnu.2017.08.029. [Epub ahead of print].

Wirth MD, Shivappa N, Burch JB, Hurley TG, Hebert JR. The dietary inflammatory index, shift work, and depression: results from NHANES. *Health Psychol.* (2017) 36:760–9. doi: 10.1037/hea00 00514

Adjibade M, Andreeva VA, Lemogne C, Touvier M, Shivappa N, Hebert JR, et al. The inflammatory potential of the diet is associated with depressive symptoms in different subgroups of the general population. *J Nutr.* (2017) 147:879–87. doi: 10.3945/jn.116.245167

Akbaraly T, Kerlau C, Wyart M, Chevallier N, Ndiaye L, Shivappa N, et al. Dietary inflammatory index and recurrence of depressive symptoms: results from the Whitehall II Study. *Clin Psychol Sci.* (2016) 4:1125–34. doi: 10.1177/2167702616645777

Shivappa N, Schoenaker DA, Hebert JR, Mishra GD. Association between inflammatory potential of diet and risk of depression in middle-aged women: the Australian Longitudinal Study on Women's Health. *Br J Nutr.* (2016) 116:1077–86. doi: 10.1017/S0007114516002853

Henry JD, Crawford JR. The short-form version of the Depression Anxiety Stress Scales (DASS-21): construct validity and normative data in a large non-clinical sample. *Br J Clin Psychol.* (2005) 44(Pt 2):227–39. doi: 10.1348/014466505X29657

Esfahani FH, Asghari G, Mirmiran P, Azizi F. Reproducibility and relative validity of food group intake in a food frequency questionnaire developed for the Tehran Lipid and Glucose Study *J Epidemiol.* (2010) 20:150–8. doi: 10.2188/jea. JE20090083

Ghaffarpour M, Houshiar-Rad A, Kianfar H. The manual for household measures, cooking yields factors and edible portion of foods. *Tehran: Nashre Olume Keshavarzy* (1999) 7:213.

Aadahl M, Jorgensen T. Validation of a new self-report instrument for measuring physical activity. *Med Sci Sports Exerc.* (2003) 35:1196–202. doi: 10.1249/01. MSS.0000074446.02192.14

Rezazadeh A, Rashidkhani B, Omidvar N. Association of major dietary patterns with socioeconomic and lifestyle factors of adult women living in Tehran, Iran. *Nutrition* (2010) 26:337–41. doi: 10.1016/j.nut.2009. 06.019

Fairburn CG, Beglin SJ. Eating Disorder Examination Questionnaire (EDE- Q 6.0). In: C. G. Fairburn editors. *Cognitive Behavior Therapy and Eating Disorders.* New York, NY: Guilford Press (2008). pp. 309–13.

Mahmoodi M, Moloodi R, Ghaderi A. persian version of eating disorder examination questionnaire and clinical impairment assessment: norms and psychometric properties for undergraduate women. *Iran J Psychiatry* (2016) 11:67–74.

Lovibond P. *Manual for the depression anxiety stress Scales.* Sydney: Sydney Psychology edition (1995).

Bayani AA. Reliability and preliminary evidence of validity of a Farsi version of the depression anxiety stress scales. *Percept Mot Skills* (2010) 111:107–14. doi: 10.2466/08.13.PMS.111.4.107-114

Rashidkhani B, Pourghassem Gargari B, Ranjbar F, Zareiy S, Kargarnovin Z. Dietary patterns and anthropometric indices among Iranian women with major depressive disorder. *Psychiatry Res.* (2013) 210:115–20. doi: 10.1016/j. psychres.2013.05.022

Albert PR. Why is depression more prevalent in women? *J Psychiatry Neurosci.* (2015) 40:219–21. doi: 10.1503/jpn.150205

Karizaki VM. Ethnic and traditional Iranian rice-based foods. *J Ethnic Foods* (2016) 3:124–34. doi: 10.1016/j.jef.2016. 05.002

Sanchez-Villegas A, Ruiz-Canela M, de la Fuente-Arrillaga C, Gea A, Shivappa N, Hebert JR, et al. Dietary inflammatory index, cardiometabolic conditions and depression in the Seguimiento Universidad de Navarra cohort study. *Br J Nutr.* (2015) 114:1471–9. doi: 10.1017/S0007114515003074

Shivappa N, Steck SE, Hurley TG, Hussey JR, Ma Y, Ockene IS, et al. A population-based dietary inflammatory index predicts levels of C-reactive protein in the Seasonal Variation of Blood Cholesterol Study (SEASONS). *Public Health Nutr.* (2014) 17:1825–33. doi: 10.1017/S13689800130 02565

Wirth MD, Burch J, Shivappa N, Violanti JM, Burchfiel CM, Fekedulegn D, et al. Association of a dietary inflammatory index with inflammatory indices and metabolic syndrome among police officers. *J Occup Environ Med.* (2014) 56:986–9. doi: 10.1097/JOM.0000000000000213

Ruiz-Canela M, Zazpe I, Shivappa N, Hebert JR, Sanchez-Tainta A, Corella D, et al. Dietary inflammatory index and anthropometric measures of obesity in a population sample at high cardiovascular risk from the PREDIMED (PREvencion con DIeta MEDiterranea) trial. *Br J Nutr.* (2015) 113:984–95. doi: 10.1017/S0007114514004401

Wood LG, Shivappa N, Berthon BS, Gibson PG, Hebert JR. Dietary inflammatory index is related to asthma risk, lung function and systemic inflammation in asthma. *Clin Exp Allergy* (2015) 45:177–83. doi: 10.1111/cea.12323

Zamora-Ros R, Shivappa N, Steck SE, Canzian F, Landi S, Alonso MH, et al. Dietary inflammatory index and inflammatory gene interactions in relation to colorectal cancer risk in the Bellvitge colorectal cancer case-control study. *Genes Nutr.* (2015) 10:447. doi: 10.1007/s12263-014-0447-x

Shivappa N, Hebert JR, Rashidkhani B. Dietary inflammatory index and risk of esophageal squamous cell cancer in a case-control study from Iran. *Nutr Cancer* (2015) 23:1–7. doi: 10.1080/01635581.2015.1082108

Lu Y, Shivappa N, Lin Y, Lagergren J, Hébert J. Diet-related inflammation and oesophageal cancer by histological type: a nationwide case–control study in Sweden. *Eur J Nutr.* (2015) 55:1683–94. doi: 10.1007/s00394-015-0987-x

Shivappa N, Zucchetto A, Serraino D, Rossi M, La Vecchia C, Hébert J. Dietary inflammatory index and risk of esophageal squamous cell cancer in a case–control study from Italy. *Cancer Causes Control* (2015) 26:1439–47 doi: 10.1007/s10552-015-0636-y

Shivappa N, Sandin S, Lof M, Hebert JR, Adami HO, Weiderpass E. Prospective study of dietary inflammatory index and risk of breast cancer in Swedish women. *Br J Cancer* (2015) 113:1099–103 doi: 10.1038/bjc. 2015.304

Shivappa N, Bosetti C, Zucchetto A, Serraino D, La Vecchia C, Hébert JR. Dietary inflammatory index and risk of pancreatic cancer in an Italian case–control study. *Br J Nutr.* (2015) 113:292–8. doi: 10.1017/S0007114514 003626

Shivappa N, Bosetti C, Zucchetto A, Montella M, Serraino D, La Vecchia C, et al. Association between dietary inflammatory index and prostate cancer among Italian men. *Br J Nutr.* (2015) 113:278–83. doi: 10.1017/S0007114514003572

Shivappa N, Jackson MD, Bennett F, Hébert JR. Increased Dietary Inflammatory Index (DII) is associated with increased risk of prostate cancer in Jamaican men. *Nutr Cancer* (2015) 67:941–8. doi: 10.1080/01635581.2015.1062117

Garcia-Arellano A, Ramallal R, Ruiz-Canela M, Salas-Salvadó J, Corella D, Shivappa N, et al. Dietary inflammatory index and incidence of cardiovascular disease in the PREDIMED study. *Nutrients* (2015) 7:4124–38. doi: 10.3390/nu7064124

Ramallal R, Toledo E, Martínez-González MA, Hernández-Hernández A, García-Arellano A, Shivappa N, et al. Dietary inflammatory index and incidence of cardiovascular disease in the SUN cohort. *PLoS ONE* (2015) 10:e0135221. doi: 10.1371/journal.pone.0135221

García-Calzón S, Zalba G, Ruiz-Canela M, Shivappa N, Hébert JR, Martínez JA, et al. Dietary inflammatory index and telomere length in subjects with a high cardiovascular disease risk from the PREDIMED-NAVARRA study: cross-sectional and longitudinal analyses over 5 y. *Am J Clin Nutr.* (2015) 102:897–904 doi: 10.3945/ajcn.115.116863

Lai JS, Hiles S, Bisquera A, Hure AJ, McEvoy M, Attia J. A systematic review and meta-analysis of dietary patterns and depression in community-dwelling adults. *Am J Clin Nutr.* (2014) 99:181–97. doi: 10.3945/ajcn.113.0 69880

Chocano-Bedoya PO, Mirzaei F, O'Reilly EJ, Lucas M, Okereke OI, Hu FB, et al. C-reactive protein, interleukin-6, soluble tumor necrosis factor alpha receptor 2 and incident clinical depression. *J Affect Disord.* (2014) 163:25–32. doi: 10.1016/j.jad.2014. 03.023

Hood KK, Lawrence JM, Anderson A, Bell R, Dabelea D, Daniels S, et al. Metabolic and inflammatory links to depression in youth with diabetes. *Diabetes Care* (2012) 35:2443–6. doi: 10.2337/dc11-2329

Doyle TA, de Groot M, Harris T, Schwartz F, Strotmeyer ES, Johnson KC, et al. Diabetes, depressive symptoms, and inflammation in older adults: results from the health, aging, and body composition study. *J Psychosomat Res.* (2013) 75:419–24. doi: 10.1016/j.jpsychores.2013.08.006

Au B, Smith KJ, Gariepy G, Schmitz N. C-reactive protein, depressive symptoms, and risk of diabetes: results from the English Longitudinal Study of Ageing (ELSA). *J Psychosomat Res.* (2014) 77:180–6. doi: 10.1016/j.jpsychores.2014.07.012

3

The Effects of Acute Moderate and High Intensity Exercise on Memory

David Marchant¹*, Sophie Hampson², Lucy Finnigan³, Kelly Marrin¹ and Craig Thorley⁴

¹ Psychology of Sport, Exercise and Movement Research Group, Department of Sport and Physical Activity, Edge Hill University, Ormskirk, United Kingdom, ² Manchester University NHS Foundation Trust, Manchester, United Kingdom, ³ School of Sport and Exercise Sciences, Liverpool John Moores University, Liverpool, United Kingdom, ⁴ Department of Psychology, James Cook University, Townsville, QLD, Australia

*Correspondence:
David Marchant
David.Marchant@edgehill.ac.uk

Acute cardiovascular exercise can enhance correct remembering but its impact upon false remembering is less clear. In two experiments, we investigated the effect of acute bouts of exercise on correct and false remembering using the Deese–Roediger–McDermott (DRM) memory test. In Experiment 1, healthy adults completed quiet rest or moderate intensity cycling prior to the memory test. In Experiment 2, a similar sample completed moderate intensity running, high intensity sprints, or a period of quiet rest prior to the memory test. In Experiment 1, acute moderate intensity exercise increased short-term correct, but not false, recall. Experiment 2 replicated these findings but also found an acute bout of high intensity exercise had no impact upon either type of short-term recall. Acute moderate intensity exercise, but not acute high intensity exercise, can improve short-term correct recall without an accompanying increase in false recall potentially through processing of contextually specific information during encoding.

Keywords: acute exercise, exercise intensity, cognition, recall, recognition, false memory

INTRODUCTION

Acute bouts of cardiovascular exercise provide moderate short-term post-exercise enhancements to several cognitive functions, including the speed of mental processing, attention, and executive function (see Chang et al., 2012; McMorris and Hale, 2012). These beneficial effects are associated with increases in arousal and available cognitive resources (e.g., Hillman et al., 2003), which are also proposed to be critical variables in efficient memory functioning. The influence of acute exercise on memory may depend on the temporal relation between the exercise bout, information encoding (the initial perceiving and learning of information), consolidation (memory trace stabilization into long-term memory formation after initial encoding) and subsequent recall (the retrieval of stored information). When exercise occurs immediately before a memory encoding task, there are moderate enhancements to the volume of studied information correctly remembered, whereas exercising during encoding appears to impair encoding (see Loprinzi et al., 2019, for a meta-analysis). Pre-encoding exercise is observed to be more beneficial than post-encoding exercise (Labban and Etnier, 2011), whilst concurrent exercise and encoding may impair subsequent recall (Soga et al., 2017). Furthermore, study characterizes in terms of exercise (intensity, duration), participants (age, fitness) and memory tasks (working memory, episodic memory, prospective memory) can moderate the potential for beneficial effects (Loprinzi, 2018). The majority of work has focused in correct recall, whilst little is known regarding acute cardiovascular exercise prior to either a short-term or long-term memory test can influence false remembering (memory of information that was not present at encoding).

Acute bouts of cardiovascular exercise, relative to rest, can enhance both short and long term explicit, declarative memory (memory that can be consciously recalled) of previously observed word lists. For example, enhancements have been observed after participants engaged in 10 min of brisk walking (e.g., English nouns: Salas et al., 2011), 40 min of moderate intensity aerobic cycling (e.g., English nouns: Coles and Tomporowski, 2008), six min of high intensity anaerobic sprints (e.g., Novel vocabulary: Winter et al., 2007), and 30 min of treadmill running above lactate threshold (e.g., Rey Auditory Verbal Learning Test: Etnier et al., 2016). In reviewing these patterns, when considering the type of memory task employed, Loprinzi (2018) suggests that whilst acute high-intensity exercise pre-memory task may impair working memory it can benefit episodic memory whilst high-intensity exercise post-encoding may not benefit long-term memory performance. These exercise-induced arousal memory benefits are thought to be associated with increased levels of brain-derived neurotrophic factor (BDNF) and catecholamines (dopamine, epinephrine, norepinephrine) (e.g., Winter et al., 2007).

The benefits of acute bouts of exercise on remembering may be of limited use if they are accompanied by increases in false remembering (e.g., recollecting events that did not happen or incorrectly recollecting events that did happen). To date, the impact of an acute bout of exercise on false remembering (as assessed using the DRM protocol) has only received limited examination. Green and Loprinzi (2018) found 15 min of self-paced brisk treadmill walking had no effect on correct or false declarative recall. Whilst Siddiqui and Loprinzi (2018) found that 20 min of brisk treadmill walking benefited accurate recall, with no differences in false recall. In contrast, Dilley et al. (2019) found 15-min high-intensity treadmill running (80%HRR) pre-encoding significantly increased correct recall over moderate intensity (50%HRR) exercise, the latter also enhanced memory over rest. False recall was not significantly impacted by exercise intensity, but the authors tentatively suggest their data indicates higher-intensity exercise may increase false recall. As such, the relationship between acute exercise pre-encoding warrants further consideration.

The Deese/Roediger-McDermott (DRM) paradigm (Roediger and McDermott, 1995) is widely used to induce false memories (see Gallo, 2010, for a review). Participants study lists of words (e.g., bed, dream, wake, snore, etc.) that are semantically associated with a non-presented critical lure word (e.g., sleep). In later assessment, participants frequently falsely recall and falsely recognize these critical lures as a previously studied word with high confidence. The Activation-Monitoring Theory (AMT, Roediger et al., 2001) and the Fuzzy Trace Theory (FTT, Brainerd and Reyna, 2002) explain why DRM word lists induce false memories. The AMT posits that, during encoding, the studied words (either consciously or unconsciously) activate the semantically associated critical lure. During subsequent memory tests, participants generate words based on their semantic activation at encoding. As the critical lure was activated at encoding, they commit a source-monitoring error and class it as a presented word (instead of an internally generated non-studied word). The FTT posits that participants generate two parallel memory traces (changes in the nervous system representing information) for studied words at encoding: verbatim traces (precise memory representations) and gist traces (vague meaning-based memory representations). The critical lures are strongly associated with gist of studied lists and are incorrectly presumed to have been studied. The AMT and FTT accounts are not mutually exclusive and both implicate the semantic association between studied lists and the non-studied critical lures in false remembering.

Currently, Loprinzi and colleagues (e.g., Siddiqui and Loprinzi, 2018) have tentatively suggested that moderate-intensity exercise may benefit accurate whilst reducing false declarative recall, whilst high-intensity exercise may elevate both accurate and false recall (Dilley et al., 2019). Consistent with this possibility, there is converging evidence from two distinct lines of research that self-reported arousal (admittedly, from other sources) can increase false remembering. Firstly, caffeine-induced arousal increased false recall of critical lures on memory tests (e.g., Mahoney et al., 2012). The second line of research demonstrates that high pre-encoding emotion-induced arousal can increase false remembering (e.g., Corson and Verrier, 2007). Taken together, self-reported arousal is often associated with increases in short-term memory false recall. Mahoney et al. (2012) and Corson and Verrier (2007) suggest that elevated arousal increases relational processing rather than item-specific processing at encoding in explain these effects. Item-specific processing focusses attention on individual studied items and how they are distinct from each other, whereas relational processing focusses participants' attention on the commonalities amongst studied items. Roediger et al. (2001) suggest that relational processing intensifies the spread of activation to the critical lures, which are more likely to be falsely remembered. These findings suggest some forms of arousal can increase false remembering and it is of interest to know whether this effect generalizes when the arousal is exercise-induced. For example, exercise-induced arousal (proposed to be associated with increases in neurotransmitters norepinephrine and dopamine) benefits speed of cognitive processing (McMorris and Hale, 2012).

The present within-subjects experiments examined the impact of a single acute bout of exercise on explicit, declarative short-term memory. Specifically, the effects of acute exercise undertaken immediately prior to encoding on subsequent short-term declarative correct and false remembering, as assessed via a DRM memory test. As exercise intensity, and therefore the degree of probable arousal, influences correct remembering, exercise intensity was manipulated here to see if it influences false remembering. More specifically, Experiment 1 examined whether engaging in an acute bout of moderate intensity aerobic exercise prior to encoding, relative to rest, impacts upon short-term declarative correct and false recall/recognition. Experiment 2 expanded this by examining whether engaging in acute moderate intensity aerobic exercise or high intensity anaerobic exercise prior to encoding, relative to rest, impacts upon short-term declarative correct and false recall/recognition. In both studies, it was anticipated that an acute bout of exercise prior to encoding would enhance short-term correct remembering. Despite previous findings (e.g., Green and Loprinzi, 2018), it is also tentatively predicted than an acute bout of exercise will elevate short-term false remembering as other forms of arousal (i.e., caffeine-induced, emotion-induced) are associated with increased false remembering (e.g., Corson and Verrier, 2007; Mahoney et al., 2012).

EXPERIMENT 1

Methods

Participants

Twenty six healthy and regularly physically active (>3 aerobic exercise sessions on three days per week for at least 30 min per session, >2 years of regular exercise participation) young adults (19M, 7F, Mage = 22.19 + 3.15 years) participated in the study after giving written informed consent. An *a priori* power analysis (using G*Power 3.1) with an α level of 5%, medium-to-large effect size (*d* = 0.6), and a power of 80%, based on effect sizes reported in previous within-subjects work (e.g., Etnier et al., 2016, *N* = 16; Labban and Etnier, 2018, *N* = 15) indicated that at least 19 participants would be required. All spoke English as their first language, had normal or corrected to normal vision, had no history of mood disorders, and were not taking any medication that would affect cognition. Participants were asked to refrain from strenuous physical exercise on the day of testing, to avoid caffeine and alcohol intake for 24 h prior to testing, to arrive appropriately hydrated, and to have not eaten for a minimum of 3 h.

Experimental Design

In a within-subjects design, participants completed two activities (rest or exercise) in a counterbalanced order. In the rest condition, participants were seated for 30 min prior to a DRM memory test. In the exercise condition, participants completed 30 min of moderate intensity exercise prior to a DRM memory test.

Activities and Measures

Rest Protocol

Participants were seated alone at a table in a quiet room and given the opportunity to read popular magazines for 30 min. This has been shown to be an acceptable rest activity the avoids boredom and does not impact memory function (Blough and Loprinzi, 2019). Participants were monitored to ensure they did not fall asleep or stand up and move around. Ratings of perceived exertion (RPE; individual's perceptions of exercise intensity) and affective valence (pleasure-displeasure) were recorded every two min.

Exercise Protocol

On a cycle ergometer (Monark, Model: 824E, Country: Sweden) participants completed a 5-min self-paced warm-up, followed by 30 min of moderate intensity cycling. Participants were asked to self-regulate a level of perceived exertion between *somewhat hard* and *hard* (within the 13–15 range on the Borg RPE scale), and were free to adjust their cadence to maintain their RPE within the target range. A reminder of the target RPE range was continuously in sight, and the researcher reminded participants every 2 min during exercise (offset from RPE measurement). RPE is a validated and practical perceptual method of directing self-selected exercise intensity, and this protocol has previously been used (e.g., Labban and Etnier, 2011) to ensure participants exercise at a moderate intensity below the ventilatory threshold. RPE, affective valence (pleasure-displeasure), and heart rate (HR) were recorded every two min. Water was available *ad libitum* throughout exercise.

Ratings of Perceived Exertion (RPE)

The Borg RPE scale (Borg, 1998) ranging from 6 (no exertion at all) to 20 (maximal exertion) was used to assess subjective interpretations of effort during exercise. The RPE scale is a widely accepted and validated method for estimating perceptions of exercise intensity, demonstrating high correlations (r = 0.80–0.90) between RPE and HR (Borg, 1998).

Affect

The Feeling Scale (FS; Hardy and Rejeski, 1989) is a single-item measure of pleasure and displeasure (how are you feeling right now?), 11-point bipolar rating scale ranging from + 5 (I feel very good), zero (neutral), to –5 (I feel very bad).

Heart Rate (HR)

Participants' HR was continuously monitored via a Polar Rate Monitor (Model A1; Polar Electro, Kempele, Finland) and recorded every 2 min.

Memory Task

The DRM paradigm (Roediger and McDermott, 1995) consisted of twelve lists of 15 word rated by Stadler et al. (1999) as producing high levels of false recognition (critical lures: Window, Doctor, Smoke, Anger, Cup, Slow, Sleep, Sweet, Rough, Soft, Cold, River). Participants were provided with standardized instructions on the task by the researcher, and this was repeated on the introductory computer screens. Two sets of 6 lists were assigned to each condition in counterbalanced order. Words were presented sequentially on a computer screen at a rate of 2s per word with a 1 s interval. Immediately after list, participants undertook a 1-min free recall test under the instruction to write as many words as possible using pen and paper. The number of correctly recalled old items (studied words), falsely recalled lures, and intrusions was totaled across the six lists. After the final free recall test, participants completed a 36-word recognition test similar to Knott and Thorley (2014). This test contained the six critical lures, 18 previously studied words (from positions one, five, and ten in each studied list), and 12 non-studied new words not semantically associated with the studied words or critical lures. On a paper response sheet, participants indicated whether the words were old (the word was previously studied) or new (the word was not previously studied). Old words were then rated as remember (recollect some contextual detail of seeing the word during encoding), know (recognized the word based on familiarity but had no recollection of any contextual information), or guess. Correct recognition of studied words, false recognition of critical lures, and incorrect recognition of non-studied new words (i.e., not critical lures) were calculated as proportions.

Procedure

Participants completed each condition activity (rest or exercise) individually on separate days at the same time of day in the same well-controlled laboratory setting led by the same researcher. There was a seven-day rest period between each session to control for factors that may affect memory performance (e.g., carry over effects). In the first session, participants read and signed an informed consent sheet, completed exercise readiness and health screening, and were familiarized with all equipment and testing procedures. On each day, participants first undertook the condition activity and then immediately completed the DRM memory tasks whilst seated in front of a computer in a distraction free testing booth situated next to the activity area. Upon completion of the activity, transition to the testing booth, reinstruction and commencing the memory task took approximately 2 min. A researcher was always present in the laboratory with the participant, and they provided the same instructions and monitoring to all participants. Following the completion of the final condition, all participants were debriefed about the aim of the experiment.

Statistical Analysis

Recall and recognition performance was analyzed with MANOVA followed by univariate ANOVAs using SPSS (version 22.0; International Business Machines Corp., Armonk, NY, United States), considering Condition (Rest vs. Exercise) as the within-subjects factor and word type (Recall: Critical Lure, Correct Recall, Other Error. Recognition: Critical Lure, Studied Word, New Word) as the dependent variables. If Mauchly's Test indicated sphericity was violated, a Greenhouse-Geisser correction was employed (εGG is reported in such cases). Partial eta-squared ($\eta p2$) proportion of variance effect size was calculated and described with Cohen's (1988) cut-off points (i.e., small = 0.0099; medium = 0.0588; large = 0.1379).

RESULTS

Exercise Intensity

To check that the self-selected approach to targeting exercise intensity was successful, HR, RPE and Affect are assessed. The mean HR during exercise was 136 bpm (±17.34), indicating exercise was undertaken at an average of 68.40% of HRmax. The mean RPE reported during exercise was 12.65 (±1.23). Taken together, exercise was at a self-selected moderate intensity (Garber et al., 2011). Average affective responses were significantly more positive in the rest condition (3.38, ±1.81) compared to the exercise condition (1.71 $\pm$ 1.12), t (25) = 4.08, $p < 0.001$.

Short-Term Free Recall

The results showed a significant multivariate effect of Condition, $\lambda = 0.70$, $F(3, 23) = 3.28$, $p = 0.038$, $\eta_p^2 = 0.30$. The follow-up univariate analyses confirmed that the difference between Rest and Exercise was significant for Correct Recall (42.69 $\pm$ 9.21 vs. 39.35 $\pm$ 7.03), $F(1, 25) = 4.81$, MSE = 145.56, $p = 0.038$, $\eta_p^2 = 0.16$. Contrary to our tentative prediction, there was no significant difference in the number of critical lures falsely recalled in the exercise (2.69 $\pm$ 1.52) and rest conditions (2.08 $\pm$ 1.44), $F(1, 25) = 3.32$, MSE = 4.92, $p = 0.08$, $\eta_p^2 = 0.12$. There was no significant main effect of condition on other recall errors (2.88 $\pm$ 3.83 vs. 1.81 $\pm$ 1.90), $F(1, 25) = 0.89$, MSE = 3.25, $p = 0.35$, $\eta_p^2 = 0.03$ (see **Table 1**).

Recognition Memory

No significant multivariate effect of Condition on the proportion of words was recognized, $\lambda = 0.99$, $F(1, 25) = 0.17$, $p = 0.68$, $\eta_p^2 = 0.01$, nor Condition x Word Type interaction $\lambda = 0.99$, $F(1, 24) = 0.03$, $p = 0.97$, $\eta_p^2 = 0.02$ (see **Table 2**). Similarly, a MANOVA with Condition (Rest vs. Exercise) and Word Type (Studied vs. Critical Lure vs. New) as within-subjects factor, and judgment type (Remember, Know, Guess) as the dependent variables showed no significant multivariate effect of Condition on the proportion of words were recognized, $\lambda = 0.97$, $F(3, 23) = 0.24$, $p = 0.87$, $\eta_p^2 = 0.03$, nor Condition x Word Type interaction $\lambda = 0.91$, $F(6, 20) = 0.34$, $p = 0.91$, $\eta_p^2 = 0.09$. An equivalent, but large, proportion of studied words were recognized and critical lures falsely recognized in both conditions, whilst participants recognized few non-studied new words across conditions. Therefore contrary to expectations, exercise did not impact upon true and false recognition.

DISCUSSION

Experiment 1 demonstrated that acute moderate intensity aerobic exercise, relative to a period of rest, prior to a DRM memory task increased short-term correct recall. This is consistent with past research showing that exercise improves the ability to retain and recall information in short-term memory (Loprinzi et al., 2019). Contrary to expectations, participants' long-term correct recognition of studied words was equivalent regardless of whether they were tested after exercise or rest. Short-term correct recall and long-term correct recognition are, therefore, differentially impacted upon by exercise in this study. In a novel comparison, we also found that moderate intensity aerobic

---

TABLE 1 | Mean (SD) number of studied words correctly recalled (max = 90), critical lures falsely recalled (max = 6), and non-studied new words incorrectly recalled following two activities (rest or moderate intensity exercise) in Experiment 1.

Activity	Studied words	Critical lures	Non-studied new words
Rest	39.35 (7.03)	2.08 (1.44)	2.89 (3.82)
Exercise	42.69 (9.21)[a]	2.69 (1.52)	1.81 (1.90)

[a]Significantly different from rest.

TABLE 2 | Mean (SD) proportion of studied words correctly recognized, critical lures falsely recognized, and non-studied new items incorrectly recognized following each activity in Experiment 1.

		Rest	Moderate exercise
Studied Words	Old (*Correct*)	0.78 (0.12)	0.77 (0.19)
	Remember	0.38 (0.27)	0.44 (0.32)
	Know	0.27 (0.26)	0.25 (0.28)
	Guess	0.12 (0.17)	0.07 (0.06)
Critical Lures	Old (*Incorrect*)	0.87 (0.17)	0.87 (0.20)
	Remember	0.47 (0.34)	0.47 (0.34)
	Know	0.31 (0.28)	0.29 (0.30)
	Guess	0.09 (0.12)	0.11 (0.14)
New Words	Old (*Incorrect*)	0.19 (0.23)	0.17 (0.25)
	Remember	0.04 (0.07)	0.05 (0.12)
	Know	0.04 (0.09)	0.02 (0.07)
	Guess	0.11 (0.18)	0.10 (0.21)

exercise, relative to rest, has no impact upon number of critical lures (or other non-studied words) falsely recalled during a short-term memory test or falsely recognized during a long-term memory test. Supporting initial observations (Siddiqui and Loprinzi, 2018) this suggests exercise-induced arousal, unlike other forms of arousal (e.g., caffeine-induced, mood-induced) does not increase false remembering. It remains to be determined whether intensity can also influence false remembering. Furthermore, as the recognition test took place several min after the exercise had finished, it is unclear whether participants arousal levels had deteriorated in the exercise condition, so they were on par with those in the rest condition. If so, that could account for the null results. Experiment 2 therefore measures participants' arousal levels prior to and after each memory test.

EXPERIMENT 2

Experiment 2 compared the impact of rest, moderate intensity aerobic exercise, and high intensity anaerobic exercise on correct and false remembering as assessed via a short-term memory free recall test and a long-term memory recognition test. Consistent with several past studies (e.g., Winter et al., 2007), we used running protocols to elicit moderate and high intensity exercise. In methodological improvements to Experiment 1, we tailored the intensity in line with participants' individual fitness level.

Methods
Participants

Twenty-five healthy, normally functioning, and physically active males volunteered for the study (M_{age} = 25.84 ± 6.46 years). Each had considerable prior experience of high intensity treadmill running. The inclusion, exclusion, and screening procedures were identical to Experiment 1. All participants were naïve to the aims of the study. Participants refrained from strenuous physical exercise on testing days, avoided caffeine and alcohol intake for 24 h prior to testing, and arrived appropriately hydrated, and having not eaten for a minimum of 3 h.

Experimental Design

In a within-subjects design modeled on that of Winter et al. (2007), participants completed three activities (rest, moderate intensity aerobic exercise, high intensity anaerobic exercise) in a counterbalanced order. In the rest condition participants rested for 40 min prior to a DRM memory test, in the moderate intensity exercise condition participants completed 40 min of steady state running prior to a DRM memory test, and in the high intensity exercise condition participants completed 2 × 3 min of sprints prior to a DRM memory test.

Activities and Measures
Rest Protocol

Similar to Study 1, participants sat quietly in the laboratory for 40 min and were given popular magazines to read, and were monitored throughout.

Exercise Protocols

Running was undertaken on a h/p/cosmos pulsar 3p treadmill (h/p/cosmos sports & medical GmbH). In the first testing session, participants' baseline fitness levels were assessed. In that session, participants completed a treadmill based graded exercise test to determine their VO2peak and HRmax. Oxygen uptake (VO2) was measured using a METAMAX cardiopulmonary exercise testing system (Cortex Biophysik GmbH) with breathing mask, pre-calibrated according to the manufacturer's instructions. A computerized indirect calorimetry system collected 30-s averages for oxygen uptake (VO2) and respiratory exchange ratio (RER). ***Moderate intensity exercise***: Participants completed 40 min of continuous moderate intensity running consisting of a 5-min warm-up (work rate at 30% of VO2peak), followed by 35 min of exercise at 60% of VVO2peak (Velocity at Vo2 Peak). ***High intensity exercise***: this condition aimed to achieve a very high intensity and high blood-lactate concentration (10 mmol/l or above) while limiting the total exercise duration, fatigue and dehydration. Participants completed a 5-min warm-up (30% of VO2peak), and then completed two incremental maximal efforts (3 min each), separated by 2 min passive recovery. In line with Winter et al. (2007) running protocol description, the treadmill speed started at 8 km/h, and increased every 10s by 2 km/h, until volitional exhaustion.

Heart Rate (HR), Affective Valence, Ratings of Perceived Exertion

These were measured in an identical manner to Experiment 1.

Arousal

Participants reported subjective arousal levels using 20-item Activation-Deactivation Adjective Checklist (ADCL), to generate four subscales; energy, tiredness, tension, and calmness. Participants rate affect adjectives on a four-point scale: definitely feel, slightly feel, cannot decide, definitely do not feel. The ADCL has acceptable reliability and validity (Thayer, 1989).

Blood-Lactate

Blood-lactate levels for moderate and high intensity running exercise was predicted to be above 10 mmol/l or below

2 mmol/l, respectively (Spurway, 1992). Blood-lactate was measured from fingertip capillary blood samples using an automated analyzer (Analox GM7 enzymatic metabolite analyzer, Analox instruments USA, Lunenburg, MA) immediately post-exercise and between recall and recognition tasks.

Memory Task

The DRM paradigm followed the same protocols from Experiment 1. Eighteen DRM lists of 15 words (critical lures: Window, Doctor, Smoke, Anger, Cup, Slow, Sleep, Sweet, Rough, Soft, Cold, River, Smell, Chair, Needle, City, Mountain, Spider) were divided into three sets of six and their assignment to each condition was counterbalanced. The recognition tests were constructed in a similar manner to Experiment 1.

Procedure

Participants individually attended four sessions (an initial screening and baseline fitness test, followed by the three activity conditions) on separate days at the same time of day (to control for diurnal variation) in the same laboratory. A seven-day rest period between each session controlled for fatigue and memory carry over effects. In the first session, participants read and signed an informed consent sheet, completed a pre-exercise health screening, the fitness test and were introduced to the memory task. In the second, third, and fourth sessions, the order of the three conditions were counterbalanced. To avoid dehydration, water was available *ad libitum* throughout exercise and participant were instructed to arrive hydrated. The same researcher provided the same instructions and monitored the participant during all activities and testing. Participants' RPE, affect, and HR were taken every 2 min during moderate intensity exercise and rest, and in the last min of each activity (sprint and recovery) of the high intensity condition. Immediately after each activity, a DRM memory test was completed in a distraction free testing booth situated next to the activity area. Upon completion of the activity, transition from the activity to the testing booth, reinstruction and commencing the memory task took approximately 2 min. A blood-lactate sample was taken and the ADCL was completed four times per experimental session: (1) before undertaking the activity (2) immediately prior to the free recall test, (3) immediately prior to the recognition test, and (4) after the recognition test. Following the final testing session, participants were debriefed regarding the aims of the experiment.

Statistical Analysis

Pre-activity blood-lactate, pre-activity arousal, average RPE, FS ratings, and HR were compared using one-way repeated measures ANOVAs. Post-activity blood-lactate was analyzed using two-way (Time × Activity) repeated-measures ANOVA. ADCL subscale ratings were analyzed using a MANOVA considering Condition (Rest vs. Moderate Exercise vs. High Intensity Exercise) and Time (Pre-Activity, Pre-free recall test, Pre-recognition test, and post-recognition test) as the within-subjects factor, and ADCL subscale (Energy, Calmness, Tiredness, Tension) as dependent variables. Mean number of studied words correctly recalled, critical lures falsely recalled, and non-studied new words incorrectly recalled in the three

activity conditions was analyzed with a MANOVA followed by univariate ANOVAs, considering Condition (Rest vs. Moderate Exercise vs. High Intensity Exercise) as the within-subjects factor, and recall type (correct recall, critical lure, and other errors) as dependent variables. For the assessment of recognition, a MANOVA with Condition (Rest vs. Moderate Intensity Exercise vs. High Intensity Exercise) as the within-subjects factor and word type (Critical Lure, Studied Word, New Word) as the dependent variables was employed. If Mauchly's Test indicated sphericity was violated, a Greenhouse-Geisser correction was employed (εGG is reported in such cases). Partial eta-squared (η_p^2) is reported as a measure of effect-size.

RESULTS

Baseline Arousal and Blood-Lactate

There were no significant multivariate effect of Condition on participants' baseline arousal levels, assessed via the four ADCL subscales, prior to each of the three activities, $\lambda = 0.91$, $F(8, 90) = 0.53$, $p = 0.83$, $\eta_p^2 = 0.05$. Similarly, there was no significant difference in their baseline blood-lactate levels prior to each activity, $F(2, 48) = 2.63$, $p = 0.08$, $\eta_p^2 = 0.10$ (see **Table 3**).

End of Activity Exertion, Heart Rate, and Affect

RPE was significantly different in the final minute of each condition, $F(1.33, 31.96) = 108.57$, $p < 0.001$, $\eta_p^2 = 0.82$, εGG = 0.67. As would be expected, participants had significantly higher average RPE during high intensity exercise (16.36 ± 3.32) compared to moderate intensity exercise (12.68 ± 2.39; $p < 0.001$) and rest (6.12 ± 0.44; $p = 0.001$) conditions, and these latter conditions were also statistically different ($p < 0.001$). HR was also significantly different in the final minute of each condition, $F(2, 48) = 632.99$, $p < 0.001$, $\eta_p^2 = 0.96$, with high intensity exercise (170bpm ± 12.55, 88.04% HRmax) producing significantly higher average HR than both moderate intensity exercise (154.08 bpm ± 15.52, 79.43% HRmax; $p < 0.001$) and rest (66.12 bpm ± 7.34, 34.03% HRmax; $p < 0.001$). The latter two activities HR were also significantly different ($p < 0.001$). Affect was significantly different between conditions, $F(2, 48) = 17.48$, $p < 0.001$, $\eta_p^2 = 0.42$, with high intensity exercise inducing less positive affect (0.24 ± 2.52) than moderate intensity exercise (2.40 ± 1.76; $p < 0.001$) and rest (3.04 ± 1.67; $p < 0.001$). End of activity affect was equivalent for the latter two activities ($p = 0.59$). Finally, self-reported arousal in the final minute of each activity condition was significantly different, $F(2, 48) = 32.91$, $p < 0.001$, $\eta_p^2 = 0.58$. High intensity exercise (4.24 ± 1.56) induced average arousal levels significantly higher than moderate intensity exercise (3.32 ± 1.38; $p = 0.02$) and rest (1.92 ± 1.19; $p < 0.001$), which were themselves different ($p < 0.001$) (see **Table 4**). Combined, the above confirm that participants felt more exerted, aroused, and less pleasurable, in the final minute of the high intensity exercise than the moderate intensity exercise and period of rest. Moreover, they felt more exerted and aroused, but no less pleasurable, toward the end of the moderate intensity exercise than the period of rest.

TABLE 3 | Blood Lactate and Arousal responses (M ± SD) before and after the three activities (rest, moderate intensity exercise, high intensity exercise) in Experiment 2.

Measure	Time	Rest	Moderate exercise	Intense exercise
Blood Lactate mmol/l	Pre-activity	1.00 (0.41)	1.13 (0.42)	1.27 (0.45)
	Post-activity	1.08 (0.42)	1.78 (0.76)	6.20 (0.55)
	Post-Recall	1.01 (0.36)	1.74 (0.58)	6.22 (1.48)
	Post-recognition	0.96 (0.29)	1.51 (0.43)	5.60 (1.35)
Energy	Pre-activity	9.84 (4.09)	11.00 (4.93)	11.44 (5.08)
	Post-activity	7.88 (4.39)	13.40 (4.74)	15.36 (4.92)
	Post-Recall	10.12 (4.60)	10.80 (4.71)	10.00 (5.33)
	Post-recognition	9.96 (4.31)	9.96 (4.78)	10.36 (5.31)
Calmness	Pre-activity	14.08 (3.55)	13.60 (5.43)	13.04 (4.06)
	Post-activity	15.80 (5.26)	10.24 (3.32)	8.56 (3.92)
	Post-Recall	14.88 (5.87)	13.08 (5.34)	13.56 (3.92)
	Post-recognition	14.24 (4.87)	13.28 (3.92)	13.64 (4.21)
Tiredness	Pre-activity	9.12 (5.59)	8.52 (4.50)	8.60 (3.98)
	Post-activity	10.28 (5.73)	6.24 (3.36)	7.48 (6.47)
	Post-Recall	9.64 (5.18)	8.16 (4.90)	9.88 (5.15)
	Post-recognition	9.76 (5.44)	8.32 (4.71)	9.32 (5.48)
Tension	Pre-activity	7.44 (3.34)	7.76 (3.11)	7.68 (3.48)
	Post-activity	7.28 (2.85)	8.68 (3.04)	8.96 (2.26)
	Post-Recall	7.80 (3.23)	7.84 (3.47)	8.00 (2.69)
	Post-recognition	7.12 (2.99)	7.64 (3.60)	7.36 (2.38)

Post-activity Blood-Lactate

Our two-way analyses of post-activity blood-lactate levels revealed a significant main effect of Activity, $F(1.33, 31.94) = 283.78$, $p < 0.001$, $\eta_p^2 = 0.92$, $\varepsilon GG = 0.67$. *Post hoc* analysis revealed that blood-lactate levels were significantly higher after high intensity exercise (6.01 ± 1.25 mmol/l) compared to moderate intensity exercise (1.68 ± 0.5 mmol/l; $p < 0.001$) and rest (1.02 ± 0.3 mmol/l; $p < 0.001$). Moreover, moderate intensity exercise resulted in higher post-exercise blood-lactate levels than rest ($p < 0.001$). There was also a main effect of Time, $F(1.24, 29.79) = 6.81$, $p = 0.002$, $\eta_p^2 = 0.22$, $\varepsilon GG = 0.62$, indicating decreasing BL post-exercise. *Post hoc* analyses showed that blood-lactate levels were lowest Post-Recognition (2.69 ± 2.5 mmol/l) compared to Post-Exercise (3.02 ± 3.0 mmol/l; $p = 0.03$) and Post-Recall (2.99 ± 2.5 mmol/l; $p < 0.001$), which were themselves not different ($p = 0.12$). There was no Activity x Time interaction, $F(1.61, 38.74) = 1.55$, $p = 0.15$, $\eta_p^2 = 0.07$, $\varepsilon GG = 0.40$. Together, this indicates exercise increased peripheral BL concentrations, and intense exercise resulted in the greatest elevation indicative of greater workload (see **Table 3**).

TABLE 4 | During-activity RPE, HR (bpm), Affect and arousal (Mean ± SD) from final section of the three activities (rest, moderate intensity exercise, high intensity exercise) in Experiment 2.

Activity	RPE	HR (bpm)	Affect	Arousal
Rest	6.12 (0.44)[b,c]	66.12 (7.34)[b, c]	3.04 (1.67)[b,c]	1.92 (1.19)[b,c]
Moderate Exercise	12.68 (2.39)[a,c]	154.08 (15.52)[a,c]	2.40 (1.76)[a,c]	3.32 (1.38)[a,c]
Intense Exercise	16.36 (3.32)[a,b]	170 12.55)[a,b]	0.24 (2.52)[a,b]	4.24 (1.56)[a,b]

[a]*Significantly different from rest,* [b]*significantly different from moderate intensity exercise,* [c]*significantly different from high intensity exercise.*

However, whilst moderate intensity BL concentrations are in line with expectations, the intense anaerobic exercise did not reach the intended threshold (e.g., lactate levels above 10 mmol/l, Spurway, 1992).

Post-activity Arousal

The results showed a significant multivariate Condition x Time interaction, $\lambda = 0.58$, $F(24, 493) = 3.45$, $p < 0.001$, $\eta_p^2 = 0.13$. The follow-up univariate analyses confirmed significant Condition x Time interactions for Energy, $F(4.55, 109.17) = 13.67$, MSE = 108.74, $p < 0.001$, $\eta_p^2 = 0.36$, $\varepsilon GG = 0.76$, Calmness, $F(4.02, 96.46) = 6.54$, MSE = 100.65, $p < 0.001$, $\eta_p^2 = 0.21$, $\varepsilon GG = 0.67$, but not Tiredness, $F(3.42, 81.97) = 1.93$, MSE = 32.56, $p = 0.12$, $\eta_p^2 = 0.07$, $\varepsilon GG = 0.57$, or Tension, $F(4.33, 103.96) = 1.14$, MSE = 5.40, $p = 0.34$, $\eta_p^2 = 0.05$, $\varepsilon GG = 0.72$. Energy levels increased post-activity for both exercise conditions when compared to rest (which had reduced from baseline), these returned to comparable levels post-recall and recognition. There were lower calmness levels post-activity for both exercise conditions compared to rest (which increased from baseline), with the lowest calmness post-intense exercise. These returned to comparable levels post-recall and recognition, albeit with calmness remaining high for the rest condition. For Tiredness, there was a significant multivariate, $\lambda = 0.63$, $F(8, 90) = 2.89$, $p < 0.01$, $\eta_p^2 = 0.20$, and univariate, $F(2, 48) = 3.30$, MSE = 89.44, $p < 0.05$, $\eta_p^2 = 0.12$, effect of Condition. Bonferroni-adjusted pairwise comparisons revealed that Tiredness was significantly lower in the Moderate Intensity Exercise condition (7.81 ± 3.62) than Rest (9.70 ± 4.74, $p = 0.02$), but not High-Intensity Exercise (8.82 ± 4.63, $p = 0.59$). The latter two conditions were also not significantly different ($p = 0.84$). Taken together, both forms of exercise resulted comparable reductions in calmness and

TABLE 5 | Mean (SD) number of studied words correctly recalled (max = 90), critical lures falsely recalled (max = 6), and non-studied new words (not critical lures) incorrectly recalled after the three activities in Experiment 2.

Activity	Studied words	Critical lures	Non-studied words
Rest	42.20 (8.36)	2.68 (1.65)	1.52 (1.66)
Moderate Exercise	47.20 (7.43)[a]	2.64 (1.47)	2.28 (2.84)
Intense Exercise	45.16 (9.87)	2.84 (1.40)	1.96 (2.17)

[a]significantly different from rest.

increases in energy post-activity, which returned to baseline post-recognition (see **Table 3**). Tiredness was lowest during all phases post-moderate intensity exercise. There was a trend for larger effects of intense exercise on energy and calmness. Rest had a smaller, yet opposite effect on these characteristics.

Short-Term Free Recall

Table 5 shows mean number of studied words correctly recalled, critical lures falsely recalled, and non-studied new words incorrectly recalled in the three activity conditions. Results showed a significant multivariate effect of Condition, $\lambda = 0.76$, $F(6, 92) = 2.28$, $p = 0.042$, $\eta_p^2 = 0.13$. The follow-up univariate analyses confirmed a significant main effect of condition for Correct Recall, $F(2, 48) = 4.96$, $MSE = 158.01$, $p = 0.011$, $\eta_p^2 = 0.17$. As expected, Bonferroni-adjusted pairwise comparisons revealed that more studied words were correctly recalled after moderate intensity $(47.20 + 8.36)$ exercise than rest $(42.20 \pm 8.36$, $p = 0.005)$. Contrary to expectations, there were no significant differences in the correct recall after moderate intensity and high intensity exercise $(45.16 \pm 9.87$, $p = 0.52)$ or after high intensity exercise and rest $(p = 0.39)$. Importantly, the activity engaged in had no impact upon the number of critical lures falsely recalled, $F(2, 48) = 0.16$, $MSE = 0.28$, $p = 0.85$, $\eta_p^2 = 0.01$, or the number of non-studied new words incorrectly recalled $F(1.22, 46.33) = 1.82$, $MSE = 37.92$, $p = 0.19$, $\eta_p^2 = 0.07$ (Greenhouse-Geisser corrections applied to the latter main effect).

Recognition Memory

The mean proportion of studied words, critical lures, and non-studied new words classed as *old* following each of the three activities, and the proportion of *remember*, *know*, and *guess* made responses to these words, are in **Table 6**. There was no significant multivariate effect of Condition on the proportion of words correctly recognized, $\lambda = 0.86$, $F(1, 25) = 0.50$, $p = 0.80$, $\eta_p^2 = 0.14$. Similarly, A MANOVA with Condition (Rest vs. Exercise) and Word Type (Studied vs. Critical Lure vs. New) as within-subjects factors, and judgment type (*Remember, Know, Guess*) as the dependent variables showed no significant multivariate effect of Condition on the proportion of words were recognized, $\lambda = 0.82$, $F(6, 19) = 0.71$, $p = 0.65$, $\eta_p^2 = 0.18$. As such, despite large proportions of studied words being accurately and critical lures falsely recognized, and few non-studied new words being recognized, exercise did not impact upon true and false recognition rates.

GENERAL DISCUSSION

The current study provides initial evidence that acute aerobic exercise can not only enhance free recall performance, but also that this benefit is not accompanied by changes in false recall. In Experiment 1, results demonstrated that moderate intensity exercise improved free recall performance compared to a rest condition, with no associated increase in false recall. In Experiment 2, moderate intensity exercise again improved memory performance, and that this benefit was also observed compared to an intense exercise condition. The intense exercise condition, however, did not result in an increase in false memory recall. This partially supports and advances the initial observations made by Loprinzi and colleagues (Dilley et al., 2019; Green and Loprinzi, 2018; Siddiqui and Loprinzi, 2018) that exercise may have beneficial effects on false memory.

By assessing both free recall and recognition memory, the data suggests that whilst free recall was benefited, recognition memory was not influenced by exercise. This supports the Dilley et al.'s (2019) findings and may be due to the different mechanisms underlying free recall and recognition (Diekelmann et al., 2010). For example, recognition tasks aid source monitoring processes through the reactivation of sensory details of the study words and their encoding context (Cabeza et al., 2001) and recognition decisions are based on inferential judgments. This can be evidenced by the similarly high levels of critical lure recognition in both experiments, but otherwise low levels in the recall test. Also, recall tests were completed before the recognition test, which has been shown to influence recognition rates (e.g., Roediger and McDermott, 1995). Similar temporal considerations are important for the impact of exercise, as the effects of exercise on self-reported arousal and blood lactate had all decreased by the recognition testing phase, reducing the effects of exercise on response bias. However, given that exercise induced arousal was elevated during encoding, this requires further consideration.

In line with FTT, these findings suggest that exercise did not influence gist based memory processes when compared to quiet rest. Concerning the increased correct recall of presented words, exercise appears to have increased verbatim processing through focusing active attention on the perceptual details of presented words (potentially through effective mental rehearsal). This suggestion is in line with the proposal that acute moderate intensity exercise facilitates attentional allocation and efficient information processing speeds during cognitive tasks (e.g., Hillman et al., 2003; Kamijo et al., 2007), also evidenced through larger P3 amplitude (Hillman et al., 2003; Kamijo et al., 2007) and shorter P3 latency (Hillman et al., 2003). This improved active attentional allocation supported the encoding of contextually specific information, and consequentially assisted the recall of presented words but not non-presented words that were merely semantically activated. It is also possible that post-exercise encoding may inhibit automatic spreading activation. Given that arousal and BL levels were highest immediately post-exercise, it is likely exercise biased the encoding phase. Indeed, researchers suggest acute exercise may primarily benefit encoding rather than consolidation (stabilization of memory

TABLE 6 | Mean (SD) proportion of studied words correctly recognized, critical lures falsely recognized, and non-studied new items incorrectly recognized following each activity in Experiment 2.

		Rest	Moderate intensity exercise	High intensity exercise
Studied Words	Old (*Correct*)	0.84 (0.15)	0.85 (0.11)	0.84 (0.12)
	Remember	0.53 (0.25)	0.59 (0.59)	0.58 (0.24)
	Know	0.21 (0.24)	0.17 (0.19)	0.15 (0.22)
	Guess	0.10 (0.08)	0.09 (0.10)	0.10 (0.13)
Critical Lures	Old (*Incorrect*)	0.85 (0.18)	0.85 (0.21)	0.86 (0.22)
	Remember	0.52 (0.30)	0.59 (0.36)	0.53 (0.35)
	Know	0.24 (0.31)	0.15 (0.20)	0.24 (0.27)
	Guess	0.09 (0.14)	0.11 (0.17)	0.09 (0.18)
New Words	Old (*Incorrect*)	0.18 (0.24)	0.10 (0.24)	0.13 (0.13)
	Remember	0.03 (0.07)	0.02 (0.04)	0.05 (0.09)
	Know	0.01 (0.03)	0.03 (0.08)	0.02 (0.06)
	Guess	0.14 (0.23)	0.05 (0.09)	0.05 (0.08)

traces post-encoding) (e.g., Labban and Etnier, 2011), although others highlight exercise benefiting consolidation (McNerney and Radvansky, 2015). These initial findings point to a limited impact of physical exercise on false memory generation.

One key limitation is that no exploration of long-term memory consolidation processes is possible, which other researchers have highlighted as a key role of exercise (e.g., Tomporowski and Pendleton, 2018). There is also the potential that as the effects of exercise remain long after exercise completion, retrieval processes may also have been influenced by exercise. In addition, the present study did not take into account baseline in memory performance. This may be an important consideration given that both propensity for false recall (e.g., Diekelmann et al., 2010) and influence of exercise on cognition (e.g., Sibley and Beilock, 2007) are sensitive cognitive capacity.

Whilst the present study addressed exercise intensity, the protocols in terms of intensity and manipulation were not without issue. For example, the American College of Sports Medicine (2013) considers moderate intensity exercise to be between 64–76% of estimated HRmax. In Experiment 1, heart rates were well within this range (68.40% HRmax), yet participants in Experiment 2 exercised on average at 79.43%HRmax in the equivalent condition. This suggests that intensity may have been higher than expected in Experiment 2, and across the sample 13 participants were above this HR range. Using perceptual data, only 6 participants rated their RPE as being above the 13 upper limit identified as indicating moderate intensity exercise. Importantly, significant differences across all conditions in Experiment 2 for RPE and HR suggest that the conditions were distinct in terms of intensity. Yet a consequence is that across the experiments, moderate intensity exercise conditions were different not only in terms of intensity, but also the resultant affective experience. With Experiment 1 participants experienced moderate intensity exercise (RPE between somewhat hard and hard, with option to adjust intensity) as more positive than in Experiment 2 (intensity set at 60% of VO2peak). This may have been a result of the self-controlled nature versus prescriptive protocols employed,

with self-selected exercise associated with more positive affective responses through perceived autonomy (Oliveira et al., 2015). Future research should explore the role of exercise intensity and its manipulation in terms of true and false memory generation. Finally, the generalizability of these findings are limited by the use of regularly physically active samples of young adults. Whilst there is limited evidence on the moderating role of fitness in the acute exercise and memory relationship (Loprinzi et al., 2019), fitness status is acknowledged an important consideration (Chang et al., 2012). Therefore, future studies are needed to explore the roles of exercise intensity and fitness, as well as other individual differences (e.g., cognitive capacity, age), proposed to moderate acute exercise and cognitive performance relationship.

In conclusion, the present study found that acute bouts of moderate intensity aerobic exercise performed before encoding and immediate retrieval of semantically associated words improved the volume of studied information correctly recalled. There were no associated increases in false memory generation, suggesting that exercise induced arousal facilitated verbatim memory traces rather than promoting gist-based processing at encoding. This is in line with Lambourne and Tomporowski (2010) meta-regression analysis observations that post-exercise exercise-induced arousal facilitates speeded mental process, as well as enhancing memory storage and retrieval, even if the exercise was intended to induce physical fatigue. This also supports initial proposals made by Loprinzi and colleagues (Green and Loprinzi, 2018; Siddiqui and Loprinzi, 2018; Dilley et al., 2019), and the encoding acute exercise benefits suggested by Labban and Etnier (2018). There may be a limitation to this arousal effect, as intense exercise did not result in improvements in free recall performance, potentially due to more negative affect during intense exercise compared to moderate intensity exercise. The beneficial effects may be associated with acute exercise's support of attentional processes and allocation, as well as arousal increasing verbatim processing of information. Research is required to address the underlying mechanisms and exercise characteristics (i.e., intensity, mode, duration and timing) that influence these false memory effects.

ETHICS STATEMENT

The studies involving human participants were reviewed and approved by Edge Hill University Department of Sport and Physical Activity Ethics Committee. The participants provided their written informed consent to participate in this study.

AUTHOR CONTRIBUTIONS

DM, CT, and KM conceived, designed, and prepared the materials. DM and KM supervised the data collection. SH and LF collected the data. DM wrote the first draft. DM, CT, KM, SH, and LF contributed to the final approval of the version to be published and agreed to be accountable for all aspects of the work. All authors contributed to revising drafts critically for important intellectual content.

ACKNOWLEDGMENTS

We would like to thank the participants for their time and efforts in this study.

REFERENCES

American College of Sports Medicine, (Ed.). (2013). *ACSM's Health-Related Physical Fitness Assessment Manual*. Philadelphia, PA: Lippincott Williams & Wilkins.

Blough, J., and Loprinzi, P. D. (2019). Experimental manipulation of psychological control scenarios: implications for exercise and memory research. *Psych* 1, 279–289. doi: 10.3390/psych1010019

Borg, G. (1998). *Borg's Perceived Exertion and Pain Scales*. Champaign, IL: Human kinetics.

Brainerd, C. J., and Reyna, V. F. (2002). Fuzzy-trace theory and false memory. *Curr. Dir. Psychol. Sci.* 11, 164–169. doi: 10.1111/1467-8721.00192

Cabeza, R., Rao, S. M., Wagner, A. D., Mayer, A. R., and Schacter, D. L. (2001). Can medial temporal lobe regions distinguish true from false? An event-related functional MRI study of veridical and illusory recognition memory. *Proc. Natl. Acad. Sci. U.S.A.* 98, 4805–4810. doi: 10.1073/pnas.081082698

Chang, Y. K., Labban, J. D., Gapin, J. I., and Etnier, J. L. (2012). The effects of acute exercise on cognitive performance: a meta-analysis. *Brain Res.* 1453, 87–101. doi: 10.1016/j.brainres.2012.02.068

Cohen, J. (1988). *Statistical Power Analysis for the Behavioral Sciences*, 2nd Edn. Hillsdale, NJ: Erlbaum.

Coles, K., and Tomporowski, P. D. (2008). Effects of acute exercise on executive processing, short-term and long-term memory. *Sports Sci.* 26, 333–344. doi: 10.1080/02640410701591417

Corson, Y., and Verrier, N. (2007). Emotions and false memories: Valence or arousal? *Psychol. Sci.* 18, 208–211. doi: 10.1111/j.1467-9280.2007.01874.x

Diekelmann, S., Born, J., and Wagner, U. (2010). Sleep enhances false memories depending on general memory performance. *Behav. Brain Res.* 208, 425–429. doi: 10.1016/j.bbr.2009.12.021

Dilley, E. K., Zou, L., and Loprinzi, P. D. (2019). The effects of acute exercise intensity on episodic and false memory among young adult college students. *Health Promot. Perspect.* 9, 143–149. doi: 10.15171/hpp.2019.20

Etnier, J. L., Wideman, L., Labban, J. D., Piepmeier, A. T., Pendleton, D. M., Dvorak, K. K., et al. (2016). The effects of acute exercise on memory and brain-derived neurotrophic factor (BDNF). *J. Sport Exerc. Psychol.* 38, 331–340. doi: 10.1123/jsep.2015-0335

Gallo, D. A. (2010). False memories and fantastic beliefs: 15 years of the DRM illusion. *Mem. Cognit.* 38, 833–848. doi: 10.3758/mc.38.7.833

Garber, C. E., Blissmer, B., Deschenes, M. R., Franklin, B. A., Lamonte, M. J., Lee, I. M., et al. (2011). Quantity and quality of exercise for developing and maintaining cardiorespiratory, musculoskeletal, and neuromotor fitness in apparently healthy adults: guidance for prescribing exercise. *Med. Sci. Sports Exerc.* 43, 1334–1359. doi: 10.1249/mss.0b013e318213fefb

Green, D., and Loprinzi, P. D. (2018). Experimental effects of acute exercise on prospective memory and false memory. *Psychol. Rep.* 122, 1313–1326. doi: 10.1177/0033294118782466

Hardy, C. J., and Rejeski, W. J. (1989). Not what, but how one feels: the measurement of affect during exercise. *J. Sport Exerc. Psychol.* 11, 304–317. doi: 10.1123/jsep.11.3.304

Hillman, C. H., Snook, E. M., and Jerome, G. J. (2003). Acute cardiovascular exercise and executive control function. *Int. J. Psychophysiol.* 48, 307–314. doi: 10.1016/s0167-8760(03)00080-1

Kamijo, K., Nishihira, Y., Higashiura, T., and Kuroiwa, K. (2007). The interactive effect of exercise intensity and task difficulty on human cognitive processing. *Int. J. Psychophysiol.* 65, 114–121. doi: 10.1016/j.ijpsycho.2007.04.001

Knott, L. M., and Thorley, C. (2014). Mood-congruent false memories persist over time. *Cogn. Emot.* 28, 903–912. doi: 10.1080/02699931.2013.860016

Labban, J. D., and Etnier, J. L. (2011). Effects of acute exercise on long-term memory. *Res. Q. Exerc. Sport* 82, 712–721. doi: 10.1080/02701367.2011.10599808

Labban, J. D., and Etnier, J. L. (2018). The effect of acute exercise on encoding and consolidation of long-term memory. *J. Sport Exerc. Psychol.* 40, 336–342. doi: 10.1123/jsep.2018-0072

Lambourne, K., and Tomporowski, P. (2010). The effect of exercise-induced arousal on cognitive task performance: a meta-regression analysis. *Brain Res.* 1341, 12–24. doi: 10.1016/j.brainres.2010.03.091

Loprinzi, P. D. (2018). Intensity-specific effects of acute exercise on human memory function: Considerations for the timing of exercise and the type of memory. *Health Promot. Perspect.* 8:255. doi: 10.15171/hpp.2018.36

Loprinzi, P. D., Blough, J., Crawford, L., Ryu, S., Zou, L., and Li, H. (2019). The temporal effects of acute exercise on episodic memory function: Systematic review with meta-analysis. *Brain Sci.* 9:87. doi: 10.3390/brainsci9040087

Mahoney, C. R., Brunyé, T. T., Giles, G. E., Ditman, T., Lieberman, H. R., and Taylor, H. A. (2012). Caffeine increases false memory in nonhabitual consumers. *J. Cogn. Psychol.* 24, 420–427. doi: 10.1080/20445911.2011.647905

McMorris, T., and Hale, B. J. (2012). Differential effects of differing intensities of acute exercise on speed and accuracy of cognition: a meta-analytical investigation. *Brain Cogn.* 80, 338–351. doi: 10.1016/j.bandc.2012.09.001

McNerney, M. W., and Radvansky, G. A. (2015). Mind racing: The influence of exercise on long-term memory consolidation. *Memory* 23, 1140–1151. doi: 10.1080/09658211.2014.962545

Oliveira, B., Deslandes, A., and Santos, T. (2015). Differences in exercise intensity seems to influence the affective responses in self-selected and imposed exercise: a meta-analysis. *Front. Psychol.* 6:1105.

Roediger, H. L., and McDermott, K. B. (1995). Creating false memories: remembering words not presented in lists. *J. Exp. Psychol. Learn Mem. Cogn.* 21, 803–814. doi: 10.1037/0278-7393.21.4.803

Roediger, H. L., Watson, J. M., McDermott, K. B., and Gallo, D. A. (2001). Factors that determine false recall: a multiple regression analysis. *Psychon. Bull. Rev.* 8, 385–407. doi: 10.3758/bf03196177

Salas, C. R., Minakata, K., and Kelemen, W. L. (2011). Walking before study enhances free recall but not judgement-of-learning magnitude. *J. Cogn. Psychol.* 23, 507–513. doi: 10.1080/20445911.2011.532207

Sibley, B. A., and Beilock, S. L. (2007). Exercise and working memory: an individual differences investigation. *J. Sport Exerc. Psychol.* 29, 783–791. doi: 10.1123/jsep.29.6.783

Siddiqui, A., and Loprinzi, P. (2018). Experimental investigation of the time course effects of acute exercise on false episodic memory. *J. Clin. Med.* 7:157. doi: 10.3390/jcm7070157

Soga, K., Kamijo, K., and Masaki, H. (2017). Aerobic exercise during encoding impairs hippocampus-dependent memory. *J. Sport Exerc. Psychol.* 39, 249–260. doi: 10.1123/jsep.2016-0254

Spurway, N. C. (1992). Aerobic exercise, anaerobic exercise and the lactate threshold. *Br. Med. Bull.* 48, 569–591. doi: 10.1093/oxfordjournals.bmb.a072564

Stadler, M. A., Roediger, H. L., and McDermott, K. B. (1999). Norms for word lists that create false memories. *Mem. Cognit.* 27, 494–500. doi: 10.3758/bf03211543

Thayer, R. E. (1989). *The Biopsychology of Mood and Arousal.* New York, NY: Oxford University Press.

Tomporowski, P. D., and Pendleton, D. M. (2018). Effects of the timing of acute exercise and movement complexity on young adults' psychomotor learning. *J. Sport Exerc. Psychol.* 40, 240–248. doi: 10.1123/jsep.2017-0289

Winter, B., Breitenstein, C., Mooren, F. C., Voelker, K., Fobker, M., Lechtermann, A., et al. (2007). High impact running improves learning. *Neurobiol. Learn. Mem.* 87, 597–609. doi: 10.1016/j.nlm.2006.11.003

4

Low Physical Activity and Cardiorespiratory Fitness in People with Schizophrenia: A Comparison with Matched Healthy Controls and Associations with Mental and Physical Health

Thomas W. Scheewe [1,2]*, Frederike Jörg [3,4], Tim Takken [5], Jeroen Deenik [6],
Davy Vancampfort [7,8], Frank J. G. Backx [9] and Wiepke Cahn [1]

[1] Department of Psychiatry, Rudolf Magnus Institute for Neuroscience, University Medical Center Utrecht, Utrecht, Netherlands, [2] Department of Human Movement and Education, Windesheim University of Applied Sciences, Zwolle, Netherlands, [3] Rob Giel Research Center, University Center of Psychiatry, University Medical Center Groningen, University of Groningen, Groningen, Netherlands, [4] Research Department, GGZ Friesland (Friesland Mental Health Services), Leeuwarden, Netherlands, [5] Child Development and Exercise Center, Wilhelmina Children's Hospital, University Medical Center Utrecht, Utrecht, Netherlands, [6] GGz Centraal, Amersfoort, Netherlands, [7] University Psychiatric Center KU Leuven, Leuven, Belgium, [8] Department of Rehabilitation Sciences, KU Leuven, Leuven, Belgium, [9] Department of Rehabilitation, Physical Therapy Science and Sports, Rudolf Magnus Institute for Neuroscience, University Medical Center Utrecht, Utrecht, Netherlands

Correspondence:
Thomas W. Scheewe
tw.scheewe@windesheim.nl

Introduction: The aim of this study was to objectively assess time spent in physical activity (PA) and sedentary behavior (SB) in patients with schizophrenia compared to healthy controls matched for age, gender and socioeconomic status. Associations between both PA and cardiorespiratory fitness (CRF) and mental and physical health parameters in patients with schizophrenia were examined.

Materials and Methods: Moderate and vigorous PA (MVPA), moderate PA, vigorous PA, total and active energy expenditure (TEE and AEE), number of steps, lying down and sleeping time was assessed with SenseWear Pro-2 body monitoring system for three 24-h bouts in patients with schizophrenia ($n = 63$) and matched healthy controls ($n = 55$). Severity of symptoms (Positive and Negative Syndrome Scale and Montgomery and Åsberg Depression Rating Scale), CRF (peak oxygen uptake, VO_{2peak}), body mass index (BMI), and metabolic syndrome were assessed.

Results: Patients with schizophrenia performed less MVPA and moderate activity had lower TEE and AEE, spent more time per day lying down and sleeping, and had poorer CRF compared to healthy controls. The amount of MVPA, but especially CRF was associated with severity of negative symptoms in patients with schizophrenia. Only CRF was associated with BMI.

Discussion: The current data offer further evidence for interventions aiming to increase physical activity and decrease sedentary behavior. Given strong associations of CRF with both negative symptoms and BMI, treatment aimed at CRF-improvement may prove to be effective.

Keywords: physical activity, sedentary behavior, cardiorespiratory fitness, schizophrenia, matched healthy controls

INTRODUCTION

The premature mortality risk in patients with schizophrenia is two to three times higher compared to the general population leading to a 7–20 year reduction in life expectancy (1–3), mainly due to cardiovascular disease (4, 5). The increased cardio-metabolic risk is partly attributable to side effects of antipsychotic medication such as weight gain, dyslipidemia, and diabetes mellitus (4, 6).

Three recent meta-analyses show patients with schizophrenia engage in less physical activity (PA) (7), have high levels of sedentary behavior (SB) in their waking day (8), and have low cardiorespiratory fitness (CRF)-levels (9). The majority of the included studies used self-report to assess PA (7) which, due to recall errors and social desirability bias, has limited validity (10, 11). Illustrative, whereas no difference in PA was found using self-report measurement, accelerometry showed a large reduction of PA in patients with schizophrenia compared to healthy controls (12). As for SB, a meta-analysis demonstrated that patients with psychosis spend 11 h of their waking day being sedentary. Again, objective measurement of SB demonstrated significantly higher levels of SB compared to self-report measurements (8).

In patients with psychosis, a limited number of studies have suggested that high levels of SB and low levels of PA are associated with an increased cardio-metabolic risk [e.g., (13, 14)]. These studies did not take CRF into account, and most of these studies assessed SB and PA using self-report (10, 11). One study examined independent associations of objectively measured SB and PA with cardio-metabolic risk in inpatients with schizophrenia as well as in age/sex/body mass index-matched healthy controls (15), but failed to take CRF into account. As far as we know, only one study (16) did include CRF when investigating associations between SB and PA with cardio-metabolic risk factors in patients with psychosis. This study showed that SB is, independently of PA and CRF, associated with the individual risk factors waist and fasting blood glucose. Strikingly, CRF, even when controlled for SB and PA, remained significantly associated with clustered cardio-metabolic risk and the individual risk factor waist. The study by Bueno-Antequera et al. (16) is mildly hampered by some limitations. For instance, they did not include healthy controls, measured CRF with a submaximal test instead of a "gold standard" cardiopulmonary exercise testing (CPET), thus limiting the validity of its results (17), and had a small sample of size of outpatients, predominantly men. Therefore, they call for more research, as well as the use of (gold standard) objective measures.

The aim of this study, therefore, is to compare objectively assessed SB and PA, as well as CRF measured by CPET, in patients with schizophrenia with matched, physically inactive, but otherwise healthy controls using data from the "The Outcome of Psychosis and Fitness Therapy" study (TOPFIT).

The second aim was to determine whether SB, PA, and CRF were associated with mental and physical health parameters in both patients with schizophrenia and matched healthy controls.

MATERIALS AND METHODS
Participants and Setting

This study included data of 63 patients with a schizophrenia spectrum disorder and 55 healthy controls, matched for gender, age, and socioeconomic status (expressed as the highest educational level of one of the parents). Patients were recruited at the University Medical Center Utrecht (Netherlands) ($n = 26$) and regional mental health care institutes (Altrecht; GGZ Duin- en Bollenstreek; GGZ Friesland) ($n = 37$). Healthy controls ($n = 55$) were recruited from the local population via advertisements. Participants were enrolled in the study between May 2007 and May 2010 and written informed consent was obtained after the procedures, and possible side effects were explained. This study was part of the TOPFIT project ("The Outcome of Psychosis and Fitness Therapy") and registered in the ISRCTN register (http://www.controlled-trials.com/ISRCTN46241817). Patients had a diagnosis of schizophrenia ($n = 45$), schizoaffective ($n = 15$), or schizophreniform disorder ($n = 3$) according to the Diagnostic and Statistical Manual of Mental Disorders, fourth edition (DSM-IV). Diagnosis was confirmed by psychiatrists using the Comprehensive Assessment of Schizophrenia and History (CASH) (18). Patients were stable on antipsychotic medication, i.e., using the same dosage for at least 4 weeks prior to inclusion. They showed no evidence for significant cardiovascular, neuromuscular, endocrine or other somatic disorders that prevented safe participation in the study (19). Patients had no primary diagnosis of alcohol or substance abuse and had an IQ $\geq$ 70, as measured with the Wechsler Adult Intelligence Scale Short Form (WAIS-III SF) (20).

The inclusion criteria for the healthy controls were no diagnosis of psychiatric disorders according to DSM-IV lifetime, no first-degree relative with a psychotic or depressive disorder, and being physically inactive before inclusion (i.e., undertaking <1 h of moderate PA weekly; based on self-report). The study was approved by the Human Ethics Committee of the University Medical Center Utrecht and research committees of participating centers.

Assessments

All measurements were assessed by a research assistant and a sports physician. Participants were asked to wear the SenseWear Pro-2 (BodyMedia, Inc., Pittsburgh, PA), body monitoring system during three 24-h time bouts (2 weekdays and 1 weekend day) except during water-based activities. This device objectively measures PA and estimates energy expenditure (21–23). The SenseWear was worn over the right arm triceps muscle and assesses minute-to-minute data through multiple sensors, namely a two-axis accelerometer and sensors measuring heat flux, galvanic skin and near body-temperature. Data are combined with gender, age, body weight, and height, to measures physical (in)activity and estimate energy expenditure using algorithms developed by the manufacturer (SenseWear Professional software, version 5.1.0.1289).

Several variables were calculated from the SenseWear data. PA was expressed in average metabolic equivalents (MET; in kcal/kg/h), an indicator of daily energy expenditure. The unit MET was used to estimate the amount of oxygen used by the body during SB and PA. Daily average time spend in total SB (<3 MET), moderate and vigorous PA (MVPA) (≥3MET), moderate (3–6 MET), vigorous (≥6 MET) were calculated from all minutes with a MET-value. Total energy expenditure (TEE; in kcals), active energy expenditure (AEE; in kcals: ≥3 MET), number of steps, lying down and sleeping time were also estimated. Data was accepted when the average on-body measuring time was at least 1,368 min per day (95% of a 24-h bout).

CRF, defined as the ability of the circulatory and respiratory systems to supply oxygen to skeletal muscles during sustained physical activity, was assessed with a cardiopulmonary exercise test (CPET), performed using a 20 watt per minute (W/min) step wise incremental protocol to exhaustion on a cycle ergometer (Lode Excalibur, Lode BV, Groningen, the Netherlands) (24). CRF was defined as the highest oxygen uptake during any 30-s interval during the test (VO2peak ml·kg^{-1}·min^{-1}) (25). Waist circumference (in cm) and anthropometric measurements (height in cm and weight in kg), using the same calibrated equipment in all participants, and metabolic syndrome (MetS), assessed according to the International Diabetes Foundation criteria (26), were obtained by the sports physician prior to the CPET.

To evaluate the severity of schizophrenia symptoms, the Positive and Negative Syndrome Scale (PANSS) total, positive, negative, and general (sub)scores were assessed (27). The Montgomery Åsberg Depression Rating Scale (MADRS) assessed co-morbid depressive symptoms (28). Detailed information on the amount and type of prescribed antipsychotic and other medication were gathered. Current antipsychotic medication prescribed was described in cumulative dosage and converted into haloperidol equivalents, conformable to a table from the Dutch National Health Service (29).

Statistical Analyses

SPSS 25.0 was used to analyze the data (Armonk, NY: IBM Corp). All statistical tests were performed two-tailed and a $p < 0.05$ was considered significant. Data were examined for outliers. All analyses were performed with and without extreme outliers to examine their influence on results. In case of non-normal distribution logarithmic transformation was applied.

Multiple analyses of variance for non-categorical variables and χ^2 analyses for categorical variables were used to examine differences between patients with schizophrenia and matched healthy controls in demographic and clinical variables. Univariate analyses were used to examine differences in SB, MVPA, moderate PA, vigorous PA, TEE, and AEE, number of steps, lying down and sleeping time, and CRF between patients and healthy controls. Gender, age, WAIS IQ-score, marital status, employment status, and Body Mass Index (BMI) were included in analyses as possible confounding factors. To investigate if differences exist between day of measurement (weekdays vs. weekend) within and between groups (patients vs. controls), repeated measures analysis of variance were performed comparing the average weekday vs. weekend day SB, MVPA, moderate PA, vigorous PA, TEE and AEE, number of steps, lying

down, and sleeping time. Correction for multiple testing was applied according to the Bonferroni-correction procedure.

In patients, backward linear regression analysis (criterion: probability of F-to-remove ≥0.10) was used to assess whether the independent variables gender, age, PANSS positive, PANSS negative, PANSS general, employment status, and MADRS-score were associated with the level of SB, MVPA, and CRF (VO$_{2peak}$ ml·kg^{-1}·min^{-1}). Similarly, we examined the association between physical health parameters (gender, age, employment status, BMI, haloperidol equivalent of antipsychotic medication prescribed, and number met criteria for the MetS) and SB, MVPA, and CRF (VO$_{2peak}$ ml·kg^{-1}·min^{-1}). We repeated the latter regression analyses in healthy controls, examining the association between physical health parameters (gender, age, employment status, BMI, number of met criteria for MetS) and SB, MVPA, and CRF.

RESULTS

Descriptive Statistics

Demographic and illness characteristics are shown in **Table 1**. Healthy controls had lower BMI ($p = 0.01$), waist circumference ($p = 0.002$), triglycerides ($p < 0.001$), and LDL-cholesterol ($p = 0.02$). Healthy controls were less likely to have MetS ($p = 0.04$), met on average less MetS criteria ($p = 0.003$), and smoked less cigarettes per day ($p \leq 0.001$). Healthy controls were more likely married ($p \leq 0.001$), had a higher IQ ($p \leq 0.001$), and higher HDL-cholesterol levels ($p < 0.001$). No significant differences in demographic and illness characteristics, except higher diastolic blood pressure ($p = 0.02$) and lower HDL-cholesterol ($p = 0.007$), were found between male and female patients. There were no differences in type [$\chi^2_{(9)} = 5.68; p = 0.77$] and dose [$F_{(1, 58)} = 1.24; p = 0.27$] of antipsychotic medication used between genders in patients.

Differences in SB, PA, and CRF

All variables, except SB, moderate PA, vigorous PA, and active energy expenditure data, complied with normality and homogeneity of variance demands. After logarithmic transformation of these variables, all data were analyzed parametrically. Average on-body percentage was below 95 percent in one patient with schizophrenia and three healthy controls. In total, 62 patients and 52 healthy controls, with an average on-body time of 98.3 (SD: 1.4) and 98.0 (SD: 1.2) percent, respectively, were thus included in further analyses. Results are presented in **Table 2**. Compared to physically inactive but otherwise healthy matched controls, patients showed significantly higher SB ($p = 0.005$), less MVPA ($p = 0.005$), and less moderate PA ($p \leq 0.001$), but equal vigorous PA ($p = 0.15$). Patients with schizophrenia had significantly lower total ($p = 0.001$) and active ($p = 0.002$) energy expenditure compared to controls. Though the average daily number of steps taken was lower in patients with schizophrenia (mean: 8040; SD: 3072) than in controls (mean: 8884; SD: 2837), this difference did not reach significance ($p = 0.16$). Patients spent significantly more time lying down ($p \leq 0.001$) and sleeping ($p < 0.001$) (expressed as minutes per day) than

TABLE 1 | Demographic and clinical characteristics for patients with schizophrenia and matched healthy controls.

Characteristic	Patients (n = 63)		Controls (n = 55)			
	N (%)		N (%)		F	p
Gender (male)	46 (73)		36 (65)		0.79	0.37
CASH: Schizophrenia	45 (71)					
Schizo-affective disorder	15 (24)					
Schizophreniform disorder	3 (5)					
Marital status (single/married/divorced)	56/4/3		30/24/1		22.71	**<0.001**
Employment status (welfare/ working/ student/ unemployed/ unknown)	51/8/1/3/0		1/27/24/2/1		81.38	**<0.001**
Treatment (inpatient/ day hospital/ out-patients/ unknown)	9/20/33/1					
Parental education level[a]:					6.79	0.34
Primary school or less	3(5)		1 (2)			
Secondary school	37 (59)		24 (44)			
College or university degree	21 (33)		30 (54)			
Unknown	2 (3)		0			
MetS (yes)[b]	22 (35)		9 (16)		5.22	**0.04**
	Mean	SD	Mean	SD	F	p
Age (year)	29.6	7.4	29.3	7.7	0.07	0.80
Height (cm)	177.9	9.2	178.2	10.1	0.03	0.86
Weight (kg)	83.0	19.2	76.3	14.3	4.51	**0.04**
BMI (kg/m^2)	26.3	6.0	23.9	3.3	6.60	**0.01**
VO$_{2peak}$ (ml/min/kg)	31.6	9.9	35.9	5.5	7.92	**<0.01**
WAIS Total IQ	87.2	15.6	108.1	13.8	58.13	**<0.001**
Nr. of MetS-criteria met[b]	2.3	1.4	1.5	1.2	9.55	**0.003**
Waist circumference (cm)	93.4	16.0	85.4	11.2	9.60	**0.002**
Systolic blood pressure (mm/hg)	125.4	12.6	122.8	12.2	1.33	0.25
Diastolic blood pressure (mm/hg)	76.2	9.1	74.6	9.1	0.99	0.32
Tryglicerides (mmol/L)	1.5	1.0	0.9	0.5	16.91	**<0.001**
HDL-cholesterol (mmol/L)	1.0	0.3	1.3	0.3	24.44	**<0.001**
LDL-cholesterol (mmol/L)	3.3	1.0	2.9	0.8	6.06	**0.02**
Smoking (cigarettes/day)	11.8	10.5	0.9	4.3	52.03	**<0.001**
Alcohol usage (glasses/week)	3.6	6.9	5.0	5.2	1.50	0.23
PANSS total score	62.6	10.7				
PANSS positive factor score	15.52	4.0				
PANSS negative factor score	17.46	5.8				
MADRS total score	15.16	8.4				
Duration of illness (years)	6.6	5.8				
Hospitalization until measurement (days)	193.7	265.3				
HEQ dose (mg/day)	8.1	5.2				

[a]Socioeconomic status, expressed as highest level of education of one of both parents according to Roick et al. (30).
[b]Assessed according to the International Diabetes Foundation criteria (26). CASH, Comprehensive Assessment of Schizophrenia and History; MetS, Metabolic Syndrome; BMI, Body Mass Index; VO2peak, maximum rate of oxygen consumption; WAIS, Wechsler Adult Intelligence Scale; HDL, High-density lipoproteins; LDL, Low-density lipoproteins; PANSS, Positive and Negative Syndrome Scale; MADRS, Montgomery and Åsberg Depression Rating Scale; HEQ, haloperidol equivalent. Significant differences at < 0.05 level are presented in bold.

controls. Patients had significantly poorer CRF than healthy controls ($p < 0.01$). Controlling for gender, age, BMI, and marital status did not change results. Controlling for WAIS IQ led to non-significance for TEE only. However, controlling for employment status led to non-significant differences in SB, PA, and TEE and AEE, but not in lying down and sleeping time. Bonferroni-correction for multiple testing did not influence the conclusions.

Differences in SB and PA on Weekdays vs. Weekend Days

Except for vigorous PA, patients and controls demonstrated significantly more SB, significantly less time on MVPA and moderate PA, had lower TEE and AEE, took fewer steps, and spent more time lying down and sleeping during the weekend compared to weekdays (Monday through Friday) (see **Table 3**). After Bonferroni-correction for multiple testing participants still

TABLE 2 | SB and PA in patients with schizophrenia and matched healthy controls, controlled for gender, age, and BMI influences.

Characteristic	Group		Test statistic	
	Patients (n = 62)	Controls (n = 52)		
	Mean ± SD	Mean ± SD	F	p
SB (<3 MET; min/day)	1303.6 ± 70.2	1254.1 ± 68.1	8.39	**0.005***
MVPA (≥3 MET; min/day)[1]	136.4 ± 70.2	185.2 ± 68.6	8.39	**0.005***
Moderate (3-6 MET; min/day)[1,a]	105.3 ± 72.1	152.1 ± 63.3	12.98	**< 0.001***
Vigorous (>6 MET; min/day)[1,a]	10.5 ± 20.3	16.1 ± 26.6	2.10	0.15
Total energy expenditure (kcal/day)[1]	2897 ± 582	3036 ± 455	10.74	**0.001***
Active energy expenditure (kcal/day)[1,a]	718 ± 595	965 ± 421	9.62	**0.002***
Steps (steps/day)[1]	8040 ± 3072	8884 ± 2837	1.97	0.16
Lying down (hours/day)[2]	11.4 ± 2.1	8.6 ± 1.2	65.95	**<0.0001***
Sleeping time (hours/day)[2]	9.2 ± 1.9	6.5 ± 1.0	68.63	**<0.0001***

[1] Higher score indicates superior physical activity.
[2] Lower score indicates superior physical activity.
[a] EXP-values of logarithmically transformed and analyzed data are presented. Significant results are presented in bold, *significant after Bonferoni correction for multiple testing.
SB, sedentary behavior; PA, physical activity; BMI, body mass index; MET, metabolic equivalent; MVPA, moderate to vigorous physical activity.

took significantly fewer steps and spent more time lying down and sleeping. No significant differences between the two 24-h weekday assessments were found in either patients or controls for any of the SB or PA variables (all $p > 0.20$). Whereas, no differences in PA or energy expenditure were found between Saturdays or Sundays in healthy controls, patients had less MVPA ($p = 0.04$) and lower TEE ($p = 0.005$), and AEE ($p = 0.009$) on Saturdays compared to Sundays.

Associations of SB, MVPA, and CRF With Mental and Physical Health

In patients, for mental health, a significant final model for SB emerged [$F_{(1, 59)} = 4.46$; $p = 0.039$; $R^2 = 0.069$] in which PANSS negative score (beta = 0.263; $p = 0.039$) was significantly associated with SB. In the final model, gender, age, employment status, WAIS IQ, PANSS positive, PANSS general, and MADRS-score were not significantly associated with SB. This means that increasing severity of negative symptoms was associated with more SB. An identical but inversed model emerged for MVPA which means that increasing severity of negative symptoms was associated with fewer MVPA. For mental health, a significant model for CRF emerged also [$F_{(4, 56)} = 17.195$; $p < 0.00000001$; $R^2 = 0.551$] in which gender (female vs. male; beta = −0.398; $p < 0.0001$), age (beta = −0.417; $p < 0.0001$), and PANSS negative score (beta = −0.502; $p < 0.00001$) MADRS score (beta = 0.198; $p = 0.040$) were significantly associated with CRF level indicating female gender, higher age, and more severe depressive and particularly negative symptoms were associated with poorer CRF.

In patients, for physical health, no significant final model for either SB nor MVPA emerged since none of the variables (gender, age, employment status, BMI, haloperidol equivalent of antipsychotic medication prescribed, and number met criteria for the MetS) were significantly associated with SB or MVPA, respectively. For physical health, a significant model for CRF did emerge [$F_{(4, 54)} = 17.566$; $p < 0.00000001$; $R^2 = 0.570$] in

which gender (female vs. male; beta = −0.255; $p = 0.011$), age (beta = −0.214; $p = 0.032$), employment status (beta = −2.04; $p = 0.032$), and BMI (beta = −0.489; $p < 0.00001$) were significantly associated with CRF level. This means female gender, higher age, being unemployed or on welfare, and higher BMI were associated with poorer CRF. When negative symptoms and BMI were combined in one regression model with CRF, both factors were equally related.

In healthy controls, a significant model emerged for MVPA [$F_{(7, 10)} = 7.095$; $p = 0.002$; $R^2 = 0.225$] in which gender (female vs. male, beta = 0.307; $p = 0.02$) and BMI (beta = −0.31, $p = 0.02$) were significantly associated with MVPA. The same holds for SB [$F_{(7, 19)} = 7.095$; $p = 0.002$; $R^2 = 0.225$; with gender −0.307, $p = 0.02$ and BMI 0.32, $p = 0.02$ being significantly associated] and CRF [$F_{(3, 48)} = 18.101$; $p < 0.00000001$; $R^2 = 0.531$, with again gender −0.638, $p < 0.0000001$, employment status (beta = −0.210; $p = 0.056$), and BMI −0.54, $p < 0.0001$ being significantly associated with CRF]. Noteworthy, females tended to have more MVPA and less SB, but poorer CRF. The latter corresponds with the model in patients, in which also female gender and higher BMI were associated with poorer CRF.

DISCUSSION

This study examined objectively measured PA and inactivity, SB and CRF in patients with schizophrenia compared to inactive healthy controls. Patients with schizophrenia performed significantly less MVPA, moderate PA, more SB, had lower total and active energy expenditure, spent more time per day lying down and sleeping, and had poorer CRF compared to healthy controls. The amount of MVPA, but more prominently CRF level, was associated with the severity of negative symptoms in patients with schizophrenia. Only CRF, and not SB or MVPA, was associated with BMI.

TABLE 3 | Differences between day of measurement (weekdays vs. weekend) within (day) and between groups (day × group; patients vs. controls).

Characteristic	Patients (n = 62)		Controls (n = 52)		Test statistic			
	Weekday	Weekend	Weekday	Weekend	Day		Day × Group	
	Mean ± SD	Mean ± SD	Mean ± SD	Mean ± SD	F	p	F	p
SB (<3 MET; min/day)	1296 ± 82	1318 ± 74	1249 ± 84	1263 ± 70	5.3	**0.02**	0.3	0.60
MVPA (≥3 MET; min/day)[1]	143.8 ± 82.2	121.6 ± 74.7	190.6 ± 84.0	174.6 ± 74.7	5.8	**0.02**	0.2	0.70
Moderate (3-6 MET; min/day)[1]	126.4 ± 75.7	106.5 ± 61.9	165.7 ± 71.2	152.6 ± 60.4	5.3	**0.02**	0.2	0.63
Vigorous (>6 MET; min/day)[1]	17.5 ± 16.6	15.2 ± 26.4	24.9 ± 23.5	21.9 ± 27.7	1.1	0.29	0.02	0.89
Total energy expenditure (kcal/day)[1]	2943 ± 634	2805 ± 621	3069 ± 522	2970 ± 475	6.5	**0.01**	0.2	0.67
Active energy expenditure (kcal/day)[1]	896 ± 546	745 ± 525	1055 ± 471	979 ± 432	4.8	**0.03**	0.5	0.47
Steps (steps/day)[1]	8565 ± 3522	6990 ± 3522	9104 ± 3251	8443 ± 3669	9.8	**0.002***	1.6	0.20
Lying down (hours/day)[2]	11.1 ± 2.2	11.9 ± 3.3	8.1 ± 1.3	9.6 ± 2.3	17.0	**<0.0001***	1.7	0.19
Sleeping time (hours/day)[2]	8.8 ± 2.1	9.8 ± 2.7	6.1 ± 0.9	7.3 ± 1.9	25.1	**<0.0001***	0.2	0.62

[1] Higher score indicates superior physical activity.
[2] Lower score indicates superior physical activity.
SB, sedentary behavior; MET, metabolic equivalent; MVPA, moderate to vigorous physical activity. Significant results are presented in bold, *significant after Bonferoni correction for multiple testing.

This study adds to current knowledge by being one of the few to include CRF in studying the relationship between PA, SB and cardiovascular disease, and, more importantly, by being the only one to use the gold standard CPET in measuring CRF. CRF indeed appeared independently related to cardio-metabolic risk, more so than SB or PA. This has two implications; it stresses the importance of taking CRF into account when assessing patients' physical health status, and it implies that the implementation of interventions aiming to increase CRF is of utmost importance in tackling the alarming cardio-metabolic health of patients with schizophrenia (31). Two previous intervention studies showed this was feasible in patients with schizophrenia (32, 33). In the current study, we found an association between CRF and severity of negative symptoms, which is in line with previous research (34). The direction of this association is as of yet not exactly known; it may seem conspicuous to think negative symptoms lead to inactivity which in turn affects CRF levels. There is however emerging evidence that a bidirectional association may be possible as well. Two studies found evidence of a direct relationship of CRF (35) on cognition and PANSS symptomatology (36), respectively. In other areas, such as depression and bipolar disorder, the effect of physical activity on mood has been widely established, even though the mechanisms through which physical activity and brain functioning (mood, cognition and symptoms) affect each other are not completely understood yet. Nonetheless, this gives hope to the idea that interventions aiming to increase CRF may also reduce negative symptoms (37). This could, on its turn, have important functional benefits as well since negative symptoms evidently impact an individual's functional capacity in daily activities (38).

Our results are furthermore consistent with previous studies which reported lower levels of PA in patients with schizophrenia compared to healthy comparison subjects (30, 39–44). In line with earlier findings, we found patients with schizophrenia spend less time on moderate PA, but not on vigorous PA (43). In accordance with the only study that used doubly labeled water,

the established criterion standard method for free-living energy expenditure assessment, we found reduced total and active energy expenditure in patients with schizophrenia (45).

Some limitations should be considered when interpreting present findings. First, SenseWear reliably assesses PA and energy expenditure in normal and overweight healthy adults (21–23, 46), yet has not been validated in patients with schizophrenia. SenseWear overestimated energy expenditure in obese subjects (46) and the current study included 15 obese patients and 2 obese healthy controls (BMI>30). Papazoglou et al. (46) used an older software version than the present study which was later shown to have an inferior accuracy (23). Second, as this is a cross-sectional study, only relationships between SB, PA, and CRF, and mental and physical health parameters could be examined, not causality. Third, we did not succeed in enrolling healthy controls fully matching the schizophrenia patient group, other than on age, socio-economic status and inactivity. In terms of cardiometabolic health, the patients were much worse off, which on the one hand stresses the seriousness of their health condition, but on the other hand impedes true comparison of the two groups. In addition, patients with schizophrenia and healthy subjects volunteered to engage in the study, which may have led to some selection bias because subjects motivated for PA and health improvement might have had greater interest in this study. Accordingly, this may have led to an overestimation of activity levels compared to the entire schizophrenia population. Also, the absence of a matched psychiatric control group is a limitation of our study. It would have been interesting to see whether activity patterns and CRF levels of patients with schizophrenia differ from patients with other psychiatric diagnoses. This might also shed light on the role of negative symptoms, which may be present in patients with other psychiatric disorders but are often more pronounced in patients with schizophrenia. Fourth, one could argue that the CPET is too strenuous for patients with schizophrenia. In our study, however, all controls and all but four patients with schizophrenia met maximal effort demand (RER peak ≥1.1), albeit that patients with schizophrenia did reach significantly lower average RER peak values than controls. This could however in part be due to poorer CRF and the fact that they are not accustomed to perform high-intensity exercise. Last, others often define SB as <1.5 MET whereas we defined it as <3 MET. This may have led to a higher estimate of SB.

In conclusion, our study shows patients with schizophrenia perform less PA, expend less total and active energy, spend more time lying down and sleeping, and have poorer CRF compared to physically inactive matched, healthy controls. Given the remarkably strong associations of CRF with both negative symptoms and BMI, improvement of CRF should be a primary treatment aim, which may affect both mental and physical health in patients with schizophrenia.

AUTHOR CONTRIBUTIONS

TS, FB, TT, and WC conceived, designed, and amended the study and wrote the protocol. TS was responsible for the acquisition of the data. TS, FJ, and TT performed the statistical analyses. TS, FJ, and TT wrote the first draft of the manuscript. All authors provided critical review of the manuscript and approved the final version.

ACKNOWLEDGMENTS

We gratefully acknowledge all participants in the TOPFIT study for their willingness to cooperate.

REFERENCES

Hayes JF, Marston L, Walters K, King MB, Osborn DPJ. Mortality gap for people with bipolar disorder and schizophrenia: UK-based cohort study 2000- 2014. *Br J Psychiatry*. (2017) 211:175–81. doi: 10.1192/bjp.bp.117.202606

Tanskanen A, Tiihonen J, Taipale H. Mortality in schizophrenia: 30- year nationwide follow-up study. *Acta Psychiatr Scand*. (2018) 138:492–9. doi: 10.1111/acps.12913

Walker ER, McGee RE, Druss BG. Mortality in mental disorders and global disease burden implications a systematic review and meta-analysis. *JAMA Psychiatry*. (2015) 72:334–41. doi: 10.1001/jamapsychiatry.2014.2502

Correll CU, Detraux J, De Lepeleire J, De Hert M. Effects of antipsychotics, antidepressants and mood stabilizers on risk for physical diseases in people with schizophrenia, depression and bipolar disorder. *World Psychiatry*. (2015) 14:119–36. doi: 10.1002/wps.20204

Laursen TM, Wahlbeck K, Hallgren J, Westman J, Osby U, Alinaghizadeh H, et al. Life expectancy and death by diseases of the circulatory system in patients with bipolar disorder or schizophrenia in the Nordic countries. *PLoS ONE*. (2013) 8:e67133. doi: 10.1371/journal.pone.0067133

Correll CU, Solmi M, Veronese N, Bortolato B, Rosson S, Santonastaso P, et al. Prevalence, incidence and mortality from cardiovascular disease in patients with pooled and specific severe mental illness: a large-scale meta- analysis of 3,211,768 patients and 113,383,368 controls. *World Psychiatry*. (2017) 16:163–80. doi: 10.1002/wps.20420

Stubbs B, Firth J, Berry A, Schuch FB, Rosenbaum S, Gaughran F, et al. How much physical activity do people with schizophrenia engage in? A systematic review, comparative meta-analysis and meta-regression. *Schizophr Res*. (2016) 176:431–40. doi: 10.1016/j.schres.2016.05.017

Stubbs B, Williams JE, Gaughran F, Craig T. How sedentary are people with psychosis? A systematic review and meta-analysis. *Schizophr Res*. (2016) 171:103–9. doi: 10.1016/j.schres.2016.01.034

Vancampfort D, Rosenbaum S, Schuch F, Ward PB, Richards J, Mugisha J, et al. Cardiorespiratory fitness in severe mental illness: a systematic review and meta-analysis. *Sports Med*. (2017) 47:343–52. doi: 10.1007/s40279-016-0574-1

Prince SA, Adamo KB, Hamel ME, Hardt J, Connor Gorber S, Tremblay M. A comparison of direct versus self-report measures for assessing physical activity in adults: a systematic review. *Int J Behav Nutr Phys Act*.(2008) 5:56. doi: 10.1186/1479-5868-5-56

Sallis JF, Saelens BE. Assessment of physical activity by self-report: status, limitations, and future directions. *Res Q Exerc Sport*. (2000) 71:1–14. doi: 10.1080/02701367.2000.11082780

Firth J, Stubbs B, Vancampfort D, Schuch FB, Rosenbaum S, Ward PB, et al. The validity and value of self-reported physical activity and accelerometry in people with schizophrenia: a population-scale study of the UK biobank. *Schizophr Bull*. (2017). 44:1293–300. doi: 10.1093/schbul/sbx149

Nyboe L, Vestergaard CH, Moeller MK, Lund H, Videbech P. Metabolic syndrome and aerobic fitness in patients with first-episode schizophrenia, including a 1-year follow-up. *Schizophr Res*. (2015) 168:381–7. doi: 10.1016/j.schres.2015.07.053

Stubbs B, Gardner-Sood P, Smith S, Ismail K, Greenwood K, Farmer R, et al. Sedentary behaviour is associated with elevated C-reactive protein levels in people with psychosis. *Schizophr Res*. (2015) 168:461–4. doi: 10.1016/j.schres.2015.07.003

Stubbs B, Chen LJ, Chung MS, Ku PW. Physical activity ameliorates the association between sedentary behavior and cardiometabolic risk among inpatients with schizophrenia: a comparison versus controls using accelerometry. *Compr Psychiatry*. (2017) 74:144–50. doi: 10.1016/j.comppsych.2017.01.010

Bueno-Antequera J, Oviedo-Caro MA, Munguia-Izquierdo D. Sedentary behaviour, physical activity, cardiorespiratory fitness and cardiometabolic risk in psychosis: the psychiactive project. *Schizophr Res*. (2018) 195:142–8. doi: 10.1016/j.schres.2017.10.012

Heyward VH, Gibson A. *Advanced Fitness Assessment and Exercise Prescription*, 7th ed. Champaign, Illinois: Human Kinetics (2014).

Andreasen NC, Flaum M, Arndt S. The Comprehensive Assessment of Symptoms and History (CASH). An instrument for assessing diagnosis and psychopathology. *Arch Gen Psychiatry*. (1992) 49:615–23. doi: 10.1001/archpsyc.1992.01820080023004

Bille K, Figueiras D, Schamasch P, Kappenberger L, Brenner JI, Meijboom FJ, et al. Sudden cardiac death in athletes: the lausanne recommendations. *Eur J Cardiovasc Prev Rehabil*. (2006) 13:859–75. doi: 10.1097/01.hjr.0000238397.50341.4a

Christensen BK, Girard TA, Bagby RM. Wechsler adult intelligence scale-third edition short form for index and IQ scores in a psychiatric population. *Psychol Assess*. (2007) 19:236–40. doi: 10.1037/1040-3590.19.2.236

Fruin ML, Rankin JW. Validity of a multi-sensor armband in estimating rest and exercise energy expenditure. *Med Sci Sports Exerc*. (2004) 36:1063–9. doi: 10.1249/01.MSS.0000128144.91337.38

Jakicic JM, Marcus M, Gallagher KI, Randall C, Thomas E, Goss FL, et al. Evaluation of the SenseWear Pro Armband to assess energy expenditure during exercise. *Med Sci Sports Exerc*. (2004) 36:897–904. doi: 10.1249/01.MSS.0000126805.32659.43

Welk GJ, McClain JJ, Eisenmann JC, Wickel EE. Field validation of the MTI actigraph and bodymedia armband monitor using the IDEEA monitor. *Obesity*. (2007) 15:918–28. doi: 10.1038/oby.2007.624

Godfrey S. *Exercise Testing in Children: Applications in Health and Disease* Philadelphia: Saunders (1974).

Astorino TA. Alterations in VOmax and the VO plateau with manipulation of sampling interval. *Clin Physiol Funct Imaging*. (2009) 29:60–7. doi: 10.1111/j.1475-097X.2008.00835.x

Alberti KGMM, Eckel RH, Grundy SM, Zimmet PZ, Cleeman JI, Donato KA, et al. Harmonizing the metabolic syndrome: a joint interim statement of the international diabetes federation task force on epidemiology and prevention; National heart, lung, and blood institute; American heart association; World heart federation; International atherosclerosis society; And international association for the study of obesity. *Circulation*. (2009) 120:1640–5. doi: 10.1161/CIRCULATIONAHA.109.192644

Kay SR, Fiszbein A, Opler LA. The positive and negative syndrome scale (PANSS) for schizophrenia. *Schizophr Bull.* (1987) 13:261–76. doi: 10.1093/ schbul/13.2.261

Montgomery SA, Asberg M. A new depression scale designed to be sensitive to change. *Br J Psychiatry.* (1979) 134:382–9. doi: 10.1192/bjp.134.4.382

Commissie Farmaceutische Hulp. *Farmacotherapeutisch Kompas.* Amstelveen: Commissie Farmacotherapeutische Hulp van het College van Zorgverzekeringen (2002).

Roick C, Fritz-Wieacker A, Matschinger H, Heider D, Schindler J, Riedel- Heller S, et al. Health habits of patients with schizophrenia. *Soc Psychiatry Psychiatr Epidemiol.* (2007) 42:268–76. doi: 10.1007/s00127-007-0164-5

Sassen B, Cornelissen VA, Kiers H, Wittink H, Kok G, Vanhees L. Physical fitness matters more than physical activity in controlling cardiovascular disease risk factors. *Eur J Cardiovasc Prev Rehabil.* (2009) 16:677–83. doi: 10.1097/ HJR.0b013e3283312e94

Heggelund J, Nilsberg GE, Hoff J, Morken G, Helgerud J. Effects of high aerobic intensity training in patients with schizophrenia: a controlled trial. *Nord J Psychiatry.* (2011) 65:269–75. doi: 10.3109/08039488.2011.560278

Scheewe TW, Backx FJG, Takken T, Jörg F, van Strater ACP, Kroes AG, et al. Exercise therapy improves mental and physical health in schizophrenia: a randomised controlled trial. *Acta Psychiatr Scand.* (2012) 127:464–73. doi: 10.1111/acps.12029

Vancampfort D, Knapen J, Probst M, Scheewe T, Remans S, De Hert M. A systematic review of correlates of physical activity in patients with schizophrenia. *Acta Psychiatr Scand.* (2012) 125:352–62. doi: 10.1111/j.1600-0447.2011.01814.x

Holmen TL, Egeland J, Andersen E, Bigseth TT, Engh JA. The association between cardio-respiratory fitness and cognition in schizophrenia. *Schizophr Res.* (2018) 193:418–22. doi: 10.1016/j.schres.2017.07.015

Curcic D, Stojmenovic T, Djukic-Dejanovic S, Dikic N, Vesic-Vukasinovic M, Radivojevic N, et al. Positive impact of prescribed physical activity on symptoms of schizophrenia: randomized clinical trial. *Psychiatr Danub.* (2017) 29:459–65. doi: 10.24869/psyd.2017.459

Rimes RR, de Souza Moura AM, Lamego MK, de Sa Filho AS, Manochio J, Paes F, et al. Effects of exercise on physical and mental health, and cognitive and

brain functions in schizophrenia: clinical and experimental evidence. *CNS Neurol Disord Drug Targets.* (2015) 14:1244–54. doi: 10.2174/1871527315666 151111130659

Aubin G, Stip E, Gelinas I, Rainville C, Chapparo C. Daily activities, cognition and community functioning in persons with schizophrenia. *Schizophr Res.* (2009) 107:313–8. doi: 10.1016/j.schres.2008.08.002

Brown S, Birtwistle J, Roe L, Thompson C. The unhealthy lifestyle of people with schizophrenia. *Psychol Med.* (1999) 29:697–701. doi: 10.1017/ S0033291798008186

Heald A, Pendlebury J, Anderson S, Narayan V, Guy M, Gibson M, et al. Lifestyle factors and the metabolic syndrome in Schizophrenia: a cross-sectional study. *Ann Gen Psychiatry.* (2017) 16:12. doi: 10.1186/s12991-017-0134-6

Kruisdijk F, Deenik J, Tenback D, Tak E, Beekman A, van Harten P, et al. Accelerometer-measured sedentary behaviour and physical activity of inpatients with severe mental illness. *Psychiatry Res.* (2017) 254:67–74. doi: 10.1016/j.psychres.2017.04.035

Lindamer LA, McKibbin C, Norman GJ, Jordan L, Harrison K, Abeyesinhe S, et al. Assessment of physical activity in middle-aged and older adults with schizophrenia. *Schizophr Res.* (2008) 104:294–301. doi: 10.1016/j. schres.2008.04.040

Ratliff JC, Palmese LB, Reutenauer EL, Liskov E, Grilo CM, Tek C. The effect of dietary and physical activity pattern on metabolic profile in individuals with schizophrenia: a cross-sectional study. *Compr Psychiatry.* (2012) 53:1028–33. doi: 10.1016/j.comppsych.2012.02.003

Ringen PA, Faerden A, Antonsen B, Falk RS, Mamen A, Rognli EB, et al. Cardiometabolic risk factors, physical activity and psychiatric status in patients in long-term psychiatric inpatient departments. *Nord J Psychiatry.* (2018) 72:1–7. doi: 10.1080/08039488.2018.1449012

Sharpe JK, Stedman TJ, Byrne NM, Wishart C, Hills AP. Energy expenditure and physical activity in clozapine use: implications for weight management. *Aust N Z J Psychiatry.* (2006) 40:810–4. doi: 10.1080/j.1440-1614.2006. 01888.x

Papazoglou D, Augello G, Tagliaferri M, Savia G, Marzullo P, Maltezos E, et al. Evaluation of a multisensor armband in estimating energy expenditure in obese individuals. *Obesity.* (2006) 14:2217–23. doi: 10.1038/oby.2006.260

5

Effect of Acute Moderate-Intensity Exercise on the Mirror Neuron System: Role of Cardiovascular Fitness Level

Zebo Xu[1,2], Zi-Rong Wang[3], Jin Li[3], Min Hu[1]* and Ming-Qiang Xiang[1]*

[1] Department of Sports and Health, Guangzhou Sport University, Guangzhou, China, [2] Department of Linguistics and Modern Languages, The Chinese University of Hong Kong, Hong Kong, China, [3] Department of Graduation, Guangzhou Sport University, Guangzhou, China

*Correspondence:
Min Hu
whoomin@aliyun.com
Ming-Qiang Xiang
xiangmq80@163.com

Objectives: The aims of this study were to use functional near-infrared spectroscopy (fNIRS) to determine whether cardiovascular fitness levels modulate the activation of the mirror neuron system (MNS) under table-setting tasks in non-exercise situation, to replicate the study that positive effect of acute moderate-intensity exercise on the MNS and investigate whether cardiovascular fitness levels modulates the effect of exercise on the activation of the MNS.

Methods: Thirty-six healthy college-aged participants completed a maximal graded exercise test (GXT) and were categorized as high, moderate, or low cardiovascular fitness. Participants then performed table-setting tasks including an action execution task (EXEC) and action observation task (OBS) prior to (PRE) and after (POST) either a rest condition (CTRL) or a cycling exercise condition (EXP). The EXP condition consisted of a 5-min warm-up, 15-min moderate-intensity exercise (65% VO_{2max}), and 5-min cool-down.

Results: No significant differences were observed for Oxy-Hb and Deoxy-Hb between different cardiovascular fitness levels in the EXEC or OBS tasks in the non-exercise session. But there were significant improvements of oxygenated hemoglobin (Oxy-Hb) in the inferior frontal gyrus (IFG) and pre-motor area (PMC) regions under the OBS task following the acute moderate exercise. Particularly, the improvements (Post-Pre) of Δ Oxy-Hb were mainly observed in high and low fitness individuals. There was also a significant improvement of deoxygenated hemoglobin (Deoxy-Hb) in the IPL region under the OBS task. The following analysis indicated that exercise improved Δ Deoxy-Hb in high fitness individuals.

Conclusion: This study indicated that the activation of MNS was not modulated by the cardiovascular fitness levels in the non-exercise situation. We replicated the previous study that moderate exercise improved activation of MNS; we also provided the first empirical evidence that moderate-intensity exercise positively affects the MNS activation in college students of high and low cardiovascular fitness levels.

Keywords: mirror neuron system, action understanding, social cognition, cardiovascular fitness level, acute moderate-intensity exercise, fNIRS

INTRODUCTION

Mirror neuron system (MNS) was activated when an individual performed action, and observed the same action performed by others (Sun et al., 2018). The first discovery of MNS was in the ventral premotor cortex (area F5) of the macaque brain; it fired when grasping food as well as when the macaque observed the experimenter grasping food. Then, the MNS was found in the rostral inferior parietal lobule (IPL) (PF/PFG), also firing when a monkey executes a goal-related action and mouth actions, as well as observing the same action in another subject (Rizzolatti et al., 1996; Gallese et al., 2004; Fogassi et al., 2005). Previous work has determined the location of the MNS in the human (Buccino et al., 2001; Gallese et al., 2004; Filimon et al., 2007; Kilner et al., 2009; Molenberghs et al., 2010) and its functions for action understanding (Johnson-Frey et al., 2003; Leslie et al., 2004) and imitation (Buccino et al., 2004; Bernier et al., 2013). A more general hypothesis was that the MNS also played a crucial role in social cognition to catch the intentions and emotions of others (Gallese, 2006; Pfeifer et al., 2008; Perkins et al., 2010). Then Language evolved became a powerful and flexible tool when humans developed a social function to exchange knowledge (Tomasello et al., 2005). However, several studies were skeptical about the role that the MNS played in social cognition, arguing that the MNS was simply the motor controller and did not include action understanding which is one of the most important basic functions in social cognition (Baird et al., 2011; Hickok et al., 2011b). Besides, other studies declared that the dorsal part of the premotor cortex in MNS did play a role in action understanding, but only the dorsomedial prefrontal of MNS which was called the mentalizing system (MENT) activated by the social relevant tasks (Spunt and Lieberman, 2012; Geiger et al., 2019).

In the field of sport psychology, cardiovascular fitness level was considered as one of the most important factors. Several studies have indicated that high fitness was associated with greater brain volume and functional connectivity (Chaddock et al., 2010; Voss et al., 2010). The role of fitness in the cognitive performance was also investigated in prior studies. Åberg et al. (2009) have shown that young adulthood with higher fitness levels would perform better in cognitive tasks. And one study researched on 877 older adults indicated that higher fitness level was associated with better motor skills, cognitive performance, and memory (Freudenberger et al., 2016). Although several studies revealed higher fitness levels related to better daily performances, there is still no study to reveal the relationship between cardiovascular fitness levels and the activation of MNS in the action understanding tasks which might be the basic neural mechanism to social function, language function, and cognitive function.

Exercise has also been shown to benefit cognition (Audiffren et al., 2009; Byun et al., 2014), the hippocampus and memory (Sayal, 2015), and improved motor control in early Parkinson's disease patients (Fisher et al., 2008), social behaviors in children with autism (Bremer et al., 2016), as well as adolescents with attention-deficit/hyperactivity disorder (ADHD) (Kamp et al., 2014). Previous work done by Drollette et al. (2012) has shown that preadolescent children had a greater performance

on the cognitive control task (Flanker task) after 15 min of moderate-intensity running at 60% maximal heart rate (HR$_{max}$) compared with resting state. Furthermore, a recent study used functional near-infrared spectroscopy (fNIRS) also demonstrated that moderate-intensity exercise could improve the activation of MNS in an action understanding social task (Xu et al., 2019), which indirectly outlined one of the neural bases of exercise improved social behaviors in children with autism. Although Xu et al. (2019) have shown the positive effect of exercise on the MNS, more studies are still needed to verify this effect.

With in-depth study, some previous studies have observed different effects of exercise on cognitive performance among different cardiovascular fitness levels. For example, Chu et al. (2015) found that acute moderate-intensity exercise can improve the performance of cognitive functions and to a specific improvement in the executive function of high and low cardiovascular fitness levels in older adults. Chang et al. (2012) also indicated the improvement of cognitive performances which are the information processing, attention, and executive function tasks after a delay of light and moderate-intensity exercise on high and low-fit younger adults in their meta-analysis study. Previous reviews also highly recommended cardiovascular fitness should be measured and analyzed in the study (Brisswalter et al., 2002; Tomporowski, 2003). Those studies mentioned above indicated that cardiovascular fitness might modulate the effect of exercise on cognitive functions, since the function of MNS was relevant with cognitive control, for example, patients with impairment of motor control and aphasia (mouth action control) after stroke were also following less activation of MNS (Small et al., 2012). However, how cardiovascular fitness level modulates the effects of acute exercise on the MNS in action understanding tasks remains less understood and warrants more explorations.

Therefore, the aims of this study were to determine whether MNS activation is related to the cardiovascular fitness level in the non-exercise situation, to replicate a study done by Xu et al. (2019), that is acute exercise can improve MNS response in the action understanding tasks and to evaluate whether the effect of moderate-intensity exercise on MNS is modulated by cardiovascular fitness, Specifically, we also made the following hypotheses.

> Hypothesis 1: Because prior studies illustrated that higher cardiovascular fitness level was related to better cognitive performance (Freudenberger et al., 2016), the MNS regions with high fitness individuals should exhibit the largest activation compare with moderate and low fitness groups in non-exercise session under our action understanding tasks.
>
> Hypothesis 2: Because the previous study has shown moderate-intensity exercise increased activation of MNS in the OBS task (Xu et al., 2019), thus, parts of MNS regions activation will be increased after exercise in the OBS task.
>
> Hypothesis 3: Because plenty of evidence indicated that the effect of exercise mainly benefits high-and low-fit individuals' cognitive performances (Chang et al., 2012), the subgroup-analyses will show the

improvements of MNS in cardiovascular high and low fitness level individuals following exercise under action understanding tasks.

MATERIALS AND METHODS

Participants

Thirty-six college-aged participants were recruited to this study (mean age 20.6 ± 1.5 years, height 169 ± 9 cm, body, weight 61.4 ± 12.5 kg; 16 females). All participants were healthy and right-handed (Edinburgh Handedness Inventory score > 0.85), and all had a normal or corrected-to-normal vision. All participants completed four sessions (body test, experimental, control, and acute exercise sessions) and were instructed to avoid any intense exercise in 24 h between each session. All participants completed a maximal oxygen consumption test and were then split into three groups based on the American College of Sports Medicine (ACSM) guidelines (American College of Sports Medicine [ACSM], 2013). The maximal oxygen consumption (VO_{2max}) of each fitness group was categorized as: low fitness group, moderate fitness group, and high fitness group (**Table 1**). According to ACSM guidelines, these groups have previously been described as having poor (35.4–43.5 ml/kg/min for male; 26.2–33.6 ml/kg/min for female), fair (43.5–49.1 ml/kg/min for male; 33.6–38.9 ml/kg/min for female), and good fitness (49.1 above ml/kg/min for male; 38.9 above ml/kg/min for female), respectively (American College of Sports Medicine [ACSM], 2013). Written informed consent was obtained from all participants in accordance with the Declaration of Helsinki. The protocol was approved by the Ethics Committee of Guangzhou Sport University.

Experimental Procedures

In the first session, participants were fully informed regarding each experimental session. Each participant gave written informed consent and filled out an International Physical Activity Questionnaire (IPAQ). Participants meeting the inclusion criteria then performed a test of cardiovascular fitness to VO_{2max} and were categorized into high, moderate, and low fitness group according to the ACSM guidelines (American College of Sports Medicine [ACSM], 2013).

The second and third sessions were the table-setting task, which has both action execution (EXEC) and action observations (OBS) tasks under experimental (EXP) and control (CTRL) conditions. By definition, acute exercise session occurred only in the EXP condition. During the acute exercise session, all participants performed 25 min of exercise on a cycle ergometer (Ergoselect 100, ergoline GmbH, Germany) that consisted of a 5 min warm-up, 15 min of exercise at moderate intensity (65% HR_{max}), and a 5 min recovery period. Heart rate (HR) was monitored by a wireless HR monitor (Acentas pulse meter, BM-CS5EU, Beijing, China). The initial cycling workload was 30 W and automatically increased in the warm-up period until HR reached 65% HR_{max}. The cycle ergometer system automatically adjusts the workload if the HR is higher than target HR to ensure

they were exercising at moderate intensity over the 15-min exercise period. Finally, participants were allowed to cool down during the recovery period at 30 W. Under the CTRL condition, participants conducted the same action execution and observation components, but rested instead of performing the exercise (**Figure 1A**).

All participants performed the table-setting task before (PRE) and after (POST) the acute exercise session or rest in the EXP and CTRL conditions. If participants individually attended exercise sessions of the experiment firstly, they performed another session on different days.

Maximal Oxygen Consumption Test

All participants had their body mass index (BMI) measured in the laboratory. The IPAQ was used to assess participants' physical activity. Cardiovascular fitness was measured using cardiopulmonary exercise testing (Jaeger-Masterscreen-CPX, Carefusion, Germany). All participants ran on a treadmill (h/p/cosmos airwalk, Germany) using the Bruce protocol for the maximal graded exercise test (GXT) (Bruce et al., 1973). VO_{2max} was determined if participants met at least three of the following four criteria: (1) respiratory exchange rate (RER) ≥ 1.15; (2) volitional exhaustion; (3) no increase in HR with increasing intensity; (4) rating of perceived exertion (RPE) ≥ 17 (Borg, 1982; Seifert et al., 2010). Participants were asked to rate their exertion on the RPE scale in the last 20 s of the GXT intensity stage before increasing workload.

The Table-Setting Task to Reflect the MNS Activity

In the initial period, participants and the experimenter (the experimenter is male in this study) sat face to face. The storage box was placed in front of the participant and the placemat placed on their right-hand side. The storage box included five table items: a plate, a saucer, a pair of chopsticks, a soupspoon, and a rice bowl. A monitor placed at a 45° angle in front of participants to presented visual cues.

In the executive (EXEC) task of the experiment, the participants were instructed to place the table items orderly onto and round the placemat with a normal, natural speed, and rhythm in 15 s after the cue was on the monitor: a picture of a cup. Participants were instructed to only use their right-hand and avoid any other movements. Then, their eyes continued to focus on the monitor that displays a cross to remind participants to remain still and avoid any movements for 20 s; this is block 1. In block 2, the four table items will be restored and placed into the storage box, with the bowl placed in front of the box in the identical order in 15 s, then with 20 s to rest. There were eight blocks in this task, block 3 and 4, block 5 and 6, block 7 and 8 were the same as block 1 and 2. The order of placement was always fixed: plate, saucer, chopsticks, soup spoon, and rice bowl (**Figure 1B**).

In the observation (OBS) task of the experiment, the table items, storage box, and placemat were turned toward to the experimenter. The visual procedures were the same as the EXEC

TABLE 1 | Participants' demographic and physiological characteristics for low, middle, and high fitness groups (mean ± SD).

Variable	High fitness	Moderate fitness	Low fitness	Total
Sample size	12	13	11	36
Gender (male)	8	7	5	20
Age (yr)	20.44 ± 1.62	20.93 ± 1.49	20.27 ± 1.27	20.58 ± 1.48
Height (cm)	171.05 ± 6.38	168.87 ± 9.54	167.64 ± 10.54	168.53 ± 8.70
Weight (kg)	62.59 ± 9.81	63.71 ± 11.92	60.06 ± 15.624	61.44 ± 12.53
BMI (kg.m^{-2})	21.27 ± 2.09	22.19 ± 2.80	21.07 ± 3.48	21.45 ± 2.92
IPAQ (METs/wk)	3342 ± 1726	3909 ± 2501	2125 ± 1286	2960 ± 1863
VO$_{2max}$ (mL.kg^{-1}.min^{-1}) for women	41.78 ± 1.68[a]	36.83 ± 0.69[b]	32.37 ± 1.65[c]	36.43 ± 3.94
VO$_{2max}$ (mL.kg^{-1}.min^{-1}) for men	55.74 ± 3.02[a]	48.01 ± 1.26[b]	41.56 ± 2.72[c]	49.49 ± 6.26
VO$_{2max}$ (mL.kg^{-1}.min^{-1}) for men and women	51.08 ± 1.80[a]	42.85 ± 1.74[b]	36.60 ± 1.88[c]	43.69 ± 8.44

BMI, body mass index; IPAQ, International Physical Activity Questionnaire; MET, metabolic equivalent; means with different superscripts a, b, and c are significantly different from one another.

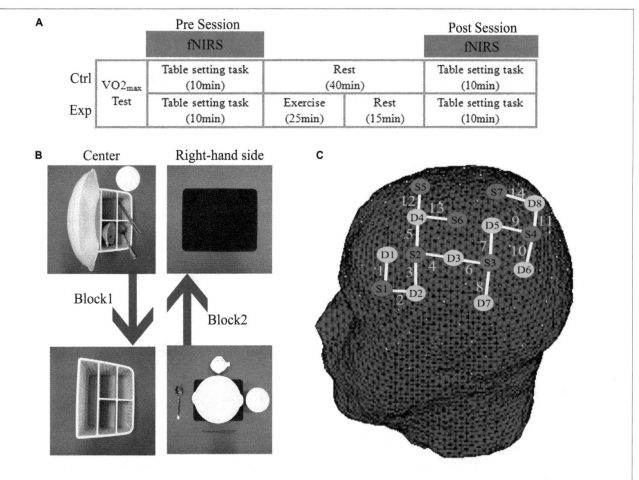

FIGURE 1 | (A) The experimental design showed the experimental (Exp) condition and the control (Ctrl) condition. Using functional near-infrared spectroscopy (fNIRS) to measure cortical hemodynamic changes while subjects performed the table-setting tasks before (Pre) and after (Post) exercise or rest. **(B)** Illustration of the design of the table-setting tasks. **(C)** fNIRS optode placement according to the 10–10 International System. Red dots represent the position of light sources. Green dots represent the position of detectors. Yellow lines depict channels.

task. The experimenter moved the table items, and participants carefully observed the movements. When the experimenter rested and watched the cross on the monitor, participants also focused on the cross and avoided any movements during the whole OBS task.

fNIRS Data Acquisition

fNIRS data were acquired using the NIRSport system (NIRx Medical Technologies, LLC, Glen Head, NY, United States). Probe-channel sets were installed with reference to the international 10/10 system into a NIRS-EEG compatible cap (EASYCAP, Herrsching, Germany) and then placed on the participant's head. The cap position was centered at the Cz point, and then thin plastic straps were inserted between probes to ensure that the distance was less than 3 cm between each source and detector. The fNIRS system consisted of eight light sources and eight detectors which formed 14 channels covering most of the MNS region on the participant's left hemisphere. Channels 1, 2, and 3 consisted of IFG (BA44/45), channels 4, 5, 12, and 13 consisted of PMC (BA6), channels 6, 7, and 8 consisted of rostral IPL (BA40), and channels 9, 10, 11, and 14 consisted of SPL (BA7) (**Figure 1C**). An already existing NIRS 10 × 10 positions were used to estimate the NMI coordinates of optodes with respect to the EEG 10/5 positions. The locations of NIRS channels were defined using the maximum probability method (**Table 2**). The ROIs were determined while three or four channels covered one Brodmann Area. We placed channels only in the left hemisphere because the left hemisphere is dominant when subjects perform a right-handed action (Filimon et al., 2007; Egetemeir et al., 2011). Prior to recording, the NIRStar acquisition software (NIRx Medical Technologies, LLC, Glen Head, NY, United States) recorded fNIRS data and verified the signal quality according to the NIRStar manual. The baseline was set while each participant was resting for 15 s prior to the table-setting test to remove irrelevant noise and signal drift (Fu et al., 2016).

Data Preprocessing

Raw data from each participant were processed within the nirsLAB analysis package (v2017.06, NIRx Medical Technologies, LLC, Los Angeles, CA, United States). Discontinuities were automatically corrected or deleted by the nirsLAB (std threshold = 5). Spikes were interpolated or manually deleted. A bandpass filter was used; 0.01 Hz was used to remove drift and 0.1 Hz was used to filter respiratory noise. We used the modified Beer–Lambert law (Cope et al., 1988) to analyze the optical data from the fNIRS system. The changes in oxygenated hemoglobin (Oxy-Hb), deoxygenated hemoglobin (Deoxy-Hb), and total hemoglobin (Total-Hb) concentration data were collected at a sampling rate set at 7.81 Hz.

Statistical Analyses

All descriptive characteristics (age, height, weight, BMI, IPAQ, and VO_{2max}) were imported into IBM SPSS Statistics 22 (SPSS Inc., Chicago, IL, United States), and then a one-way ANOVA was used to compared characteristics between cardiovascular fitness levels (high, moderate, and low).

The statistical parametric mapping (SPM) level 1 (within-subject) package incorporated into nirsLAB was based on the canonical hemodynamic function (parameters in nirsLAB = [6 16 1 1 6 0 32]) to determine event-related changes in Oxy-Hb, Deoxy-Hb, and total-Hb during action execution and observation. Finally, the *beta* values of the Oxy-Hb and Deoxy-Hb were exported from each participant for statistical analysis. Second-level analyses (SPM 2) level 2 assessed differences in groups to export brain activation maps.

The *beta* values of the Oxy-Hb and Deoxy-Hb from each ROI of the participant as the dependent variable were imported to IBM SPSS Statistics 22 (SPSS Inc., Chicago, IL, United States). The one-way ANOVA was applied to compare Oxy-Hb and Deoxy-Hb between levels in non-exercise session (CTRL PRE, CTRL POST, and EXP PRE sessions). Then Oxy-Hb and Deoxy-Hb were subjected to three-way repeated measure ANOVA under different tasks (EXEC and OBS) with three factors: conditions (EXP and CTRL), time sessions (PRE and POST) as within-subject factors, cardiovascular fitness levels (high, moderate, and low) as a between-subject factor. Then when it exhibited main effect on conditions and three-way interaction was significantly different, following two-way repeated measure ANOVA used Bonferroni correction method was applied to the [Post–Pre] Oxy-Hb or Deoxy-Hb contrast (Δ Oxy-Hb and Δ Deoxy-Hb) of EXP and CTRL conditions in these ROIs to compare the effect of exercise on the MNS-related regions that were known as activated by action execution and action observation. We used contrast value of Oxy-Hb or Deoxy-Hb because it would help to eliminate potential variations as different MNS activation may be caused by doing the tasks on different days. All values are presented as mean ± SE. An alpha of 0.05 was used as the statistical significance level for all comparisons.

RESULTS

Participant Characteristics

We summarize the basic descriptive characteristics for the three-fitness level. One-way ANOVA indicated no significant difference among fitness levels on the demographic variables of age, height, weight, BMI, and IPAQ. As expected, VO_{2max} was significantly different between fitness levels [$F(2, 33) = 15.73$, $P < 0.001$], and *post hoc* analyses revealed that all three groups were significantly different from each other. The high fitness level group showed the highest VO_{2max} value, the moderate fitness group followed, and the low fitness group had the lowest value (**Table 1**).

Cortical Hemodynamic Change in OBS Task

In the OBS task, the one-way ANOVA was conducted on each ROI to determine whether the Oxy-Hb and Deoxy-Hb were significant differences between levels in non-exercise session (CTRL PRE, CTRL POST, and EXP PRE sessions). However, it revealed no significant differences between cardiovascular fitness levels with regard to Oxy-Hb and Deoxy-Hb.

The three-way repeated measures ANOVA was performed on each of the ROI of the Oxy-Hb and Deoxy-Hb. It revealed a significant main effect on conditions [$F(2,33) = 9.30$, $P < 0.05$, $\eta^2 = 0.22$], a significant interaction between conditions, time sessions, and cardiovascular fitness levels [$F(2,33) = 3.42$, $P < 0.05$, $\eta^2 = 0.17$] in IFG region. It also revealed a significant main effect on conditions [$F(2,33) = 4.70$, $P < 0.05$, $\eta^2 = 0.13$] and a marginal significant interaction [$F(2,33) = 2.70$, $P = 0.08$, $\eta^2 = 0.14$] in the PMC region. However, there was

TABLE 2 | The MNI coordinate of each channel, the source, and detector positions are in the 10-10 system.

| Channel | Source—Detector | MNI coordinate | | | Brodmann area and anatomical label (percentage overlap) |
		X	Y	Z	
1	F5–F3	−46	39	26	45—Pars triangularis Broca's area (72.56%)
2	F5–FC5	−56	24	20	45—Pars triangularis Broca's area (53.08%)
3	FC3–FC5	−55	12	34	44—Pars opercularis, part of Broca's area (47.81%)
4	FC3–C3	−50	−3	50	6—Pre-motor and supplementary motor cortex (61.71%)
5	FC3–FC1	−38	12	55	6—Pre-motor and supplementary motor cortex (37.52%)
6	CP3–C3	−52	−34	52	40—Supramarginal gyrus part of Wernicke's area (43.32%)
7	CP3–CP1	−39	−48	60	40—Supramarginal gyrus part of Wernicke's area (41.82%)
8	CP3–CP5	−57	−48	38	40—Supramarginal gyrus part of Wernicke's area (65.46%)
9	P1–CP1	−24	−62	62	7—Somatosensory association cortex (82.72%)
10	P1–P3	−32	−73	47	7—Somatosensory association cortex (69.67%)
11	P1–PZ	−13	−73	56	7—Somatosensory association cortex (91.59%)
12	FCZ–FC1	−13	12	67	6—Pre-motor and supplementary motor cortex (73.21%)
13	C1–FC1	−26	−5	68	6—Pre-motor and supplementary motor cortex (81.78%)
14	CPZ–PZ	2	−61	66	7—Somatosensory association cortex (58.83%)

The Brodmann area with maximum probability was used in final location of each channel.

no significant interaction in the IPL and SPL regions. In order to determine which fitness level of activation of these two ROIs were increased by exercise, two-way repeated measure ANOVA was used to compare the contrast value (Δ Oxy-Hb) of EXP and CTRL conditions. It indicated that was a significant difference in the low fitness level [$F_{(2,33)}$ = 5.11, $P < 0.05$, $\eta^2 = 0.13$, Bonferroni-corrected] in IFG region. Also, it exhibited significant difference in the high fitness level [$F_{(2,33)} = 17.36$, $P < 0.001$, $\eta^2 = 0.35$, Bonferroni-corrected] and low fitness level [$F_{(2,33)} = 7.62$, $P < 0.05$, $\eta^2 = 0.19$, Bonferroni-corrected] in the PMC region. However, there was no significant difference in PMC and IFG regions in the moderate fitness level (**Figure 2**).

With regard to Deoxy-Hb, there was a significant main effect in conditions [$F_{(2,33)} = 7.92$, $P < 0.05$, $\eta^2 = 0.19$], a significant interaction between conditions, time sessions, and cardiovascular fitness levels [$F_{(2,33)} = 3.33$, $P < 0.05$, $\eta^2 = 0.17$] in IPL region. In order to determine which fitness level of activation of this ROI was increased by exercise, two-way repeated measure ANOVA was used to compare the contrast value (Δ Deoxy-Hb) of EXP and CTRL conditions. It indicated that was a significant difference in the high fitness level [$F_{(2,33)} = 6.14$, $P < 0.05$, $\eta^2 = 0.16$, Bonferroni-corrected] in IPL region. There was no significant difference in the IPL region in the moderate and low fitness levels.

Cortical Hemodynamic Change in EXEC Task

In the EXEC condition, the one-way ANOVA was also conducted to each ROI determine whether the Oxy-Hb and Deoxy-Hb were significantly different between levels of fitness in the non-exercise session, which were not affected by exercise. The results revealed no significant differences between cardiovascular fitness levels for Oxy-Hb and Deoxy-Hb.

The three-way repeated measures ANOVA was also performed on each of the ROI of Oxy-Hb and Deoxy-Hb, it revealed no significant main effect on conditions or interaction

between conditions, time sessions, and cardiovascular fitness levels for both Oxy-Hb and Deoxy-Hb. The data that support the findings of this study are openly available in Mendeley at http://dx.doi.org/10.17632/s8tp7d75dw.1.

DISCUSSION

Our study indicated that there was no significant difference between fitness levels with EXEC or OBS task under non-exercise session, which implied different cardiovascular fitness levels could not reflect different activation of MNS under this table-setting social task and denied Hypothesis 1. Wright et al. (2019) evidenced that physical development is positively correlated with cognitive performance, language ability, and social-emotional state. Higher fitness level has been shown that was associated with better average accuracy and response time across all level of spatial memory tasks, lower switch cost in elderly adults, these higher fitness older adults also showed a greater functional connectivity which was related to better cognitive function (Voss et al., 2010; Prakash et al., 2011). Some investigations have shown that physical fitness level was relevant to language development. One study indicated that compared with typical developmental children, children with developmental language disorders showed worse performance on vertical jump (Muursepp et al., 2014). Also, the physical fitness performance of children with developmental language disorders was significantly lower than those of typical children (van der Niet et al., 2014). Although our study showed that there was no significant difference between cardiovascular fitness levels and MNS activation, it does not conflict with previous works because the cognitive function, social cognition, and language function are still different functions in the human brain, and participants were both college students which generally excluded language developmental disorders. And the most crucial point is that the values of VO_{2max} in the low level of our participants were also higher than those with language developmental disorders

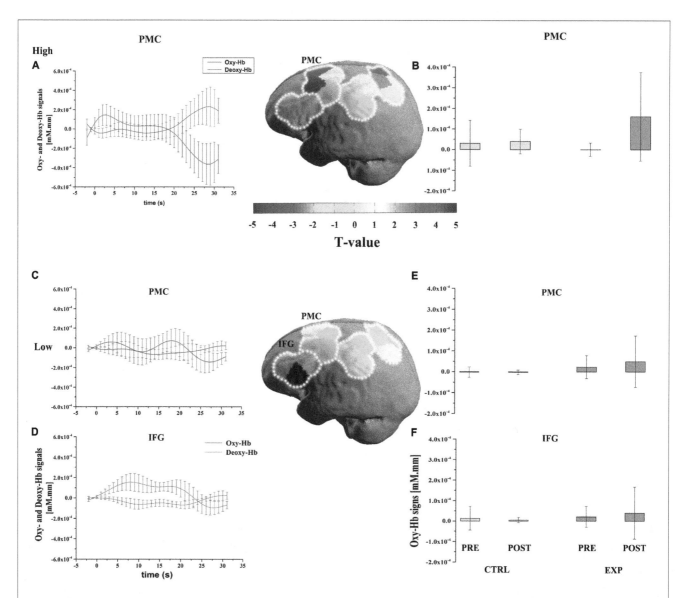

FIGURE 2 | Figures describe the significant improvement of oxygenated hemoglobin Δ Oxy-Hb response after exercise during the OBS task. The upper part is the cortical activation patterns with high cardiovascular fitness level (high: **A,B**) and the lower part is the cortical activation patterns with low cardiovascular fitness level (low: **C–F**). Three graphs of first column depict the timelines for the significant Δ Oxy-Hb (red) and Δ Deoxy-Hb (blue) signal which are shown in arbitrary units (mM·mm) **(A,C,D)**. Significant Oxy-Hb signal changes in ROIs during the OBS task in all conditions are shown in the last column. Error bars indicate standard error **(B,E,F)**. Middle figures are t-map of oxy-Hb signal contrast activation in the OBS task. T-values are shown according to the color bar.

relatively. More studies are needed to determine whether cardiovascular fitness level reflects social and language cognition.

Mirror neuron system has been reported to be an action execution and observation matching system. It also played a crucial role in the development of motor and language functions (Nishitani and Hari, 2000; Tettamanti et al., 2005). Our study illustrated that moderate-intensity exercise has a positive effect on the functions of MNS by increasing the Oxy-Hb during an OBS task. This result was consistent with Hypothesis 2 and other similar studies, which have shown the beneficial effect of moderate-intensity exercise on executive functions as indexed by the increasing Oxy-Hb (Yanagisawa et al., 2010; Byun et al., 2014). Therefore, the result of this study implied

that moderate exercise might be an effective way to improve social cognition by activating the MNS. Our result was consistent with recent studies showed that moderate exercise benefited those who have social cognition deficits social behaviors such as autism spectrum disorder (ASD) (Magnusson et al., 2012; Schmitz et al., 2017), in whom an MNS deficit has been described (Theoret et al., 2005; Hadjikhani et al., 2006). fMRI studies have also suggested no mirror neuron activity in the inferior frontal gyrus (pars opercularis in children with autism during imitation of emotional expressions (Dapretto et al., 2005), as well as during observation of human motion (Martineau et al., 2010). Our study indirectly provided one of the first pieces of neural basic evidence that exercise can improve the social behaviors of children with autism by improving the activation of MNS.

In addition, the subgroup analysis also showed that moderate exercise benefited people with high and low fitness levels, but not at moderate fitness level. Thus, Hypothesis 3 was supported. Specifically, it revealed the improvement of MNS activation in high fitness levels of the PMC region and improved the MNS activation of low fitness level individuals in IFG and PMC regions under OBS task. AS we can find plenty evidence to support acute exercise improved human brain functions of high and low fit individuals, recent studies have demonstrated the positive effect of acute exercise on cognitive performance of high and low fitness group in old adults (Chang et al., 2012, 2015; Chu et al., 2015). For instance, Chu et al. (2015) recruited forty-six healthy older adults to do a reading control and Stroop tasks after 30 min aerobic exercise training, the results revealed that acute exercise improved the performance of these two types of cognitive functions in both high and low fitness level old adults. Moreover, Hogan et al. (2013) demonstrated that unfit group has lower error rates in the flanker task under the exercise condition compared with rest condition and faster RTs were observed in fit participants after exercise. Although a previous meta-analysis has reported that fitness level significantly modulated the positive effects of exercise for low fit and high fit participants after a delay following exercise (Chang et al., 2012), In contrast, Chang et al. (2014) indicated acute exercise can improve performance in the congruent condition of Stroop task in all levels of cardiovascular fitness, but individuals of high cardiovascular fitness level demonstrated longer response times under incongruent condition. More research is needed since particularly in the context that social cognition and executive function are two different brain functions. Possible explanations for this result is the different values of VO_{2max} were used in different studies to categorized different fitness levels (Chang et al., 2014), the intensity of exercise and possibly different durations of exercise protocol led to different results (Chang et al., 2012). In addition, we hypothesized that social cognition is more sensitive to the stimulation of exercise when individuals are of low cardiovascular fitness, which can be easily aroused in a short period of time. However, individuals of moderate fitness are accustomed to moderate exercise, such that they experience marginal returns on social cognition improvement. Only when individuals reach a high fitness level in a long-term training program, can social cognition enjoy the greatest benefits from exercise since our body is in an optimal condition. There were few studies that have used neuroimaging methods to investigate the effect of exercise on different aerobic fitness levels participants' cognition (Pesce, 2009). Therefore, more research is required to determine how and why moderate-intensity exercise benefits MNS in high and low fitness individuals.

Besides, PMC area as one of important MNS regions, it showed improvements of activation in both high and low fit individuals under the action understanding task (OBS). This result can be supported by previous study demonstrated the positive effect of exercise intervention on Parkinson's disease patients, they showed that exercise increased motor control in early Parkinson's disease patients (Fisher et al., 2008; Shah et al., 2016). In Petzinger et al. (2013)'s review, they summarized exercise intervention to enable the goal-based motor skill training to engage the cognitive circuit to motor learning. Exercise increased the blood flow and facilitated the neuroplasticity in elderly adults, so this has the potential to result in the improvement of both cognitive and automatic components of motor control. Thus, our study indirectly explained why exercise intervention increased the self-perceived capability through instruction and feedback (reinforcement) in Parkinson's elderly adults, which can be explained by improving the action understanding function after exercise.

We also discuss whether the exercise only improved one of the functions of MNS which is motor control. Or exercise only improved action understanding but not to reach the social cognition function. Hickok et al. (2011b) suggest that MNS was merely a motor control or action selection function, and does not include understanding action performing by oneself or others. They provided much evidence to show that information flowing down into the temporal lobes was used to connect our visual and auditory experience with memories of conceptual objects and the dorsal stream processes that same visual information to integrate with the PMC region to generate movement. As the MNS was part of this dorsal stream, the output of motor (Hickok et al., 2011a). However, previous studies also indicated perform social tasks could activate PMC regions (Buccino et al., 2001; Molnar-Szakacs et al., 2006; Perkins et al., 2015), this evidence supported MNS function involves action understanding to social recognition. Moreover, our study implied that the MNS basic function is not only a motor controller since participants remained still and simply observed the action will not requiring any extra motor control function in this process (OBS tasks), the result indicated improvements in Oxy-Hb and Deoxy-Hb in action observation task after exercise to support moderate exercise was indeed stimulating the action understanding function. Similar to the argument mentioned above, some researchers also argued that parts of MNS (dorsal part of PMC) was responded by the action understanding, but the theory of mind or social cognition function is control by MENT (dorsal part of mPFC and the IFG as another part of MNS) (Geiger et al., 2019), even this statement is true, the result from our study indicated that exercise might benefit social cognition is still valid. Since in IFG region, the activation of low-level participants was still improved.

LIMITATION AND FUTURE RESEARCH

The present study might be limited because the Oxy-Hb and Deoxy-Hb values within each fitness level between men and women were not categorized identically, this issue due to the limit number of participants in each fitness level. Therefore, these issues may limit the generalizability of our findings and future research should identify the role of sex on exercise and the MNS. However, since the factor of gender has already been counter-balanced in this study (four out of 12 were female in high fitness, six out of 13 were female in moderate, and six out of 11 were female in low fitness), we can assume that effect of gender would not bias the results.

Another question is whether we should use measures of Oxy-Hb or Deoxy-Hb to represent behavioral data. Some studies have indicated that the Oxy-Hb signal is often observed to have a higher amplitude than the Deoxy-Hb signal (Strangman et al., 2002; Yanagisawa et al., 2010), which means that Oxy-Hb is more sensitive to the task response (Cheng et al., 2015). Our study also illustrated more amplitude changes using Oxy-Hb signal compared with Deoxy-Hb. However, we were still able to observe some trace when using Deoxy-Hb in our study, which suggests that Deoxy-Hb data from fNIRS is still necessary to include in the analysis for a more comprehensive picture.

As our study only used the acute aerobic exercise protocol, and different protocols of exercise have indicated different effects on cognitive performances, expanded researches into effect of long-term exercise, and different exercise protocols of training programs are necessary to determine the effect of exercise on MNS. And more task protocols involve behavioral index associate with social cognition performance should be included into neuroimaging studies since we only used the Oxy-Hb and Deoxy-Hb as the index to indicate the effect of exercise on the MNS.

ETHICS STATEMENT

The studies involving human participants were reviewed and approved by the Ethics Committee of Guangzhou Sport University. The patients/participants provided their written informed consent to participate in this study. Written informed consent was obtained from the individual(s) for the publication of any potentially identifiable images or data included in this article.

AUTHOR CONTRIBUTIONS

ZX, MH, and M-QX contributed to conception and design of the study. ZX, Z-RW, and JL organized the database. ZX and M-QX analyzed the data. ZX wrote the first draft of the manuscript. MH and M-QX contributed to manuscript revision and read and approved the submitted version.

ACKNOWLEDGMENTS

The authors wish to thank the study participants for their involvement. The authors would like to thank Xiaocong Chen for his help with revising this article. ZX would like to thank Wanshan for inspiring him with love and accompanying him on the road of life.

REFERENCES

Åberg, M., Pedersen, N., Torén, K., Svartengren, M., Bäckstrand, B., Johnsson, T., et al. (2009). Cardiovascular fitness is associated with cognition in young adulthood. *Proc. Natl. Acad. Sci. U.S.A.* 106, 20906–20911. doi: 10.1073/pnas. 0905307106

American College of Sports Medicine [ACSM] (2013). *ACSM's Guidelines for Exercise Testing and Prescription*, 9th Edn. Philadelphia, PA: Lippincott Williams & Wilkins.

Audiffren, M., Tomporowski, P. D., and Zagrodnik, J. (2009). Acute aerobic exercise and information processing: modulation of executive control in a random number generation task. *Acta Psychol. (Amst.)* 132, 85–95. doi: 10.1016/ j.actpsy.2009.06.008

Baird, A. D., Scheffer, I. E., and Wilson, S. J. (2011). Mirror neuron system involvement in empathy: a critical look at the evidence. *Soc. Neurosci.* 6, 327–335. doi: 10.1080/17470919.2010.547085

Bernier, R., Aaronson, B., and McPartland, J. (2013). The role of imitation in the observed heterogeneity in EEG mu rhythm in autism and typical development. *Brain Cogn.* 82, 69–75. doi: 10.1016/j.bandc.2013.02.008

Borg, G. A. V. (1982). Psychophysical bases of perceived exertion. *Med. Sci. Sports Exerc.* 14, 377–381. doi: 10.1249/00005768-198205000-00012

Bremer, E., Crozier, M., and Lloyd, M. (2016). A systematic review of the behavioural outcomes following exercise interventions for children and youth with autism spectrum disorder. *Autism* 20, 899–915. doi: 10.1177/ 1362361315616002

Brisswalter, J., Collardeau, M., and René, A. (2002). Effects of acute physical exercise characteristics on cognitive performance. *Sports Med.* 32, 555–566. doi: 10.2165/00007256-200232090-00002

Bruce, R. A., Kusumi, F., and Hosmer, D. (1973). Maximal oxygen intake and nomographic assessment of functional aerobic impairment in cardiovascular disease. *Am. Heart J.* 85, 546–562. doi: 10.1016/0002-8703(73)90502-4

Buccino, G., Binkofski, F., Fink, G. R., Fadiga, L., Fogassi, L., Gallese, V., et al. (2001). Action observation activates premotor and parietal areas in a somatotopic manner: an fMRI study. *Eur. J. Neurosci.* 13, 400–404. doi: 10. 1111/j.1460-9568.2001.01385.x

Buccino, G., Vogt, S., Ritzl, A., Fink, G. R., Zilles, K., and Freund, H. J.

(2004). Neural circuits underlying imitation learning of hand actions: an event-related fMRI study. *Neuron* 42, 323–334. doi: 10.1016/s0896-6273(04)00 181-3

Byun, K. H., Hyodo, K., Suwabe, K., Ochi, G., Sakairi, Y., and Kato, M. (2014). Positive effect of acute mild exercise on executive function via arousal-related prefrontal activations: an fNIRS study. *Neuroimage* 98, 336–345. doi: 10.1016/j. neuroimage.2014.04.067

Chaddock, L., Erickson, K. I., Prakash, R. S., Kim, J. S., Voss, M. W., and VanPatter, M. (2010). A neuroimaging investigation of the association between aerobic fitness, hippocampal volume, and memory performance in preadolescent children. *Brain Res.* 1358, 172–183. doi: 10.1016/j.brainres.2010. 08.049

Chang, Y. K., Chi, L., Etnier, J. L., Wang, C. C., Chu, C. H., and Zhou, C. L. (2014). Effect of acute aerobic exercise on cognitive performance: role of cardiovascular fitness. *Psychol. Sport Exerc.* 15, 464–470. doi: 10.1016/j.psychsport.2014. 04.007

Chang, Y. K., Chu, C. H., Wang, C. C., Song, T. F., and Wei, G. X. (2015). Effect of acute exercise and cardiovascular fitness on cognitive function: an event–related cortical desynchronization study. *Psychophysiology* 52, 342–351. doi: 10.1111/psyp.12364

Chang, Y. K., Labban, J. D., Gapin, J. I, and Etnier, J. L. (2012). The effects of acute exercise on cognitive performance: a meta-analysis. *Brain Res.* 1453, 87–101. doi: 10.1016/j.brainres.2012.02.068

Cheng, X., Li, X., and Hu, Y. (2015). Synchronous brain activity during cooperative exchange depends on gender of partner: a fNIRS–based hyperscanning study. *Hum. Brain Mapp.* 36, 2039–2048. doi: 10.1002/hbm.22754

Chu, C.-H., Chen, A.-G., Hung, T.-M., Wang, C.-C., and Chang, Y.-K. (2015). Exercise and fitness modulate cognitive function in older adults. *Psychol. Aging* 30, 842–848. doi: 10.1037/pag0000047

Cope, M., Delpy, D. T., Reynolds, E. O., Wray, S., Wyatt, J., and van der Zee, P. (1988). Methods of quantitating cerebral near infrared spectroscopy data. *Adv. Exp. Med. Biol.* 222, 183–189. doi: 10.1007/978-1-4615-9510-6_21

Dapretto, M., Davies, M. S., Pfeifer, J. H., Scott, A. A., Sigman, M., and Bookheimer, S. Y. (2005). Understanding emotions in others: mirror neuron dysfunction in children with autism spectrum disorders. *Nat. Neurosci.* 9, 28–30. doi: 10.1038/nn1611

Drollette, E. S., Shishido, T., Pontifex, M. B., and Hillman, C. H. (2012). Maintenance of cognitive control during and after walking in preadolescent children. *Med. Sci. Sports Exerc.* 44, 2017–2024. doi: 10.1249/MSS.0b013e318258bcd5

Egetemeir, J., Stenneken, P., Koehler, S., Fallgatter, A. J., and Herrmann, M. J. (2011). Exploring the neural basis of real-life joint action: measuring brain activation during joint table setting with functional near-infrared spectroscopy. *Front. Hum. Neurosci.* 5:95. doi: 10.3389/fnhum.2011.00095

Filimon, F., Nelson, J. D., Hagler, D. J., and Sereno, M. I (2007). Human cortical representations for reaching: mirror neurons for execution, observation, and imagery. *Neuroimage* 37, 1315–1328. doi: 10.1016/j.neuroimage.2007.06.008

Fisher, B. E., Wu, A. D., Salem, G. J., Song, J., Lin, C. H., and Yip, J. (2008). The effect of exercise training in improving motor performance and corticomotor excitability in people with early Parkinson's disease. *Arch. Phys. Med. Rehabil.* 89, 1221–1229. doi: 10.1016/j.apmr.2008.01.013

Fogassi, L., Ferrari, P. F., Gesierich, B., Rozzi, S., Chersi, F., and Rizzolatti, G. (2005). Parietal lobe: from action organization to intention understanding. *Science* 308, 662–667. doi: 10.1126/science.1106138

Freudenberger, P., Petrovic, K., Sen, A., Toglhofer, A. M., Fixa, A., Hofer, E., et al. (2016). Fitness and cognition in the elderly the Austrian stroke prevention study. *Neurology* 86, 418–424. doi: 10.1212/wnl.0000000000002329

Fu, G., Wan, N. J. A., Baker, J. M., Montgomery, J. W., Evans, J. L., and Gillam, R. B. (2016). A proof of concept study of function-based statistical analysis of fNIRS data: syntax comprehension in children with specific language impairment compared to typically-developing controls. *Front. Behav. Neurosci.* 10:108. doi: 10.3389/fnbeh.2016.00108

Gallese, V. (2006). Intentional attunement: a neurophysiological perspective on social cognition and its disruption in autism. *Brain Res.* 1079, 15–24. doi: 10.1016/j.brainres.2006.01.054

Gallese, V., Keysers, C., and Rizzolatti, G. (2004). A unifying view of the basis of social cognition. *Trends Cogn. Sci.* 8, 396–403. doi: 10.1016/j.tics.2004.07.002

Geiger, A., Bente, G., Lammer, S., Tepest, R., Roth, D., and Bzdok, D. (2019). Distinct functional roles of the mirror neuron system and the mentalizing system. *Neuroimage* 202:116102. doi: 10.1016/j.neuroimage.2019.116102

Hadjikhani, N., Joseph, R. M., Snyder, J., and Tager-Flusberg, H. (2006). Anatomical differences in the mirror neuron system and social cognition network in autism. *Cereb. Cortex* 16, 1276–1282. doi: 10.1093/cercor/bh069

Hickok, G., Costanzo, M., Capasso, R., and Miceli, G. (2011a). The role of Broca's area in speech perception: evidence from aphasia revisited. *Brain Lang.* 119, 214–220. doi: 10.1016/j.bandl.2011.08.001

Hickok, G., Houde, J., and Rong, F. (2011b). Sensorimotor integration in speech processing: computational basis and neural organization. *Neuron* 69, 407–422. doi: 10.1016/j.neuron.2011.01.019

Hogan, M., Kiefer, M., Kubesch, S., Collins, P., Kilmartin, L., and Brosnan, M. (2013). The interactive effects of physical fitness and acute aerobic exercise on electrophysiological coherence and cognitive performance in adolescents. *Exp. Brain Res.* 229, 85–96. doi: 10.1007/s00221-013-3595-0

Johnson-Frey, S. H., Maloof, F. R., Newman-Norlund, R., Farrer, C., Inati, S., and Grafton, S. T. (2003). Actions or hand-object interactions? Human inferior frontal cortex and action observation. *Neuron* 39, 1053–1058. doi: 10.1016/S0896-6273(03)00524-5

Kamp, C. F., Sperlich, B., and Holmberg, H. C. (2014). Exercise reduces the symptoms of attention–deficit/hyperactivity disorder and improves social behaviour, motor skills, strength and neuropsychological parameters. *Acta Paediatr.* 103, 709–714. doi: 10.1111/apa.12628

Kilner, J. M., Neal, A., Weiskopf, N., Friston, K. J., and Frith, C. D. (2009). Evidence of mirror neurons in human inferior frontal gyrus. *J. Neurosci.* 29, 10153–10159. doi: 10.1523/jneurosci.2668-09.2009

Leslie, K. R., Johnson-Frey, S. H., and Grafton, S. T. (2004). Functional imaging of face and hand imitation: towards a motor theory of empathy. *Neuroimage* 21, 601–607. doi: 10.1016/j.neuroimage.2003.09.038

Magnusson, J. E., Cobham, C., and McLeod, R. (2012). Beneficial effects of clinical exercise rehabilitation for children and adolescents with autism spectrum disorder (ASD). *J. Exerc. Physiol. Online* 15, 71–79.

Martineau, J., Andersson, F., Barthelemy, C., Cottier, J. P., and Destrieux, C. (2010). Atypical activation of the mirror neuron system during perception of hand motion in autism. *Brain Res.* 1320, 168–175. doi: 10.1016/j.brainres.2010.01.035

Molenberghs, P., Brander, C., Mattingley, J. B., and Cunnington, R. (2010). The role of the superior temporal sulcus and the mirror neuron system in imitation. *Hum. Brain Mapp.* 31, 1316–1326. doi: 10.1002/hbm.20938

Molnar-Szakacs, I., Kaplan, J., Greenfield, P. M., and Iacoboni, M. (2006). Observing complex action sequences: the role of the fronto-parietal mirror neuron system. *Neuroimage* 33, 923–935. doi: 10.1016/j.neuroimage.2006.07.035

Muursepp, I., Aibast, H., Gapeyeva, H., and Paasuke, M. (2014). Sensorimotor function in preschool-aged children with expressive language disorder. *Res. Dev. Disabil.* 35, 1237–1243. doi: 10.1016/j.ridd.2014.03.007

Nishitani, N., and Hari, R. (2000). Temporal dynamics of cortical representation for action. *Proc. Natl. Acad. Sci. U.S.A.* 97, 913–918. doi: 10.1073/pnas.97.2.913

Perkins, T., Stokes, M., McGillivray, J., and Bittar, R. (2010). Mirror neuron dysfunction in autism spectrum disorders. *J. Clin. Neurosci.* 17, 1239–1243. doi: 10.1016/j.jocn.2010.01.026

Perkins, T. J., Bittar, R. G., McGillivray, J. A., Cox, I. I., and Stokes, M. A. (2015). Increased premotor cortex activation in high functioning autism during action observation. *J. Clin. Neurosci.* 22, 664–669. doi: 10.1016/j.jocn.2014.10.007

Pesce, C. (2009). "An integrated approach to the effect of acute and chronic exercise on cognition: the linked role of individual and task constraints," in *Exercise and Cognitive Function*, eds T. McMorris, P. D. Tomporowski, and M. Audiffren, (Hoboken, NJ: Wiley-Heinrich), 211–226. doi: 10.1002/9780470740668.ch11

Petzinger, G. M., Fisher, B. E., McEwen, S., Beeler, J. A., Walsh, J. P., and Jakowec, M. W. (2013). Exercise-enhanced neuroplasticity targeting motor and cognitive circuitry in Parkinson's disease. *Lancet Neurol.* 12, 716–726. doi: 10.1016/S1474-4422(13)70123-6

Pfeifer, J. H., Iacoboni, M., Mazziotta, J. C., and Dapretto, M. (2008). Mirroring others' emotions relates to empathy and interpersonal competence in children. *Neuroimage* 39, 2076–2085. doi: 10.1016/j.neuroimage.2007.10.032

Prakash, R. S., Voss, M. W., Erickson, K. I., Lewis, J., Chaddock, L., Malkowski, E., et al. (2011). Cardiorespiratory fitness and attentional control in the aging brain. *Front. Hum. Neurosci.* 4:229. doi: 10.3389/fnhum.2010.00229

Rizzolatti, G., Fadiga, L., Gallese, V., and Fogassi, L. (1996). Premotor cortex and the recognition of motor actions. *Cogn. Brain Res.* 3, 131–141. doi: 10.1016/0926-6410(95)00038-0

Sayal, N. (2015). Exercise training increases size of hippocampus and improves memory PNAS (2011) vol. 108 | no. 7 | 3017-3022. *Ann. Neurosci.* 22:107. doi: 10.5214/ans.0972.7531.220209

Schmitz, S. O., Mcfadden, B. A., Golem, D. L., Pellegrino, J. K., Walker, A. J., Sanders, D. J., et al. (2017). The effects of exercise dose on stereotypical behavior in children with autism. *Med. Sci. Sports Exerc.* 49, 983–990. doi: 10.1249/mss.0000000000001197

Seifert, T., Brassard, P., Wissenberg, M., Rasmussen, P., Nordby, P., and Stallknecht, B. (2010). Endurance training enhances BDNF release from the human brain. *Am. J. Physiol. Regul. Integr. Comp. Physiol.* 298, R372–R377. doi: 10.1152/ajpregu.00525.2009

Shah, C., Beall, E. B., Frankemolle, A. M., Penko, A., Phillips, M. D., Lowe, M. J., et al. (2016). Exercise therapy for Parkinson's disease: pedaling rate is related to changes in motor connectivity. *Brain Connect.* 6, 25–36. doi: 10.1089/brain.2014.0328

Small, S. L., Buccino, G., and Solodkin, A. (2012). The mirror neuron system and treatment of stroke. *Dev. Psychobiol.* 54, 293–310. doi: 10.1002/dev.20504

Spunt, R. P., and Lieberman, M. D. (2012). An integrative model of the neural systems supporting the comprehension of observed emotional behavior. *Neuroimage* 59, 3050–3059. doi: 10.1016/j.neuroimage.2011.10.005

Strangman, G., Boas, D. A., and Sutton, J. P. (2002). Non-invasive neuroimaging using near-infrared light. *Biol. Psychiatry* 52, 679–693. doi: 10.1016/s0006-3223(02)01550-0

Sun, P. P., Tan, F. L., Zhang, Z., Jiang, Y. H., Zhao, Y., and Zhu, C. Z. (2018). Feasibility of functional near-infrared spectroscopy (fNIRS) to investigate the mirror neuron system: an experimental study in a real-life situation. *Front. Hum. Neurosci.* 12:86. doi: 10.3389/fnhum.2018.00086

Tettamanti, M., Buccino, G., Saccuman, M. C., Gallese, V., Danna, M., and Scifo, P. (2005). Listening to action-related sentences activates fronto-parietal motor circuits. *J. Cogn. Neurosci.* 17, 273–281. doi: 10.1162/0898929053124965

Theoret, H., Halligan, E., Kobayashi, M., Fregni, F., Tager-Flusberg, H., and Pascual-Leone, A. (2005). Impaired motor facilitation during action observation in individuals with autism spectrum disorder. *Curr. Biol.* 15, R84–R85. doi: 10.1016/j.cub.2005.01.022

Tomasello, M., Carpenter, M., Call, J., Behne, T., and Moll, H. (2005).

Understanding and sharing intentions: the origins of cultural cognition. *Behav. Brain Sci.* 28, 675–691. doi: 10.1017/s0140525x05000129

Tomporowski, P. D. (2003). Effects of acute bouts of exercise on cognition. *Acta Psychol. (Amst.)* 112, 297–324. doi: 10.1016/s0001-6918(02)00134-8

van der Niet, A. G., Hartman, E., Moolenaar, B. J., Smith, J., and Visscher, C. (2014). Relationship between physical activity and physical fitness in school-aged children with developmental language disorders. *Res. Dev. Disabil.* 35, 3285–3291. doi: 10.1016/j.ridd.2014.08.022

Voss, M. W., Erickson, K. I., Prakash, R. S., Chaddock, L., Malkowski, E., Alves, H., et al. (2010). Functional connectivity: a source of variance in the association between cardiorespiratory fitness and cognition? *Neuropsychologia* 48, 1394–1406. doi: 10.1016/j.neuropsychologia.2010.01.005

Wright, P. M., Zittel, L. L., Gipson, T., and Williams, C. (2019). Assessing relationships between physical development and other indicators of school readiness among preschool students. *J. Teach. Phys. Educ.* 38, 388–392. doi: 10.1123/jtpe.2018-0172

Xu, Z., Hu, M., Wang, Z.-R., Li, J., Hou, X.-H., and Xiang, M.-Q. (2019). The positive effect of moderate-intensity exercise on the mirror neuron system: an fNIRS Study. *Front. Psychol.* 10:986. doi: 10.3389/fpsyg.2019.00986

Yanagisawa, H., Dan, I., Tsuzuki, D., Kato, M., Okamoto, M., and Kyutoku, Y. (2010). Acute moderate exercise elicits increased dorsolateral prefrontal activation and improves cognitive performance with Stroop test. *Neuroimage* 50, 1702–1710. doi: 10.1016/j.neuroimage.2009.12.023

6

The Impact of Hypomania on Aerobic Capacity and Cardiopulmonary Functioning

Aura Shoval[1], Hilary F. Armstrong[1], Julia Vakhrusheva[2], Jacob S. Ballon[3], Matthew N. Bartels[4] and David Kimhy[5]*

[1] Department of Rehabilitation and Regenerative Medicine, Columbia University, New York, NY, United States, [2] Department of Psychiatry, Columbia University, New York, NY, United States, [3] Department of Psychiatry and Behavioral Science, Stanford University, Stanford, CA, United States, [4] Department of Rehabilitation Medicine, Albert Einstein College of Medicine, Bronx, NY, United States, [5] Department of Psychiatry, Icahn School of Medicine at Mount Sinai, New York, NY, United States

*Correspondence:
David Kimhy
david.kimhy@mssm.edu

Background: Hypomanic episodes are characterized by increased goal-directed behavior and psychomotor agitation. While the affective, cognitive, and behavioral manifestations of such episodes are well-documented, their physiological influence on aerobic capacity and cardiopulmonary functioning are unknown.

Methods: We describe a case report of an individual with schizophrenia who experienced a hypomanic episode while serving as a control participant (wait list) in a single-blind, randomized clinical trial examining the impact of aerobic exercise (AE) on neurocognition in people schizophrenia. As part of the trial, participants completed two scheduled clinical assessments and cardiopulmonary exercise tests (VO_2max) at baseline and 12 weeks later at end of study. All participants received standard psychiatric care during the trial. Following a baseline assessment in which he displayed no evidence of mood lability, the subject returned on Week-12 for his scheduled follow-up assessment displaying symptoms of hypomania. He was able to complete the follow-up assessment, as well as third assessment 2 weeks later (Week-14) when his hypomanic symptoms ebbed.

Results: While not engaging in AE, the subject's aerobic capacity, as indexed by VO_2max, increased by 33% from baseline to Week-12. In comparison, participants engaged in the aerobic exercise training increased their aerobic capacity on average by 18%. In contrast, participants in the control group displayed a small decline (−0.5%) in their VO_2max scores. Moreover, the subject's aerobic capacity increased even further by Week-14 (49% increase from baseline), despite the ebbing of his hypomania symptoms at that time. These changes were accompanied by increases in markers of aerobic fitness including peak heart rate, respiratory exchange rate, peak minute ventilation, watts, and peak systolic blood pressure. Resting systolic and diastolic blood pressure, and peak diastolic blood pressure remained unchanged.

Conclusions: Our findings suggest that hypomania produce substantial increase in aerobic capacity and that such elevations may remain sustained following the ebbing of hypomanic symptoms. Such elevations may be attributed to increased mobility and goal-directed behavior associated with hypomania, as individuals in hypomanic states may ambulate more frequently, for longer duration, and/or at higher intensity. Our results provide a first and unique view into the impact of hypomania on aerobic capacity and cardiopulmonary functioning.

Keywords: Schizophrenia, hypomania, aerobic fitness (VO$_2$max), cardiopulmonary, mania and bipolar disorder, cardiopulmonar exercise testing, cardiopulmonary activity

BACKGROUND

Hypomanic episodes are characterized by increased goal-directed behavior and psychomotor agitation manifested by more frequent pacing, fidgeting, and hand-wringing. While the cognitive, affective, and behavioral manifestations of such episodes have been documented extensively (1, 2), their influence on the physiological functioning of afflicted individuals is unknown. Specifically, the impact of hypomania on aerobic capacity and cardiopulmonary functioning is undetermined.

To address this issue, we describe a case report of an individual with schizophrenia, subject AA, who experienced a hypomanic episode while serving as a control participant in a single-blind, randomized clinical trial examining the impact of aerobic exercise (AE) on neurocognition in individuals with schizophrenia. As part of this study, participants were randomized to receive 12 weeks of regular psychiatric care (Treatment as Usual; TAU) or AE training in addition to TAU (3, 4). In this article, we report on subject AA's aerobic capacity and cardiopulmonary functioning before the trial (baseline), during the hypomanic episode (week 12), as well as 2 weeks later (week 14) when his hypomania symptoms ebbed. We characterized his performance and reviewed and contrasted it with the other study participants.

METHODS

The study was approved by the Columbia University's New York State Psychiatric Institute Institutional Review Board (NYSPI-IRB) and all participants signed a consent form. A written informed consent was obtained from the participant (subject AA) for the publication of this case report. All participants completed scheduled clinical, cognitive, and cardiopulmonary exercise tests (CPET) at baseline and follow-up (12 Weeks). Following approval by the NYSPI-IRB, subject AA completed a third CPET 2 weeks later (week 14).

Measures

Detailed descriptions of the study rationale and procedures have been reported elsewhere (4–7). Briefly, aerobic capacity was determined by CPET to establish VO$_2$max, considered the "gold standard" index of aerobic capacity. VO$_2$max is an index of the maximum capacity of an individual's body to transport and use oxygen during incremental aerobic exercise, reflecting the individual's aerobic capacity level. All tests were completed on weekdays at ~10 a.m. and were performed on an electronically braked cycle ergometer (Ergometrics 800, SensorMedics Inc., Yorba Linda, CA) with a Viasys Encore metabolic cart (Viasys Corporation, Loma Linda, CA). Continuous 12-lead

telemetry was monitored via CardioSoft electrocardiogram software (GE/CardioSoft, Houston, TX). Participants completed measurements of a 5-min resting baseline, 3-min of no-resistance warm-up, ramping exercise protocol of 10–15 watts to peak exercise with a target of exercise for 8–12 min. Exercise was terminated when the subject reached maximum capacity (VO$_2$ plateau; 85% of maximal heart rate (HRmax; 220-age) (8); respiratory quotient ≥1.1; or self-reported exhaustion) (9). A 3-min active recovery period completed the test. We used VO$_2$peak (ml/kg/min) scores in all analyses.

Additional cardiopulmonary variables were collected including heart rate (HR), respiratory exchange ratio (RER), resting and peak systolic and diastolic blood pressure (SBP, DBP), peak minute ventilation (VE), peak tidal volume (Vt), end tidal carbon dioxide pressure (PetCO$_2$), rate of carbon dioxide production at peak (VCO$_2$ L/min), and peak work rate (Watts). The clinical raters and technicians administering the CPET were blinded to the subjects intervention assignment and clinical status.

RESULTS

Subject AA is a slender 20-year-old, never married, male of Asian descent with a DSM-IV diagnosis of schizophrenia (onset at age 19). At the time of the study, he lived with relatives and had no family history of psychosis. At study entry his body mass index was 21.8 and he was prescribed Proloxin 37.5 mg injection every other week, lamotrigine 100 mg twice a day, hydroxyzine 50 mg twice a day, and benztropine 1 mg twice a day. He denied smoking. Subject AA endorsed moderately severe auditory hallucinations and religious delusions, but was clinically stable and reported to function well, just completing his freshman year in a local community college. Subject AA completed his baseline CPET, clinical, and cognitive assessments with no difficulties and was randomized to receive TAU. He displayed no mood lability during his baseline assessment. On week 12, upon arriving for the scheduled follow-up CPET, he displayed symptoms consistent with hypomania including elevated mood, flight of ideas, psychomotor agitation, and poor impulse control. Despite his condition, he completed his CPET, but given his clinical status, he was tested again 2 weeks later (Week 14), at which point his hypomanic symptoms were no longer present and he returned to his clinical baseline. His urine toxicology tests at baseline, Week 12, and Week 14 were all negative.

Examination of changes in aerobic capacity from baseline to follow-up (Week 12) among all participants indicated the AE group increased their VO$_2$max on average by 18%, compared to

TABLE 1 | Subject AA cardiopulmonary functioning before, during, and post-hypomania.

	Baseline (before hypomania)	Week 12 (during hypomania)	Week 14 (post-hypomania)
VO_2 Peak (ml/kg/min)	26.1	34.8	39.1
Resting heart rate (RHR)	77	86	70
Peak heart rate (PHR)	122	170	161
Respiratory exchange ratio (RER)	0.9	1.1	1.0
Peak minute ventilation (L/min)	42.6	65.8	73.4
Peak end tidal carbon dioxide pressure ($PetCO_2$)	43.3	42.4	41.4
Peak wattage (watts)	100	154	155
Resting systolic blood pressure (RSBP)	115	118	121
Peak systolic blood pressure (PSBP)	157	198	183
Resting diastolic blood pressure (RDBP)	72	86	74
Peak diastolic blood pressure (PDBP)	75	78	80

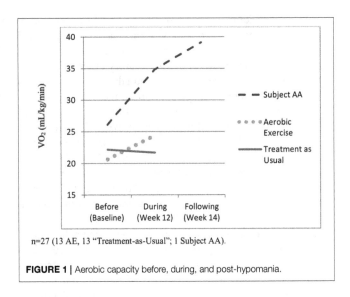

n=27 (13 AE, 13 "Treatment-as-Usual"; 1 Subject AA).

FIGURE 1 | Aerobic capacity before, during, and post-hypomania.

a small decline in the TAU group (−0.5%) (4). In comparison, Subject AA's VO_2max increased by 33% during this period, although he denied engaging in any aerobic exercises in the preceding weeks. At Week 14, his aerobic capacity was elevated even further (49% increase from baseline), despite the ebbing of hypomania symptoms at that point (see **Table 1** and **Figure 1**). His resting heart rate increased from 77 to 86 beats/min during hypomania and then went down to 70 beats/min following the hypomanic episode. A number of other cardiopulmonary variables increased from baseline to hypomania and post-hypomania periods including peak HR, respiratory exchange rate, peak minute ventilation, watts, and peak systolic blood pressure. $PetCO_2$ decreased. These trends are all consistent with markers of increased aerobic fitness. In contrast, other parameters including resting systolic and diastolic blood pressure, as well as peak diastolic blood pressure remained unchanged.

To ensure that Subject AA's increase in VO_2max was not related to higher workload, we examined his VO_2 at the same workload (100 watts) to control for potential effort-related variability across sessions. His VO_2 at 100 watts was lowest prior to the hypomanic episode (1.66 L/min), higher during (1.75 L/min), and highest following the episode (2.03 L/min). Examination of the performance at the same workload (100 watts) show that for Peak VO_2, there was a larger component of volitional effect on conditioning. This view is corroborated by the similar trend in VO_2max showing the lowest prior (26.1 kg L/min), higher during (34.8 kg L/min), and highest following the hypomanic episode (39.1 L/min). Likewise, VE also rose in a similar fashion and peak HR were elevated more at both follow up evaluations (Weeks 12 and 14).

DISCUSSION

To the best of our knowledge, the present report is the first characterization of the impact of hypomania on aerobic capacity

and cardiopulmonary functioning. Our results suggest that episodes of hypomania produce substantial increases in aerobic capacity and that such elevations may be present even following the ebbing of hypomanic symptoms. Such increases may be attributed to heightened mobility and goal-directed behavior associated with hypomania, as individuals in hypomanic states may ambulate more frequently, for longer durations, and/or at higher intensity, resulting in increased VO_2, peak wattage, as well as higher anaerobic threshold. Such episodes may also be associated with a greater ability to push harder on CPET, as indicated by higher workload (watts) with higher peak HR and VE in the latter tests. Thus, volitional aspects may also play a greater role in performance, necessitation careful review of CPET results of patients assessed during hypomanic states.

Overall, the improvement in subject AA's aerobic capacity, while not engaging in aerobic exercise, surpassed study participants engaging in a formal AE training program with a trainer (3 60-min sessions per week over 12 weeks). The improvement in other parameters such as workload and peak HR, support the view of hypomanic state-related increases in aerobic capacity, with the caveat that subject AA also gave a far higher effort with increased HR and minute ventilation. These indicators were even more elevated at Week 14. Overall, these findings are consistent with results from studies in the general population that indicate that increases in incidental physical activity (e.g., increased tapping of foot, pacing) correlate with higher VO_2 max. For example, McGuire and Ross (10) have found that duration and intensity of incidental activities indexed by accelerometers were associated with higher VO_2 max. Other authors have reported similar results, finding "fidgeting" and incidental physical activity increasing VO_2max (11, 12).

VO_2 is an important marker of physical health, as increased VO_2 has been linked to early lower mortality (13, 14). Previous reports have documented significant lower aerobic fitness in individuals with schizophrenia (4) along with prevalence of early mortality among individuals diagnosed with schizophrenia, schizoaffective disorder, as well as bipolar disorder (15, 16). Thus, our findings of hypomanic episodes resulting in VO_2max elevations provoke an intriguing question–does the experience of manic episodes and the resulting VO_2 increases confer potential long-term protection with regard to early mortality risk? A recent meta-analysis has found no cardiorespiratory fitness differences between diagnostic subgroups of individuals with severe mental illness (e.g., schizophrenia, bipolar disorder, and major depressive disorder) (17). Previous reports have also documented significant elevations in early mortality among individuals with severe mental illness including those diagnosed with schizophrenia, schizoaffective disorder, and bipolar disorder (15, 16). Consistent with these findings, a review of medical records of 326 patients with a psychotic disorder treated at the Mayo Clinic in Minnesota between 1950 and 1980 found no significant difference in median survival for patients with schizophrenia vs. those with schizoaffective disorder (18). However, a population cohort study in Denmark (5,558,959 persons of which 261,887 persons had been admitted to a psychiatric hospital) found both females and males admitted with a diagnosis of schizophrenia had a higher mortality rate ratio of natural causes of death, compared to persons admitted with unipolar, bipolar, and schizoaffective disorders (19). Of note, natural causes of mortality comprised of cardiovascular diseases, respiratory diseases, endocrine and metabolic conditions, as well as old age and apoplexy, and malignant neoplasms. Thus, given the complexity of the longitudinal relationship between cardiopulmonary fitness and early mortality risk, the research literature at present does not provide conclusive support for the potential of manic episodes to confer protection for early mortality risk via temporal VO_2 increases. Future studies should aim to elucidate this potential link, as it may inform the mechanisms associated with increased early mortality in individuals with severe mental illness.

The present report has a number of limitations. One limitation is the focus on a single individual. Secondly, the appraisal of (lack of) AE by Subject AA during the period prior to the follow-up assessments was based on his self-report, rather than via actigraph. Another limitation is the lack of follow-up assessments post the Week 14 assessment. Such information would have been valuable to characterize the timeline and long-term impact of hypomania on cardiopulmonary indicators. Finally, the changes in aerobic capacity and cardiopulmonary functioning may reflect, in part, Subject AA's young age, lower BMI, and relatively higher baseline aerobic capacity. Thus, the results should be interpreted with caution and future studies should aim to confirm our findings in larger and more diverse samples, including individuals who are older and have higher BMI. In contrast, the present report has a number of strengths including evaluation of naturally occurring hypomania that developed and resolved during "real world" functioning, a rigorous research assessment of clinical symptoms, as well as the use of CPET, a "gold standard" of aerobic capacity and cardiopulmonary functioning assessment.

In summary, the present report is the first characterization of changes in aerobic capacity and cardiopulmonary functioning associated with hypomanic episodes. Our results indicate that hypomanic episodes lead to substantial increases in aerobic capacity and improvements in cardiopulmonary functioning, and such increases may last for weeks and well-beyond the period of active hypomanic symptoms.

AUTHOR CONTRIBUTIONS

DK designed the study and wrote the protocol. MB and HA conducted the aerobic fitness and cardiopulmonary analyses, as well as provided the statistical data. JV conducted the diagnostic and clinical assessments. JB served as a medical director of the study and assisted with the monitoring of the participants' health. AS managed the literature searches, and along with DK, wrote the first draft of the manuscript. All authors contributed to and have approved the final version of the manuscript.

REFERENCES

Benazzi F. Bipolar II disorder : epidemiology, diagnosis and management. *CNS Drugs* (2007) 21:727–40. doi: 10.2165/00023210-200721090-00003

Cassidy F., Yatham LN, Berk M, Grof P. Pure and mixed manic subtypes: a review of diagnostic classification and validation. *Bipolar Dis.* (2008) 10:131–43. doi: 10.1111/j.1399-5618.2007.00558.x

Kimhy D, Vakhrusheva J, Bartels MN, Armstrong HF, Ballon JS, Khan S, et al. Aerobic fitness and body mass index in individuals with schizophrenia: Implications for neurocognition and daily functioning. *Psychiatr Res.* (2014) 220:784–91. doi: 10.1016/j.psychres.2014.08.052

Kimhy D, Vakhrusheva J, Bartels MN, Armstrong HF, Ballon JS, Khan S, et al. The impact of aerobic exercise on brain-derived neurotrophic factor and neurocognition in individuals with schizophrenia: a single-blind, randomized clinical trial. *Schizophr Bull.* (2015) 41:859–68. doi: 10.1093/schbul/sbv022

Armstrong HF, Bartels MN, Paslavski O, Cain D, Shoval HA, Ballon JS, et al. The impact of aerobic exercise training on cardiopulmonary functioning in individuals with schizophrenia. *Schizophr Res.* (2016) 173:116–7. doi: 10.1016/j.schres.2016.03.009

Kimhy D, Khan S, Ayanrouh L, Chang RW, Hansen MC, Lister A, et al. Use of active-play video games to enhance aerobic fitness in schizophrenia: feasibility, safety, and adherence. *Psychiatr Serv.* (2016) 67:240–3. doi: 10.1176/appi.ps.201400523

Kimhy D, Lauriola V, Bartels MN, Armstrong HF, Vakhrusheva J, Ballon JS, et al. Aerobic exercise for cognitive deficits in schizophrenia - The impact of frequency, duration, and fidelity with target training intensity. *Schizophr Res.* (2016) 172:213–5. doi: 10.1016/j.schres.2016.01.055

Medicine ACOs Clinical Exercise Testing. In: Thompson WR, editor. *ACSM's Guidelines for Exercise Testing and Supervision.* 8th ed. Philadeplhia, PA: Woulters Kluwer; Lippincott; Williams and Wilkins (2009). pp. 105–35.

Borg G. *Borg's Perceived Exertion and Pain Scales.* Champaign, IL:Human Kinetics (1998).

McGuire KA, Ross R. Incidental physical activity and sedentary behavior are not associated with abdominal adipose tissue in inactive adults. *Obesity* (20112) 20:576–82. doi: 10.1038/oby.2011.278

Hagger-Johnson G, Gow AJ, Burley V, Greenwood D, Cade JE. Sitting time, fidgeting, and all-cause mortality in the UK women's cohort study. *Am J Prev Med.* (2016) 50:154–60. doi: 10.1016/j.amepre.2015.06.025

Pavey TG, Pulsford R. Fidgeting is associated with lower mortality risk. *Evid Based Med.* (2016) 21:109. doi: 10.1136/ebmed-2016-110410

Sui X, LaMonte MJ, Laditka JN, Hardin JW, Chase N, Hooker SP, et al. Cardiorespiratory fitness and adiposity as mortality predictors in older adults. *JAMA* (2007) 298:2507–16. doi: 10.1001/jama.298.21.2507

Wei M, Kampert JB, Barlow CE, Nichaman MZ, Gibbons LW, Paffenbarger RS, et al. Relationship between low cardiorespiratory fitness and mortality in normal-weight, overweight, and obese men. *JAMA* (2007) 282:1547–53. doi: 10.1001/jama.282.16.1547

Osby U, Correia N, Brandt L, Ekbom A, Sparen P. Mortality and causes of death in schizophrenia in Stockholm county, Sweden. *Schizophr Res.* (2000) 45:21– 8. doi: 10.1016/S0920-9964(99)00191-7

Weiner M, Warren L, Fiedorowicz JG. Cardiovascular morbidity and mortality in bipolar disorder. *Ann Clin Psychiatry* (2011) 23:40–7.

Vancampfort D, Firth J, Schuch F, Rosenbaum S, De Hert M, Mugisha J, et al. Physical activity and sedentary behavior in people with bipolar disorder: a systematic review and meta-analysis. *J Affect Dis.* (2016) 201:145–52. doi: 10.1016/j.jad.2016.05.020

Capasso RM, Lineberry TW, Bostwick JM, Decker PA, St Sauver J. Mortality in schizophrenia and schizoaffective disorder: an Olmsted County, Minnesota cohort: 1950-2005. *Schizophr Res.* (2008) 98:287–94. doi: 10.1016/j.schres.2007.10.005

Laursen TM, Munk-Olsen T, Nordentoft M, Mortensen PB. Increased mortality among patients admitted with major psychiatric disorders: a register-based study comparing mortality in unipolar depressive disorder, bipolar affective disorder, schizoaffective disorder, and schizophrenia. *J Clin Psychiatry* (2007) 68:899–907. doi: 10.4088/JCP. v68n0612

7

The Effect of Spatial Ability in Learning from Static and Dynamic Visualizations: A Moderation Analysis in 6-Year-Old Children

Anis Ben Chikha[1†], Aïmen Khacharem[2†], Khaled Trabelsi[3] and Nicola Luigi Bragazzi[4]*

[1] Ksar-Saïd, Manouba University, ECOTIDI UR16ES10, Tunis, Tunisia, [2] LIRTES (EA 7313), UFR SESS-STAPS, Paris-East Créteil University, Créteil, France, [3] Research Laboratory: Education, Motricité, Sport et Santé, EM2S, LR19JS01, High Institute of Sport and Physical Education of Sfax, University of Sfax, Sfax, Tunisia, [4] Laboratory for Industrial and Applied Mathematics, Department of Mathematics and Statistics, York University, Toronto, ON, Canada

*Correspondence:
Nicola Luigi Bragazzi
bragazzi@yorku.ca

[†] These authors have contributed equally to this work and share first authorship

Previous studies with adult human participants revealed mixed effects regarding the relation between spatial ability and visual instructions. In this study, we investigated this question in primary young children, and particularly we explored how young children with varying levels of spatial abilities integrate information from both static and dynamic visualizations. Children ($M = 6.5$ years) were instructed to rate their invested mental effort and reproduce the motor actions presented from static and dynamic 3D visualizations. The results indicated an interaction of spatial ability and type of visualization: high spatial ability children benefited particularly from the animation, while low spatial ability learners did not, confirming therefore the ability-as-enhancer hypothesis. The study suggests that an understanding of children spatial ability is essential to enhance learning from external visualizations.

Keywords: multimedia learning, spatial ability, young children, animation, cognitive abilities

INTRODUCTION

Issues of spatial ability and learning achievement have been an underlying topic of psychological and educational discussions for many years (e.g., Presmeg, 1986; Wanzel et al., 2002; Unal et al., 2009). Concerning the spatial ability and its influence on learning from static and dynamic visualizations, numerous research has been conducted (e.g., Höffler, 2010; Höffler and Leutner, 2011; Nguyen et al., 2012; Berney et al., 2015; Castro-Alonso et al., 2018; de Koning et al., 2019; Kühl et al., 2018; Castro-Alonso et al., 2019a; Castro-Alonso et al., 2019b). However, studies investigating the effect of visualization type and spatial ability on children learning performances are lacking. Our study is, therefore, an attempt to directly examine this issue in the context of multimedia learning. Two principal research questions oriented this investigation: First, what external visualization will lead to the best understanding of a 3D game sequence in 6-year-old children? Second, does the efficiency of an external visualization depend upon children spatial ability?

Dynamic visualizations such as animations and videos can nowadays be easily integrated into a multitude of learning and training environments (Sherer and Shea, 2011; Kay, 2012; Khacharem et al., 2015a; Berney and Bétrancourt, 2016). It has been known that dynamic visualizations may facilitate learning as the learner can explicitly (and directly) perceive spatiotemporal changes in the depicted system/procedure. In the case of static visualizations, on the other hand, the learners have to mentally imagine spatiotemporal changes, which is assumed to be more challenging. Another argument suggests that the unequivocal depiction of a dynamic event through an animation can help the learner avoid misinterpretations of motion indicators used in static pictures, such as arrow symbols. Khacharem et al. (2015b) give the example of a diagram of play in which arrow symbols are used to depict players' motion. Learners might incorrectly interpret/understand the significance and the amplitude of the depicted arrows. This may impose significant levels of cognitive load and lead to misunderstanding and consequently, to a deficient mental model (Lewalter, 2003; Khacharem et al., 2020). Additionally, the external depiction of a movement by a dynamic visualization is considered to be more entertaining and engaging than equivalent static visualizations, which may, in turn, lead to better learning results (e.g., Lepper and Malone, 1987; Rieber, 1991; Khacharem, 2017). Recently, some evidence has demonstrated that dynamic visualizations seem to be particularly efficient for teaching procedures/contents that are realistic, based on human movements, and involving procedural-motor knowledge (Höffler and Leutner, 2007).

However, it has been shown that the fleeting nature of dynamic visualizations generates transient information that can slow down their learning effectiveness (Ayres and Paas, 2007). The transient information effect is a loss of learning due to information disappearing before the learner has time to adequately process it or link it with new information (Sweller et al., 2011). Cognitive Load Theory (Sweller, 1994; Van Merrienboer and Sweller, 2005) suggests that the transitory nature of animations may impose extraneous cognitive load due to the temporal limits of working memory. When learning with dynamic visualizations, one frame is displayed at a time, and once the dynamic visualization has advanced beyond a given frame, that frame is no longer available to the learner. In this case, learners are required to process current information and integrate it with previous information at the same time. Such cognitive-perceptual processing may impose a higher cognitive load on working memory resources. Another argument suggests that animations may generate an illusion of understanding (Hegarty et al., 2003; Rebetez et al., 2010). An animation that provides the succession of steps and transformations over time from beginning to end (without interactivity) does not mobilize cognitive investment, but rather promotes passive rather than active learning.

Learning from external visualizations is considered to be an active process that is influenced by the prerequisites of the learner. One crucial factor mediating the effectiveness of such processes is learner spatial ability (e.g., Hegarty and Kriz, 2008; Schnotz and Rasch, 2008). Spatial ability refers to a group of cognitive functions and aptitudes that is crucial in manipulating and processing visuospatial information (Lajoie, 2008; Castro-Alonso and Atit, 2019). Spatial visualization ability is a measure of the ability to mentally rotate or fold objects and to imagine the changes in location and form due to this manipulation (e.g., Mayer and Sims, 1994). This ability varies significantly within humans; some individuals have a facility for transforming spatial information, while others find these processes very challenging (Caroll, 1993; Hegarty and Waller, 2005). Currently, two different

hypotheses are employed to explain the relation between spatial abilities and presentations formats.

The ability-as-compensator hypothesis (Mayer and Sims, 1994; Höffler, 2010; Höffler and Leutner, 2011) posits that dynamic visualizations can assist low spatial ability learners by offering an explicit representation of temporal aspects of the system, thus reducing the need to mentally animating the static information. However, high spatial ability learners do not gain particular benefit from dynamic visualization because they are more cognitively equipped to generate an adequate mental representation of the depicted content regardless of the presentation format (Mayer, 2001). For example, Höffler and Leutner (2011) investigated the respective role of spatial ability and type of visualization (animation versus a series of static pictures) on learning of chemistry concepts. Spatial ability was measured using the Paper Folding test and the Card Rotation test (Ekstrom et al., 1976). The results indicated that low-spatial ability learners showed poor learning outcome when learning from static pictures while high-spatial learners did not. Conversely, when learning from animation, spatial ability did not moderate learning outcome as low and high spatial ability learners performed equally (Lee and Shin, 2012; Berney et al., 2015; Sanchez and Wiley, 2017).

On the other hand, the enhancer hypothesis (Hegarty and Sims, 1994; Hegarty, 2005; Huk, 2006; Höffler, 2010) claims that high spatial ability learners should uniquely benefit from the dynamic visualizations as they have enough cognitive capabilities left for mental model building of the content to-be-learned (Mayer, 2001; Huk, 2006). However, spatial ability learners experience an increase of unnecessary cognitive load while learning with static visualizations because their ability to mentally animate spatio-temporal information is limited (Hegarty and Sims, 1994; Hegarty, 2005; Huk, 2006; Keller et al., 2006; Höffler, 2010). Huk (2006) found that the incorporation of dynamic 3D models depicting a plant/animal cell enhance learning outcomes only in high spatial ability learners who are cognitively better ready to process dynamic visualizations since they have enough cognitive capacity left for building a coherent representation of the content to be learned. In contrast, low spatial ability learners are cognitively loaded by dynamic visualizations; therefore, they performed better with static visualizations.

A closer look at the aforementioned studies reveals that relatively little attention has been devoted to understanding the role of spatial abilities when learning from external visualizations in young children. Terlecki and Newcombe (2005) noted that young children have greater experience with modern multimedia technologies such as videos and computerized animations and, as a result, spatial ability could play an important role in learning processes. Previous research on spatial acquisition has indicated that mental paper folding emerges at 5.5 years of age and develops through early primary school (Harris et al., 2013). Similarly, it has been shown that enhancement in the ability to perform the object-based spatial transformations that necessitate spatial manipulation of mental image occurs from 5 years-old, although at a slower speed than adults (e.g., Frick et al., 2009; Funk et al., 2005; Kosslyn et al., 1990; Marmor, 1977; Crescentini et al., 2014). The purpose of this study was to explore the relative effects of spatial ability and type of visualization on children ability to learn a 3-D game sequence. This study employed the Mental Folding Test for Children (MFTC; Harris et al., 2013) and the Children's Mental Transformation Task (CMTT; Levine et al., 1999; Ehrlich et al., 2006) in which adequate validity and reliability on assessing spatial visualization ability in children have been established. First, we hypothesized that watching an animation that explicitly depicted learning contents would result in better learning outcomes than watching a series of static pictures (Hypothesis 1). Second, based on the ability-as-compensator hypothesis, we expected that children with low spatial ability would principally benefit from animation, whereas children with high spatial would benefit equally from both static pictures and animation (Hypothesis 2).

MATERIALS AND METHODS

Participants

A sample of 64 children (M = 6.5 years; SD = 0.23; 50% girls) in Grade 1 participated in this study. Children with intellectual disability, neurological disorder and/or uncorrectable hearing and/or visual impairment were excluded. They had not previously taken part in any similar research. The parents were required to consent to the inclusion of their child in the study and provide basic information on the child's developmental history. The study was conducted according to the Declaration of Helsinki and fully approved by the Sfax University Ethics Committee (approval code CPP 0076/2017)" before the commencement of the study.

Material Learning

A 3-D game sequence titled "the passing game" was designed and developed using Macromedia Flash MX Professional 2004. The game contained 10 players positioned as follows: seven players on the bottom line (attackers) and one player on each sideline (playmaker). It started with the teacher designing the number of an attacker (from 1 to 7) and ended with the designed attacker grounding the ball over the goal line. The game consisted of 11 steps. During each step, the attacker carried a set of actions: dribbling, hand passing, walking and accelerating. The game sequence of 47*sec* was presented via either an animation or a series of 12 static pictures representing the key moments of the sequence. Both versions were accompanied by the same verbal commentary. The learning and output stimuli were presented on a 17-inch LCD computer screen with a 1,280 × 1,024-pixel display. **Figure 1** gives a screenshot from the 3D game sequence used in the study.

Measures
Spatial Ability
Children's individual spatial ability was evaluated by two different tests. The MFTC (Harris et al., 2013) is a test developed for measuring the 4–7 years old children's ability to fold 2D shapes in their mind. It is a multiple-choice test where both sides of the shapes are presented in different colors. **Figure 2** shows one of the test items of the MTFC.

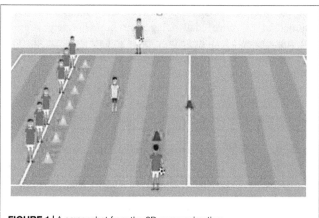

FIGURE 1 | A screenshot from the 3D game animation.

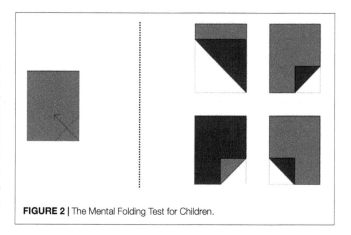

FIGURE 2 | The Mental Folding Test for Children.

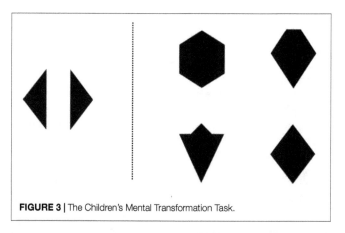

FIGURE 3 | The Children's Mental Transformation Task.

Another measure was the CMTT (Ehrlich et al., 2006; Levine et al., 1999) which consists of a multiple-choice test asking 4–7 years old children to point out the shape that will come into being when the previously presented two shapes are combined. **Figure 3** shows one of the test items of the CMTT.

For each test the percentage of correctly solved items related to the total number of items was calculated; the mean of the two scores represented each participant's spatial abilities. **Figure 4** shows the distribution of the 6 years-children's spatial ability in

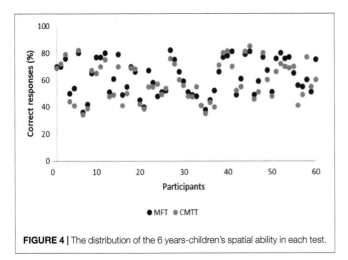

FIGURE 4 | The distribution of the 6 years-children's spatial ability in each test.

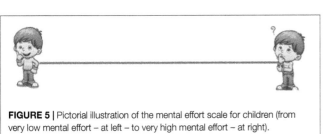

FIGURE 5 | Pictorial illustration of the mental effort scale for children (from very low mental effort – at left – to very high mental effort – at right).

each test. The correlation of MFT and CMTT was significant with $r = 0.88$.

Self-Report of Mental Effort

The experimenter explained to the children that he would like to know how they were feeling after the learning phase. In particular, they instructed them to indicate "*How much thinking did you do to complete the task; did you do a lot of thinking or only a little?*" Subsequently, the experimenter presented a picture and said: "*In this picture, the little boy seems to be thinking very hard.*" Then the experimenter pointed to the other picture and said, "*In this picture, he does not seem to be thinking hard at all. How did you feel in the task you just performed*? Finally, the experimenter asked children to place a hash mark between the two pictures (100-mm) and encouraged them to use the full range of the line. Scores were determined by measuring the placement of the hash mark on the 100-mm line. The children were reassured that there were no right or wrong answers. **Figure 5** provides a pictorial illustration of the mental effort scale.

Motor Recall Performance

Children were asked to accurately recall and execute – in a well-arranged area form the schoolyard – the game sequence. To ensure a smooth running of the situation an individual was instructed to intervene – by providing an oral corrective feedback – each time the children performed a wrong action. For each correct action in the recall test, the participants were assigned one point with a maximum score of 15 points, otherwise, they received zero points.

Hesitation Time

This variable represents the time that elapses between the end and the start of a new action made by the participant. It corresponds to the moments of immobility or steps backward (recall of already executed actions).

Procedure

The session lasted about 30 min, and only one child was tested in each session. First, children completed the spatial ability tests. Afterward, each child was randomly assigned to one experimental condition and was instructed to memorize as precisely as possible the evolution of the game sequence after viewing it one time only. Finally, after the learning task, the computer was switched off, and the post-tests were administered.

Statistical Analysis

To test the mediating effect of spatial ability, we performed mediation analysis using the pre-specified Model 1 of PROCESS macro (Hayes, 2013). PROCESS application developed by Preacher and Hayes (2008) which is an SPSS procedure (PROCESS, v2.13) that facilitates path analysis and mediation analysis by using ordinary least squares regression (Hayes et al., 2017). An analysis using 5,000 bootstrap samples with 95% confidence levels of the CIs was performed after mean-centering the continuous predictor variables. Three separate moderation analyses were performed in which spatial ability served as moderator variable and recall performance, hesitation time or subjective ratings of cognitive load were used as dependent variables. Significance was accepted for all analyses at the level of $p \leq 0.05$.

RESULTS

The results for motor recall performance show a significant regression model, $R^2 = 0.57$, $p < 0.01$. The regression analysis showed significant main effects of both spatial ability [$\beta = 0.419$, se(HC4) = 0.094, $p < 0.001$] and condition [$\beta = -1.004$, se(HC4) = 0.218, $p < 0.001$] on recall, and an interaction effect between spatial ability and condition [$\beta = -0.088$, se(HC4) = 0.06, $p = 0.04$]. Children with high level of spatial ability performed significantly better in the animation condition than in the static condition, while children with low spatial ability achieved the same performance regardless the experimental condition (**Figure 6**).

The results for cognitive load showed a non-significant regression model, $R^2 = 0.078$, $p = 0.137$. The regression analysis showed no main effect for spatial ability [$\beta = 0.048$, se(HC4) = 0.159, $p > 0.05$], a marginal main effect of condition [$\beta = 0.467$, se(HC4) = 0.261, $p = 0.06$], and no interaction of spatial ability and condition [$\beta = -0.060$, se(HC4) = 0.093, $p > 0.05$].

The results for hesitation time showed a regression model, $R^2 = 0.191$, $p = 0.002$, that was significant. The regression analysis showed a significant main effect for spatial ability [$\beta = -0.507$, se(HC4) = 0.181, $p = 0.007$], no main effect of condition [$\beta = 0.703$, se(HC4) = 0.399, $p = 0.10$], and a marginally

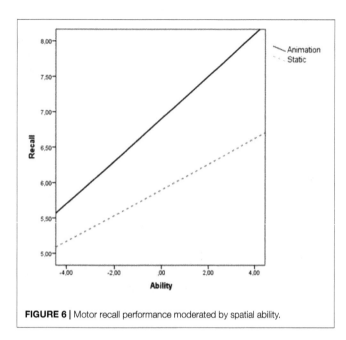

FIGURE 6 | Motor recall performance moderated by spatial ability.

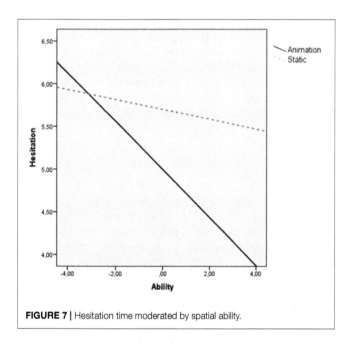

FIGURE 7 | Hesitation time moderated by spatial ability.

significant interaction effect between spatial ability and condition [β = 0.224, se(HC4) = 0.123, p = 0.07]. Children with high level of spatial ability reduce their hesitation time in the animation condition compared to the static condition, while children with low spatial ability keep the same hesitation time regardless the type of visualization (**Figure 7**).

DISCUSSION

In the current study, a group of primary school children were asked to remember and execute 12 elements of play, shown from static and dynamic 3D visualizations. The moderating role

of spatial ability was investigated with respect to motor recall performance, hesitation time and experienced cognitive load.

In line with Hypothesis 1, the results of this study showed that children receiving animations performed better compared to children receiving the static pictures (i.e., they achieved higher motor recall, invested less mental load, and needed less time). This indicates that the explicit presentation of the dynamic aspect of the game such as trajectory and motion helped children in constructing a deeper understanding of the game sequence. Thereby, this dynamic information can directly be read off from the animation, which in turn reduces extraneous cognitive load and incertitude (expressed by the hesitation time before each motor recall). In contrast, with static pictures, this dynamic information needs to be inferred by children via an animation mental process, which is generally assumed to be a more demanding cognitive task than merely perceiving temporal changes (Hegarty et al., 2003). Moreover, previous research have revealed that dynamic visualizations can be more effective form of instruction if they are realistic and involve procedural knowledge (Höffler and Leutner, 2007; Ayres et al., 2009; Wong et al., 2009; Garland and Sanchez, 2013; Castro-Alonso et al., 2015). In this research, we used animations that followed the prescriptions of this earlier research.

Another important finding of this study was the significant interaction found between spatial ability and type of visualization indicating an ability—as—enhancer hypothesis. Children with high spatial ability performed better from animation rather than static pictures (i.e., they achieved higher motor recall, needed less hesitation time and invested the same amount of mental load). It seems that these learners had already developed cognitive capabilities that enabled them to fluently process the fleeting dynamic information without a cognitive overload. However, in the static presentation, they would need to reconcile their cognitive resources with instructional details that were for them redundant and superfluous, which might impose additional extraneous cognitive load and reduce relative general performance. On the other hand, the results revealed that children with low spatial ability do not gain particular benefit from animation (i.e., they achieved the same recall motor score, they invested same amount of mental load and needed the same hesitation time). Because animations change continuously over time, these learners may not be able to process and integrate specific key elements of information that occur within the flow of information (e.g., Lowe, 1999; Rasch and Schnotz, 2009). In contrast, learning from static pictures is self-paced in the sense that learners were allowed as much time as they needed to reinspect a particular information. Therefore, it is likely that interactive animations, which allow children to control the progress of the animation, might be more helpful than animations that play at a fixed rate.

As is the case for all experimental studies, there are some limitations to the generalizability of our results. The limiting variables include the participants used for this research, which included primary school children (in Grade 1); the subject matter area, which focused on motor-procedural learning; and the design of learning materials used, which consisted of a computer-based projection with restricted interactivity.

Further research needs to investigate whether our findings can be applied to younger or older children, other subject matter areas, and types of learning materials. Another limitation of the present study is that we did not controlled some moderating variables frequently encountered in animation research (Castro-Alonso et al., 2016), such as the quantity of elements depicted (number bias, i.e., number of images depicted is different in static and animated format), and the visualization format size (size bias, i.e., the animation is larger than the 12 static pictures). Future research could test whether eliminating/minimizing these biases (e.g., by designing all visualizations with the same dimensions) actually influence the learning outcomes. In this study, it was demonstrated that even children with high spatial abilities failed to effectively learn from static pictures. Further research should examine the effect of some external supports considered as helpful in adults (e.g., arrows-indicating motion; Imhof et al., 2013) on children mental animation abilities. Previous studies (e.g., Jarodzka et al., 2010; Mehigan et al., 2011) showed that the way of gazing at the external visualizations is strongly related to individual differences. It would be interesting therefore to employ eye tacking measurements to assess how children with different levels of spatial abilities gaze at animations and static pictures while learning.

CONCLUSION

In sum, these results suggest caution in the use of static pictures to convey dynamic information to young children. The static format is considered as the basic visual tool to communicate explicit visual movement may, but this study offers no reason to conclude that static format inherently provides more educational value than animation format. The difficulty to learn from static pictures is noticeable among both low and high spatial abilities children. In the end, casting more light on the way in which children use static and dynamic information will hopefully provide valuable input to teaching, learning, and the design of effective learning materials.

ETHICS STATEMENT

The studies involving human participants were reviewed and approved by the parents were required to consent to the inclusion of their child in the study and provide basic information on the child's developmental history. The study was conducted according to the Declaration of Helsinki and fully approved the Sfax University Ethics Committee (approval code CPP 0076/2017). Written informed consent to participate in this study was provided by the participants' legal guardian/next of kin.

AUTHOR CONTRIBUTIONS

All authors listed have made a substantial, direct and intellectual contribution to the work, and approved it for publication.

ACKNOWLEDGMENTS

The authors wish to thank Anis Haddadi and Julien Gerald who created the required situations, as well as Monique Chedid for her technical assistance. The authors would also express their sincere gratitude to participants involved for their efforts, commitment, and enthusiasm throughout the study.

REFERENCES

Ayres, P., and Paas, F. (2007). Making instructional animations more effective: A cognitive load approach. *Appl. Cogn. Psychol.* 21, 695–700.

Ayres, P., Marcus, N., Chan, C., and Qian, N. (2009). Learning hand manipulative tasks: When instructional animations are superior to equivalent static representations. *Comput. Hum. Behav.* 25, 348–353. doi: 10.1016/j.chb.2008.12.013

Berney, S., and Bétrancourt, M. (2016). Does animation enhance learning? A meta-analysis. *Comput. Educ.* 101, 150–167. doi: 10.1016/j.compedu.2016.06.005

Berney, S., Bétrancourt, M., Molinari, G., and Hoyek, N. (2015). How spatial abilities and dynamic visualizations interplay when learning functional anatomy with 3D anatomical models. *Anat. Sci. Educ.* 8, 452–462. doi: 10.1002/ase.1524

Caroll, J. B. (1993). *Human Cognitive Abilities: A Survey of Factor-analytic Studies.* Cambridge: Cambridge University Press.

Castro-Alonso, J. C., and Atit, K. (2019). "Different abilities controlled by visuospatial processing," in *Visuospatial processing for education in health and natural sciences,* ed. J. C. Castro-Alonso (Cham: Springer), 23–51. doi: 10.1007/978-3-030-20969-8_2

Castro-Alonso, J. C., Ayres, P., and Paas, F. (2015). Animations showing Lego manipulative tasks: Three potential moderators of effectiveness. *Comput. Educ.* 85, 1–13. doi: 10.1016/j.compedu.2014.12.022

Castro-Alonso, J. C., Ayres, P., and Paas, F. (2016). Comparing apples and oranges? A critical look at research on learning from statics versus animations. *Comput. Educ.* 102, 234–243. doi: 10.1016/j.compedu.2016.09.004

Castro-Alonso, J. C., Ayres, P., and Sweller, J. (2019a). "Instructional visualizations, cognitive load theory, and visuospatial processing," in *Visuospatial processing for education in health and natural sciences,* ed. J. C. Castro-Alonso (Cham: Springer), 111–143. doi: 10.1007/978-3-030-20969-8_5

Castro-Alonso, J. C., Ayres, P., Wong, M., and Paas, F. (2018). Learning symbols from permanent and transient visual presentations: Don't overplay the hand. *Comput. Educ.* 116, 1–13. doi: 10.1016/j.compedu.2017.08.011

Castro-Alonso, J. C., Wong, M., Adesope, O. O., Ayres, P., and Paas, F. (2019b). Gender imbalance in instructional dynamic versus static visualizations: A meta-analysis. *Educ. Psychol. Rev.* 31, 361–387. doi: 10.1007/s10648-019-09 469-1

Crescentini, C., Fabbro, F., and Urgesi, C. (2014). Mental spatial transformations of objects and bodies: Different developmental trajectories in children from 7 to 11 years of age. *Dev. Psychol.* 50:370. doi: 10.1037/a0033627

de Koning, B. B., Marcus, N., Brucker, B., and Ayres, P. (2019). Does observing hand actions in animations and static graphics differentially affect learning of hand-manipulative tasks? *Comput. Educ.* 141:103636. doi: 10.1016/j.compedu.2019.103636

Ehrlich, S. B., Levine, S. C., and Goldin-Meadow, S. (2006). The importance of gesture in children's spatial reasoning. *Dev. Psychol.* 42:1259. doi: 10.1037/0012-1649.42.6.1259

Ekstrom, R. B., French, J. W., and Harman, H. H. (1976). *Manual for Kit of Factor Referenced Cognitive Tests.* Princeton, NJ: Educational Testing Service.

Frick, A., Daum, M. M., Walser, S., and Mast, F. W. (2009). Motor processes in children's mental rotation. *J. Cognit. Dev.* 10, 18–40. doi: 10.1080/15248370902966719

Funk, M., Brugger, P., and Wilkening, F. (2005). Motor processes in children's imagery: The case of mental rotation of hands. *Dev. Sci.* 8, 402–408.

doi: 10.1111/j.1467-7687.2005.00428.x

Garland, T. B., and Sanchez, C. A. (2013). Rotational perspective and learning procedural tasks from dynamic media. *Comput. Educ.* 69, 31–37. doi: 10.1016/j.compedu.2013.06.014

Harris, J., Hirsh-Pasek, K., and Newcombe, N. S. (2013). Understanding spatial transformations: Similarities and differences between mental rotation and mental folding. *Cogn. Process.* 14, 105–115. doi: 10.1007/s10339-013-0544-6

Hayes, A. F. (2013). *The PROCESS macro for SPSS and SAS (version 2.13)*.

Hayes, A. F., Montoya, A. K., and Rockwood, N. J. (2017). The analysis of mechanisms and their contingencies: PROCESS versus structural equation modeling. *Australas. Mark. J.* 25, 76–81. doi: 10.1016/j.ausmj.2017.02.001

Hegarty, M. (2005). "Multimedia learning about physical systems," in *The Cambridge Handbook of Multimedia Learning*, ed. R. E. Mayer (Cambridge: Cambridge University Press), 447–465. doi: 10.1017/CBO9780511816819.029

Hegarty, M., and Kriz, S. (2008). "Effects of knowledge and spatial ability on learning from animation," in *Learning with animation: research implications for design*, eds R. Lowe and W. Schnotz (Cambridge: Cambridge University Press), 3–29.

Hegarty, M., and Sims, V. K. (1994). Individual differences in mental animation during mechanical reasoning. *Mem. Cogn.* 22, 411–430. doi: 10.3758/bf03200867

Hegarty, M., and Waller, D. A. (2005). "Individual differences in spatial abilities," in *The Cambridge handbook of visuospatial thnking*, eds P. Shah and A. Miyake (Cambridge: Cambridge University Press), 121–169. doi: 10.4324/9780203641583-17

Hegarty, M., Kriz, S., and Cate, C. (2003). The roles of mental animations and external animations in understanding mechanical systems. *Cogn. Instr.* 21, 209–249. doi: 10.1207/s1532690xci2104_1

Höffler, T. N. (2010). Spatial ability: Its influence on learning with visualizations—a meta-analytic review. *Educ. Psychol. Rev.* 22, 245–269. doi: 10.1007/s10648-010-9126-7

Höffler, T. N., and Leutner, D. (2007). Instructional animation versus static pictures: A meta-analysis. *Learn. Instr.* 17, 722–738. doi: 10.1016/j.learninstruc.2007.09.013

Höffler, T. N., and Leutner, D. (2011). The role of spatial ability in learning from instructional animations–Evidence for an ability-as-compensator hypothesis. *Comput. Hum. Behav.* 27, 209–216. doi: 10.1016/j.chb.2010.07.042

Huk, T. (2006). Who benefits from learning with 3D models? The case of spatial ability. *J. Comput. Assist. Learn.* 22, 392–404. doi: 10.1111/j.1365-2729.2006.00180.x

Imhof, B., Scheiter, K., Edelmann, J., and Gerjets, P. (2013). Learning about locomotion patterns: Effective use of multiple pictures and motion-indicating arrows. *Comput. Educ.* 65, 45–55. doi: 10.1016/j.compedu.2013.01.017

Jarodzka, H., Scheiter, K., Gerjets, P., and Van Gog, T. (2010). In the eyes of the beholder: How experts and novices interpret dynamic stimuli. *Learn. Instr.* 20, 146–154. doi: 10.1016/j.learninstruc.2009.02.019

Kay, R. H. (2012). Exploring the use of video podcasts in education: A comprehensive review of the literature. *Comput. Hum. Behav.* 28, 820–831. doi: 10.1016/j.chb.2012.01.011

Keller, T., Gerjets, P., Scheiter, K., and Garsoffky, B. (2006). Information visualizations for knowledge acquisition: The impact of dimensionality and color coding. *Comput. Hum. Behav.* 22, 43–65. doi: 10.1016/j.chb.2005.01.006

Khacharem, A. (2017). Top-down and bottom-up guidance in comprehension of schematic football diagrams. *J. Sports Sci.* 35, 1204–1210. doi: 10.1080/02640414.2016.1218034

Khacharem, A., Trabelsi, K., Engel, F. A., Sperlich, B., and Kalyuga, S. (2020). The Effects of Temporal Contiguity and Expertise on Acquisition of Tactical Movements. *Front. Psychol.* 11:413. doi: 10.3389/fpsyg.2020.00413

Khacharem, A., Zoudji, B., and Kalyuga, S. (2015a). Expertise reversal for different forms of instructional designs in dynamic visual representations. *Br. J. Educat. Technol.* 46, 756–767. doi: 10.1111/bjet.12167

Khacharem, A., Zoudji, B., and Kalyuga, S. (2015b). Perceiving versus inferring movements to understand dynamic events: The influence of content complexity. *Psychol. Sport. Exerc.* 19, 70–75. doi: 10.1016/j.psychsport.2015.03.004

Kosslyn, S. M., Margolis, J. A., Barrett, A. M., Goldknopf, E. J., and Daly, P. F. (1990). Age differences in imagery abilities. *Child Dev.* 61, 995–1010. doi: 10.2307/1130871

Kühl, T., Stebner, F., Navratil, S. C., Fehringer, B. C. O. F., and Münzer, S. (2018). Text information and spatial abilities in learning with different visualizations

formats. *J. Educ. Psychol.* 110, 561–577. doi: 10.1037/edu0000226

Lajoie, S. P. (2008). Metacognition, self regulation, and self-regulated learning: A rose by any other name? *Educ. Psychol. Rev.* 20, 469–475. doi: 10.1007/s10648-008-9088-1

Lee, D. Y., and Shin, D. H. (2012). An empirical evaluation of multi-media based learning of a procedural task. *Comput. Hum. Behav.* 28, 1072–1081. doi: 10.1016/j.chb.2012.01.014

Lepper, M. R., and Malone, T. W. (1987). "Intrinsic motivation and instructional effectiveness in computer-based education," in *Aptitude, learning, and instruction: Vol. 3. Conative and affective process analyses*, eds R. E. Snow and M. J. Farr (Hillsdale, NJ: Lawrence Erlbaum), 255–286.

Levine, S., Huttenlocher, J., Taylor, A., and Langrock, A. (1999). Early sex differences in spatial skill. *Dev. Psychol.* 35, 940–949. doi: 10.1037/0012-1649.35.4.940

Lewalter, D. (2003). Cognitive strategies for learning from static and dynamic visuals. *Learn. Instr.* 13, 177–189. doi: 10.1016/s0959-4752(02)00019-1

Lowe, R. K. (1999). Extracting information from an animation during complex visual learning. *Eur. J. Psychol. Educ.* 14, 225–244. doi: 10.1007/BF03172967

Marmor, G. S. (1977). Mental rotation and number conservation: are they related? *Dev. Psychol.* 13:320. doi: 10.1037/0012-1649.13.4.320

Mayer, R. E. (2001). *Multimedia learning*. New York: Cambridge University Press.

Mayer, R. E., and Sims, V. K. (1994). For whom is a picture worth a thousand words? Extensions of a dual-coding theory of multimedia learning. *J. Educ. Psychol.* 86:389. doi: 10.1037//0022-0663.86.3.389

Mehigan, T. J., Barry, M., Kehoe, A., and Pitt, I. (2011). "Using eye tracking technology to identify visual and verbal learners," in *2011 IEEE International Conference on Multimedia and Expo*, (New York, NY: IEEE), 1–6.

Nguyen, N., Nelson, A. J., and Wilson, T. D. (2012). Computer visualizations: Factors that influence spatial anatomy comprehension. *Anat. Sci. Educ.* 5, 98–108. doi: 10.1002/ase.1258

Preacher, K. J., and Hayes, A. F. (2008). Asymptotic and resampling strategies for assessing and comparing indirect effects in multiple mediator models. *Behav. Res. Methods* 40, 879–891. doi: 10.3758/BRM.40.3.879

Presmeg, N. C. (1986). Visualization in high school mathematics. *Learn. Math.* 6, 42–46.

Rasch, T., and Schnotz, W. (2009). Interactive and non-interactive pictures in multimedia learning environments: effects on learning outcomes and learning efficiency. *Learn. Instr.* 19, 411–422. doi: 10.1016/j.learninstruc.2009.02.008

Rebetez, C., Bétrancourt, M., Sangin, M., and Dillenbourg, P. (2010). Learning from animation enabled by collaboration. *Instr. Sci.* 38, 471–485. doi: 10.1007/s11251-009-9117-6

Rieber, L. P. (1991). Effects of visual grouping strategies of computer-animated presentations on selective attention in science. *Educ. Technol. Res. Dev.* 39, 5–15. doi: 10.1007/bf02296567

Sanchez, C. A., and Wiley, J. (2017). "Dynamic visuospatial ability and learning from dynamic visualizations," in *Learning from Dynamic Visualization*, eds R. Lowe and R. Ploetzner (Cham: Springer), 155–176. doi: 10.1007/978-3-319-56204-9_7

Schnotz, W., and Rasch, T. (2008). "Functions of animation in comprehension and learning," in *Learning with Animation: Research Implications for Design*, eds L. Richard and W. Schnotz (New York, NY: Cambridge UP), 92–113.

Sherer, P., and Shea, T. (2011). Using online video to support student learning and engagement. *Coll. Teach.* 59, 56–59. doi: 10.1080/87567555.2010.511313

Sweller, J. (1994). Cognitive load theory, learning difficulty, and instructional design. *Learn. Instr.* 4, 295–312. doi: 10.1016/0959-4752(94)90003-5

Sweller, J., Ayres, P., and Kalyuga, S. (2011). "Measuring cognitive load," in *Cognitive load theory*, eds J. Sweller, S. Kalyuga, and P. Ayres (New York, NY: Springer), 71–85. doi: 10.1007/978-1-4419-8126-4_6

Terlecki, M. S., and Newcombe, N. S. (2005). How important is the digital divide? The relation of computer and videogame usage to gender differences in mental rotation ability. *Sex Roles* 53, 433–441. doi: 10.1007/s11199-005-6765-0

Unal, H., Jakubowski, E., and Corey, D. (2009). Differences in learning geometry among high and low spatial ability pre-service mathematics teachers. *Int. J. Math. Educ. Sci. Technol.* 40, 997–1012. doi: 10.1080/00207390902912852

Van Merrienboer, J. J., and Sweller, J. (2005). Cognitive load theory and complex learning: Recent developments and future directions. *Educ. Technol. Rev.* 17, 147–177. doi: 10.1007/s10648-005-3951-0

Wanzel, K. R., Hamstra, S. J., Anastakis, D. J., Matsumoto, E. D., and Cusimano, M. D. (2002). Effect of visual-spatial ability on learning of spatially-complex surgical skills. *Lancet* 359, 230–231. doi: 10.1016/s0140-6736(02)07441-x

Wong, A., Marcus, N., Ayres, P., Smith, L., Cooper, G. A., Paas, F., et al. (2009). Instructional animations can be superior to statics when learning human motor skills. *Comput. Hum. Behav.* 25, 339–347. doi: 10.1016/j.chb.2008.12.012

8

Is Obesity in Young People with Psychosis a Foregone Conclusion? Markedly Excessive Energy Intake is Evident Soon after Antipsychotic Initiation

Scott B. Teasdale [1,2], Philip B. Ward [2,3]*, Rebecca Jarman [1], Tammy Wade [1], Elisa Rossimel [1], Jackie Curtis [1,2], Julia Lappin [2], Andrew Watkins [1,4] and Katherine Samaras [5,6,7]

[1] Keeping the Body in Mind Program, South Eastern Sydney Local Health District, Sydney, NSW, Australia, [2] School of Psychiatry, UNSW Sydney, Sydney, NSW, Australia, [3] Schizophrenia Research Unit, South Western Sydney Local Health District, Ingham Institute for Applied Medical Research, Liverpool, NSW, Australia, [4] Faculty of Health, University of Technology Sydney, Ultimo, NSW, Australia, [5] Department of Endocrinology, St Vincent's Hospital, Sydney, NSW, Australia, [6] Diabetes and Metabolism Division, Garvan Institute of Medical Research, Sydney, NSW, Australia, [7] St Vincent's Clinical School, UNSW Sydney, Sydney, NSW, Australia

*Correspondence:
Philip B. Ward
p.ward@unsw.edu.au

Introduction: Antipsychotic medication (APM) initiation is associated with rapid and substantial weight-gain and high rates of obesity. Obesity leads to premature onset of cardiometabolic diseases and contributes to the 15–20 year shortfall in life expectancy in those experiencing severe mental illness. Dietary energy intake excess is critical to weight management but is yet to be quantified in youth with first episode psychosis (FEP) receiving APM. This study aimed to describe the degree of energy overconsumption and the food sources contributing to this in youth with FEP.

Materials and Methods: People aged 15–30 years with FEP receiving APM completed diet histories through qualified dietitians to assess energy imbalance and food sources. Outcome measures were: (i) energy balance; and (ii) intake of core and discretionary foods.

Results: Participants ($n = 93$) were aged 15–29 years (mean $= 21.4 \pm 2.9$ years) and exposed to APMs for a median for 8 months (Interquartile Range (IQR) 11 months). Energy balance was exceeded by 26%, by a median 1,837 kJ per day (IQR 5,365 kJ). APM polypharmacy and olanzapine were linked to larger excesses in dietary energy intake. The greatest contributors to energy intake were refined grain foods (33%) and discretionary foods (31%).

Conclusion: Young people with FEP receiving APMs appear to have markedly excessive energy consumption, likely contributing to rapid weight-gain, and thereby seeding future poor physical health. Larger, prospective studies are needed to gain a greater understanding of dietary intake, and its effects on health, in people with FEP.

Keywords: weight gain, psychosis, antipsychotics, early intervention, diet

INTRODUCTION

People receiving antipsychotic medication (APM) for first-episode of psychosis (FEP) experience rapid, excessive weight gain and acquire risk factors for cardiometabolic disease (1, 2). Weight-gain is most rapid in the first few months of APM treatment, and accompanied by central obesity (3). Longitudinal data shows that mean weight gain is 12 kg over the first 2 years of APM treatment, increasing to a mean 19 kg over the first 4 years (4). The higher rates of abdominal obesity (OR 4.43), hypertriglyceridemia (OR 2.73), metabolic syndrome (OR 2.35), low HDL (OR 2.35), diabetes (OR 1.99), and hypertension (OR 1.36) compared to controls (5), culminates in a 20-year life expectancy gap compared to the general population (6, 7). Each of these drivers ill health are preventable lifestyle factors relating to dietary intake.

A recent prospective study followed people from their first episode of psychosis, and found that after 20 years, 62% of people with schizophrenia and 50% of people with bipolar disorder were obese, substantially higher than national averages (8). Interestingly, those with SCZ gained significantly more weight in the first 10 years compared to the subsequent 10 years, whereas those with bipolar disorder gained less weight in the first 10 years compared to years 10–20. Critically, this study monitored weight change for 20 years, significantly longer than other prospective studies, and showed for the first time that weight gain may not being to plateau until between 10 and 20 years post first hospitalization. The authors also suggested that participants could continue to gain weight, even after the 20-year observation period.

Appropriate dietary energy intake is fundamental to weight stability, management of weight excess, and managing cardiometabolic risk. It is yet to be explored, however, in people with FEP. APM are associated with increased appetite (9), unhealthy dietary intake (10), disordered eating behaviors (11) and sedentary behavior (reduced energy expenditure) (12), however mechanisms are not clearly understood. Dopamine, serotonin, muscarinic, and histamine receptors have all been implicated in APM-induced hunger changes, with APM with a high affinity for the $5-HT_{2C}$ and muscarinic receptors associated with the greatest risk for weight-gain (13). Evidence also suggests weight-gain mechanisms innate to the psychiatric illness, such as brain structural damages (14). The eating process in those experiencing psychosis is made difficult due to impaired executive functioning, which complicates restrained eating and facilitates disinhibition (15). It appears that both drug-naïve and those receiving APM treatment have insensitive rewards systems shifting the preference to less nutritious foods high in sugar, salt, and fat (14).

Whilst APM-induced changes in appetite, weight and obesity have been well-documented, the energy intakes, food preferences and dietary quality of youth with FEP receiving APM have yet to be clearly quantitated. Limited published data highlight unhealthy dietary habits in severe mental illness (10), with diets lower in fruit and fiber, and higher intake of sweet foods and drinks compared to the general population. Much remains to be delineated, including quantitation of energy excess, dietary quality, and shortfalls to national dietary guidelines.

In addition to energy consumption, diet quality also importantly contributes to health. Quality is inferred from the inclusion of essential fatty acids, protein, vitamins, minerals, and fiber, typically found in "core food groups" such as vegetables, fruit, wholegrains, milk, cheese, and yogurt, and protein-rich foods (meat, poultry, seafood, eggs, nuts, and legumes). On the other hand, "discretionary foods" are low- or non- nutritious foods typically found in "Westernized" diets, which are generally high in added sugars, salt and/or fat, and are identified risk factors for poor cardiometabolic health (16).

Understanding these food choices and preferences is fundamental to the development of dietary strategies to reverse and/or prevent APM-induced obesity in youth with psychosis. To the authors' knowledge no study has yet examined energy intake relative to individual energy requirement in order to estimate energy excess, in the early stage of APM-treatment when weight gain occurs most rapidly. Further, comparisons of diet quality against national standards are lacking.

AIMS OF THE STUDY

In youth with FEP receiving APM, this study aimed to (i) quantify energy intake against energy requirements to determine the degree of energy intake imbalance, and (ii) examine diet quality, compared to Australian national dietary recommendations.

METHODS

Design

We undertook a cross-sectional analysis of dietary intake in youth experiencing FEP. Inclusion criteria were: (i) 15–30 years of age, (ii) within 2 years of first onset of psychotic symptoms, and (iii) receiving APM. Exclusion criteria were having received dietary education and/or intervention since commencing APM. The treating psychiatrists provided data on psychotropic medications and Diagnostic and Statistical Manual for Mental Disorders (DSM-V) diagnoses (17). This study received ethical approval from the South Eastern Sydney Local Health District Human Research Ethics Committee (HREC ref no: 14/276; LNR/14/POWH/614). This study was reported using the Strengthening the Reporting of Observational Studies in Epidemiology–Nutritional Epidemiology (STROBE-nut) guidelines (18).

Participants/Setting

Participants were patients who were referred, as part of routine care, to the *Keeping the Body in Mind* program between January 2015 and December 2017, from three allied community youth mental health services in urban Sydney. *Keeping the Body in Mind* is a lifestyle program involving a dietitian, exercise physiologist, and mental health nurse consultant, targeting the physical health of people with mental illness. On referral to the program, dietary intake was assessed by a dietitian using a comprehensive diet history (19), accounting for usual intake and variation. A food checklist was included to ensure all food categories were evaluated. Portion size was estimated using food models and measuring cups. The frequency of various foods was evaluated, including the typical composition of meals (20). Individual diet histories were completed in a private consulting room, over 30–60 min. This dietary assessment formed part of a broader cardiometabolic lifestyle assessment (21), including anthropometric and physical activity measures and was conducted prior to the delivery of *Keeping the Body in Mind* intervention (22).

Outcome Measures

Estimated energy intake (EEI) was derived from kilojoule values assigned to food groups described in the Australian Guide to Healthy Eating (AGHE) (23). To determine energy balance, estimated energy requirement (EER) was calculated for each participant using the Schofield equation (24), adjusting for physical activity level (sedentary 1.3–1.4x BMR, light-moderate 1.5–1.6x BMR, active 1.7–1.8x BMR) (25) and using adjusted ideal body weight for participants with a body mass index (BMI) $\geq$25 kg/m^2 (see **Supplementary Material 1**) (26). Using Goldberg et al. cut-off limit for plausible intake, participants were considered to be underreporting if the EEI:BMR ratio was <0.9 (27).

Diet quality was measured by estimating serves of core food groups: (i) vegetables (separately for starch and non-starch vegetables), (ii) fruit, (iii) milk, cheese, yogurt, and alternatives, (iv) grain foods, (v) protein foods such as meat, poultry, fish, eggs, nuts and seeds, and (vi) discretionary foods as defined in the AGHE (23). These estimated intakes of food group servings were compared to the recommended serves, based on age and sex, also defined in the AGHE (23). Grain foods were further categorized into mostly wholegrain ($\geq$50% wholegrain products) or refined (<50% wholegrain products).

Weight (kg) was measured with participants barefoot in light street clothing. Height (m) was measured using a stadiometer with participants barefoot. Body mass index (BMI) was calculated using weight/ height x height, kg/m^2. Waist circumference (cm) was measured horizontally at the navel using a measuring tape to the nearest 0.1 cm. BMI was categorized using the World Health Organization classification (28). Central obesity was categorized using waist circumference and the International Diabetes Federation classification (29).

Statistical Analyses

We compared (i) estimated energy intake and recommended energy intakes, and (ii) estimated food group intake and recommended food group intakes. The Shapiro-Wilk test was run as a test of normality. Paired sample and/or independent samples t-tests were run to test for significance between variables for normally distributed data, and reported as mean and standard deviation. The Wilcoxon Signed Ranks Test was used to test for statistical significance for non-normally distributed data. Non-normally distributed data were reported as median and range. Chi-squared tests examined the weight and waist circumference status of participants. Kruskal-Wallis Tests with Pairwise Comparisons were used for subgroup analyses of excess energy intake by diagnosis and APM prescription. A

Spearman's Rho correlation was run between excess energy intake and: (i) chlorpromazine equivalents, and (ii) duration of APM treatment. Statistical significance was set at $p < 0.05$. A Bonferroni correction was incorporated for t-test comparisons across multiple food groups, with a new statistical significance level set at $p < 0.007$. Analyses were performed using SPSS Version 24 (Chicago, IL, United States).

RESULTS

There were 93 participants (58 males, 62%), mean age 21.4 $\pm$ 2.9 years. Participants were predominantly Europids ($n = 52$, 56%) and, in decreasing frequency, Asian ($n = 27$, 29%), Maori/Pacific Islander ($n = 6$, 7%), Aboriginal/Torres Strait Islander ($n = 3$, 3%), Middle Eastern ($n = 3$, 3%), South American ($n = 1$, 1%), and African ($n = 1$, 1%). DSM-V diagnoses were: schizophrenia ($n = 32$), bipolar affective disorder ($n = 16$), psychosis not otherwise specified ($n = 15$), major depressive disorder with psychosis ($n = 10$), schizoaffective disorder ($n = 10$), substance-induced psychosis ($n = 4$), schizophreniform disorder ($n = 2$), delusional disorder ($n = 1$), organic psychosis ($n = 1$), brief reactive psychosis ($n = 1$), and psychosis due to another medical condition ($n = 1$). Demographic, diagnostic and medication data are provided in **Table 1**.

The majority of participants received APM monotherapy ($n = 81$, 88%): risperidone ($n = 28$), aripiprazole ($n = 19$), olanzapine ($n = 16$), quetiapine ($n = 8$), paliperidone ($n = 4$), clozapine ($n = 3$), amisulpride ($n = 2$), ziprasidone ($n = 2$). Eleven participants were prescribed dual APM: aripiprazole with olanzapine ($n = 5$), risperidone ($n = 1$), or quetiapine ($n = 2$); clozapine with amisulpride ($n = 1$), aripiprazole and quetiapine ($n = 1$); and quetiapine with paliperidone ($n = 1$). Mean dosage prescribed was 242 $\pm$ 186 mg chlorpromazine equivalents. Median APM exposure was 8 months (IQR 7 months). A range of mood stabilizer, antidepressant and benzodiazepine medications were also prescribed to some participants.

The mean BMI was 25.7 $\pm$ 5.0 kg/m^2 (males: 26.1 $\pm$ 4.4 kg/m$^{2;}$ females 24.9 $\pm$ 5.7 kg/m^2). Forty three participants had healthy BMI (48%), with large proportions overweight ($n = 31$, 33%) or obese ($n = 16$, 17%). One participant was underweight. Males (60%) were more frequently overweight or obese compared to females (34%), ($X^2 = 5.9$, $p = 0.01$). The percent of females with central obesity was numerically higher than for males ($n = 22$, 63% vs. $n = 30$, 52%), but this difference was not statistically significant, $X^2 = 1.1$, $p = 0.2$).

All participants met Goldberg's criteria for plausible energy intake reporting. Estimated energy intake (EEI) was significantly and substantively higher than estimated energy requirements (EER) ($Z = -5.1$, $P < 0.001$), with a median energy intake excess of 1,837 kJ per day (IQR 5,365 kJ). Median energy intake excess for males was 1,771 kJ per day (IQR 5,355 kJ), and for females 1,837 kJ per day (IQR 5,196 kJ) (**Table 2**). There was a significant difference for mean excess energy between different APM ($H = 15.7$, $p < 0.05$). Excess energy consumption was significantly higher in those prescribed APM polypharmacy when compared to those prescribed amisulpride ($p < 0.01$)

TABLE 1 | Demographic and clinical measures in young people with first episode psychosis.

		Males(n = 58)	Females (n = 35)	Total(n = 93)
DEMOGRAPHIC				
Age	mean (SD)	21.5 (2.8)	21.2 (3.2)	21.4 (2.9)
Ethnicity	n (%)			
Europid		37 (64)	15 (42)	52 (56)
Asian		13 (21)	14 (40)	27 (29)
Maori/Pacific Islander		5 (9)	1 (3)	6 (7)
Aboriginal/Torres Strait Islander		1 (2)	2 (6)	3 (3)
Middle Eastern		1 (2)	2 (6)	3 (3)
African		0 (0)	1 (3)	1 (1)
South American		1 (2)	0 (0)	1 (1)
PHYSICAL ACTIVITY LEVEL				
Sedentary		36 (62)	24 (68)	60 (64)
Light-Moderate		14 (24)	10 (29)	24 (26)
Active		8 (14)	1 (3)	9 (10)
ANTHROPOMETRIC MEASURES				
Weight	kg (SD)	82.4 (15.4)	66.8 (16.2)	76.5 (17.4)
BMI	kg/m^2 (SD)	26.1 (4.4)	24.9 (5.7)	25.7 (5.0)
BMI classification	n (%)			
Underweight (<18.5 kg/m^2)		1 (2)	0 (0)	1 (1)
Ideal weight (18.5–24.9 kg/m^2)		22 (38)	23 (66)	45 (49)
Overweight (25–29.9 kg/m^2)		27 (46)	4 (11)	31 (33)
Obese (≥30.0 kg/m^2)		8 (14)	8 (23)	16 (17)
Waist circumference	cm (SD)	93.7 (12.6)	86.7 (12.8)	91.0 (13.0)
Waist circumference classification	n (%)			
Ideal		28 (48)	13 (37)	41 (44)
Increased risk		30 (52)	22 (63)	52 (56)
DSM-V Diagnosis	n (%)			
Schizophrenia		25 (43)	7 (20)	32 (34)
Schizoaffective disorder		5 (8)	5 (14)	10 (11)
Schizophreniform disorder		0 (0)	2 (6)	2 (2)
Bipolar affective disorder		9 (16)	7 (20)	16 (17)
Substance-induced psychosis		3 (5)	1 (3)	4 (5)
Psychosis not otherwise specified		6 (10)	9 (25)	15 (16)
Major depression with psychosis		9 (16)	1 (3)	10 (11)

(Continued)

TABLE 1 | Continued

		Males(n = 58)	Females (n = 35)	Total(n = 93)
Delusion disorder		0 (0)	1 (3)	1 (1)
Organic psychosis		1 (2)	0 (0)	1 (1)
Brief reactive psychosis		0 (0)	1 (3)	1 (1)
Psychosis due to another medical Condition		0 (0)	1 (3)	1 (1)
PSYCHOTROPIC MEDICATIONS				
Antipsychotic	n (%)			
Risperidone		18 (31)	10 (29)	28 (30)
Aripiprazole		12 (21)	9 (26)	19 (20)
Quetiapine		4 (7)	4 (11)	8 (9)
Olanzapine		11 (19)	5 (14)	16 (17)
Clozapine		3 (5)	0 (0)	3 (3)
Amisulpride		1 (2)	1 (3)	2 (2)
Ziprasidone		1 (2)	1 (3)	2 (2)
Paliperidone		2 (3)	2 (6)	4 (4)
Antipsychotic polypharmacy		6 (10)	5 (14)	11 (12)
Chlorpromazine equivalent	mg (SD)	261 (208)	209 (138)	242 (186)
Duration of antipsychotic (months)	median (IQR)	8.7 (7.5)	7.0 (5.7)	8.1 (6.9)
Antidepressant	n (%)			
Yes		15 (26)	12 (34)	27 (29)
Mood stabilizer				
Yes		15 (26)	5 (14)	20 (22)
Benzodiazepine				
Yes		4 (7)	1 (3)	5 (5)
ADDITIONAL MEDICATION				
Metformin		1 (2)	1 (3)	2 (2)

and those prescribed risperidone ($p < 0.05$); those prescribed olanzapine reported significantly higher excess energy intake when compared to amisulpride ($p < 0.01$), risperidone ($p = 0.02$) and aripiprazole ($p = 0.04$). There was no relationship between medication dosage (chlorpromazine equivalents), or duration of treatment with APM, and excess energy intake in this sample ($r = -0.004$, $p = 0.97$; $r = 0.02$, $p = 0.85$). There was no significant difference between those prescribed: one APM only, APM polypharmacy, APM and mood stabilizer, APM and antidepressant, or APM, mood stabilizer and antidepressant ($X^2 = 3.8, p = 0.44$). There was no significant difference between all diagnoses within this sample ($H = 2.3$, $p = 0.81$), or major subgroups: (i) schizophrenia spectrum, (ii) bipolar affective and (iii) major depression with psychosis ($H = 0.6, p = 0.90$).

The sources of energy intake were, in descending order of magnitude: grain foods (33%); discretionary foods (31%); protein-rich foods (17%); added unsaturated fats and oils including spreads (6%); dairy (milk, cheese and yogurt) (6%); fruit (4%); and vegetables (3%). Mean daily serves of food groups

TABLE 2 | Energy intake in young people with first episode psychosis.

	Mean energy intake kJ/day (SD)	Mean energy requirement kJ/day (SD)	Median difference kJ/day (IQR)	Wilcoxon signed ranks test
GROUP				
Male	13,651 (4,517)	11,167 (1,320)	1,771 (5,355)	$Z=-3.6$, $p < 0.001$
Female	11,513 (4,326)	8,479 (1,132)	1,837 (5,196)	$Z=-3.8$, $p < 0.001$
Total	12,846 (4,544)	10,155 (1,808)	1,837 (5,365)	$Z=-5.1$, $p < 0.001$

were: grain foods 7.2 ± 3.7, discretionary foods 6.6 ± 5.8, protein foods 3.7 ± 2.2, dairy foods 1.7 ± 1.4, fruit 1.7 ± 1.8, and vegetables 2.8 ± 1.8 (**Table 3**).

Reported intakes were compared to Australian national dietary recommendations. There was a significantly higher than recommended intake of discretionary [$t_{(92)} = 6.4$, $p < 0.001$]. In contrast, there were shortfalls in recommended intakes of vegetables [$t_{(92)} = -13.4$, $p < 0.001$], dairy [$t_{(92)} = -6.5$, $p < 0.001$], and unsaturated oils/spreads [$t_{(34)} = -14.9$, $p < 0.001$]. The majority of participants consumed grain-containing foods as refined/processed products (81%); only 19% consumed predominantly wholegrain products. The majority of participants had shortfalls in the recommended intakes of vegetables (86%), dairy (73%), and fruit (61%). The recommended intake of discretionary food intake was exceeded in 72% of participants.

DISCUSSION

To our knowledge, this is the first study to demonstrate that youth with severe mental illness receiving APM and other psychotropic medications have energy intakes that exceed individual requirements by some 26% on average. Further, excessive intakes of discretionary foods and refined grain-based foods were evident, along with insufficient intakes of vegetables, dairy and fruit. In combination with the sedentariness already documented in people with psychosis (12), this excessive energy intake is likely to contribute substantially to the rapid and excessive weight-gain observed in the years after APM initiation. The weight change dynamics paradigm of Hall and co-workers' (30) predicts that every 100 kJ (24 kcal) intake excess will have an eventual bodyweight change of 1 kg, with half this weight change occurring within 1 year, and 95% weight change occurring within 3 years. Applying this model to the excess daily energy intake of 1,837 kJ (439 kcal) found in our study an eventual bodyweight change of approximately 18 kg would be expected. This can help explain the mean 20 kg weight gain that has been observed in people receiving APM over the first 4 years of treatment (4).

Whilst increasing physical activity is important for reducing cardiovascular risk, and symptoms of depression and possibly psychosis (31, 32), increased physical activity alone is unlikely

to adequately address this excessive energy imbalance: the hypothetical 70 kg person would need to walk an additional 3.5 h at 4 km/h or run for 1 h at 10 km/h each day to expend the observed energy surplus (33). Therefore, reduction of energy intake will be essential for preventing or reducing the weight gain that follows APM initiation and their long-term use.

The higher excess in dietary energy intake found for both APM polypharmacy and olanzapine is congruent with the literature, with both of these having higher weight gain potential compared to other second-generation APM (34, 35). Treatment with a mood stabilizer and some antidepressant medications can result in weight-gain. Given that our inclusion criteria were young people with FEP receiving APM, with no restriction on additional psychotropic medication prescription, it was difficult to disentangle the effects of mood stabilizer and antidepressant medication on dietary intake. Larger studies, with set psychotropic medication criteria would allow greater exploration of the effects of mood stabilizer and antidepressant medications (with and without APM) on food and dietary energy intake. Our study did not find a relationship between APM dosage and excess dietary energy intake, although it is conceivable that higher APM dosage would be associated with greater appetite and therefore higher dietary energy intake. Larger, appropriately designed studies would be needed to confirm the effect that APM dosage has on dietary intake.

Study limitations include the following: First, the cross-sectional design means that prospective studies that measure dietary intake at multiple time points are needed to confirm these findings. Second, while the program aims to assess all young people with FEP attending local health district services, there is potential for more health conscious consumers to engage in a dietary assessment. Third, there would be value in including a matched comparison group of youth not receiving APMs. Ideally, the comparator group would comprise sociodemographically-matched youth with mental health disorders that do not require treatment with APMs, such as depression and/or anxiety. Though it is worthy to note that the reported energy intake was substantially higher for both males and females in this study compared to data from the general population aged 19–30 years (36); 13,651 vs. 11,004 kJ/day for males, and 11,513 vs. 7,863 kJ/day for women. This reinforces the effects that impairments in executive function/reward system and increased appetite have on energy intake in people with psychosis. Fourth, important covariables such as symptom level/functioning, economic status, education, marital status, and metabolic/cardiovascular comorbidities, were not able to be included in this analysis and should be considered for future studies. Fifth, we could not determine if the nutritional issues predated APM use. Dietary data in pre-medicated FEP are required, but there are significant pragmatic obstacles to collecting such data pre-treatment, due to the nature of untreated severe mental illness and compliance with nutritional assessment. Sixth, dietary intake was estimated using the diet history method, a subjective measure that could lead to selective underreporting. The gold-standard objective biomarkers and the doubly labeled water technique are expensive and intensive for both the

TABLE 3 | Description of dietary patterns in young people with first episode psychosis.

	Percent of energy intake	Recommended servings/day*		Mean intake servings/day (SD)		Statistical test **	Percent of participants meeting national nutrition recommendations [11].
		Male	Female	Male (n = 22)	Females (n = 13)		
FOOD GROUPS							
Grain foods	33	6	6	7.1 (3.8)	7.4 (3.8)	$t_{(92)} = 2.5, p = 0.013$	19% choosing predominantly wholegrain
Protein-based foods	17	3	2.5	4.0 (3.2)	3.2 (1.9)	$t_{(92)} = 2.8, p = 0.009$	
Dairy and alternatives	6	2.5	2.5	1.8 (1.5)	1.6 (1.2)	$t_{(92)} = -6.5, p < 0.001^{***}$	27%
Vegetables	3	6	5	2.6 (1.8)	3.3 (1.8)	$t_{(92)} = -13.4, p < 0.001^{***}$	14%
Fruit	4	2	2	1.8 (2.2)	1.5 (1.2)	$t_{(92)} = 1.6, p = 0.103$	39%
Oils/spreads	6	4	2	2.0 (1.3)	1.8 (1.5)	$t_{(92)} = -14.9, p < 0.001^{***}$	28%
Discretionary foods	31	0–3	0–2.5	7.6 (6.6)	4.8 (3.3)	$t_{(92)} = 6.4, p < 0.001^{***}$	27%

* Recommended serves per day including serving sizes are described in the Australian Guide to Healthy Eating [11].
** Mean intake of all participants compared to recommended serves/day.
*** Statistically significant after applying Bonferroni correction, with statistical significance set at $p < 0.007$.

researcher and participant, and therefore not feasible in all studies. Studies that include these objective measures would help confirm findings using subjective measures. The final limitation is the conservative model used to calculate discretionary food consumption; the benchmark was set at the upper limit recommended, which would generally be reserved for those with higher energy requirements. This may have underestimated discretionary food intake. The dietary methodology did not enable us to estimate intake of trans and saturated fats, and free sugars, particularly relevant given the high intakes of discretionary foods.

Comprehensive care of youth with severe mental illness should incorporate lifestyle interventions to ameliorate cardiometabolic risk factors. Weight-gain prevention interventions implemented after APM initiation have larger effect sizes, compared to weight-loss interventions in people with enduring severe mental illness (37). Recognition of rapid weight-gain and cardiometabolic health decline soon after APM-initiation, together with evidence that lifestyle interventions in early psychosis programs prevent such outcomes (22), underpin the Healthy Active Lives (HeAL) Declaration (38), that defines 5-year targets for key lifestyle factors contributing to poor cardiometabolic health in severe mental illness (www.iphys. org.au). These include specific dietitian-led interventions for weight management, which have been shown to be effective in severe mental illness (37). Further exploration is also needed for the use of adjunctive nutrients in people experiencing FEP as a potential method of improving symptoms and functioning (39).

While not explored in this study, it is important to note that people at ultra-high risk for psychosis and APM naïve people (with FEP also have high rates of cardiometabolic abnormalities

40). This may be explained, at least in part, by the impaired executive functioning and reward system complicating the eating process and increasing the preference for non-nutritious foods high in sugar, salt and fat (14). Further exploration of the effectiveness of weight-gain preventative measures in those at ultra-high risk for psychosis and APM naïve people with FEP are needed.

In summary, this cross-sectional study suggests excessive consumption of discretionary and processed foods and numerous shortfalls in essential quality requirements are likely contributing not only to rapid weight gain, but also to other longer-term health sequelae in people in the early stages of APM treatment. Addressing the energy intake excesses observed in people with FEP receiving APM may assist in preventing weight-gain in the early stages of APM treatment. Larger, prospective studies, measuring dietary intake at multiple time points would assist in providing a greater understanding of the dietary intake, and its effects on health, in people with FEP.

AUTHOR CONTRIBUTIONS

ST, PW, AW, JC, and KS conceived the study and sought ethical approval. ST, RJ, TW, and ER completed the assessments. JC and JL provided psychiatry input and confirmed diagnoses. ST, PW, and KS analyzed the data. ST led manuscript preparation. PW, JC, JL, and KS added scientific intellect. RJ, TW, ER, and AW assisted with clinically relevant components. All authors approved the final version of the manuscript.

ACKNOWLEDGMENTS

We acknowledge the *Keeping the Body in Mind* teams, as well as staff and clients of youth mental health programs across SESLHD for their assistance with this study.

REFERENCES

Correll CU, Robinson DG, Schooler NR, Brunette MF, Mueser KT, Rosenheck RA, et al. Cardiometabolic risk in patients with first-episode schizophrenia spectrum disorders: baseline results from the RAISE-ETP study. *JAMA Psychiatry* (2014) 71:1350–63. doi: 10.1001/jamapsychiatry.20 14.1314

Curtis J, Henry C, Watkins A, Newall H, Samaras K, Ward PB. Metabolic abnormalities in an early psychosis service: a retrospective, naturalistic cross-sectional study. *Earl Interv Psychiatry* (2011) 5:108–14. doi: 10.1111/j.1751-7893.2011.00262.x

Zhang Q, Deng C, Huang X-F. The role of ghrelin signalling in second-generation antipsychotic-induced weight gain. *Psychoneuroendocrinology* (2013) 38:2423–38. doi: 10.1016/j.psyneuen.2013.07.010

Álvarez-Jiménez M, González-Blanch C, Crespo-Facorro B, Hetrick S, Rodriguez-Sánchez JM, Pérez-Iglesias R, et al. Antipsychotic-induced weight gain in chronic and first-episode psychotic disorders. *CNS Drugs* (2008) 22:547–62. doi: 10.2165/00023210-200822070-00002

Vancampfort D, Wampers M, Mitchell AJ, Correll CU, Herdt A, Probst M, et al. A meta-analysis of cardio-metabolic abnormalities in drug naïve, first-episode and multi-episode patients with schizophrenia versus general population controls. *World Psychiatry* (2013) 12:240–50. doi: 10.1002/wps.20069

Brown S, Kim M, Mitchell C, Inskip H. Twenty-five year mortality of a community cohort with schizophrenia. *Br J Psychiatry* (2010) 196:116–21. doi: 10.1192/bjp.bp.109.067512

Newcomer JW. Antipsychotic medications: metabolic and cardiovascular risk. *J Clin Psychiatry* (2007) 68:8–13.

Strassnig M, Kotov R, Cornaccio D, Fochtmann L, Harvey PD, Bromet EJ. 20- year progression of BMI in a county-wide cohort of people with schizophrenia and bipolar disorder identified at their first episode of psychosis. *Bipolar Disord.* (2017) 19:336–43. doi: 10.1111/bdi.12505

Fountaine RJ, Taylor AE, Mancuso JP, Greenway FL, Byerley LO, Smith SR, et al. Increased food intake and energy expenditure following administration of olanzapine to healthy men. *Obesity* (2010) 18:1646–51. doi: 10.1038/oby.2010.6

Dipasquale S, Pariante CM, Dazzan P, Aguglia E, McGuire P, Mondelli V. The dietary pattern of patients with schizophrenia: a systematic review. *J Psychiatr Res.* (2013) 47:197–207. doi: 10.1016/j.jpsychires.2012.10.005

Kluge M, Schuld A, Himmerich H, Dalal M, Schacht A, Wehmeier PM, et al. Clozapine and olanzapine are associated with food craving and binge eating: Results from a randomized double-blind study. *J Clin Psychopharmacol.* (2007) 27:662–6. doi: 10.1097/jcp.0b013e31815a8872

Stubbs B, Williams J, Gaughran F, Craig T. How sedentary are people with psychosis? a systematic review and meta-analysis. *Schizophr Res.* (2016) 171:103–9. doi: 10.1016/j.schres.2016.01.034

Lett TAP, Wallace TJM, Chowdhury NI, Tiwari AK, Kennedy JL, Müller DJ. Pharmacogenetics of antipsychotic-induced weight gain: review and clinical implications. *Mol Psychiatry* (2012) 17:242–66. doi: 10.1038/mp.2011.109

Minichino A, Francesconi M, Salatino A, Delle Chiaie R, Cadenhead K. Investigating the link between drug-naive first episode psychoses (FEPs), weight gain abnormalities and brain structural damages: relevance and implications for therapy. *Prog Neuropsychopharmacol Biol Psychiatry* (2017) 77:9–22. doi: 10.1016/j.pnpbp.2017.03.020

Knolle-Veentjer S, Huth V, Ferstl R, Aldenhoff JB, Hinze-Selch D. Delay of gratification and executive performance in individuals with schizophrenia: Putative role for eating behavior and body weight regulation. *J Psychiatric Res.* (2008) 42:98–105. doi: 10.1016/j.jpsychires.2006.10.003

Bauer UE, Briss PA, Goodman RA, Bowman BA. Prevention of chronic disease in the 21st century: elimination of the leading preventable causes of premature death and disability in the USA. *Lancet* (2014) 384:45–52. doi: 10.1016/S0140-6736(14)60648-6

American Psychiatric Association. *Diagnostic and Statistical Manual of Mental Disorders (DSM-5)*. Washington DC: American Psychiatric Pub (2013).

Lachat C, Hawwash D, Ocké MC, Berg C, Forsum E, Hörnell A, et al. Strengthening the reporting of observational studies in epidemiology- nutritional epidemiology (STROBE-nut): An extension of the STROBE statement. *Nutr Bull.* (2016) 41:240–51. doi: 10.1371/journal.pmed.1002036

Burrows TL, Martin RJ, Collins CE. A systematic review of the validity of dietary assessment methods in children when compared with the method of doubly labeled water. *J Am Diet Assoc.* (2010) 110:1501–10. doi: 10.1016/j.jada.2010.07.008

Thompson FE, Subar AF. Dietary assessment methodology. In: Coulston ACB, editors. *Nutrition in the Prevention and Treatment of Disease.* 2nd edn. London: Elsevier (2008).

Curtis J, Newall HD, Samaras K. The heart of the matter: cardiometabolic care in youth with psychosis. *Earl Interv Psychiatry* (2012) 6:347–53. doi: 10.1111/j.1751-7893.2011.00315.x

Curtis J, Watkins A, Rosenbaum S, Teasdale S, Kalucy M, Samaras K, et al. Evaluating an individualized lifestyle and life skills intervention to prevent antipsychotic-induced weight gain in first-episode psychosis. *Earl Interv Psychiatry* (2016) 10:267–76. doi: 10.1111/eip.12230

National Health and Medical Research Council. *Australian Dietary Guidelines.* Canberra: NHMRC (2013). Available online from: http://www.eatforhealth.gov.au. Schofield WN. Predicting basal metabolic rate, new standards and review of previous work. *Hum Nutr Clin Nutr.* (1984) 39:5–41.

Black AE. Critical evaluation of energy intake using the Goldberg cut-off for energy intake: basal metabolic rate. A practical guide to its calculation, use and limitations. *Int J Obesity* (2000) 24:1119. doi: 10.1038/sj.ijo.0801376

Krenitsky J. Adjusted body weight, pro: evidence to support the use of adjusted body weight in calculating calorie requirements. *Nutr Clin Pract.* (2005) 20:468–73. doi: 10.1177/0115426505020004468

Goldberg G, Black A, Jebb S, Cole T, Murgatroyd P, Coward W, et al. Critical evaluation of energy intake data using fundamental principles of energy physiology: 1. Derivation of cut-off limits to identify under-recording. *Eur J Clin Nutr* (1991) 45:569–81.

World Health Organisation. *Global Database on Body Mass Index.* Geneva: WHO (2018) Available online at: https://www.who.int/gho/ncd/risk_factors/ bmi_text/en/

Alberti KGMM, Zimmet P, Shaw J. Metabolic syndrome - a new world-wide definition. A consensus statement from the international diabetes federation. *Diabet Med.* (2006) 23:469–80. doi: 10.1111/j.1464-5491.2006.01858.x

Hall KD, Sacks G, Chandramohan D, Chow CC, Wang YC, Gortmaker SL, et al. Quantification of the effect of energy imbalance on bodyweight. *Lancet* (2011) 378:826–37. doi: 10.1016/S0140-6736(11)60812-X

Rosenbaum S, Tiedemann A, Sherrington C, Curtis J, Ward PB. Physical activity interventions for people with mental illness: a systematic review and meta-analysis. *J Clin Psychiatry* (2014) 75:964–74. doi: 10.4088/JCP.13r08765

Firth J, Carney R, Elliott R, French P, Parker S, McIntyre R, et al. Exercise as an intervention for first-episode psychosis: a feasibility study. *Earl Interv Psychiatry* (2016) 12:307–15. doi: 10.1111/eip.12329

McArdle WD, Katch FI, Katch VL. Energy expenditure at rest and during physical activity. In: McArdle WD, Katch FI, Katch VL, editors. *Essentials of Exercise Physiology.* 5th edn. Philidelphia, PA: Wolters Kluwer (2016).

Rummel-Kluge C, Komossa K, Schwarz S, Hunger H, Schmid F, Lobos CA, et al. Head-to-head comparisons of metabolic side effects of second generation antipsychotics in the treatment of schizophrenia: a systematic review and meta-analysis. *Schizophr Res.* (2010) 123:225–33. doi: 10.1016/j.schres.2010.07.012

Maayan L, Correll CU. Weight gain and metabolic risks associated with antipsychotic medications in children and adolescents. *J Child Adolesc Psychopharmacol.* (2011) 21:517–35. doi: 10.1089/cap.2011.0015

Australian Bureua of Statistics (ABS). *Australian Health Survey: Nutrition First Results - Foods and Nutrients 2011-12.* Canberra: ABS (2014). Availableonlineat:http://www.abs.gov.au/ausstats/abs@.nsf/lookup/4364.0.55.007main$+$features12011-12

Teasdale SB, Ward PB, Rosenbaum S, Samaras K, Stubbs B. Solving a weighty problem: systematic review and meta-analysis of nutrition interventions in severe mental illness. *Br J Psychiatry* (2017) 210:110–8. doi: 10.1192/bjp.bp.115.177139

Shiers D, Curtis J. Cardiometabolic health in young people with psychosis. *Lancet Psychiatry* (2014) 1:492–4. doi: 10.1016/S2215-0366(14) 00072-8

Firth J, Rosenbaum S, Ward PB, Curtis J, Teasdale SB, Yung AR, et al. Adjunctive nutrients in first episode psychosis: a systematic review of efficacy, tolerability and neurobiological mechanisms. *Early Interv Psychiatry* (2018) 12:774–83. doi: 10.1111/eip.12544

Cadenhead KS, Minichino A, Kelsven S, Addington J, Bearden C, Cannon TD, et al. Metabolic abnormalities and low dietary Omega 3 are associated with symptom severity and worse functioning prior to the onset of psychosis:i findings from the North American Prodrome Longitudinal Studies Consortium. *Schizophr Res.* (2018) doi: 10.1016/j.schres.2018.09.022. [Epub ahead of print].

9

Comparing the Psychological Effects of Meditation- and Breathing-Focused Yoga Practice in Undergraduate Students

Xin Qi[1†], Jiajin Tong[2†], Senlin Chen[3†], Zhonghui He[1] and Xiangyi Zhu[2]*

[1] Department of Physical Education and Research, Peking University, Beijing, China, [2] Beijing Key Laboratory of Behavior and Mental Health, School of Psychological and Cognitive Sciences, Peking University, Beijing, China, [3] School of Kinesiology, Louisiana State University, Baton Rouge, LA, United states

Correspondence:
Zhonghui He
hezhh@pku.edu.cn

[†] These authors share first authorship

Objectives: The present study aimed to compare the psychological effects of meditation- and breathing-focused yoga practice in undergraduate students.

Methods: A 12-weeks yoga intervention was conducted among a group of undergraduate students enrolled in four yoga classes at an academically prestigious university in Beijing, China. Four classes were randomized to meditation-focused yoga or breathing-focused yoga. A total of 86 participants finished surveys before and after the 12-weeks intervention, measuring work intention, mindfulness, and perceived stress. The repeated-measure multivariate analysis of covariance (MANCOVA) followed by univariate analyses were conducted to examine the differences in work intention, mindfulness, and stress between the two yoga intervention groups over the semester, after controlling for age and gender.

Results: The repeated-measure MANCOVA revealed significant group differences with a median effect size [Wilks' lambda, $\Lambda = 0.90$, $F(3, 80) = 3.10$, $p = 0.031$, $\eta^2 = 0.104$]. Subsequent univariate analyses showed that students in the breathing-focused yoga group had significant higher work intentions [$F_{(1, 82)} = 5.22$; $p = 0.025$; $\eta^2_p = 0.060$] and mindfulness [$F_{(1, 82)} = 6.33$; $p = 0.014$; $\eta^2_p = 0.072$] but marginally lower stress [$F_{(1, 82)} = 4.20$; $p = 0.044$; $\eta^2_p = 0.049$] than students in the meditation-focused yoga group.

Conclusion: Yoga practice with a focus on breathing is more effective than that with a focus on meditation for undergraduates to retain energy for work, keep attention and awareness, and reduce stress.

Keywords: meditation, breathing, yoga, work intention, mindfulness, stress

INTRODUCTION

Yoga has different components including postures, movements, meditation, and breathing (pranayama) (Brown and Gerberg, 2005). The current literature has seen a general consensus of yoga's function in retaining energy and vitality (Bowden et al., 2012; Tyagi et al., 2016) and reducing stress (Riley and Park, 2015). However, little is known of the relative importance of specific components of yoga practices, especially between the most revisited practices of meditation and breathing. Prior research has shown that yoga postures and movements can reduce depression (Carter and Byrne, 2004), but meditation and breathing may be more important to other mental health outcomes including stress and mood (Wheeler et al., 2019), sustained attention (Schmalzl et al., 2018), working memory capacity (Quach et al., 2016) posttraumatic stress disorder, hyperarousal symptoms of sleep disturbance, flashbacks, or anger outbursts (Carter and Byrne, 2004). Moreover, there are evidences for potential differences between meditation and breathing in literature such as the levels of energy (Joshi and Telles, 2009; Zaccaro et al., 2018), attention, and practice difficulty (Brown and Gerbarg, 2009). Thus, the yoga practices of meditation and breathing may function differently in a group of novices with daily mental activities. Our findings may help disclose the nature of yoga components and provide unique guidance for novices with mental work in yoga practices.

Meditation refers to engagement of mental exercise to reach a heightened level of spiritual awareness (Clarke et al., 2018). Meditation is frequently reported to have significant impacts on biological and psychological outcomes. For example, Hendriks (2018) systematically reviewed 11 research studies to examine the effects of yoga meditation on mental health outcomes such as anxiety, depression, stress, and well-being. Meditation also has been studied as an independent practice beyond the scope of yoga such as Buddhist meditation, compassion meditation, mindfulness meditation, and sound meditation. For example, one study showed that meditation was associated with molecular changes in cerebral cortex, prefrontal area, autonomic nervous system, hormones, etc. (Jindal et al., 2013). Meditation is beneficial to cognitive outcomes (Chiesa et al., 2011) and can facilitate stress management (Borchardt and Zoccola, 2018). Specifically, traditional Buddhist meditation programs led to improvement in stress levels and mood (Shonin et al., 2014). Gallegos et al.'s (2017) and Hilton et al.'s (2017) meta-analysis found that mindfulness meditation alleviated the symptoms of posttraumatic stress. Wielgosz et al.'s (2019) review summarized the efficacious applications of mindfulness meditation to many specific domains of psychopathology. Philips et al. (2019) found that sound meditation was better than silence meditation to relax and reduce acute stress.

Breathing as a mental practice has received increasing research interest. During yoga exercise, an individual can practice different patterns of breathing and use specialized techniques to enhance breathing skills such as inhaling deeply into the abdomen, holding the breath at certain parts of the breathing cycle (Brown and Gerbarg, 2009), breathing at varying rates, such as *Sudarshan Kriya* yogic breathing (Brown and Gerbarg, 2005), and/or high-frequency yoga breathing (Joshi and Telles, 2009). Brandani et al.'s (2017) review of 13 studies showed that yoga breathing had a hypotensive effect. Joshi and Telles (2009) found that high-frequency yoga breathing improved selective attention and that breath awareness increased available neural resources by examining event-related potentials (i.e., the P300). Besides biological impacts, breathing, as an important component of yoga practice, can bring upon dramatic

psychological and mental benefits. For example, Telles et al. (2011) found that high-frequency yoga breathing significantly decreased the optical illusion, an indicator of improved attention and visual perception. Janakiramaiah et al. (1998) found that yoga breathing functioned as effectively as medical treatment for dysthymic disorder. Shastri et al. (2017) showed that yoga breathing reduced aggression, improved mindfulness, and emotion regulation in undergraduate students. Saoji et al. (2018) also found that yoga breathing enhanced psychological functions such as state mindfulness. Further, Tellhed et al. (2019) found mindfulness mediated the relationship between yoga breathing and mental health. Kizhakkeveettil et al. (2019) summarized that yoga breathing improved the quality of life in individuals with chronic disease by reducing stress, pain, anxiety, depression and fatigue, and improving sleep and emotion. Breathing, as an independent practice, was also found to impact on both autonomic and central nervous systems and psychological status such as increased comfort, vigor and alertness, and reduced symptoms of anxiety, anger, and confusion (Zaccaro et al., 2018).

As summarized above, both meditation and breathing have significant effects on biological and mental outcomes. Despite the usefulness of meditation and breathing, prior research suggests that they may function differently in influencing mental health outcomes such as energy (Joshi and Telles, 2009; Zaccaro et al., 2018) and attention (Brown and Gerbarg, 2009). First, breathing may be related to higher levels of energy, improved attention (Telles et al., 2011), increased available neural resources (Joshi and Telles, 2009), vigor and alertness (Zaccaro et al., 2018), while meditation is usually related to serenity (calmness of mind and body) and relaxation (Koopmann-Holm et al., 2013; Jones et al., 2018; Philips et al., 2019). The increased mental resources and alertness by breathing may stimulate active engagement and improve readiness for tasks, which coincides with work intention. Work intention refers to a guide to purposeful action as it is a mental representation of the behavior an employee chooses to manifest (Ajen and Fishbein, 1980). Intention to continue one's work reflects one's energy level at work, so breathing-focused yoga practice may retain higher levels of work intention than meditation-focused yoga practice. Second, while both meditation and breathing could help achieve mindfulness (Saoji et al., 2018; Wielgosz et al., 2019), breathing may be more practical in achieving mindfulness, a state of consciousness emphasizing attention and awareness in the present (Brown and Ryan, 2003). For example, "many people who try to learn meditation cannot focus their minds," "some find the practices difficult and austere...lack the patience to persist," and "trying to meditate while under severe stress sometimes magnifies the subjective sense of distress" (Brown and Gerbarg, 2009, p. 56). However, "one can affect the mind and consciousness through manipulation of the breath" (Brown and Gerbarg, 2009, p. 55). Thus, breathing-focused yoga practice may be more effective to improve mindfulness (i.e., attention and awareness) in a group of yoga novices. Since higher energy levels and mindfulness can help people decrease stress (Tong et al., 2020), breathing-focused yoga practice may be also better to reduce stress than meditation in a group of yoga novices.

Furthermore, a few researches have simultaneously compared the functions of meditation and breathing as yoga components (Ross et al., 2012). Only one study to our knowledge has compared between these yoga practices (Wheeler et al., 2019), which found that yoga manipulation (i.e., poses, breathing, meditation, or listening to a lecture about yoga) was equally effective in reducing anxiety and improving mood but did not affect responses to stressors in a group of yoga novices. This study utilized only a 20-min intervention, which is not a full yoga session and may be not enough to show any different effects of meditation and breathing. A longer intervention with multiple sessions over several weeks is needed to indicate any potential difference and show whether this difference can be retained.

Therefore, the current research aims to explore the potential differences between yoga practices of meditation and breathing in energy and stress-related outcomes in undergraduates, novices with daily mental activities. We hypothesize that breathing-focused yoga practice would be more effective than meditation-focused yoga to promote work intention (1a), and mindfulness (1b), and to reduce stress perception (1c). The varying effects of meditation and breathing may be evident in novice yoga exercisers such as undergraduate students; however, this assumption needs to be tested through empirical evidence. Most undergraduate students have little to no experience of practicing yoga exercise, and they are considered a vulnerable population for mental health (Balon et al., 2015). Engaging in considerable mental work daily, undergraduates would need to accumulate mental resources and alertness at work and to focus. Examining undergraduate students' work intention, mindfulness, and perceived stress, as a function of yoga practices (breathing- or meditation-focused), is important to their academic performance and mental health. We chose to study undergraduate students in this study also because prior yoga research has shown success in recruiting and retaining a relatively large sample of undergraduate students as participants (Shastri et al., 2017; Wheeler et al., 2019); thus we felt confident to recruit a sample of undergraduate students in this study.

MATERIALS AND METHODS

Experimental Design and Procedure

A 12-weeks yoga intervention was conducted among undergraduate students with no prior experience with yoga. Participants were assigned into two groups of meditation- and breathing-focused yoga practice, randomly by class. During the semester, students attended a morning yoga class per week for 12 consecutive weeks following the prescribed intervention. Participants were asked to dress in comfortable clothing and avoid a meal after getting up before attending the class. Baseline surveys were conducted before intervention, and post-training surveys were conducted after the 12th session. Surveys were requested to be finished before leaving the class.

Baseline and posttraining data on work intention, mindfulness, and perceived stress were collected. Age, gender, and other medication, health, and previous exercise information were collected at baseline. Surveys were delivered online by Wechat link or QR-code. It is a research design with a between-subject variable (meditation-focused group, breathing-focused group) and a within-subject variable (pre, post).

Participants

Undergraduate students ($N = 120$) from four yoga classes at an academically prestigious Chinese university completed a survey measuring their current work intention, mindfulness, and stress, both at the beginning and the end of one semester. There were 27–32 students in each class. Participants were invited by survey links and made decisions to participate in this study by their own. Students received course credit for their participation. Before data collection, the university's institutional review board approved the research protocol for human subjects.

Power analysis showed that the repeated ANOVA with within-between interaction needed a sample size of 90 at the power level of 0.80 ($\alpha = 0.05$ with effect size of 0.15 and correlation among repeated measures of 0.50). Survey invitations were delivered to 120 participants. Individuals who have regular practice of yoga or similar techniques in the previous year were excluded (Tong et al., 2020), and there were 101 valid data for pre-survey. The final sample, with matched pre- and post-intervention measures, included 86 students (with five males) aged between 19 and 23 $M = 20.79; SD = 1.00$). The attrition rate is 71.7%, and there is no significant difference on age or gender between the attrition and remained group. A total of 46 participants from two yoga classes were designated into the breathing-focused yoga group, while 40 participants from the other two yoga classes were designated into the meditation-focused yoga group. These two groups did not differ on demographic (i.e., age, gender) or pre-intervention measures (i.e., work intention, mindfulness, stress), based on -tests analyses.

Hatha Yoga Intervention Program

Usually, one-time breathing intervention lasts for 1–20 min Joshi and Telles, 2009; Telles et al., 2011; Saoji et al., 2018; Tellhed et al., 2019), and yoga exercise may be more effective when different parts function together. Thus, our study aimed to utilize a normal 80-min yoga session with a valid 10-min practice of meditation/breathing and compare the relative importance of meditation and breathing across 12 sessions of yoga practices. To conduct a fair comparison, the participants would be requested to breathe at a low rate similar to mediation, but breathing deeply into the abdomen, and pursue and develop awareness of in-and-out breathing (Brown and Gerbarg, 2009). Although meditation can be divided into two categories as focusing on mental processes or focusing on bodily processes (Hendriks, 2018), meditation-focused yoga practice in this study focused on the mental processes including focused attention, open monitoring, and visualization (Jindal et al., 2013).

(Participants performed 80 min of Hatha yoga exercise Riley and Park, 2015) in a morning yoga class per week for 12 weeks. Each class comprised of three main stages, including meditation or breathing (10 min, Stage 1), posture-holding exercise (60 min, Stage 2), and relaxation (10 min, Stage 3), as shown in **Table 1**. Students were directed to do meditations in the meditation-focused yoga group ("Please adjust

TABLE 1 | Hatha Yoga intervention program.

Stage (time)	Breathing-focused group	Meditation-focused group
1. Intervention (10 min)	Breathing: Participants were instructed to engage in slow and rhythmic breathing performed deeply into the abdomen and through the nostrils (Brown and Gerbarg, 2009), as indicated as initial breath regulation in Hatha yoga, focus attention on the breathing (Kabat-Zinn, 2003) and pursue and develop awareness of in-and-out breathing (Brown and Gerbarg, 2009)...."Please adjust your posture and close your eyes...Continue to breathe slowly and deeply...Observe breathing deep into your chest, into your abdomen...Feel the movement of diaphragm and abdomen wall and the extension of the spine...Visualize the breath moving up and down and in and out your body...Feel the temperature of our breath in and out...Feel the steady rhythm of smooth breathing..."	Mediation: Participants were instructed to engage in imagination of nice and vivid pictures in mind with voluntarily focused attention and non-reactive open monitoring of the contents of own experience (Jindal et al., 2013). "Please adjust your posture and close your eyes...Imagine some pictures you like...Gaze at the picture in details and keep focused...Draw back your attention when realizing you are distracted...Feel your inner calm state..."
2. Posture (60 min)	Posture-holding includes 10–12 postures after warm-up such as forward folding, bridge pose, cobra, bow, waist rotating, downward facing dog, cat stretch, warrior, triangle, tree. Practice 6–10 times for each posture. Stay in each posture for 30–60 s.	
3. Relaxation (10 min)	Relaxation means to lie in tranquil, stop any physical and mental activities, and relax each part of the body. The instructor speaks out names of specific body parts to lead the scanning relaxation. Finally, the instructor describes one or two pictures with relaxation and calm.	

your posture and close your eyes...Imagine some pictures you like...Gaze at the picture in details and keep focused...Draw back your attention when realizing you get distracted...Feel your inner calm state...") while doing breathing in the breathing-focused yoga group ("Please adjust your posture and close your eyes...Keep breathing slowly and deeply...Observe your own breathing deep into your chest, into your abdomen...Feel the movement of diaphragm and abdomen wall and the extension of the spine...Visualizing the breath moving up and down and in and out your body...Feel the temperature of our breath in and out...Feel the steady rhythm of smooth breathing...") during Stage 1 for each class. Participants in the meditation-focused yoga group were instructed to engage in imagination of nice and vivid pictures in mind with voluntarily focused attention and non-reactive open monitoring of the contents of own experience (Jindal et al., 2013). Participants in the breathing-focused yoga group were instructed to engage in a slow and rhythmic breathing performed deeply into the abdomen and through the nostrils (Brown and Gerbarg, 2009), indicated as initial breath regulation in Hatha yoga, focus their own attention on the breath (Kabat-Zinn, 2003), and pursue and develop awareness of in-and-out breathing (Brown and Gerbarg, 2009).

The intervention plan was strictly followed in each session. The participants had full participation and involvement in each session of the yoga practices. The attendance rate for all sessions was 100%.

The Instructor

These interventions were provided by the same instructor using the same instructions and the same music across the two conditions each week. The instructor was the first author of this paper, who designed the schema for yoga intervention. She was a female tenured professor in the department of physical education with more than 13 years of experiences teaching and coaching yoga to undergraduate students. She was a senior fitness yoga trainer certified by the Federation of University Sports of China. She also held certification in instructing Yogi Yoga, a registered yoga school by Yoga Alliance USA. Additionally, her massive open online yoga course (MOOC) achieved the national

online open course certification from the National Department of Education, which is also listed in the global online course platform of Coursera and is selected by over 220,000 students.

Instrumentations
Demographic Survey

Participants were requested to fill in the blanks with their student ID and age. They were asked to choose the class they took and their gender.

Work Intention

Work intention was measured by six items in both pre- and post-training surveys. It was developed for this research according to the definition of work intention (Ajen and Fishbein, 1980). Participants were requested to rate on a seven-point scale ranging from 1 (very much unwilling) to 7 (very much willing) about their willingness to complete the survey. A sample item is phrased as "please indicate how much you want to continue completing the remaining survey right now." The reliabilities are αs = 0.97 and 0.98 for pre- and post-interventions, respectively.

Mindfulness

Mindfulness was measured by Brown and Ryan's (2003) 15-item Mindful Attention and Awareness Scale on a seven-point scale ranging from 1 (never) to 7 (always). Participants were requested to rate how frequently each situation occurs recently, rather than whether they generally agree. A sample item is stated as "It seems I am 'running on automatic' without much awareness of what I'm doing" (reverse scored). The reliabilities are αs = 0.86 and 0.91 for pre- and post-interventions, respectively.

Perceived Stress

Stress was measured by seven items adopted from the Depression Anxiety Stress Scale (Lovibond and Lovibond, 1995) on a seven-point scale ranging from 1 (never) to 7 (always). The instruction for administering this survey was the same with the mindfulness measure. It was used in previous yoga literature (Tong et al., 2020). Sample items include, "I found it difficult to relax" and "I tended to over-react to situations." The reliabilities are αs = 0.89 and 0.90 for pre- and post-interventions, respectively.

Data Analysis

We conducted a repeated-measure multivariate analysis of covariance (MANCOVA), followed by univariate analyses, to examine the differences between meditation-focused and breathing-focused yoga interventions over the semester, in terms of ratings of work intention, mindfulness, and stress. Many previous yoga researches focused on a designated group of age and sex (such as middle-aged women, adolescence, undergraduates, see Quach et al., 2016; Philips et al., 2019). Some research explored how age or sex were related to yoga practice effect (Savita, 2006; Cahn et al., 2017; Rojiani et al., 2017) and some controlled demographic variables in empirical studies (Fishbein et al., 2016; Cahn et al., 2017; Tong et al., 2020). Moreover, age and/or sex were found to be significantly related to outcomes of work motivation (Boumans et al., 2012), mindfulness (Edwards, 2019), and stress (Folkman et al., 1987). Thus, age and gender were included as covariates[1] in this model. Pre- and post-measures were analyzed as within-group variables, and the intervention type was the between-group variable.

RESULTS

Table 2 presents the descriptive statistical results for all research variables over time for each intervention group, and **Table 3** presents the correlation matrix. The intra-class correlations (ICCs) for all focal variables were small (ranging 0.01–0.03), indicating that there was none to minimal clustering effect and that the data observations for these focal constructs were independent despite class memberships.

The test of homogeneity of covariance matrices was not significant [Box's $M = 25.81$, $F_{(21, 24883)} = 1.13$, $p = 0.30$], indicating that the observed covariance matrices of the dependent variables were equal across groups. Results from the pre-post training MANCOVA revealed significant group differences with a median effect size [Wilks' lambda, $\Lambda = 0.90$, $F(3, 80) = 3.10$, $p = 0.031$, $\eta^2 = 0.104$]. Subsequently, significant group by time interaction effects were observed for work intention [$F_{(1, 82)} = 5.22$, $p = 0.025$, $\eta^2_p = 0.060$), mindfulness [$F_{(1, 82)} = 6.33$, $p = 0.014$, $\eta^2_p = 0.072$], and stress [$F_{(1, 82)} = 4.20$, $p = 0.044$, $\eta^2_p = 0.049$], respectively. To characterize the meaning of these interactions, marginal means of the models were estimated for each group at pre and post measures, as shown in **Figures 1–3**. Simple effect analyses showed that between-group differences emerged at post-intervention for work intention [$t(84) = 2.30$, $p = 0.024$], mindfulness [$t(84) = 2.00$, $p = 0.049$], and stress [$t(84) = -1.68$, $p = 0.096$]. Students in the breathing-focused group had significant higher work intentions and mindfulness but marginally lower stress than students in

[1] Since there were no age and gender differences between groups in this research, we also analyzed the data without any controls. Without controlling for age and gender, the MANOVA and ANOVAs results are very similar. Results from the pre-post training MANOVA revealed significant group differences with a median effect size (Wilks' lambda, $\Lambda = 0.91$, F(3.82) = 2.81, p = 0.045, $\eta^2 = 0.093$). Subsequently, group by time interaction effects were observed significant for work intention ($F_{1,84} = 4.74$, p = 0.032, $\eta^2_p = 0.053$), mindfulness (F $_{1,84} = 5.72$, p = 0.019, $\eta^2_p = 0.064$), and marginally for stress (F$_{1,84} = 3.81$, p = 0.054, $\eta^2_p = 0.043$), respectively.

TABLE 2 | Descriptive statistics for each group, mean (SD).

Variable	Breathing-focused group	Meditation-focused group
Age	20.63 (1.10)	20.98 (0.83)
Gender (% women)	95.65%	92.50%
N	46	40
Pre-intervention		
Work intention	4.48 (1.49)	4.36 (1.49)
Mindfulness	4.50 (0.89)	4.50 (0.91)
Stress	3.87 (1.26)	3.73 (1.33)
Post-intervention		
Work intention	4.36 (1.59)	3.56 (1.64)
Mindfulness	4.90 (1.04)	4.45 (1.04)
Stress	3.29 (1.21)	3.74 (1.26)

TABLE 3 | Correlations between research variables.

Variable	1	2	3	4	5	6	7	8	9
1 Intervention group	–								
2 Pre-work intention	−0.04	–							
3 Pre-mindfulness	0.001	0.15	–						
4 Pre-stress perception	−0.06	0.03	−0.56**	–					
5 Post-work intention	−0.24*	0.56**	0.15	0.02	–				
6 Post-mindfulness	−0.21*	0.07	0.59**	−0.32**	0.32**	–			
7 Post-stress perception	0.18	0.05	−0.42**	0.36**	−0.24*	−0.72**	–		
8 Age	0.17	0.02	−0.15	0.03	−0.01	−0.07	−0.04	–	
9 Sex	0.07	−0.29**	−0.03	0.01	−0.17	−0.06	0.06	−0.30**	–

$N = 86$. *$p < 0.05$, **$p < 0.01$.

the meditation-focused group. Examination of the change for each intervention group also supported the function of breathing-focused yoga intervention. Comparatively, the breathing-focused group had significant increase in mindfulness ($B_{breathing} = 0.42 \pm 0.13$, $p = 0.002$; $B_{meditation} = -0.07 \pm 0.14$, $p = 0.64$) and decrease in stress ($B_{breathing} = -0.61 \pm 0.21$, $p = 0.005$; $B_{meditation} = 0.04 \pm 0.23$, $p = 0.87$) over the semester. The meditation-focused group significantly decreased work intention ($B_{breathing} = -0.09 \pm 0.22$, $p = 0.66$; $B_{meditation} = -0.83 \pm 0.23$, $p = 0.001$).

DISCUSSION

The aim of this research was to compare the relative importance of meditation-focused and breathing-focused yoga practice in energy retention and related stress reduction in a group of undergraduate students. Major findings are: (1) Students in the breathing-focused yoga group reported significant increase in mindfulness and significant decrease in stress, while students in the meditation-focused yoga group reported significant decrease in work intention; (2) Students in the breathing-focused yoga

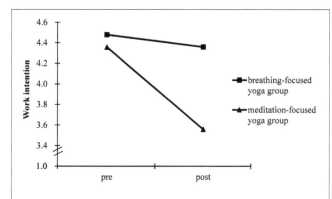

FIGURE 1 | Marginal means estimated for work intention before and after intervention by group.

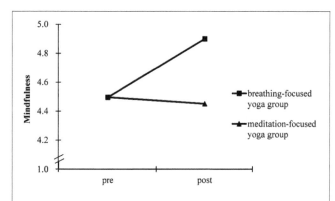

FIGURE 2 | Marginal means estimated for mindfulness before and after intervention by group.

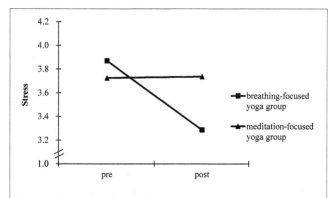

FIGURE 3 | Marginal means estimated for stress before and after intervention by group.

group had significant higher work intentions and mindfulness and had marginally less stress than students in the meditation-focused yoga group at post-intervention.

It was found that students in the meditation-focused yoga group reported significant decrease in work intention, while the breathing-focused group did not have any significant changes in terms of work intention. It may be due to the time for the post-training survey was in the end of a normal semester, and students were busy coping with the final exams. With much

resources invested into the final exams, students may have limited energy to spend in other tasks such as filling out a survey. It can be indicated as lower levels of purposeful action (Ajen and Fishbein, 1980).

We found that breathing-focused yoga practice is more effective than meditation-focused yoga practice in increasing mindfulness and reducing stress. It is different from previous no-difference findings (Wheeler et al., 2019). As discussed in the Introduction section, a 20-min intervention without a full yoga intervention (combined with postures) and without an intervention of multiple sessions may limit the function of breathing and meditation (Wheeler et al., 2019). Our findings are consistent with previous literature supporting that breathing directly increase oxygenation to strengthen the physical body (Brown and Gerbarg, 2005) and achieves energy and resources (Joshi and Telles, 2009; Telles et al., 2011; Zaccaro et al., 2018), while meditation achieves serenity and relaxation (Koopmann-Holm et al., 2013; Jones et al., 2018; Philips et al., 2019). When people more easily achieve energy and resources through breathing-focused yoga practice, they would not frequently feel stressed, compared to meditation-focused practice. Moreover, breathing may be more practical and is related to vigor and alertness (Zaccaro et al., 2018), while meditation may be not easily learned and practiced for undergraduates (Brown and Gerbarg, 2009). Thus, breathing may easily help undergraduates achieve better attention and awareness (i.e., mindfulness), which also leads to lower stress. Although our findings may be due to the relatively easily achieved benefits of yoga breathing and biological energy enhancement by better oxygenation, it may be also due to the difference between awareness of inner body and outer imagination. When people are inexperienced yoga practitioners, practice of mental attention on inner body may be easier to heighten the level of spiritual awareness than through outer imagination. However, all the mentioned benefits of mediation (Hendriks, 2018) may be achieved when people are experienced.

The present research contributes to the yoga literature by going further in disclosure the nature of important yoga components. It provided evidence showing the advantage of breathing-focused yoga over meditation-focused yoga practice in terms of energy retention, attention and awareness, and stress reduction, which confirms the value to direct a nuanced examination of separate yoga components. This stream of research would indicate the relative importance of yoga components and disclose the nature of these components. Practically, our findings would help novices find a quick and easy way to achieve benefits of yoga, as breathing is easier than meditation (Brown and Gerbarg, 2009). Practitioners can take into separate yoga components into detailed consideration when designing a new yoga program. For example, postures with more breathing and less meditation may be an effective yoga program for young and inexperienced people.

Besides the above strengths, there are some limitations. First, all the indicators were self-reported. The benefits of yoga components may be subjective rather than objective. Future research may use other ratings or biological indicators such as cortisol and event-related potentials (P300) to better support the function of individual yoga components. Since breathing regulation involves both biological techniques and mental awareness (Ramdev, 2005) and meditation involves both mental and bodily processes (Hendriks, 2018), the biological indicators may also help to examine detailed components of breathing and meditation. Second, meditation may be better conducted in older adults such as the working population with richer personal experience than undergraduate students. Future research needs to explore whether our findings can be generalized into other groups.

Another limitation of the study is with the measurement of work intention. Work intention is an indication of energy, which was hypothesized to be an important psychological benefit of yoga practice, especially of breathing-focused yoga practice. The measure showed sound internal consistency reliability in this current study. However, asking the participants to reference to an immediate cognitive task (i.e., completing the survey) as representation of work may not thoroughly capture undergraduate students' work or occupation in general, although completing the survey was the immediate task they were asked to perform. Future research may examine whether yoga would energize undergraduate students' work intention in other tasks (e.g., studying in a course, working for a part-time job, cramming for an exam).

Finally, lack of quality of delivery data should be recognized as an area of weakness for fidelity check in this study. Future research is encouraged to collect data about participants' effort and attentions.

CONCLUSION

Yoga breathing is an important component and can achieve better benefits than yoga mediation in undergraduate students. Designing a yoga program with combination of breathing and postures facilitates psychological resources and stress coping.

ETHICS STATEMENT

The studies involving human participants were reviewed and approved by the Committee for Protecting Human and Animal Subjects, School of Psychological and Cognitive Sciences, Peking University. The ethics committee waived the requirement of written informed consent for participation.

AUTHOR CONTRIBUTIONS

XQ, JT, ZH, and SC contributed to conception and design of the study. XQ conducted the experiment. JT, XZ, and SC analyzed the data. JT wrote the first draft of the manuscript. All authors contributed to manuscript revision and read and approved the submitted version.

REFERENCES

Ajen, I., and Fishbein, M. (1980). *Understanding Attitudes and Predicting Social Behavior*. Englewood Cliffs, NJ: Prentice-Hall.

Balon, R., Beresin, E. V., Coverdale, J. H., Louie, A. K., and Roberts, L. W. (2015). College mental health: a vulnerable population in an environment with systemic deficiencies. *Acad. Psychiatry*. 39, 495–497. doi: 10.1007/s40596-015-0390-1

Borchardt, A. R., and Zoccola, P. M. (2018). Recovery from stress: an experimental examination of focused attention meditation in novices. *J. Behav. Med.* 41, 836–849. doi: 10.1007/s10865-018-9932-9

Boumans, N. P. G., de Jong, A. H. J., and Janssen, S. M. (2012). Age-differences in work motivation and job satisfaction: the influence of age on the relationship between work characteristics and workers' outcomes. *Int. J. Aging Hum. Dev.* 73, 331–350. doi: 10.2190/ag.73.4.d

Bowden, D., Gaudry, C., An, S. C., and Gruzelier, J. (2012). A comparative randomised controlled trial of the effects of brain wave vibration training, iyengar yoga, and mindfulness on mood, well-being, and salivary cortisol. *Evid. Based Complement Alternat. Med.* 2012:234713. doi: 10.1155/2012/234713

Brandani, J. Z., Mizuno, J., Ciolac, E. G., and Monteiro, H. L. (2017). The hypotensive effect of Yoga's breathing exercises: a systematic review. *Complement Ther. Clin. Pract.* 28, 38–46. doi: 10.1016/j.ctcp.2017.05.002

Brown, K. W., and Ryan, R. M. (2003). The benefits of being present: mindfulness and its role in psychological well-being. *J. Pers. Soc. Psychol.* 84, 822–848. doi: 10.1037/0022-3514.84.4.822

Brown, R. P., and Gerbarg, P. L. (2005).). Sudarshan Kriya Yogic breathing in the treatment of stress, anxiety, and depression. Part II–clinical applications and guidelines. *J. Altern. Complement Med.* 11, 711–717. doi: 10.1089/acm.2005.11.711

Brown, R. P., and Gerbarg, P. L. (2009). Yoga breathing, meditation, and longevity. *Ann. N. Y. Acad. Sci.* 1172, 54–62. doi: 10.1111/j.1749-6632.2009.04394.x

Cahn, B. R., Goodman, M. S., Peterson, C. T., Maturi, R., and Mills, P. J. (2017). Yoga, meditation and mind-body health: increased BDNF, cortisol awakening response, and altered inflammatory marker expression after a 3-month yoga and meditation retreat. *Front. Hum. Neurosci.* 11:315. doi: 10.3389/fnhum.2017.00315

Carter, J., and Byrne, G. (2004). *A Two Year Study of the use of Yoga in a Series of Pilot Studies as an Adjunct to Ordinary Psychiatric Treatment in a Group of Vietnam War Veterans Suffering From Post Traumatic Stress Disorder*. Available at: https://www.Therapywithyoga.com (Accessed November 27, 2004).

Chiesa, A., Calati, R., and Serretti, A. (2011). Does mindfulness training improve cognitive abilities? A systematic review of neuropsychological findings. *Clin. Psychol. Rev.* 31, 449–464. doi: 10.1016/j.cpr.2010.11.003

Clarke, T. C., Barnes, P. M., Black, L. I., Stussman, B. J., and Nahin, R. L. (2018). Use of yoga, meditation, and chiropractors among U.S. adults aged 18 and over. *NCHS Data Brief.* 325, 1–8.

Edwards, D. J. (2019). Age, pain intensity, values-discrepancy, and mindfulness as predictors for mental health and cognitive fusion: hierarchical regressions with mediation analysis. *Front. Psychol.* 10:517. doi: 10.3389/fpsyg.2019.00517

Fishbein, D., Miller, S., Herman-Stahl, M., Williams, J., Lavery, B., Markovitz, L., et al. (2016). Behavioral and psychophysiological effects of a yoga intervention on high-risk adolescents: a randomized control trial. *J. Child. Fam. Stud.* 25, 518–529. doi: 10.1007/s10826-015-0231-6

Folkman, S., Lazarus, R. S., Pimley, S., and Novacek, J. (1987). Age differences in stress and coping processes. *Psychol. Aging* 2, 171–184. doi: 10.1037/0882-7974.2.2.171

Gallegos, A. M., Crean, H. F., Pigeon, W. R., and Heffner, K. L. (2017). Meditation and yoga for posttraumatic stress disorder: a meta-analytic review of randomized controlled trials. *Clin. Psychol. Rev.* 58, 115–124. doi: 10.1016/j.cpr.2017.10.004

Hendriks, T. (2018). The effects of Sahaja Yoga meditation on mental health: a systematic review. *J. Complement Integr. Med.* 15:20160163. doi: 10.1515/jcim-2016-0163

Hilton, L., Maher, A. R., Colaiaco, B., Apaydin, E., Sorbero, M. E., and Booth, M. (2017). Meditation for posttraumatic stress: systematic review and meta-analysis. *Psychol. Trauma* 9, 453–460. doi: 10.1037/tra0000180

Janakiramaiah, N., Gangadhar, B. N., Murthy, P., Harish, M. G., Shetty, K. T., and Subbakrishna, D. K. (1998). Therapeutic efficacy of sudarshan kriya yoga (sky) in dysthymic disorder. *Nimhans J.* 16, 21–28.

Jindal, V., Gupta, S., and Das, R. (2013). Molecular mechanisms of meditation. *Mol. Neurobiol.* 48, 808–811. doi: 10.1007/s12035-013-8468-9

Jones, D. R., Graham-Engeland, J. E., Smyth, J. M., and Lehman, B. J. (2018). Clarifying the associations between mindfulness meditation and emotion: daily high- and low-arousal emotions and emotional variability. *Appl. Psychol. Health Well Being* 10, 504–523. doi: 10.1111/aphw.12135

Joshi, M., and Telles, S. (2009). A nonrandomized non-naive comparative study of the effects of kapalabhati and breath awareness on event-related potentials in trained yoga practitioners. *J. Altern. Complement Med.* 15, 281–285. doi: 10.1089/acm.2008.0250

Kabat-Zinn, J. (2003). Mindfulness-based interventions in Context: past, present, and future. *Clin. Psychol. Sci. Pract.* 10, 144–156. doi: 10.1093/clipsy.bpg016

Kizhakkeveettil, A., Whedon, J., Schmalzl, L., and Hurwitz, E. L. (2019). Yoga for quality of life in individuals with chronic disease: a systematic review. *Altern. Ther. Health Med.* 25, 36–43.

Koopmann-Holm, B., Sze, J., Ochs, C., and Tsai, J. L. (2013). Buddhist-inspired meditation increases the value of calm. *Emotion* 13, 497–505. doi: 10.1037/a0031070

Lovibond, P. F., and Lovibond, S. H. (1995). The structure of negative emotional states: comparison of the depression anxiety stress scales (DASS) with the beck depression and anxiety inventories. *Behav. Res. Ther.* 33, 335–343. doi: 10.1016/0005-7967(94)00075-u

Philips, K. H., Brintz, C. E., Moss, K., and Gaylord, S. A. (2019). Didgeridoo sound meditation for stress reduction and mood enhancement in undergraduates: a randomized controlled trial. *Glob. Adv. Health Med.* 8, 1–10. doi: 10.1177/2164956119879367

Quach, D., Jastrowski Mano, K. E., and Alexander, K. (2016). A randomized controlled trial examining the effect of mindfulness meditation on working memory capacity in adolescents. *J. Adolesc. Health* 58, 489–496. doi: 10.1016/j.jadohealth.2015.09.024

Ramdev, S. (2005). *Pranayama: Its Philosophy and Practice.* Haridwar: Divya Prakashan.

Riley, K. E., and Park, C. L. (2015). How does yoga reduce stress? A systematic review of mechanisms of change and guide to future inquiry. *Health Psychol. Rev.* 9, 379–396. doi: 10.1080/17437199.2014.981778

Rojiani, R., Santoyo, J. F., Rahrig, H., Roth, H. D., and Britton, W. B. (2017). Women benefit more than men in response to college-based meditation training. *Front. Psychol.* 8:551. doi: 10.3389/fpsyg.2017.00551

Ross, A., Friedmann, E., Bevans, M., and Thomas, S. (2012). Frequency of yoga practice predicts health: results of a national survey of yoga practitioners. *Evid. Based Complement Altern. Med.* 2012:983258. doi: 10.1155/2012/983258

Saoji, A. A., Raghavendra, B. R., Madle, K., and Manjunath, N. K. (2018). Additional practice of yoga breathing with intermittent breath holding enhances psychological functions in yoga practitioners: a randomized controlled trial. *Explore* 14, 379–384. doi: 10.1016/j.explore.2018.02.005

Savita, R. K. (2006). *Comparehensive Training of Astang Yoga on Reaction Time and Selected Physiological Variables in Relation to Age and Sex of School Children.* Doctroal thesis, Lakshmibai National Institute of Physical Education, Gwalior.

Schmalzl, L., Powers, C., Zanesco, A. P., Yetz, N., Groessl, E. J., and Saron, C. D. (2018). The effect of movement-focused and breath-focused yoga practice on stress parameters and sustained attention: a randomized controlled pilot study. *Conscious Cogn.* 65, 109–125. doi: 10.1016/j.concog.2018.07.012

Shastri, V. V., Hankey, A., Sharma, B., and Patra, S. (2017). Investigation of yoga pranayama and vedic mathematics on mindfulness, aggression and emotion regulation. *Int. J. Yoga* 10, 138–144. doi: 10.4103/0973-6131.213470

Shonin, E., Van Gordon, W., and Griffiths, M. D. (2014). Meditation awareness training (MAT) for improved psychological well-being: a qualitative examination of participant experiences. *J. Relig. Health* 53, 849–863. doi: 10.1007/s10943-013-9679-0

Telles, S., Maharana, K., Balrana, B., and Balkrishna, A. (2011). Effects of high-frequency yoga breathing called kapalabhati compared with breath awareness on the degree of optical illusion perceived. *Percept. Mot. Skills* 112, 981–990. doi: 10.2466/02.20.22.PMS.112.3.981-990

Tellhed, U., Daukantaitë, D., Maddux, R. E., Svensson, T., and Melander, O. (2019). Yogic breathing and mindfulness as stress coping mediate positive health outcomes of yoga. *Mindfulness* 10, 2703–2715. doi: 10.1007/s12671-019-01225-4

Tong, J., Qi, X., He, Z., Chen, S., Pederson, S. J., Cooley, P. D., et al. (2020). The immediate and durable effects of yoga and physical fitness exercises on stress. *J. Am. Coll. Heath* 1–9. doi: 10.1080/07448481.2019.1705840

Tyagi, A., Cohen, M., Reece, J., Telles, S., and Jones, L. (2016). Heart rate variability, flow, mood and mental stress during yoga practices in yoga practitioners, non-yoga practitioners and people with metabolic syndrome. *Appl. Psychophysiol. Biofeedb.* 41, 381–393. doi: 10.1007/s10484-016-9340-2

Wheeler, E. A., Santoro, A. N., and Bembenek, A. F. (2019). Separating the "limbs" of yoga: limited effects on stress and mood. *J. Relig. Health* 58, 2277–2287. doi: 10.1007/s10943-017-0482-1

Wielgosz, J., Goldberg, S. B., Kral, T. R. A., Dunne, J. D., and Davidson, R. J. (2019). Mindfulness meditation and psychopathology. *Annu. Rev. Clin. Psychol.* 15, 285–316. doi: 10.1146/annurev-clinpsy-021815-093423

Zaccaro, A., Piarulli, A., Laurino, M., Garbella, E., Menicucci, D., Neri, B., et al. (2018). How breath-control can change your life: a systematic review on psycho-physiological correlates of slow breathing. *Front. Hum. Neurosci.* 12:353. doi: 10.3389/fnhum.2018.00353

10

Objectively Assessed Daily Steps—Not Light Intensity Physical Activity, Moderate-to-Vigorous Physical Activity and Sedentary Time—Is Associated with Cardiorespiratory Fitness in Patients with Schizophrenia

John A. Engh [1]*, Jens Egeland [1,2], Ole A. Andreassen [3,4], Gry Bang-Kittilsen [1], Therese T. Bigseth [1], Tom L. Holmen [1], Egil W. Martinsen [4], Jon Mordal [1] and Eivind Andersen [5]

[1] Division of Mental Health and Addiction, Vestfold Hospital Trust, Tønsberg, Norway, [2] Department of Psychology, University of Oslo, Oslo, Norway, [3] NORMENT, KG Jebsen Centre for Psychosis Research, Oslo, Norway, [4] Division of Mental Health and Addiction, Institute of Clinical Medicine, University of Oslo, Oslo, Norway, [5] Faculty of Humanities, Sports and Educational Science, University of South-Eastern Norway, Horten, Norway

*Correspondence:
John A. Engh
john.engh@medisin.uio.no

People with schizophrenia often have an unhealthy sedentary lifestyle with low level of physical activity and poor cardiorespiratory fitness—an important predictor of cardiovascular disease. We investigated the relations between cardiorespiratory fitness and both sedentary time and different aspects of physical activity, such as daily steps, light intensity physical activity, and moderate-to-vigorous physical activity. Using accelerometer as an objective measure of sedentary time and physical activity we estimated their relations to cardiorespiratory fitness in 62 patients with schizophrenia with roughly equal gender distribution, mean age of 36 and 15 years illness duration. We found a significant association between daily steps and cardiorespiratory fitness when accounting for gender, age, sedentary time, light intensity physical activity, and respiratory exchange ratio (maximal effort). Moderate-to-vigorous physical activity was not significantly associated with cardiorespiratory fitness. In conclusion, the amount of steps throughout the day contributes to cardiorespiratory fitness in people with schizophrenia, independently of light intensity physical activity and sedentary time. We did not find a significant relationship between moderate-to-vigorous physical activity and cardiorespiratory fitness. This may have implications for the choice of strategies when helping patients with schizophrenia improve their cardiorespiratory fitness.

Keywords: schizophrenia, lifestyle, cardiovascular disease, daily steps, physical activity, cardiorespiratory fitness, accelerometer, sedentary time

INTRODUCTION

People with schizophrenia are prone to overweight, diabetes and chronic metabolic disease (1) and often have a deleterious lifestyle, including low levels of moderate-to-vigorous physical activity (MVPA) and high levels of sedentary time (2). The average life expectancy is 15–20 years shorter than the general population, and cardiovascular disease (CVD) is the largest contributing factor to the increase in mortality (3). Low cardiorespiratory fitness (CRF) is a strong independent risk factor for all-cause mortality (4, 5) associated with low life expectancy and increased risk for CVD in the general population (4–6) and in schizophrenia (7, 8). Thus, knowledge on how to effectively improve CRF in schizophrenia is urgently needed. The beneficial effects of MVPA and the smaller effects of light intensity physical activity (PA) on CRF in the general population are well documented (9, 10). Less is known about the relations in people with schizophrenia. Another aspect of interest is the extent sedentary time influences CRF in the patient group. Sedentary time refers to the time spent for any duration or in any context in sedentary behaviors, defined as any waking behavior characterized by an energy expenditure equal to or less than 1.5 the resting metabolic rate while in a sitting, reclining or lying posture (11–13). Recent studies suggest that sedentary time is an important determinant of CRF levels, which is independent of physical activity (14, 15) A third aspect of interest is the total PA level. The number of daily steps have been associated with positive health effects in the general population (16) and in individuals with high cardiovascular risk (17). Studies on healthy overweight persons have indicated that reduced total daily PA causes reduction in CRF as well as worsening of other cardiometabolic health outcomes (18, 19). Increasing the total PA by walking (i.e., daily steps), as well as breaking the sedentary habit could be a path to improved CRF distinct from light intensity PA and MVPA (20, 21). It is not known whether the potential health effects facilitated by daily steps in people with schizophrenia are cumulative, increasing with the amount of total PA. The aim of the current study was to examine whether objectively assessed light intensity PA, MVPA, total daily steps, and sedentary time, exert *independent* influences on CRF in people with schizophrenia.

MATERIALS AND METHODS

Participants

Sixty-two patients were recruited from the main study Effects of physical activity in psychosis (EPHAPS) from August 2014 through September 2016 in catchment area-based and publicly funded outpatient psychiatric clinics in Vestfold County, Norway. A subgroup of the patients was referred from primary health care to the outpatient clinics for specific participation in the project. Patients diagnosed with schizophrenia spectrum disorder established using SCID I (22) who were aged 18–67 and understood and spoke a Scandinavian language were eligible for the study. Interviews were conducted by a clinical psychologist or a specialist in psychiatry. For further details on study design see Engh et al. (23) and on patient

TABLE 1 | Demographic and clinical characteristics, physical activity and sedentary time of the participants.

	N	Value	SD
Age (years), mean	62	36.3	13.7
Gender (women, %)	62	27 (43.5)	–
Duration illness (years)	61	14.9	12.2
Smokers (%)	62	40 (64.5)	–
Body mass index (kg*m^{-2})	62	29.2	5.7
PANSS positive subscale* (score range 7–42)	62	15.2	5.1
PANSS negative subscale* (score range 7–42)	61	17.9	7.0
PANSS total score* (score range 30–210)	61	65.3	17.5
Antipsychotic medication DDD**	62	1.7	0.9
Light intensity Physical activity (min/day^{-1})	62	216	92.4
Moderate/vigorous physical activity (min/day^{-1})	62	28.7	31.0
Steps/day (steps*day^{-1})	62	5685.0	3641.0
Sedentary time (h*day^{-1})	62	8.6	1.6
VO$_{2peak}$ (mL*kg^{-1}*min^{-1}), all participants	62	30.2	11.6
VO$_{2peak}$ (mL*kg^{-1}*min^{-1}), participants fulfilling maximal effort criteria***	52	31.5	11.8
VO$_{2peak}$ (mL*kg^{-1}*min^{-1}), participants not fulfilling maximal effort criteria****	10	33.9	7.7

*Data presented in % or mean. *PANSS, Positive and Negative Syndrome Scale; **DDD, defined daily dose, dose equivalence estimate based on total intake of antipsychotics per day; ***Respiratory exchange ratio≥ 1.00. ****Respiratory exchange ratio < 1.00.*

recruitment, study eligibility and data collection see Engh et al. (23) and Andersen et al. (24). All except one patient received antipsychotic treatment. Demographic and clinical characteristics are presented in **Table 1**.

Assessments

For further details on measurement of physical activity, sedentary time, and oxygen uptake see (24). PA and sedentary time was assessed using the ActiGraph GT3X+ (ActiGraph, LLC, Pensacola, FL, USA) worn over the left hip while awake for four consecutive days. Analyses were restricted to participants who wore the accelerometer for a minimum of 10 h per day for 2 days or more. To identify different intensities of PA, count thresholds corresponding to the energy cost of the given intensity were applied to the data set. Sedentary time was defined as all activity <100 counts per minute (CPM), a threshold that corresponds with sitting, reclining, or lying down (25). Light intensity PA was defined as 100–2019 CPM, moderate as 2020–5998 CPM, and vigorous as CPM $\geq$ 5999 (26). The amount of minutes per day at different intensities was based on summing the time where the activity count met the criteria for the specific intensity. Cardiorespiratory fitness (CRF) was operationalized as VO$_{2peak}$ measuring the highest oxygen uptake in a maximum exercise test on a treadmill (Woodway, Würzburg, Germany). Some individuals may fail to reach true VO$_{2max}$, and for the sake of conservative reporting, we therefore use the term VO$_{2peak}$ (mL*kg^{-1}*min^{-1}). We used a modified Balke protocol (27), where speed was held constant at 5 km·h^{-1} and the inclination angle was increased by one degree every minute until exhaustion within 6–12 min. Gas exchange was continuously sampled in a

TABLE 2 | Correlation coefficients between physical activity measures, sedentary time, and VO_{2peak}.

	Gender	Age	Light intensity physical activity	Moderate/vigorous physical activity	Steps/day	Sedentary time
Light intensity physical activity	0.11	0.18	–	–	–	–
Moderate/vigorous physical activity	−0.11	−0.35**	0.09	–	–	–
Steps/day	0.16	−0.25	0.45**	0.73**	–	–
Sedentary time	−0.09	0.01	−0.44**	−0.31*	0.42**	–
VO_{2peak}	−0.22	−0.64**	−0.002	0.28*	0.34**	0.02

*$p < 0.05$; **$p < 0.001$.

TABLE 3 | Regression analysis presenting explained variance in VO_{2peak}.

	R	R^2	Unstand-ardized coefficie-nt (B)	Standard error	Standar-dized coefficient (Beta)	t-value	Variance inflation factor (VIF)	P- value
Gender	−0.164	0.027	−3.914	2.270	−0.169	−1.724	1.068	0.090
Age	−0.510	0.260	−0.481	0.090	−0.568	−5.368	1.243	<0.001**
Light intensity physical activity	0.054	0.0008	0.008	0.015	0.067	0.569	1.535	0.572
Steps/day	0.206	0.042	11.747	5.404	0.262	2.174	1.615	0.034*
Sedentary time	0.134	0.018	0.018	0.013	0.156	1.412	1.346	0.163

$N = 62$ for all variables. All physical activity variables and sedentary time were assessed by accelerometer.
Partial correlation to VO_{2peak} (R), uniquely explained variance (R^2) by each of the predictors, unstandardized coefficients (B), standard error of the coefficients, standardized coefficients (Beta), t-values, variance inflation factors (VIF), and p-values are presented in the standard regression model. *$p < 0.05$; **$p < 0.001$.

mixing chamber every 30 s by breathing into a two-way breathing valve (2700 series, Hans Rudolph Inc., Kansas City, USA). The breathing valve was connected to a Jaeger Oxycon Pro used to analyze the oxygen and carbon content. Maximal effort was assessed by the respiratory exchange ratio (RER). Participants reached the criteria when RER ≥ 1.00. Participants' psychotropic drugs prescription was presented as defined daily dose (DDD) based on approved dose recommendations. DDD provides a rough estimate of participants' drugs consumption utilizing the assumed average maintenance dose per day for each specific drug used independent of dosage form for its main indication on adults (i.e., schizophrenia for antipsychotics). For example, the DDDs for chlorpromazine and risperidone are 300 mg and 5 mg respectively. DDD were calculated in accordance with guidelines from the World Health Organization Collaborating Center for Drug Statistics Methodology (http://www.whocc.no/atcdd). Information on smoking, illness duration and medication was obtained through interview and the use of hospital records. Weight was measured without shoes in light clothing by a SECA electronic scale to the nearest 0.5 kg. Height was measured without shoes with a transportable stadiometer and set to the nearest 0.5 cm.

Statistics

Variables that were not normally distributed (*steps/day; MVPA*) were log-transformed in the statistical analyses. Multiple regression analyses (all covariates entered concomitantly in the model) were employed to examine the relationships between independent variables and VO_{2peak}. VO_{2peak} was used to represent the outcome, cardiorespiratory fitness. Selection of variables in the regression model was based on Pearson

correlation tests between VO_{2peak}, measures of physical activity and sedentary time and other variables with assumed clinical importance. Correlation coefficients are shown in **Table 2**. Due to high correlation between the independent variables MVPA and steps/day ($r = 0.73$) two separate regression analyses were employed using each of these two independent variables and all other selected variables. The independent variable steps/day, and not MVPA, was included in the final regression model. When testing for multicollinearity correlations between independent variables were sufficiently low ($r < 0.70$) and the variation inflation factor fell within the criteria (VIF < 10). All statistical analyses were performed using IBM SPSS (Statistical Pack- age for the Social Sciences for Windows, version 24, IBM, Inc., Chicago, IL, USA).

RESULTS

As shown in **Table 3**, VO_{2peak} was significantly associated with gender, age and steps/day when all other covariates were controlled. Regression coefficients and standard errors can be found in the table. In a separate regression analysis encompassing MVPA in addition to the independent variables gender, age, light intensity PA and sedentary time, MVPA did not contribute to VO_{2peak}. Eighty-four percent of the participants obtained the criteria for RER. The main results were unaltered in a multiple regression analysis with participants attaining RER ≥ 1.00.

DISCUSSION

The main finding in the current study was that total daily steps was significantly associated with VO_{2peak}, independently of light intensity physical activity, the amount of time spent sedentary and maximal effort during testing of oxygen consumption. Moderate-to-vigorous physical activity was not significantly associated with VO_{2peak}. Our findings suggest that the amount of daily walking activity is of importance for patients with schizophrenia by contributing to the established health indicator VO_{2peak}. As a measure of the total physical activity daily steps differs from the measures of physical activity at defined levels of activity. VO_{2peak} may reflect the individual's participation in physical activity of different intensity. The influence of physical activity at specific intensity levels on VO_{2peak} has been focus of previous research. A meta-regression of moderators of physical activity showed that low VO_{2peak} was associated with low levels of moderate-to-vigorous physical activity (2). In a recent study of patients with psychosis using a 6 min-walking test as a proxy for CRF, both MVPA and total PA showed significant moderate positive correlations with CRF (28). The findings in the current study indicate that repeated or prolonged sequences of walking could have favorable health effects in schizophrenia. However, the current study investigating the relations between VO_{2peak} and physical activity at different intensity levels, sedentary behavior and daily steps in patients with schizophrenia needs to be replicated.

A comparison of studies using objective assessments of PA and sedentary behavior with studies based on self-reports suggests that people with schizophrenia underestimate the amount of sedentary time and overestimate the duration of their PA (2). The objective assessment of PA is a strength of the current study. A limitation is the cross sectional design without the opportunity to draw inferences concerning causal effects. The encouragement of repeated indoor, as well as outdoor physical activity, could be organized according to personal preference and implemented as part of treatment in community-based mental health care. In conclusion, the amount of steps throughout the day contributes to VO_{2peak} in people with schizophrenia, independently of light intensity physical activity and sedentary time. Moderate-to-vigorous physical activity was not significantly associated with VO_{2peak}. This may have implications for the choice of strategies when helping patients with schizophrenia improve their cardiorespiratory fitness.

ETHICS STATEMENT

This study was carried out in accordance with the recommendations of Regional Ethics Committee of Southern and Eastern Norway (REK Sør-Øst) under file number 2014/372/REK Sør-Øst C with written informed consent from all subjects. All subjects gave written informed consent in accordance with the Declaration of Helsinki. The protocol was approved by the Regional Ethics Committee of Southern and Eastern Norway (REK Sør-Øst).

AUTHOR CONTRIBUTIONS

JAE and EA conceived the study. JAE, JE, EA, and JM acquired funding and approval of the ethics committee. These four researchers, in addition to EWM and OAA, contributed to study design. TLH, TTB, GB-K and JM carried out parts of the clinical testing. The manuscript has been drafted by JAE, EA, JE, OAA, GB-K, TTB, TLH, EWM, and JM. All authors read, worked on and approved the final manuscript.

ACKNOWLEDGMENTS

The investigators would like to thank the patients participating in the study, and the members of the EPHAPS study group who participated in the data collection and data management. We also give special thanks to Helge Bjune, Ole-Jakob Bredrup, Ellen Gurine Færvik, Jan-Freddy Hovland, Camilla Lahn-Johannessen, and Bjørn-Einar Oscarsen for conducting the measurements.

REFERENCES

Ringen PA, Engh JA, Birkenaes AB, Dieset I, Andreassen OA. Increased mortality in schizophrenia due to cardiovascular disease - a non-systematic review of epidemiology, possible causes, and interventions. *Front Psychiatry* (2014) 5:137. doi: 10.3389/fpsyt.2014.00137

Vancampfort D, Firth J, Schuch FB, Rosenbaum S, Mugisha J, Hallgren M, et al. Sedentary behavior and physical activity levels in people with schizophrenia, bipolar disorder and major depressive disorder: a global systematic review and meta-analysis. *World Psychiatry* (2017) 16:308–15. doi: 10.1002/wps.20458

Correll CU, Solmi M, Veronese N, Bortolato B, Rosson S, Santonastaso P, et al. Prevalence, incidence and mortality from cardiovascular disease in patients with pooled and specific severe mental illness: a large-scale meta- analysis of 3,211,768 patients and 113,383,368 controls. *World Psychiatry* (2017) 16:163–80. doi: 10.1002/wps.20420

Blair SN, Kampert JB, Kohl HW III, Barlow CE, Macera CA, Paffenbarger RS, et al. Influences of cardiorespiratory fitness and other precursors on cardiovascular disease and all-cause mortality in men and women. *JAMA* (1996) 276:205–10. doi: 10.1001/jama.1996.03540030039029

Lee DC, Sui X, Artero EG, Lee IM, Church TS, McAuley PA, et al. Long-term effects of changes in cardiorespiratory fitness and body mass index on all-cause and cardiovascular disease mortality in men: the Aerobics Center Longitudinal Study. *Circulation* (2011) 124:2483–90. doi: 10.1161/CIRCULATIONAHA.111.038422

Kodama S, Saito K, Tanaka S, Maki M, Yachi Y, Asumi M, et al. Cardiorespiratory fitness as a quantitative predictor of all-cause mortality and cardiovascular events in healthy men and women: a meta-analysis. *JAMA* (2009) 301:2024–35. doi: 10.1001/jama.2009.681

Hayes JF, Marston L, Walters K, King MB, Osborn DPJ. Mortality gap for people with bipolar disorder and schizophrenia, UK-based cohort study 2000– 2014. *Br J Psychiatry.* (2017) 211:175–81. doi: 10.1192/bjp.bp.117.202606

Samaras K, Correll CU, Curtis J. Premature mortality and schizophrenia- the need to heal right from the start. *JAMA Psychiatry* (2016) 73:535–6. doi: 10.1001/jamapsychiatry.2015.3432

Oja P. Dose response between total volume of physical activity and health and fitness. *Med Sci Sports Exerc.* (2001) 33 (6 Suppl):S428–37; discussion S452–3.

McGuire KA, Ross R. Incidental physical activity is positively associated with cardiorespiratory fitness. *Med Sci Sports Exerc.* (2011) 43:2189–94. doi: 10.1249/MSS.0b013e31821e4ff2

Yates T, Wilmot EG, Davies MJ, Gorely T, Edwardson C, Biddle S, et al. Sedentary behavior: what's in a definition? *Am J Prev Med.* (2011) 40:e33–4; author reply e34. doi: 10.1016/j.amepre.2011.02.017

Pate RR, O'Neill JR, Lobelo F. The evolving definition of "sedentary." *Exerc Sport Sci Rev.* (2008) 36:173–8. doi: 10.1097/JES.0b013e3181877d1a

Tremblay MS, Aubert S, Barnes JD, Saunders TJ, Carson V, Latimer-Cheung AE, et al. Sedentary Behaviour Research Network (SBRN) - terminology consensus project process and outcome. *Int J Behav Nutr Phys Act.* (2017) 14:75. doi: 10.1186/s12966-017-0525-8

Kulinski JP, Khera A, Ayers CR, Das SR, de Lemos JA, Blair SN, et al. Association between cardiorespiratory fitness and accelerometer-derived physical activity and sedentary time in the general population. *Mayo Clin Proc.* (2014) 89:1063–71. doi: 10.1016/j.mayocp.2014.04.019

Bouchard C, Blair SN, Katzmarzyk PT. Less sitting, more physical activity, or higher fitness? *Mayo Clin Proc.* (2015) 90:1533–40. doi: 10.1016/j.mayocp.2015.08.005

Dwyer T, Pezic A, Sun C, Cochrane J, Venn A, Srikanth V, et al. Objectively measured daily steps and subsequent long term all-cause mortality, the tasped prospective cohort study. *PLoS ONE* (2015) 10:e0141274. doi: 10.1371/journal.pone.0141274

Yates T, Haffner SM, Schulte PJ, Thomas L, Huffman KM, Bales CW, et al. Association between change in daily ambulatory activity and cardiovascular events in people with impaired glucose tolerance (NAVIGATOR trial): a cohort analysis. *Lancet* (2014) 383:1059–66. doi: 10.1016/S0140- 6736(13)62061-9

Olsen RH, Krogh-Madsen R, Thomsen C, Booth FW, Pedersen BK. Metabolic responses to reduced daily steps in healthy nonexercising men. *JAMA* (2008) 299:1261–3. doi: 10.1001/jama.299.11.1259

Krogh-Madsen R, Thyfault JP, Broholm C, Mortensen OH, Olsen RH, Mounier R, et al. A 2-wk reduction of ambulatory activity attenuates peripheral insulin sensitivity. *J Appl Physiol.* (1985) (2010) 108:1034–40. doi: 10.1152/japplphysiol.00977.2009

Bjørgaas M, Vik JT, Saeterhaug A, Langlo L, Sakshaug T, Mohus RM, et al. Relationship between pedometer-registered activity, aerobic capacity and self-reported activity and fitness in patients with type 2 diabetes. *Diabetes Obes Metab.* (2005) 7:737–44. doi: 10.1111/j.1463-1326.2004.00464.x

Cao ZB, Miyatake N, Higuchi M, Ishikawa-Takata K, Miyachi M, Tabata Prediction of VO2max with daily step counts for Japanese adult women. *Eur J Appl Physiol.* (2009) 105:289–96. doi: 10.1007/s00421-008- 0902-8

Spitzer RL, Williams JB, Gibbon M, First MB. The structured clinical interview for DSM-III-R (SCID) I: History, rationale, and description. *Arch Gen Psychiatry* (1992) 49:624–9.

Engh JA, Andersen E, Holmen TL, Martinsen EW, Mordal J, Morken G, et al. Effects of high-intensity aerobic exercise on psychotic symptoms and neurocognition in outpatients with schizophrenia: study protocol for a randomized controlled trial. *Trials* (2015) 16:557. doi: 10.1186/s13063-015- 1094-2

Andersen E, Holmen TL, Egeland J, Martinsen EW, Bigseth TT, Bang-Kittilsen G, et al. Physical activity pattern and cardiorespiratory fitness in individuals with schizophrenia compared with a population-based sample. *Schizophr Res.* (2018) 201:98–104. doi: 10.1016/j.schres.2018.05.038

Matthews CE, Chen KY, Freedson PS, Buchowski MS, Beech BM, Pate RR, et al. Amount of time spent in sedentary behaviors in the United States, 2003– 2004. *Am J Epidemiol.* (2008) 167:875–81. doi: 10.1093/aje/ kwm390

Troiano RP. A timely meeting: objective measurement of physical activity. *Med Sci Sports Exerc.* (2005) 37(11 Suppl.):S487–9. doi: 10.1249/01.mss.0000185473.32846.c3

Balke B, Ware RW. An experimental study of physical fitness of air force personnel. *U S armed forces Med J.* (1959) 10:675–88.

Bueno-Antequera J, Oviedo-Caro M, Munguía-Izquierdo D. Sedentary behaviour, physical activity, cardiorespiratory fitness and cardiometabolic risk in psychosis, The PsychiActive project. *Schizophr Res.* (2018) 195:142–8. doi: 10.1016/j.schres.2017.10.012

11

The Mediating Role of Non-reactivity to Mindfulness Training and Cognitive Flexibility

Yingmin Zou[1], Ping Li[1], Stefan G. Hofmann[2] and Xinghua Liu[1]*

[1] Beijing Key Laboratory of Behavior and Mental Health, School of Psychological and Cognitive Sciences, Peking University, Beijing, China, [2] Department of Psychological and Brain Sciences, Boston University, Boston, MA, United States

*Correspondence:
Xinghua Liu
xinghua_liu@pku.edu.cn

Mindfulness training has been shown to have a beneficial effect on cognitive flexibility. However, little is known about the mediators that produce this effect. Cross-sectional studies show that there might be a link between Non-judgment, Non-reactivity and cognitive flexibility. Longitudinal studies examining whether Non-judgment or Non-reactivity mediate the effectiveness of mindfulness training on improving cognitive flexibility are lacking. The present study aims to test the effect of mindfulness training on increasing cognitive flexibility and to test whether this effect is mediated by Non-judgment or Non-reactivity. We conducted a single-blind randomized controlled trial in 54 nonclinical high-stress participants between October 2018 and January 2019. Participants were randomly assigned to a Mindfulness Based Stress Reduction (MBSR) group or a waitlist control group. The experimenters were blind to the group assignment of participants. The MBSR group received 8-weekly sessions (2.5-h per week) and a one-day retreat (6-h), and was required to accomplish a 45-min daily formal practice during the intervention. The waitlist control group did not receive any intervention during the waiting period and received a 2-day (6-h per day) mindfulness training after the post-intervention. The primary outcome was self-report cognitive flexibility and perceived stress administered before and after MBSR. The secondary outcome was self-report mindfulness skills (including Non-reactivity and Non-judgment) measured at pre-treatment, Week 3, Week 6, and post-intervention. For cognitive flexibility, mixed-model repeated-measure ANOVA results showed that there were significant main effects of Time, Group and a significant interaction of Time by Group. Follow-up ANOVA indicated that the MBSR group was associated with greater improvements in cognitive flexibility than the waitlist. Path analysis results showed that the effect of the treatment on cognitive flexibility at post-treatment was fully mediated by Non-reactivity at Week 6. The mediation effects of Non-reactivity at Week 3, and Non-judgment at Week 3 and Week 6 were not significant. Our findings support the efficacy of MBSR on improving cognitive flexibility. Non-reactivity is an important element of the effectiveness of MBSR training on cognitive flexibility.

Keywords: Mindfulness Based Stress Reduction, cognitive flexibility, non-reactivity, mediation, mechanism

INTRODUCTION

Mindfulness has been defined as attention or awareness to present-moment experiences with acceptance (Baer, 2003; Kabat-Zinn, 2003; Bishop et al., 2004). Importantly, mindfulness is an innate capacity of humans. At the same time, it can be fostered and deepened by mindfulness based interventions (MBIs) (Lindsay and Creswell, 2017), such as the Mindfulness Based Stress Reduction Program (MBSR) (Kabat-Zinn, 1990) and Mindfulness Based Cognitive Therapy (MBCT) (Segal et al., 2012). MBI alleviates psychological distress (e.g., stress, anxiety, mood symptoms) with medium effect sizes compared to waitlist controls (Hedge's gs = 0.41−0.53), and active treatment controls (Hedge's gs = 0.33−0.5) (Hofmann et al., 2010; Khoury et al., 2013). Additionally, preliminary evidence supports that MBI enhances cognitive abilities (e.g., cognitive flexibility, attention, and executive functioning), which might affect social functioning (Lutz et al., 2015; Li et al., 2018; Wielgosz et al., 2019). Some studies suggest that cognitive flexibility promotes effective management of stressful life events, and is associated with good mental health (Kashdan and Rottenberg, 2010; Logue and Gould, 2014).

Cognitive flexibility is conceptualized as the ability to flexibly and adaptively respond to the environments, as opposed to the rigid or automatic thinking style, triggered by prior experience (Hayes et al., 1999; Shapiro et al., 2006; Dennis and Vander Wal, 2010). Lack of cognitive flexibility, or cognitive rigidity, is an important vulnerability for the development and maintenance of psychological distress (Morris and Mansell, 2018). When confronted with difficult life situations, individuals with a rigid thinking style tend to perceive the situation as unchangeable and uncontrollable and tend to engage in rumination, leading to distress in the long term. If individuals see only one solution to a difficult life situation, they might perceive themselves as incapable of problem solving. That might interfere with their long-term goals, which might further increase emotional distress. As part of cognitive behavioral therapy (CBT), psychological distress is alleviated by targeting maladaptive and rigid automatic cognitions with more adaptive cognitions (Derubeis et al., 1991; Chambless and Gillis, 1993). In this context, Dennis and Vander Wal (2010) developed a self-report instrument, the Cognitive Flexibility Inventory (CFI), to measure cognitive flexibility. The CFI consists of two factors, namely the Control factor and the Alternative factor. Items on the Control factor measure the degree to which individuals perceive the difficult life situation as controllable. Items on the Alternative factor denote the extent to which individuals perceive multiple explanations and solutions to the difficult life situation. It seems likely that individuals with flexible and adaptive cognitions experience less psychological distress than those with rigid thinking styles. In fact, a greater level of perceived control has been shown to be associated with higher tendency to adapt coping strategies to different stressful life situations (Cheng and Cheung, 2005). Furthermore, individuals with higher levels of perceived control tend to accommodate with life stressors including economic difficulties, unemployment and care-given burdens (Zautra et al., 2012). Less dichotomous

thinking (e.g., If I fail at my work, then I am a failure as a person), was indicative of alleviated perceived stress (Otto et al., 1997; Ford and Shook, 2018). Meanwhile, it is evident that an increase in perceived problem solving capability predicted less perceived stress longitudinally (Otto et al., 1997), suggesting that flexible cognitions contribute to successful management of life event stress.

Mindfulness has long been proposed to be associated with cognitive flexibility. Some researchers have proposed that cognitive flexibility is a component of mindfulness (Bishop et al., 2004; Chanowitz and Langer, 1981; Feldman et al., 2007; Frewen et al., 2008; Moore and Malinowski, 2009). For example, Chanowitz and Langer (1981) defined mindfulness as a consciousness state or a mode of cognitive functions that would allow individuals to get actively involved in reframing the environment. This, in turn, might enable individuals to draw voluntary attention on contextual cues, leading to flexible and adaptive cognitions or behaviors. Bishop et al. (2004) suggested that mindfulness is operationally defined as the self-regulation of attention and orientation to the experience. Being cognitive flexible is considered an important component of self-regulation of attention. However, relatively little is known about the role of cognitive flexibility in mindfulness (Kee and Wang, 2008). Moore (2013) has shown that cognitive flexibility is positively associated with mindfulness and contributed to flow experiences when controlled for mindfulness, suggesting that cognitive flexibility and mindfulness are independent but correlated constructs. Similar to cognitive flexibility, mindfulness was found to be associated with lower levels of perceived stress (Senders et al., 2014; Gustafsson et al., 2015). Shapiro et al. (2006) proposed that mindfulness trainings might facilitate awareness of one's habitual reactions and enable individuals to see the present situation as it is and respond adaptively and flexibly. So far, only one study has shown that MBI improves self-report cognitive flexibility. Shapero et al. (2018) found that for depressed individuals, participants receiving MBCT training reported higher levels of cognitive flexibility than a waitlist group. In sum, mindfulness is positively associated with cognitive flexibility and both of them are associated with lower emotional distress. On top of that, emerging evidence suggests that MBIs might be effective for improving cognitive flexibility.

Although mindfulness has been shown to cultivate adaptive and flexible responses, the mechanism producing this effect requires further exploration. Theoretical models have provided fundamental insights for the underlying mechanism. The mindfulness stress-buffering theory (Creswell and Lindsay, 2014) proposes that acceptance is the main ingredient of mindfulness training on adaptive responses for stress. Acceptance is often defined as openness toward emotion and experience (Campbell-Sills et al., 2006). The ability to accept stressors buffers the habitual appraisals and responses, which in turn facilitates new appraisals and coping strategies. Studies have shown that the association between trait mindfulness with peace of mind was mediated by acceptance (Xu et al., 2015), and the positive link between mindfulness and subjective well-being was significantly mediated by self-acceptance only (Xu et al., 2016). Moreover, accepting pain increased pain endurance and tolerance after training than simply paying attention to the pain without accepting it (Wang et al., 2019).

It has been suggested that accepting an experience might be cultivated by approaches that encourage individuals to fully experience their bodily sensations, emotions, and thoughts without changing or avoiding them (Hayes et al., 1999). However, little is known about the specific mindfulness-based approach that fosters this acceptance attitude. Lindsay and Creswell (2017) proposed that mindfulness training might foster acceptance through non-judgmental (without judging them as good or bad) and non-reactive (without reacting to change them) attitudes toward internal and external experiences. Mindfulness practices emphasize Non-judgment by allowing for any experience arising in our mind, without evaluating them as good or bad. Thus, this process may be presumed to shift habitual stress appraisal sets. Non-reactivity is accomplished through allowing experiences to come and go without reacting in an effort to change them. Non-reactivity is important in explaining the reduction of mood symptoms gained by mindfulness training. After a 3-month training, Non-reactivity predicted more reduction of mood symptoms in a present awareness mindfulness training group as compared to a progressive muscle relaxation training group (Gao et al., 2018). Theoretically, Non-reactivity may buffer the stress reactivity, which in turn would permit the generation of new responses, thus increasing cognitive flexibility (Kuyken et al., 2010; Dajani and Uddin, 2015; Van Der Velden and Roepstorff, 2015). Baer et al. (2012) reported that Non-judgment and Non-reactivity both showed significant improvements from baseline to Week 3 and Week 6 of a mindfulness intervention. Therefore, Week 3 and 6 might be two critical time points when changes in Non-judgment and Non-reactivity during mindfulness training occurs. Although theoretical models make reasonable assumptions, empirical evidence is relatively lacking. Currently, the pathways linking mindfulness training, Non-judgment/Non-reactivity and cognitive flexibility are poorly understood.

The present study aims to examine the effect of MBSR on cognitive flexibility and the mediating role of Non-judgment and Non-reactivity among them. Based on the previous studies, we hypothesized that: (1) Compared to a waitlist control group, the MBSR group will show elevated cognitive flexibility scores at post-intervention; (2) Non-reactivity scores during the intervention will mediate the treatment-induced changes in cognitive flexibility at the post-treatment assessment point; and (3) Non-judgment scores during the intervention will significantly mediate the relationship between intervention group and cognitive flexibility scores at post-intervention.

MATERIALS AND METHODS

Participants
One hundred and two participants were recruited via social media advertisement. The inclusion criteria were: (a) a score on the Chinese Perceived Stress Scales (CPSS; Yang and Huang, 2003) ≥26; (b) having no prior experience with the 8-week MBSR or MBCT protocol; (c) a practice frequency of yoga, meditation,

or Tai chi less than 20 min per week in the past six months; (d) absence of severe or unstable physical illness that would prevent one from attending trainings; and (e) a commitment to the group setting (e.g., randomization, no schedule conflicts, no attendance to other MBI or experiments during training). Participants were excluded if they met the DSM-IV-TR criteria (American Psychiatric Association [APA], 1994) for any diagnosis in the past six months. They were excluded if they had any self-injury or suicidal risks, aggression or destructive behaviors. The trial was conducted between October 2018 and January 2019, at the Peking University, Beijing, China.

Procedure
Participants were invited to complete a survey attached to the advertisement. The survey included questions about personal experiences and information (e.g., the prior experience about MBSR or MBCT; the practice frequency of yoga, meditation, or Tai chi; the physical condition), and the CPSS. A study staff member subsequently telephoned to confirm the participant was able to commit to the group setting. Meanwhile, they were invited to attend the Structured Clinical Interview for DSM-IV-TR (First et al., 2002) conducted by a psychiatrist. The CONSORT checklist (Schulz et al., 2010) of this clinical trial is displayed in **Supplementary Material**.

After eligibility assessment, 54 participants were included. To match the gender and age between the MBSR group and waitlist group, a research assistant used a stratified random method to allocate participants. First, the age range was calculated. Then, the potential number of strata was assigned an integer that could be divided by the age range. The optimal number of strata was reached when the gender ratio within each strata became approximately 1:1. In our study, eight was chosen as the final strata number. The randomization was carried out within each strata. The random number sequence from 1 to 100 was generated by Excel. Each participant was allocated to a random number. This random number was divided by 2. If the remainder was 0, the corresponding participant was allocated to the MBSR group. If the remainder was 1, the participant was allocated to the waitlist group.

Twenty-six participants were allocated to the MBSR group, and 28 were allocated to the waitlist group (allocation ratio = 13:14). Group assignment was done by the research assistant. The participants would not be informed of their assignment until they completed the pre-test. Before the pre-test, all participants gave their informed consent. The intervention started on November 2018 and ended on January 2019. The MBSR group received the 8-week (2.5-h per week) sessions and a one-day retreat (a weekend between Week 6 and Week 7), led by two instructors adhering to the MBSR developed by Kabat-Zinn (1990). Meanwhile, participants were asked to practice guided meditation for 45 min daily. The waitlist group was not offered any kind of intervention during the waiting period, but they had access to a 2-day mindfulness training after the post-intervention. Participants were asked to complete the self-report questionnaires at 4 time points based on the timeline of MBSR group: pre-treatment (pre randomization, T1), Week 3 test (T2), Week 6 test (T3), and post-treatment (the week following week

8, T4) (for the flowchart of the participants, see **Figure 1**). The questionnaires were delivered to the participants via an online link before the session. Participants had 40 min for completing the measures. Within the training period, the participants and the instructors were not blind to the group assignment, only the experimenters were blind. Participants who finished all the tests were thanked and received 100 RMB as compensation. Our study protocol was approved by the Association for Ethics and Human and Animal Protection in School of Psychological and Cognitive Sciences, Peking University (No. 2018-10-02).

Measures

The Chinese version (Deng et al., 2011) of the Five Facet Mindfulness Questionnaire (FFMQ; Baer et al., 2008) was used to assess the tendency to be mindful. The FFMQ consists of 39 items with a 5-point Likert rating scale (1 = never or very rarely true, 5 = very often or always true). Its five-factor construct is reliable and valid in English and Chinese settings, which refers to Observing (e.g., "I notice the smells and aromas of things"), Describing (e.g., "I am good at finding words to describe my feelings"), Acting with awareness (e.g., "I find myself doing things without paying attention," reverse coding), Non-reactivity to inner experiences (e.g., "I perceive my feelings and emotions without having to react to them"), and Non-judging of inner experiences (e.g., "I think some of my emotions are bad or inappropriate and I should not feel them," reverse coding). A higher score indicates that one is more mindful in everyday life. If the mediating role of Non-judgment and Non-reactivity is to be verified, their changes have to emerge prior to the changes of outcome variables (Kazdin, 2007). Thus, the FFMQ was evaluated during the MBSR intervention in addition to the pre- and post-treatment. In the present study, the Cronbach's αs of the FFMQ, and the five subscales across 4 time points ranged from 0.84 to 0.93.

The Chinese version (Wang et al., 2016) of the CFI (Dennis and Vander Wal, 2010) was utilized to assess the ability to generate alternative explanations and solutions to difficult situations. The CFI is comprised of 20 items utilizing a 1–5 point Likert rating scale (1 = never, 5 = always). It assesses two aspects of cognitive flexibility: the proneness to perceive difficulties as controllable (e.g., "When I encounter difficult situations, I feel like I am losing control," "I am capable of overcoming the difficulties in life that I face"), and the capability to generate multiple explanations and solutions when confronted with life events and difficulties (e.g., "I consider multiple options before making a decision," "I like to look at difficult situations from many different angles"). The original CFI has good internal consistency (Cronbach's αs = 0.84−0.92), 7-weeks test-retest reliability ($r = 0.81$) and construct validity for clinical and non-clinical samples (Dennis and Vander Wal, 2010). The Chinese version showed good internal consistency (Cronbach's αs = 0.81) and revealed a two-factor structure, consistent with the original scale. Higher scores indicate more flexibility in cognitive appraisal and problem solving when encountering difficult situations. To examine the efficacy of MBSR on cognitive flexibility, the CFI was administered at pre- and post-treatment. The Standardized Response Mean (SRM)

(the mean difference between pre- and post-treatment divided by the standard deviation of the difference), was 0.93, indicating large sensitivity to change (Cohen, 1992). In the present study, the Cronbach's αs of CFI were at 0.75 pre-intervention, and 0.91 at post-intervention.

The CPSS (Cohen et al., 1983; Yang and Huang, 2003) was administered to evaluate the degree to which individuals perceived their situations as uncontrollable, unpredictable, and unresolvable in the past month. The CPSS includes 14 items (e.g., "I feel intense and stressful," "I feel that the problem is constantly accumulating and cannot be solved") with a 5-ponit Likert rating scale (0 = never, 4 = always). It exhibits great internal consistency and construct validity in English and Chinese settings (Cohen et al., 1983; Yang and Huang, 2003). A higher score indicates a higher level of perceived stress. The CPSS was conducted at pre and post-treatment in order to capture the stress reduction effect of MBSR. In the present study, the Cronbach's αs of CPSS were 0.72 at pre-treatment, and 0.86 at post-treatment.

Data Analyses

First, we utilized G*power 3.1 (Faul et al., 2007) to compute the required sample size. Based on a previous study (Shapero et al., 2018), we considered a between-group effect size (η^2) of 0.24 regarding the mindfulness training effect on cognitive flexibility. To obtain power of 0.8 with two measurement points, the total sample size of 50 would be sufficient to detect a significant Group × Time interactions by repeated-measure ANOVAs at $p < 0.05$.

Second, we conducted the missing value analysis with the Statistical Package for Social Sciences (version 17.0 for Windows; SPSS Inc., Chicago, IL, United States). All data were analyzed using multivariate intention-to-treat analyses. For FFMQ, CFI, and CPSS, Little's MCAR (Missing Completely At Random) tests showed that data were missed at random ($ps > 0.05$). We used the expectation-maximization method suggested by Newgard and Lewis (2015) to impute the missing data. We compared group differences in age, gender, educational years, FFMQ, CFI, and CPSS scores at pre-treatment, using independent sample t-tests for continuous variables, and the chi-square test for the categorical variable. If significant, those would be co-varied in analysis.

Third, effects of MBSR on improvement in perceived stress and cognitive flexibility were examined using mixed-model repeated-measure ANOVAs using SPSS. A series of follow-up ANOVAs or t-tests were conducted following significant main effects and interactions.

Latent growth curve modelings (LGCMs) were conducted to explore the longitudinal trajectories of FFMQ total score and factor scores, and to investigate whether individuals or groups would differ in the initial levels and longitudinal changes in these scores. We estimated two latent factors (intercept and slope) across four waves (T1–T4). The intercept was defined by fixing the four parameters with a loading of 1.0, representing constant initial levels across four waves. The slope was fixed at loadings with 0, 3, 6, 8, representing the time spaces with T1. Group (0 = MBSR, 1 = waitlist) was incorporated as a covariate to test for the treatment effect on trajectories of mindfulness skills.

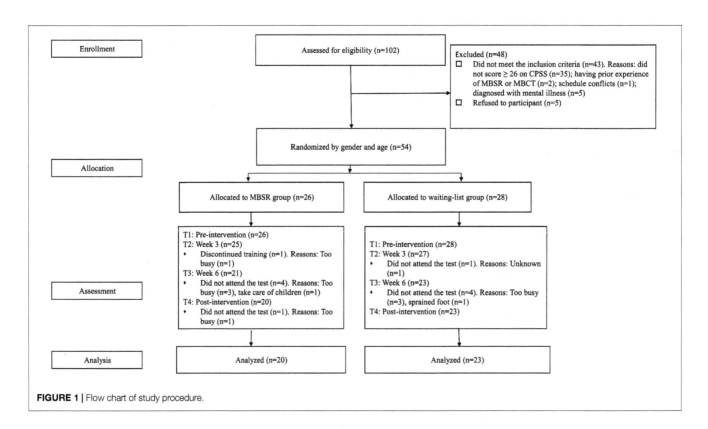

FIGURE 1 | Flow chart of study procedure.

LGCMs were administered using the Lavaan package (Rosseel, 2012) in R. Based on the criteria by Hu and Bentler (1999), CFI > 0.9, RMSEA < 0.08, and SRMR < 0.1 suggest a good fit of the model.

The mediation analyses were performed with Mplus version 5.2 (Muthén and Muthén, 2007). Adopting the method recommended by Baron and Kenny (1986), a mediation effect was determined by calculating the product of path coefficients constituting the indirect effect (e.g., path coefficient of the independent variable to mediator, and path coefficient of mediator to outcome variable) divided by bootstrapped standard error of this product. A bootstrap procedure was used to increase the statistical power (MacKinnon et al., 2002). We ran four separate mediation models to determine whether Non-reactivity at Week 3 or Week 6 and/or Non-judgment at Week 3 or Week 6, mediate the relationship between MBSR training and post-treatment cognitive flexibility. In each model, intervention group, which was transformed into dummy variable (0 = MBSR group, 1 = waitlist group), served as the independent variable. Post-treatment CFI scores served as the outcome variable. Thus, each model comprised of a path ("a" path coefficient) from group (MBSR or waitlist group) to mediator (Non-reactivity at Week 3 or Week 6, Non-judgment at Week 3 or Week 6), a path ("b" path coefficient) from mediator to outcome variable (post-intervention CFI score), and a direct path ("c'" path coefficient) from group to outcome variable controlling for mediator. The indirect effect of MBSR training on cognitive flexibility via the mediator is calculated by "a" multiplied by "b" ("ab" coefficient), the MODEL INDIRECT command was utilized in Mplus 5.2. A mediation effect was

marked by a significant *ab* coefficient. In addition, goodness of fit parameters included comparative fit index (CFI), root-mean-square error of approximation (RMSEA), standardized root mean square residual (SRMR). According to the criteria by Hu and Bentler (1999), CFI > 0.9, RMSEA < 0.08, SRMR < 0.1 indicates good fit.

To examine the statistical power, we used Cohen's d to calculate the effect size of t-tests. Cohen (1988) defined a small, medium, and large effect size as 0.2, 0.5, and 0.8. We also used partial η^2 (Cohen's f) to calculate the effect size of the main effects and interactions. A value of η^2 ranging from 0.01 to 0.059 indicates a small, between 0.059 and 0.138 indicates a medium, and values ≥ 0.138 a large effect size (Cohen, 1988). We adopted the Monte Carlo method to calculate the power of mediation tests (Schoemann et al., 2017). The number of replication was set to 1000. For each replication, 200 times of random draws from the distribution of regression coefficients were used. As suggested by Cohen (1988), for the proportion of a variable explained by another variable, a small, medium, and large effect size was 0.01, 0.09, and 0.25, respectively.

RESULTS

Demographical and Descriptive Data
The two groups were demographically matched and showed no significant difference in age ($t_{(52)} = 0.24$, $p = 0.81$, Cohen's $d = 0.07$, 95% Confidence Interval (CI): -0.48 to 0.61), gender ($X^2_{(52)} = -0.26$, $p = 0.8$), educational years ($t_{(52)} = -0.2$, $p = 0.84$, Cohen's $d = -0.05$, 95% CI: -0.49 to 0.6), or per capita monthly

income ($t_{(52)} = 0.54$, $p = 0.6$, Cohen's $d = 0.15$, 95% CI: -0.49 to 0.6). There were no significant group differences in pre-treatment FFMQ ($t_{(52)} = -0.82$, $p = 0.41$, Cohen's $d = -0.22$, 95% CI: -0.77 to 0.32), CFI ($t_{(52)} = 1.36$, $p = 0.18$, Cohen's $d = 0.37$, 95% CI: -0.18 to 0.92) or CPSS ($t_{(52)} = -0.67$, $p = 0.51$, Cohen's $d = -0.18$, 95% CI: -0.73 to 0.37) (see **Table 1**). Thus, no pre-treatment variables were co-varied in the follow-up analysis.

In total, the drop-out rate was 20.37%. Six participants dropped out of the MBSR group (23.08%). Among them, one participant discontinued training at Week 3 because he was too busy, four participants did not attend the Week 6, for the reason of being too busy ($n = 3$) or taking care of children ($n = 1$). 1 participant did not complete the post-intervention, reporting being too busy. For the waitlist group, five participants dropped out (17.86%). Among them, one participant did not attend the Week 3 test, reason unknown. Four participants did not complete Week 6 test, for the reasons of being too busy ($n = 3$) or having a sprained foot ($n = 1$) (see **Figure 1**).

Trajectory of Change in Mindfulness at Pre-treatment, Week 3, Week 6, and Post-treatment

The LGCMs analyses showed that only the Non-reactivity model had acceptable fit indices (CFI = 1, TLI = 1, RMSEA<0.001, SRMR = 0.067), whereas FFMQ total score and the other subscale models did not fit well (see **Table 2**). For Non-reactivity, the mean initial score was 21.75. The mean slope was 0.85, which was significantly different from zero ($p < 0.001$), suggesting a steady increase of Non-reactivity over time in the full sample. The value 0.85 can be interpreted as an average of 0.85 increase of Non-reactivity subscale score per unit of time. The variance of the intercept was 7.78 ($p = 0.002$), indicating significant individual variability of initial Non-reactivity score. The variance of slope and its covariance with intercept was not significant ($p = 0.12$ and $p = 0.701$, respectively). There was no significant group difference on the initial Non-reactivity subscale score ($\beta = -1.36$, $p = 0.169$). However, the factor Group (0 = MBSR, 1 = waitlist) showed

a significant effect on the slope for Non-reactivity ($\beta = -0.34$, $p = 0.019$), indicating that the MBSR group increased faster than the waitlist group on Non-reactivity subscale score. Taken together, there was individual variability in Non-reactivity at the initial level, but the groups did not differ in the initial Non-reactivity score. On average, the slope grew over time. There was no individual difference in the growth rate. Group had a significant effect on the growth rate. The MBSR group increased at a faster speed than the waitlist control on the Non-reactivity score (see **Table 3**).

The Effect of MBSR on Perceived Stress and Cognitive Flexibility

For the CPSS scores, there was a significant main effect of Time ($F_{(1,52)} = 313.78$, $p < 0.001$, partial $\eta^2 = 0.86$, 95% CI: 0.78–0.9), but the Group effect ($F_{(1)} = 0.001$, $p = 0.99$, partial $\eta^2 = 0.001$, 95% CI: -0.55 to 0.55) and Time by Group interaction effects were not significant ($F_{(1,52)} = 1.17$, $p = 0.29$, partial $\eta^2 = 0.02$, 95% CI: 0–0.15).

For the CFI scores, the Time effect ($F_{(1,52)} = 59.86$, $p < 0.001$, partial $\eta^2 = 0.53$, 95% CI: 0–0.15), Group effect ($F_{(1)} = 7.03$, $p = 0.01$, partial $\eta^2 = 0.12$, 95% CI: 1.25–2.57) and Time by Group interaction effect were significant ($F_{(1,52)} = 4.27$, $p = 0.04$,

TABLE 2 | Model fits based on the latent growth curve model of FFMQ scales.

Variables	χ^2	df	CFI	TLI	RMSEA	SRMR
NR	5.16	7.00	1.00	1.02	0.001	0.07
FT	35.54***	7.00	0.72	0.61	0.30	0.40
NJ	35.13***	7.00	0.74	0.63	0.30	0.23
OB	18.12**	7.00	0.91	0.87	0.19	0.12
DE	38.69***	7.00	0.68	0.54	0.32	0.18
AW	74.86***	7.00	0.45	0.21	0.47	0.49

*NR = the Non-reactivity subscale score, FT = the FFMQ total score, NJ = the Non-judgment subscale score, OB = the Observing subscale score, DE = the Describing subscale score, AW = the Acting with Awareness subscale score. **p < 0.01, ***p < 0.001.*

TABLE 1 | Demographical and descriptive data for the MBSR and waiting-list group at baseline.

Variables	MBSR ($n = 26$)	Waiting-list controls ($n = 28$)	t/X^2	p	Cohen's d
Age	34.12 (7.63)	33.6 (8.24)	0.24	0.81	0.07
Gender (% Female)	69.23%	72.41%	−0.26	0.8	/
Educational years	17.82 (2.29)	17.93 (1.92)	−0.2	0.84	−0.05
Per capita monthly income (RMB)	21, 653.94 (30, 479.14)	17, 975.95 (19, 968.86)	0.54	0.6	0.15
FFMQ total score	107.88 (13.79)	110.95 (13.73)	−0.82	0.41	−0.22
Observing	24.65 (5.96)	25.67 (5.42)	−0.66	0.52	−0.18
Describing	23.12 (2.98)	23.25 (2.69)	−0.17	0.86	−0.05
Acting with awareness	17.73 (3.98)	18.63 (6.58)	−0.6	0.55	−0.16
Non-reactivity	20.35 (2.8)	19.62 (4.26)	0.74	0.46	0.2
Non-judgment	22.04 (5.42)	23.79 (6.13)	−1.12	0.27	−0.31
CFI	68.92 (4.46)	66.96 (5.87)	1.36	0.18	0.37
CPSS	43.96 (4.35)	44.74 (4.27)	−0.67	0.51	−0.18

Gender was presented with Percentage, the other variables were presented with Mean (SD). MBSR = The Mindfulness Based Stress Reduction; FFMQ = The Five Facet Mindfulness Questionnaire, CFI = The Cognitive Flexibility Inventory, CPSS = The Chinese Perceived Stress Scale.

TABLE 3 | Parameter estimates based on latent growth curve model of FFMQ scales.

	Estimate	SE	t	p
NR				
Mean				
Intercepts	21.75	1.60	13.59	<0.001***
Slope	0.85	0.23	3.67	<0.001***
Variances				
NR1	3.56	1.79	1.99	0.047*
NR2	4.24	1.21	3.52	<0.001***
NR3	4.06	1.34	3.03	0.002**
NR4	7.64	2.40	3.19	0.001**
Intercepts	7.78	2.52	3.09	0.002**
Slope	0.09	0.06	1.56	0.12
Covariance				
Intercept with slope	−0.12	0.31	−0.38	0.701
Regression				
Intercept on group	−1.36	0.99	−1.38	0.169
Slope on group	−0.34	0.14	−2.34	0.019*
FT				
Mean				
Intercepts	117.87	5.26	22.43	<0.001***
Slope	5.17	0.79	6.54	<0.001***
Variances				
FT1	422.34	87.08	4.85	<0.001***
FT2	46.84	16.23	2.89	0.004**
FT3	56.08	20.30	2.76	0.006**
FT4	277.43	56.44	4.92	<0.001***
Intercepts	−16.67	38.65	−0.43	0.666
Slope	−2.97	1.01	−2.93	0.003**
Covariance				
Intercept with slope	26.79	5.22	5.13	<0.001***
Regression				
Intercept on group	−0.41	3.24	−0.13	0.9
slope on group	−2.02	0.49	−4.16	<0.001***
NJ				
Mean				
Intercepts	24.04	1.48	16.23	<0.001***
Slope	1.55	0.45	3.45	0.001**
Variances				
NJ1	37.09	7.90	4.69	<0.001***
NJ2	24.76	5.04	4.91	<0.001***
NJ3	25.34	5.49	4.62	<0.001***
NJ4	−5.78	4.98	−1.16	0.246
Intercepts	−12.12	4.32	−2.81	0.005**
Slope	0.69	0.25	2.71	0.007**
Covariance				
Intercept with slope	0.33	0.75	0.43	0.665
Regression				
Intercept on group	0.32	0.91	0.35	0.725
Slope on group	−0.70	0.28	−2.52	0.012**
OB				
Mean				
Intercepts	25.29	2.82	8.96	<0.001***
Slope	0.84	0.29	2.95	0.003**

(Continued)

TABLE 3 | Continued

	Estimate	SE	t	p
Variances				
OB1	16.45	4.29	3.83	<0.001***
OB2	3.51	1.60	2.20	0.028*
OB3	7.57	2.24	3.38	0.001**
OB4	16.37	4.29	3.82	<0.001***
Intercepts	25.43	7.21	3.53	<0.001***
Slope	−0.03	0.09	−0.28	0.783
Covariance				
Intercept with slope	−0.14	0.61	−0.22	0.823
Regression				
Intercept on group	−0.69	1.74	−0.40	0.693
Slope on group	−0.33	0.18	−1.90	0.057
DE				
Mean				
Intercepts	22.86	1.49	15.37	<0.001***
Slope	0.98	0.21	4.64	<0.001***
Variances				
DE1	8.66	2.63	3.29	0.001**
DE2	13.69	3.25	4.22	<0.001***
DE3	10.40	2.88	3.61	<0.001***
DE4	9.49	3.02	3.14	0.002**
Intercepts	2.15	2.69	0.80	0.424
Slope	−0.07	0.07	−0.95	0.342
Covariance				
Intercept with slope	1.35	0.35	3.81	<0.001***
Regression				
Intercept on group	0.47	0.92	0.51	0.607
Slope on group	−0.13	0.13	−1.01	0.315
AW				
Mean				
Intercepts	19.76	0.93	21.21	<0.001***
Slope	1.24	0.36	3.45	001**
Variances				
AW1	54.16	10.44	5.19	<0.001***
AW2	16.21	3.25	4.99	<0.001***
AW3	2.79	2.51	1.11	0.226
AW4	32.54	6.29	5.17	<0.001***
Intercepts	−23.22	4.92	−4.72	<0.001***
Slope	−0.28	0.17	−1.63	0.104
Covariance				
Intercept with slope	4.21	0.83	5.10	<0.001***
Regression				
Intercept on group	0.80	0.57	1.40	0.163
Slope on group	−0.36	0.22	−1.60	0.109

NR = the Non-reactivity subscale score, FT = the FFMQ total score, NJ = the Non-judgment subscale score, OB = the Observing subscale score, DE = the Describing subscale score, AW = the Acting with Awareness subscale score. 1–4 = time points, *p < 0.05, **p < 0.01, ***p < 0.001.

partial $\eta^2 = 0.08$, 95% CI: 0–0.23). Follow-up t-tests showed that CFI scores increased significantly from pre- to post-treatment for both groups ($ps < 0.001$). However, the MBSR group scored higher than the waitlist control group at post-treatment ($p = 0.003$) (see **Figure 2**).

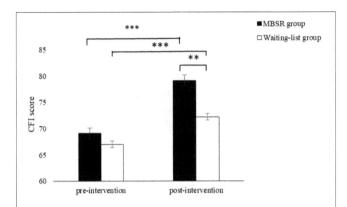

FIGURE 2 | The Cognitive Flexibility Inventory scores as a function of Time and Group. Error bars represent standard error of the mean. **$p < 0.01$ and ***$p < 0.001$.

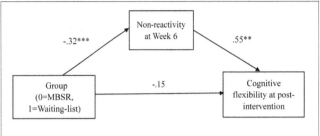

FIGURE 3 | Path analysis illustrating the mediation effect of Non-reactivity at Week 6 on the relationship of MBSR training and cognitive flexibility. **$p < 0.01$ and ***$p < 0.001$.

The Mediating Effects of Non-reactivity and Non-judgment on the Relationship of MBSR and Cognitive Flexibility

The effect of MBSR on cognitive flexibility was not mediated by Non-reactivity at Week 3. The corresponding fit indices were reasonably good ($\chi^2_{(3)}$ = 16.08, $p < 0.001$, CFI = 1, RMSEA < 0.001, SRMR < 0.001). However, the indirect effect was not significant ($ab = -0.07$, SE = 0.05, $p = 0.14$), despite a trend toward improved Non-reactivity at Week 3 via MBSR ($a = -0.24$, SE = 0.14, $p = 0.08$), and a statistically significant prediction on cognitive flexibility via Non-reactivity at Week 3 ($b = 0.28$, SE = 0.09, $p = 0.002$). The power of the indirect effect of Non-reactivity at Week 3 was 0.23.

There was a full mediation effect of Non-reactivity at Week 6. The model fit the data well ($\chi^2_{(3)}$ = 39, $p < 0.001$, CFI = 1, RMSEA < 0.001, SRMR < 0.001). A significant intervention effect of MBSR on Non-reactivity at Week 6 was found ($a = -0.32$, SE = 0.11, $p = 0.003$), suggesting that MBSR improved Non-reactivity at Week 6. Furthermore, Non-reactivity at Week 6 positively predicted cognitive flexibility at post-treatment ($b = 0.55$, SE = 0.09, $p < 0.001$). The improvement of cognitive flexibility at post-treatment accounted by MBSR via Non-reactivity at Week 6 was significant ($ab = -0.18$, SE = 0.07, $p = 0.008$). Controlling for the mediating effect of Non-reactivity at Week 6, there was no significant association between group and cognitive flexibility at post-treatment ($c' = -0.15$, SE = 0.08, $p = 0.06$), indicating a full mediation effect by Non-reactivity at Week 6 (see **Figure 3**). The mediating effect of Non-reactivity at Week 6 accounted for 53.94% of the total effect between group and cognitive flexibility. The power of the indirect effect of Non-reactivity at Week 6 was 0.69.

The effect of MBSR on cognitive flexibility was not mediated by Non-judgment at Week 3. Despite the good model fit ($\chi^2_{(3)}$ = 24.62, $p < 0.001$, CFI = 1, RMSEA < 0.001, SRMR < 0.001), the indirect effect of Non-judgment at Week 3 was not significant ($ab = -0.01$, SE = 0.06, $p = 0.82$). The power of the indirect effect of Non-judgment at Week 3 was 0.04. The failure to find a significant mediating effect might be due to the disassociation between group and Non-judgment at Week 3 ($a = -0.03$, SE = 0.13, $p = 0.82$), indicating that there were no differentiated effects of MBSR training or waitlist assignment on Non-judgment at Week 3. There was a significant association between Non-judgment at Week 3 and cognitive flexibility at post-treatment ($b = 0.45$, SE = 0.07, $p < 0.001$).

Similar to Week 3, there was no mediating effect of Non-judgment at Week 6 on group and cognitive flexibility at post-treatment. The model fit the data well ($\chi^2_{(3)}$ = 13.48, $p < 0.001$, CFI = 1, RMSEA < 0.001, SRMR < 0.001), but the indirect effect did not reach a significant level ($ab = -0.09$, SE = 0.08, $p = 0.27$). The power of the indirect effect of Non-judgment at Week 6 was 0.17. Despite the fact that Non-judgment at Week 6 predicted cognitive flexibility at post-treatment ($b = 0.66$, SE = 0.11, $p < 0.001$), improvements in Non-judgment at Week 6 could not be differentiated from waitlist group ($a = -0.13$, SE = 0.11, $p = 0.24$). Model fit indices please see **Table 4**.

DISCUSSION

The present work examined the efficacy of MBSR on cognitive flexibility in non-clinical stressed populations and the mediating effects of Non-reactivity and Non-judgment in explaining this effect. We put forward three hypotheses. First, we hypothesized that MBSR would be effective in improving cognitive flexibility, which was supported by the data. MBSR training had an immediate effect on cognitive flexibility with a medium effect size. Results also showed that compared with waitlist controls, MBSR training did not have incremental effect on stress reduction. Our second hypothesis was that Non-reactivity during intervention mediated the relationship between intervention group and cognitive flexibility. This hypothesis was partly supported. Non-reactivity at Week 3 did not mediate the association between Group and cognitive flexibility. However, Non-reactivity at Week 6 fully mediated the relationship between group and cognitive flexibility, which explained 53.94% of overall variances. Third, we hypothesized that Non-judgment during intervention mediated the relationship between group and cognitive flexibility, which was not supported by the data. Neither Non-judgment at Week 3 nor that at Week 6 mediated the association between MBSR training and cognitive flexibility.

TABLE 4 | Model fit indices and standardized path coefficients for hypothesized mediation models.

Model	χ^2/df	CFI[2]	RMSEA	SRMR	Standardized path coefficients	IND %
IV: Group	5.36	1	< 0.001	< 0.001	$a = -0.24$, SE = 0.14, $p = 0.08$	20.3
Mediator: Week 3 Non-reactivity					$b = 0.28$, SE = 0.09, $p = 0.002$**	
Outcome: Post-test CFI[1]					$c' = -0.26$, SE = 0.09, $p = 0.004$**	
					$ab = -0.07$, SE = 0.05, $p = 0.14$	
IV: Group	13	1	< 0.001	< 0.001	$a = -0.32$, SE = 0.11, $p = 0.003$**	53.94
Mediator: Week 6 Non-reactivity					$b = 0.55$, SE = 0.09, $p < 0.001$**	
Outcome: Post-test CFI[1]					$c' = -0.15$, SE = 0.08, $p = 0.06$	
					$ab = -0.18$, SE = 0.07, $p = 0.008$**	
IV: Group	8.2	1	< 0.001	< 0.001	$a = -0.03$, SE = 0.13, $p = 0.82$	4.24
Mediator: Week 3 Non-judgment					$b = 0.45$, SE = 0.07, $p < 0.001$**	
Outcome: Post-test CFI[1]					$c' = -0.32$, SE = 0.08, $p < 0.001$***	
					$ab = -0.01$, SE = 0.06, $p = 0.82$	
IV: Group	4.49	1	< 0.001	< 0.001	$a = -0.13$, SE = 0.11, $p = 0.24$	26.97
Mediator: Week 6 Non-judgment					$b = 0.66$, SE = 0.11, $p < 0.001$***	
Outcome: Post-test CFI[1]					$c' = -0.24$, SE = 0.09, $p = 0.005$**	
					$ab = -0.09$, SE = 0.08, $p = 0.27$	

IV = Independent variable, CFI[1] = The Cognitive Flexibility Inventory, CFI[2] = The Comparative fit index, RMSE a = Root-mean-square error of approximation, SRMR = Standardized root mean square residual, a = The path coefficient from IV to mediator, b = The path coefficient from mediator to outcome, c' = The path of IV to outcome controlling for mediator, ab = a*b (the indirect effect), IND% = The percentage of the indirect effect on the total effect. **$p < 0.01$, ***$p < 0.001$.

Using a randomized controlled trial, we provided evidence that the MBSR program is effective in cultivating ability to generate alternative explanations. First, MBSR training lead to a significantly greater improvement in cognitive flexibility than waitlist controls. Second, the MBSR group achieved approximately 10 points increase in CFI from pre- to post-treatment, with a medium effect size. Our finding is consistent with another study that reported an 11-point increase in CFI for MBCT training group (Shapero et al., 2018). This finding is consistent with the general idea that MBI should improve the tendency to be mindful in everyday life, which might result in improvements in psychological outcomes, including responding adaptively to life events. Taken together, MBSR appears to be particularly effective in cultivating ability to perceive stressful life events as controllable and to form alternative explanations for stressful situations.

Unexpectedly, we did not replicate MBSR's well-documented effect on psychological distress reduction (Chiesa and Serretti, 2009; Khoury et al., 2015; Ma et al., 2018), which is surprising. Four explanations are possible. First, demographical characteristics and baseline mindfulness might have confounded the treatment effect on the results. We conducted follow-up repeated-measure ANOVAs to include each of the potential covariates (e.g., age, gender, education, family income, initial level of FFMQ). The results showed that the Time by Group interaction was not significant ($ps = 0.14$–0.21), indicating that demographics and initial mindfulness level did not confound the training effect on stress. Second, participants in the MBSR group might have had a low basic stress level, which might lead to limited health benefits from the mindfulness training (Yu et al., 2019). We compared the baseline stress level with previous studies in stressed population without psychiatric disorders (Marcus et al., 2003; Chang et al., 2004; Yu et al., 2019). The abovementioned studies reported that the MBSR

group had an average item score ranging from 1.8 to 2.7 points approximately at pre-treatment, whereas our sample in the MBSR group had an average item score of about 3 points, indicating a relative higher stress level, which did not support this explanation. Third, it is possible that participants in the waitlist group also experienced stress reduction over time. In fact, the waitlist controls in our study experienced substantially reduced stress from pre- to post-treatment (average item scores, pre-treatment: 3.2 points, post-treatment: 2.2 points). However, Yu et al. (2019) reported that waitlist controls perceived slightly higher stress from pre- to post-treatment (average item scores, pre-treatment: 1.8 points, post-treatment: 1.9 points). It is possible that the stress reduction effect for the waitlist controls in our study was driven by natural decay of stress or self-regulation, which warrants further investigations. Fourth, our assessment of stress (CPSS) emphasized the cognitive appraisal (e.g., uncontrollable, unpredictable, and unresolvable) of difficult situations, which did not include other aspects of stress responses (e.g., somatization). Therefore, it is possible that our assessment method was not sensitive enough to capture the severity of stress. These speculations warrant further investigations.

Non-reactivity at Week 6 during intervention had a full mediation effect on intervention group and cognitive flexibility. Our finding suggests that through 6 weeks of mindfulness practice, the Non-reactivity skill, which is about allowing experiences to come and go by themselves, without being attached to or changing them, was a successful and critical means to foster cognitive flexibility. These findings are in accordance with neuroimaging studies. For example, Creswell et al. (2007) found that individuals who showed less openness and acceptance to experiences, exhibited stronger activation in limbic systems when labeling negative thoughts and experiences. Whereas individuals who processed high openness and acceptance to experience exhibited stronger activation in prefrontal regions and inhibition of the limbic responses, suggesting successful inhibiting of habitual responses.

It is important to note that Non-reactivity at Week 3 did not mediate the relationship between intervention group and cognitive flexibility. This finding is not surprising. From path analysis statistics, failure to detect a mediation effect might be due to a disassociation between group and Non-reactivity at Week 3, which indicates the change of Non-reactivity was not attributed to the lack of effectiveness of MBSR. Tracing back to the 8-week MBSR program (Kabat-Zinn, 1990), the first three weeks introduced a small part of Non-reactivity skills. For example, participants were guided to experience bodily sensations, including exploring pain feelings and letting go of the reaction of changing the feeling of pain. In addition, participants were gradually guided to explore and experience emotional experiences, and to not take immediate action. But the most important exercises of Non-reactivity skills were introduced starting in Week 5. For instance, participants were guided to face the life stress, accept their own stress response, and temporarily not react so that they can get rid of the habitual reactions and eventually create a new way of coping. Therefore, for the MBSR group, the improvement of Non-reactivity from pre-treatment to Week 3 was far more subtle (mean at pre-treatment: 20.35, mean at Week 3: 21.56) than Week 6.

Our findings are consistent with the notions that Non-reactivity, cultivated by mindfulness, would alter the association between the perception and appraisal for the environmental stimuli (Lutz et al., 2015). Furthermore, this finding is convergent with growing evidence that non-reaction to emotion leads to beneficial psychological outcomes. For example, after a 3-month training, only Non-reactivity in FFMQ predicted greater reduction in mood symptoms in a present awareness mindfulness training group as compared to a progressive muscle relaxation training group (Gao et al., 2018). It has been suggested that adopting accepting-emotion strategies reduced negative affect (Campbell-Sills et al., 2006), and alleviated anxiousness and avoidance reactions (Levitt et al., 2004). In addition, prior research indicated that the improvement of the Non-reactivity facet from pre- to post-treatment mediated the effect of mindfulness training on decreasing depression symptoms from pre- to post-treatment in clinical samples (Heeren et al., 2015). These findings suggest that Non-reactivity may be a powerful mechanism of mindfulness. The underlying process might be that higher levels of Non-reactivity make it easier for people to disengage from established but unhelpful responses (Malinowski, 2013; Makowski et al., 2019), switch mental states adaptively, inhibit habitual responses, and thus have time to improve the ability to generate new appraisals and solutions to difficult situations. It is possible that the treatment targeted aspects directly linked to the content of the items included in the CFI. The CFI had a moderately positive correlation with the FFMQ at baseline ($r = 0.35$, $p = 0.008$), indicating a link between them. These speculations warrant further investigation. In summary, Non-reactivity is one important component of the effectiveness of MBSR training on cognitive flexibility.

For the longitudinal trajectories of FFMQ scales across four time points, we found the only the Non-reactivity scale fitted the latent curve model well. There was substantial individual variability in the initial score. All individuals increased on Non-reactivity at the same rate. However, the inclusion of group as a covariate resulted in a statistically significant growth rate. Specifically, the MBSR group increased at a faster speed than the waitlist controls.

Contrary to our hypothesis, Non-judgment during intervention did not mediate the effect of intervention group and cognitive flexibility. We make two speculations in explaining this finding. First, because some participants missed some assessment points, results might be biased. This is especially true for the waitlist control group, because those participants who persisted might have had greater interests in mindfulness than those who discontinued. Therefore, they might have been motivated to learn more about mindfulness from reading books or other materials, in which Non-judgment might be mentioned frequently. Over time, they would report a higher level Non-judgment skills, making the MBSR training effect of Non-judgment less notable. Second, improvements of Non-judgment at Week 3 and Week 6 were not explained by the efficacy of MBSR training. This speculation is supported by the fact that "a" path coefficients were not significant (for Non-judgment at Week 3: $a = -0.03$, SE = 0.13, $p = 0.82$; for Non-judgment at Week 6: $a = -0.13$, SE = 0.11, $p = 0.24$).

Several limitations should be considered. The present study had a small sample size, which might lower the statistical power. Our sample comprised of mostly women and highly educated participants, therefore conclusions should be taken with caution if generalizing to heterogeneous samples. We recruited participants without DSM-diagnosed mental illness, which may weaken the motivation of engagement with MBSR. In terms of practice duration, previous literatures showed that college students practiced 1.5 times/week (13 min/time) on average (Solhaug et al., 2019), whereas the mean practice durations in smokers were 20.89 min/day (Goldberg et al., 2014). Unfortunately, we did not collect the data of practice duration in this study to examine this issue. We used waitlist group (without any treatment) as controls, which could not explore the specific effect of mindfulness training. Measures were self-report instruments, which might be biased by retrospective memory and we did not assess actual life events. Future studies should consider measuring stressful life events, because cognitive flexibility may not only be trait-like stable but also context dependent (Schultz and Searleman, 2002). Furthermore, the missing outcome data might have biased the estimation of the treatment effect. Follow-up data were not collected, thus the maintenance effect remains in question. Future studies should use larger samples to test the replicability of this finding. Samples should include larger proportions of men and low-educated populations to test the generalization of the conclusion. Active controls such as psycho-education or relaxation training should be taken into account to test the specific effect of MBSR. Follow-up assessments would be needed to explore the maintenance effect, or the long-term benefits of improving cognitive flexibility. Finally, future studies are needed to examine other facets of mindfulness and their specific effects on stress and emotions (Carpenter et al., 2019).

Despite the abovementioned limitations, our findings exhibit sufficient statistical power and indicated that MBSR training is effective in improving flexible cognitions (perceived control and alternative explanations and solutions) confronting stressful life events, with a medium effect size. Furthermore, our findings suggest that Non-reactivity is the primary focus for MBSR training to increase cognitive flexibility. Our findings bridge knowledge gaps in prior studies by elucidating that Non-reactivity mediated the efficacy of mindfulness training on cognitive flexibility.

ETHICS STATEMENT

This research involves human participants. All procedures performed in studies involving human participants were in accordance with the ethical standards of the research committee (the Association for Ethics and Human and Animal Protection in School of Psychological and Cognitive Sciences, Peking University, 2018-10-02) and with the 1964 Helsinki Declaration and its later amendments or comparable ethical standards. Informed consent was obtained from all individual participants included in the study.

AUTHOR CONTRIBUTIONS

YZ collected, analyzed, and interpreted the data, and wrote the drafts of the manuscript. PL collected the data. SH collaborated in the commenting on and editing the drafts of the manuscript. XL designed the study, taught part of the MBSR program, interpreted the findings, and commented critically on the drafts of the manuscript.

ACKNOWLEDGMENTS

We are grateful for all the participants. We would like to thank Xiaoming Wang who taught part of the MBSR programs, Ruixiang Cao who administered clinical assessment, Mengyao He who helped with data collection, and Pinaire Megan who helped improve the overall English language.

REFERENCES

American Psychiatric Association [APA] (1994). *Diagnostic and Statistical Manual of Mental Disorders*, 4th Edn. Washington, DC: American Psychiatric Association.

Baer, R. A. (2003). Mindfulness training as a clinical intervention: a conceptual and empirical review. *Clin. Psychol. Sci. Pract.* 10, 125–143. doi: 10.1093/clipsy.bpg015

Baer, R. A., Carmody, J., and Hunsinger, M. (2012). Weekly change in mindfulness and perceived stress in a mindfulness-based stress reduction program. *J. Clin. Psychol.* 68, 755–765. doi: 10.1002/jclp.21865

Baer, R. A., Smith, G. T., Lykins, E., Button, D., Krietemeyer, J., Sauer, S., et al. (2008). Construct validity of the five facet mindfulness questionnaire in meditating and nonmeditating samples. *Assessment* 15, 329–342. doi: 10.1177/1073191107313003

Baron, R. M., and Kenny, D. A. (1986). The moderator-mediator variable distinction in social psychological research: conceptual, strategic, and statistical considerations. *J. Pers. Soc. Psychol.* 51, 1173–1182. doi: 10.1037//0022-3514.51.6.1173

Bishop, S. R., Lau, M., Shapiro, S., Carlson, L., Anderson, N. D., Carmody, J., et al. (2004). Mindfulness: a proposed operational definition. *Clin. Psychol. Sci. Pract.* 11, 230–241. doi: 10.1093/clipsy.bph077

Campbell-Sills, L., Barlow, D. H., Brown, T. A., and Hofmann, S. G. (2006). Effects of suppression and acceptance on emotional responses of individuals with anxiety and mood disorders. *Behav. Res. Ther.* 44, 1251–1263. doi: 10.1016/j.brat.2005.10.001

Carpenter, J. K., Conroy, K., Gomez, A. F., Curren, L. C., and Hofmann, S. G. (2019). The relationship between trait mindfulness and affective symptoms: a meta-analysis of the five facet mindfulness questionnaire (FFMQ). *Clin. Psychol. Rev.* 74:101785. doi: 10.1016/j.cpr.2019.101785

Chambless, D. L., and Gillis, M. M. (1993). Cognitive therapy of anxiety disorders. *J. Consult. Clin. Psychol.* 61, 248–260.

Chang, V. Y., Palesh, O., Caldwell, R., Glasgow, N., Abramson, M., Luskin, F., et al. (2004). The effects of a mindfulness-based stress reduction program on stress, mindfulness self-efficacy, and positive states of mind. *Stress Health* 20, 141–147. doi: 10.1002/smi.1011

Chanowitz, B., and Langer, E. J. (1981). Premature cognitive commitment. *J. Pers. Soc. Psychol.* 41, 1051–1063. doi: 10.1037/0022-3514.41.6.1051

Cheng, C., and Cheung, M. (2005). Cognitive processes underlying coping flexibility: differentiation and integration. *J. Pers.* 73, 859–886. doi: 10.1111/j.1467-6494.2005.00331.x

Chiesa, A., and Serretti, A. (2009). Mindfulness-based stress reduction for stress management in healthy people: a review and meta-analysis. *J. Altern. Complement. Med.* 15, 593–600. doi: 10.1089/acm.2008.0495

Cohen, J. (1988). *Statistical Power Analysis for the Behavioral Sciences*. New York, NY: Routledge.

Cohen, J. (1992). A power primer. *Psychol. Bull.* 112, 155–159.

Cohen, S., Kamarck, T., and Mermelstein, R. (1983). A global measure of perceived stress. *J. Health Soc. Behav.* 24, 385–396.

Creswell, J. D., and Lindsay, E. K. J. C. D. I. P. S. (2014). How does mindfulness training affect health? A mindfulness stress buffering account. *Curr. Dir. Psychol. Sci.* 23, 401–407. doi: 10.1177/0963721414547415

Creswell, J. D., Way, B. M., Eisenberger, N. I., and Lieberman, M. D. (2007). Neural correlates of dispositional mindfulness during affect labeling. *Psychosom. Med.* 69, 560–565. doi: 10.1097/PSY.0b013e3180f6171f

Dajani, D. R., and Uddin, L. Q. (2015). Demystifying cognitive flexibility: implications for clinical and developmental neuroscience. *Trends Neurosci.* 38, 571–578. doi: 10.1016/j.tins.2015.07.003

Deng, Y. Q., Liu, X. H., Rodriguez, M. A., and Xia, C. Y. (2011). The five facet mindfulness questionnaire: psychometric properties of the Chinese version. *Mindfulness* 2, 123–128. doi: 10.1177/1073191113485121

Dennis, J. P., and Vander Wal, J. S. (2010). The cognitive flexibility inventory: instrument development and estimates of reliability and validity. *Cogn. Ther. Res.* 34, 241–253. doi: 10.1007/s10608-009-9276-4

Derubeis, R. J., Evans, M. D., Hollon, S. D., Garvey, M. J., and Tuason, V. B. (1991). How does cognitive therapy work? Cognitive change and symptom change in cognitive therapy and pharmacotherapy for depression. *J. Consult. Clin. Psychol.* 58, 862–869. doi: 10.1037//0022-006x.58.6.862

Faul, F., Erdfelder, E., Lang, A. G., and Buchner, A. (2007). G*Power 3: a flexible statistical power analysis program for the social, behavioral, and biomedical sciences. *Behav. Res. Methods* 39, 175–191. doi: 10.3758/bf03193146

Feldman, G., Hayes, A., Kumar, S., Greeson, J., and Laurenceau, J.-P. (2007). Mindfulness and emotion regulation: the development and initial validation of the cognitive and affective mindfulness scale-revised (CAMS-R). *J. Psychopathol. Behav. Assess.* 29, 177–190. doi: 10.1007/s10862-006-9035-8

First, M. B., Spitzer, R. L., Gibbon, M., and Williams, J. B. W. (2002). *Structured Clinical Interview for DSM-IV-TR Axis I Disorders, Research Version, Patient Edition. (SCID-I/P)*. New York, NY: New York State Psychiatric Institute.

Ford, C., and Shook, N. (2018). Negative cognitive bias and perceived stress: independent mediators of the relation between mindfulness and emotional distress. *Mindfulness* 10, 100–110. doi: 10.1007/s12671-018-0955-7

Frewen, P. A., Evans, E. M., Maraj, N., Dozois, D. J. A., and Partridge, K. (2008). Letting go: mindfulness and negative automatic thinking. *Cogn. Ther. Res.* 32, 758–774. doi: 10.1007/s10608-007-9142-1

Gao, L., Curtiss, J., Liu, X., and Hofmann, S. G. (2018). Differential treatment mechanisms in mindfulness meditation and progressive muscle relaxation. *Mindfulness* 9, 1268–1279. doi: 10.1007/s12671-017-0869-9

Goldberg, S. B., Del Re, A. C., Hoyt, W. T., and Davis, J. M. (2014). The secret ingredient in mindfulness interventions? A case for practice quality over quantity. *J. Couns. Psychol.* 61, 491–497. doi: 10.1037/cou000 0032

Gustafsson, H., Davis, P., Skoog, T., Kenttä, G., and Haberl, P. (2015). Mindfulness and its relationship with perceived stress, affect, and burnout in elite junior athletes. *J. Clin. Sport Psychol.* 9, 263–281. doi: 10.1123/jcsp.2014-0051

Hayes, S. C., Strosahl, K. D., and Wilson, K. G. (1999). *Acceptance and Commitment Therapy: An Experiential Approach to Behavior Change.* New York, NY: Guilford Press.

Heeren, A., Deplus, S., Peschard, V., Nef, F., Kotsou, I., Dierickx, C., et al. (2015). Does change in self-reported mindfulness mediate the clinical benefits of mindfulness training? A controlled study using the French translation of the five facet mindfulness questionnaire. *Mindfulness* 6, 553–559. doi: 10.1007/s12671-014-0287-1

Hofmann, S. G., Sawyer, A. T., Witt, A. A., and Oh, D. (2010). The Effect of mindfulness-based therapy on anxiety and depression: a meta-analytic review. *J. Consult. Clin. Psychol.* 78, 169–183. doi: 10.1037/a0018555

Hu, L. T., and Bentler, P. M. (1999). Cutoff criteria for fit indexes in covariance structure analysis: conventional criteria versus new alternatives. *Struct. Equ. Model.* 6, 1–55. doi: 10.1080/10705519909540118

Kabat-Zinn, J. (1990). *Full Catastrophe Living: Mindfulness Meditation in Everyday Life.* New York, NY: Delacorte.

Kabat-Zinn, J. (2003). Mindfulness-based interventions in context: past, present, and future. *Clin. Psychol. Sci. Pract.* 10, 144–156. doi: 10.1093/clipsy.bpg016

Kashdan, T. B., and Rottenberg, J. (2010). Psychological flexibility as a fundamental aspect of health. *Clin. Psychol. Rev.* 30, 865–878. doi: 10.1016/j.cpr.2010.03.001

Kazdin, A. E. (2007). Mediators and mechanisms of change in psychotherapy research. *Annu. Rev. Clin. Psychol.* 3, 1–27. doi: 10.1016/j.cpr.2016.09.004

Kee, Y. H., and Wang, J. C. K. (2008). Relationships between mindfulness, flow dispositions and mental skills adoption: a cluster analytic approach. *Psychol. Sport Exerc.* 9, 393–411. doi: 10.1016/j.psychsport.2007.07.001

Khoury, B., Lecomte, T., Fortin, G., Masse, M., Therien, P., Bouchard, V., et al. (2013). Mindfulness-based therapy: a comprehensive meta-analysis. *Clin. Psychol. Rev.* 33, 763–771. doi: 10.1016/j.cpr.2013.05.005

Khoury, B., Sharma, M., Rush, S. E., and Fournier, C. (2015). Mindfulness-based stress reduction for healthy individuals: a meta-analysis. *J. Psychosom. Res.* 78, 519–528. doi: 10.1016/j.jpsychores.2015.03.009

Kuyken, W., Watkins, E., Holden, E., White, K., Taylor, R. S., Byford, S., et al. (2010). How does mindfulness-based cognitive therapy work? *Behav. Res. Ther.* 48, 1105–1112. doi: 10.1016/j.brat.2010.08.003

Levitt, J. T., Brown, T. A., Orsillo, S. M., and Barlow, D. H. (2004). The effects of acceptance versus suppression of emotion on subjective and psychophysiological response to carbon dioxide challenge in patients with panic disorder. *Behav. Ther.* 35, 747–766. doi: 10.1016/s0005-7894(04)80018-2

Li, Y., Liu, F., Zhang, Q., Liu, X., and Wei, P. (2018). The effect of mindfulness training on proactive and reactive cognitive control. *Front. Psychol.* 9:1002. doi: 10.3389/fpsyg.2018.01002

Lindsay, E. K., and Creswell, J. D. (2017). Mechanisms of mindfulness training: monitor and acceptance theory (MAT). *Clin. Psychol. Rev.* 51, 48–59. doi: 10.1016/j.cpr.2016.10.011

Logue, S. F., and Gould, T. J. (2014). The neural and genetic basis of executive function: attention, cognitive flexibility, and response inhibition. *Pharmacol. Biochem. Behav.* 123, 45–54. doi: 10.1016/j.pbb.2013.08.007

Lutz, A., Jha, A. P., Dunne, J. D., and Saron, C. D. (2015). Investigating the phenomenological matrix of mindfulness-related practices from a neurocognitive perspective. *Am. Psychol.* 70, 632–658. doi: 10.1037/a003 9585 doi: 10.1037/a0039585

Ma, Y., She, Z. Z., Siu, A. F. Y., Zeng, X. L., and Liu, X. H. (2018). Effectiveness of online mindfulness-based interventions on psychological distress and the mediating role of emotion regulation. *Front. Psychol.* 9:2090. doi: 10.3389/fpsyg.2018.02090

MacKinnon, D. P., Lockwood, C. M., Hoffman, J. M., West, S. G., and Sheets,

V. (2002). A comparison of methods to test mediation and other intervening variable effects. *Psychol. Methods* 7, 83–104. doi: 10.1037/1082-989x.7.1.83

Makowski, D., Sperduti, M., Lavallée, S., Nicolas, S., and Piolino, P. (2019). Dispositional mindfulness attenuates the emotional attentional blink. *Conscious. Cogn.* 67, 16–25. doi: 10.1016/j.concog.2018.11.004

Malinowski, P. (2013). Neural mechanisms of attentional control in mindfulness meditation. *Front. Neurosci.* 7:8. doi: 10.3389/fnins.2013.00008

Marcus, M. T., Fine, P. M., Moeller, F. G., Khan, M. M., Pitts, K., Swank, P. R., et al. (2003). Change in stress levels following mindfulness-based stress reduction in a therapeutic community. *Addict. Disord. Their Treat.* 2, 63–68. doi: 10.1097/00132576-200302030-00001

Moore, A., and Malinowski, P. (2009). Meditation, mindfulness and cognitive flexibility. *Conscious. Cogn.* 18, 176–186. doi: 10.1016/j.concog.2008.12.008

Moore, B. A. (2013). Propensity for experiencing flow: the roles of cognitive flexibility and mindfulness. *Humanist. Psychol.* 41, 319–332. doi: 10.1080/08873267.2013.820954

Morris, L., and Mansell, W. (2018). A systematic review of the relationship between rigidity/flexibility and transdiagnostic cognitive and behavioral processes that maintain psychopathology. *J. Exp. Psychopathol.* 9, 1–40.

Muthén, L. K., and Muthén, B. O. (2007). *Mplus User's Guide*, 5th Edn. Los Angeles, CA: Muthén & Muthén.

Newgard, C. D., and Lewis, R. J. (2015). Missing data: how to best account for what is not known. *JAMA* 314, 940–941. doi: 10.1001/jama.2015.10516

Otto, M. W., Fava, M., Penava, S. J., Bless, E., Muller, R. T., and Rosenbaum, J. F. (1997). Life event, mood, and cognitive predictors of perceived stress before and after treatment for major depression. *Cogn. Ther. Res.* 21, 409–420.

Rosseel, Y. (2012). Lavaan: an R package for structural equation modeling. *J. Stat. Softw.* 48, 1–36. doi: 10.3389/fpsyg.2014.01521

Schoemann, A. M., Boulton, A. J., and Short, S. D. (2017). Determining power and sample size for simple and complex mediation models. *Soc. Psychol. Pers. Sci.* 8, 379–386. doi: 10.1177/1948550617715068

Schultz, P. W., and Searleman, A. (2002). Rigidity of thought and behavior: 100 years of research. *Genet. Soc. Gen. Psychol. Monogr.* 128, 165–207.

Schulz, K. F., Altman, D. G., Moher, D., and Consort Group (2010). CONSORT 2010 statement: updated guidelines for reporting parallel group randomised trials. *BMC Med.* 8:18. doi: 10.1186/1741-7015-8-18

Segal, Z. V., Williams, M. G., and Teasdale, J. D. (2012). *Mindfulness-Based Cognitive Therapy for Depression*, 2nd Edn. New York, NY: The Guilford Press.

Senders, A., Bourdette, D., Hanes, D., Yadav, V., and Shinto, L. (2014). Perceived stress in multiple sclerosis: the potential role of mindfulness in health and well-being. *J. Evid. Based Complementary Altern. Med.* 19, 104–111. doi: 10.1177/2156587214523291

Shapiro, S. L., Carlson, L. E., Astin, J. A., and Freedman, B. (2006). Mechanisms of mindfulness. *J. Clin. Psychol.* 62, 373–386.

Shapero, B. G., Greenberg, J., Mischoulon, D., Pedrelli, P., Meade, K., and Lazar, S. W. (2018). Mindfulness-based cognitive therapy improves cognitive functioning and flexibility among individuals with elevated depressive symptoms. *Mindfulness* 9, 1457–1469. doi: 10.1007/s12671-018-0889-0 doi: 10.1007/s12671-018-0889-0

Solhaug, I., de Vibe, M., Friborg, O., Sorlie, T., Tyssen, R., Bjorndal, A., et al. (2019). Long-term mental health effects of mindfulness training: a 4-year follow-up study. *Mindfulness* 10, 1661–1672. doi: 10.1007/s12671-019-01100-2

Van Der Velden, A. M., and Roepstorff, A. (2015). Neural mechanisms of mindfulness meditation: bridging clinical and neuroscience investigations. *Nat. Rev. Neurosci.* 16, 439–439. doi: 10.1038/nrn3916-c1 doi: 10.1038/nrn3916-c1

Wang, Y., Yang, Y., Xiao, W. T., and Su, Q. (2016). Validity and reliability of the Chinese version of the cognitive flexibility inventory in college students. *Chin. Ment. Health J.* 30, 58–63.

Wang, Y. Z., Qi, Z. Z., Hofmann, S. G., Si, M., Liu, X. H., and Xu, W. (2019). Effect of acceptance versus attention on pain tolerance: dissecting two components of mindfulness. *Mindfulness* 10, 1352–1359. doi: 10.1007/s12671-019-1091-8

Wielgosz, J., Goldberg, S. B., Kral, T. R. A., Dunne, J. D., and Davidson, R. J. (2019). Mindfulness meditation and psychopathology. *Annu. Rev. Clin. Psychol.* 15, 285–316. doi: 10.1146/annurev-clinpsy-021815-093423

Xu, W., Oei, T. P., Liu, X., Wang, X., and Ding, C. (2016). The moderating and mediating roles of self-acceptance and tolerance to others in the relationship between mindfulness and subjective well-being. *J. Health Psychol.* 21, 1446–1456. doi: 10.1177/1359105314555170

Xu, W., Rodriguez, M. A., Zhang, Q., and Liu, X. J. M. (2015). The mediating effect of self-acceptance in the relationship between mindfulness and peace of mind. *Mindfulness* 6, 797–802. doi: 10.1007/s12671-014-0319-x

Yang, T. Z., and Huang, H. T. (2003). An epidemiological study on stress among urban residents in social transition period. *Chin. J. Epidemiol.* 24, 760–764.

Yu, S. T., Xu, W., Liu, X. H., and Xiao, L. C. (2019). A controlled study of mindfulness training intervening negative emotions and perceived stress in individuals. *Chin. Ment. Health J.* 33, 40–45.

Zautra, A. J., Davis, M. C., Reich, J. W., Sturgeon, J. A., Arewasikporn, A., and Tennen, H. (2012). Phone-based interventions with automated mindfulness and mastery messages improve the daily functioning for depressed middle-aged community residents. *J. Psychother. Integr.* 22, 206–228. doi: 10.1037/a0029573

12

Harnessing the Four Elements for Mental Health

Jerome Sarris[1,2]*, Michael de Manincor[1], Fiona Hargraves[1] and Jack Tsonis[1,3]

[1] NICM Health Research Institute, Western Sydney University, Westmead, NSW, Australia, [2] Professorial Unit, The Melbourne Clinic, Department of Psychiatry, Melbourne University, Melbourne, VIC, Australia, [3] THRI, Western Sydney University, Campbelltown, NSW, Australia

*Correspondence:
Jerome Sarris
j.sarris@westernsydney.edu.au

Humans are intimately connected to nature, and our physical and mental health is influenced strongly by our environment. The "elements," classically described in humoral theory as Fire, Water, Earth, and Air, all may impact our mental health. In a contemporary sense, these elements reflect a range of modifiable factors: UV light or heat therapy (Fire); sauna, hydrotherapy, and balneotherapy (Water); nature-based exposure therapy and horticulture (Earth); oxygen-rich/clean air exposure; and breathing techniques (Air). This theoretical scoping review paper details the emerging evidence for a range of these elements, covering epidemiological and interventional data, and provides information on how we can engage in "biophilic" activities to harness their potential benefits. Interventional examples with emerging evidentiary support include "forest-bathing," heat therapy, sauna, light therapy, "greenspace" and "bluespace" exercise, horticulture, clay art therapy activities, and pranayamic yoga breathing exercises. Further robust research is however required to firmly validate many of these interventions, and to establish their therapeutic applications for the benefit of specific mental health disorders.

Keywords: lifestyle, mental health, mood, anxiety, psychological, well-being, nature, lifestyle medicine

INTRODUCTION

Humans have an intimate connection to nature, and by our very being, we are part of nature (1). Several distinguished clinicians and historians in centuries past have posited that primordial elements construct a person and that imbalances are the cause of ill health. While scientific advancement has moved well beyond such rudimentary medical theory, there may still be merit in considering some of the basic tenets of the philosophy underpinning the humors for potential application in maintaining or enhancing mental health. At the very least, it should be recognized that some aspects of modernity have had a deleterious effect on mental health (2, 3). While a range of medications have been invented, these have had only modest effects for most psychiatric disorders, and concerns have increased over the impact of negative psychosocial changes such as the breakdown of family units, stressful jobs and a challenging work–life balance, a more sedentary life, poorer nutrition, declining air quality, and a decreased connection with nature. In respect to the diminishing interface with our biosphere than was evident with our ancestors, this is also affecting our microbiome, which is modified by exposure to nature (4).

The classical understanding of the elements and their relationship with human health was advanced by physicians such as Hippocrates and Galen (5). This was characterized as the "four humors," which each pertained to an element with distinct qualities: Melancholic [Earth (dry)], Sanguine [Air (cold)], Choleric [Fire (hot)], and Phlegmatic [Water (moist)]. An imbalance of these elements internally was considered to be responsible for disease. There was also appreciation that external exposure to these elements could modify health *via* redressing imbalance. For example, if a person had signs of melancholia (dry skin, feeling cold, emotionally withdrawn, reduced mobility, and depressed mood), then exposure to warmth, moisture, and activity may be considered to be of assistance. Traditional medicine models including Unani, Ayurveda, and Traditional Chinese Medicine also embodied similar elemental constructs and are still practiced in modern times, with health conditions treated by addressing elemental imbalances and deficiencies (6).

Firstly, *we are not proposing that therapeutic use of "the elements" should replace mainstream pharmacotherapy or psychological techniques.* We are, however, suggesting that enhanced contemporary understanding (and requisite robust research) of this interplay may inform a potential use within an integrative treatment model for mental disorders. This may provide an additional avenue to enhance general mental health and perceived well-being. In the most basic form, as humans, to survive (and indeed thrive) we need clean air, fresh water, a regulated body temperature, and the nutrients that are ultimately derived from the earth. As our understanding of the importance of these aspects on mental health is advancing, so is the consideration of harnessing their benefits for use as potential health-enhancing interventions.

To our knowledge, no academic paper to date has covered a review of the evidence for the mental health applications of all "the elements" in this classic sense; thus, we conducted a broad scoping review of the area. We reviewed pertinent literature from Medline, EBSCO, and Web of Science databases, and selected key literature that best fitted thematically within the domains of "Earth," "Fire," "Water," and "Air." **Figure 1** details the therapeutic interventions covered under these domains. We specifically cover the key literature on 1) the relationship between these elements and mental health (in respect to underlying epidemiological data) and 2) any clinical trials utilizing interventions that fitted thematically under one of the four elements.

EARTH

We categorized this domain to encapsulate aspects pertaining to the influence of direct exposure to earth/soil and flora, time spent in nature (in particular wilderness environments) and the application of "greenspace exercise," interactions with animals, and novel interventions such as clay art therapy.

Adequate exposure to nature (greenspace) may provide benefits for general health, and data support that increased urbanization and exposure to excessive industrialization may negatively impact health (7). The benefits of spending time in nature for mental

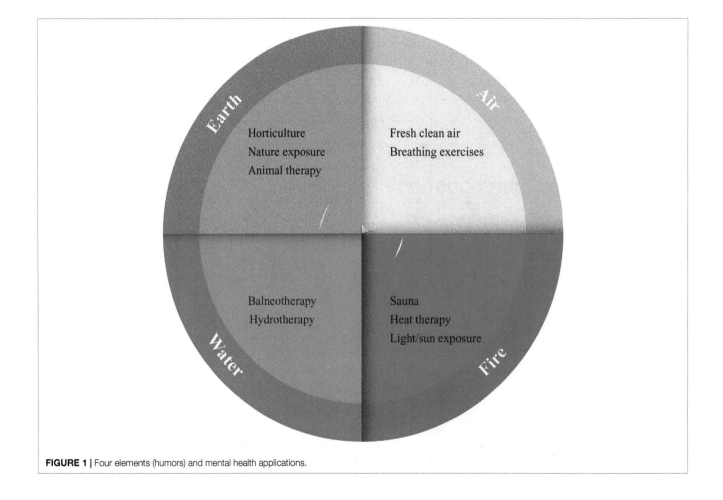

FIGURE 1 | Four elements (humors) and mental health applications.

health are evident (8), including increased exposure to sunlight and fresh air, in addition to a range of beneficial psychosocial elements in some situations. Aside from these benefits, direct interaction with nature (and biodiversity) also impacts the development of the microbiome, which may also have mental health influences (9, 10). While this may be beneficial, when interacting with soil, some caution is needed in terms of potential contaminants (e.g., chemicals and harmful pathogens).

In respect to interventions within this domain, a novel study involving "clay art" therapy conducted a short-term intervention (six 2.5-h sessions) assessing its effects on a range of mental health outcomes for 106 depressed individuals (11). Compared to the visual art group control, depressive symptoms decreased, in addition to improvements in general health and perceived well-being. The therapeutic effects of sufficient greenspace may involve a range of factors, and it is of note that, in children, it also stimulates cognitive development *via* increased scope for risk-taking, imagination, and self-discovery (12).

Actively engaging in horticulture may also improve mental health. A nature-assisted rehabilitation program in a group of general patients ($n = 118$) with noted severe stress levels and/or mild to moderate depression was assessed for changes in sick-leave status and healthcare consumption (13). These patients were compared to matched controls ($n = 678$). Results showed that there were benefits in reduced healthcare consumption for those participating in the rehabilitation garden compared to the control, but no change in sick-leave status.

In respect to being a potential adjunctive intervention in people with a range of psychiatric disorders, a Serbian study was conducted involving 30 patients who participated in a horticultural therapy (HT) program or a control group (occupational art therapy) (14). The results indicated that HT had a positive influence on the mental health and well-being of the participants. Furthermore, a difference was revealed in the test results of the stress subscale before and after the intervention, with a stronger effect for anxious males. Another HT project involving 49 participants undergoing a Veterans Affairs substance abuse treatment program showed that 5 h/day of HT for 3 weeks had a reduction in cortisol levels and a trend for improvement in depressed mood and quality of life compared to usual occupational therapy (15). Other uncontrolled research involving a 12-week HT program ($n = 46$) for people with clinical depression confirmed significant beneficial change in mental health variables during the intervention (16). A reduction in depression severity persisted at 3-months follow-up, and most interesting, an increase in social activity and social cohesion was reported after the intervention. An 8-week indoor gardening program has also revealed beneficial social connectedness and a reduction in loneliness in the elderly confined to nursing homes (17). Further research has shown that compared to a sedentary activity, such as reading, it can even have acute stress-reducing effects, as seen in salivary cortisol reductions (18).

To increase a mental health benefit from exposure to nature, physical activity may also be coupled with this (e.g., nature walks). Such exercise may synergistically increase well-being beyond physical activity in an urban setting (19). While the evidence of specific health benefits from nature-assisted therapy (e.g., wilderness treks) is unclear due to a current lack of rigorous

studies, overall the evidence is supportive of a therapeutic effect. A meta-analytic analysis of 10 UK studies involving a clinical population of participants ($n = 1,252$) with a range of mental disorders found moderate effect sizes for green exercise in improving mood and self-esteem in healthy samples (19). This result also mirrored a systematic review by Annerstedt and Wahrborg (20) who found that for studies of moderate to low evidence grade, health improvements were reported in 26 out of 29 studies. Finally, a systematic review of 11 studies ($n = 833$) on participation in physical activity and exercise in natural environments (versus indoor activity) revealed that 9 out of 11 trials showed some improvement in mental well-being (21). Compared to exercising indoors, exercising in natural environments was associated with decreases in tension, confusion, anger, and depression, and a perceived increase in energy and feelings of positive engagement. Specific examples of nature-based physical activity, with a direct connection to soil or flora, that have shown to enhance mental health outcomes include sailing, gardening, horse-riding, wilderness hiking, and running in nature (19). Green exercise has also been found to be an effective way to reduce the stress of workers, showing an improvement on positive affect and blood pressure beyond urban indoor exercise, in a small-scale acute pilot study ($n = 14$) (22).

One interesting public health application found to occur in Japan (23) is the prescriptive recommendation of "forest bathing," known as "*Shinrin-yoku.*" In simple terms, this involves advising people to spend time in forests. Preliminary evidence reveals that such exposure (compared to time spent in urban settings) can improve general mental health while altering physiological stress and immune biomarkers. Studies have, for example, revealed that short-term exposure to forests reduces levels of malondialdehyde, interleukin-6, tumor necrosis factor alpha, and cortisol, and enhances mental health indices (24). The same research group found a similar beneficial effect in elderly people with chronic heart failure (25). Forest-based therapy has also been found to be beneficial for treating depression and anxiety symptoms in patients with chronic stroke (26). One study involving 55 patients with chronic stroke were randomly assigned to either a stay at a recreational forest site or at an urban hotel. The results revealed lower depression, anxiety, and stress scores in favor of the forest stay group.

Humans commonly have close relationships with animals, and they can provide physical affection and a feeling of unconditional love, assist in the maintenance of a routine, and also provide responsibility and an additional sense of life purpose. Formalized animal-assisted therapy may involve horses (equine therapy), dogs, or even interactions with mammals such as dolphins. Time spent with farm animals by people with a range of psychiatric disorders may reduce depression and state anxiety and increase a sense of self-efficacy (27).

FIRE

We categorized this domain to encapsulate aspects pertaining to the influence of direct exposure to light (sunlight or artificial light) or heat (*via* vectors including sauna, or heated objects applied to the body, e.g., hot rocks).

It is a commonly held transcultural anecdotal belief that one's mood improves when the sun is out, and inclement weather is at bay. While acute exposure to sunshine (and a pleasant temperature according to the individual) may enhance mood, there is an inconsistent relationship with seasonal variations with the prevalence of mood disorders (28, 29). The effects of sunshine exposure on mental health may in part be mediated by vitamin D. However, while low levels of vitamin D appear to be associated with depression risk, there is conflicting evidence as to the effects of supplementation on improving mood (30–32). In fact, one study involving 198 participants with multiple sclerosis who were followed prospectively for an average of 2.3 years revealed that reported sun exposure was inversely associated with depression and fatigue scores (33). Interestingly, only high levels of vitamin D (> 80 nm) were inversely associated with depression scores, but this was not significant after adjustment for reported sun exposure. In other words, the sun exposure, not the vitamin D levels, reflected improvement in mood and energy.

Another facet of "light-based therapy" for mood modulation is in the application of simulating dawn in order to stimulate serotonin and cortisol secretion and to regulate circadian rhythm (34, 35). Several clinical trials have shown that this may be particularly beneficial for seasonal affective disorder (SAD). Randomised controlled trials (RCTs) of 2 to 8 weeks in duration have assessed the differential effectiveness between simulating dawn (half an hour prior to waking between 100 and 300 lux) versus high 1,500–10,000 lux bright light therapy (36–38). Results are conflicting, and both may be potentially effective in SAD, with stronger support for general bright light therapy.

One of the most common health interventions involving the targeted use of heat is sauna, which includes the traditional variety (using radiant heat and hot rocks to create moisture) and the modern infrared variety (which typically uses far-infrared light). To date, significantly more research exists with regard to traditional sauna (39), although emerging evidence suggests that infrared sauna promotes similar physiological benefits (40). While evidence remains preliminary with only a very small number of controlled studies having been conducted on the health effects of regular sauna bathing (40), the basic physiological effects have been known for some time (41).

More recently, the first longitudinal studies have been conducted on a large Finnish cohort ($n = 2315$), with results that show positive outcomes in a range of health domains, such a cardiovascular disease (42), hypertension (43), respiratory illness (44), and even dementia (45). The authors of these studies outline how the physiological response to sauna bathing corresponds to low- and moderate-intensity physical exercise and suggest that "these proposed functional improvements associated with sauna bathing correspond to similar benefits seen with regular physical exercise" (p. 546) (42). Although a current breadth of research is lacking (especially for mental health applications), because the general benefits appear to be associated with increasing activity of the thermoregulatory system, it is reasonable to assume that similar benefits are obtained from other modalities of atmosthermic bathing from different cultural traditions. These include the Islamic "hammam," the Native American "sweat lodge," and the Japanese "onsen," all of which enjoy long-held reputations for their regenerative capacity (46).

One particular aspect of classic sauna practice that requires further interrogation for general and mental health effects is the common adoption of cold exposure after heat exposure (cold showers/air/snow after the sauna). A 2015 study involving 3,018 participants (aged 18–65 years) without severe comorbidity and no routine experience of cold showering were randomized to hot and cold shower cycles (or a control group) during 30 consecutive days followed by 60 days of showering cold at their own discretion for the intervention groups (47). The primary outcome was illness days and related sickness absence from work. Results revealed a 29% reduction in sickness absence for hot to cold showers compared to the control group, but not illness days in adults without severe comorbidity. These results suggest that further investigation into cold exposure and sauna bathing is an important area of research, especially considering the prevalence of the practice at a global level.

At least one small study exists ($n = 9$), but this examined acute body temperatures rather than longer-term effects and did not investigate qualitative differences in perception of sauna enjoyment as a result of cold exposure (48). Another study from 2016 ($n = 37$) found that cold water immersion after sauna may be safe for patients with chronic heart failure, but that the practice should be conducted with caution (49). The study likewise did not consider qualitative aspects of cold exposure, which has been described as eliciting perceived regeneration in recent ethnographic literature (50). While outside the focus of this review (and in direct contrast to heat based therapies), there is also a recognized potential use of cold therapy alone (cryotherapy) for a range of health applications.

In respect to specific effects on mental health outcomes from sauna, there is overwhelming anecdotal evidence from traditional folklore (46), but minimal scientific or sociological evidence. In the same Finnish cohort discussed above, there was found to be a strong association between frequent sauna bathing and a reduction of psychotic disorders after a median follow-up of 25 years (51), but this is the only longitudinal evidence currently available. Other studies have suggested a positive effect of mood from a Korean "jjimjilbang" sauna (52, 53), as well as reduction of pain intensity in chronic conditions such as hypertension headaches (54). Given the prevalence of anecdotal reports about the relationship between sauna and improved mental health, this is another promising line of investigation that requires sustained attention from the global scientific community, especially in light of recent positive results concerning the use of whole body hyperthermic (WBH) therapy to alleviate major depressive disorder (55). WBH involves the use of sustained heat for 1–2 h to raise core body temperature (sometimes via a device that heats the inside of a tent that covers the body).

A prior uncontrolled study found that a single session of WBH reduced depressive symptoms in people experiencing depression, and thus researchers sought to test whether this effect would outperform a sham control condition (a matched procedure but with no heat). They assessed a single acute treatment in a 6-week, randomized, double-blind study involving 34 adults with major depressive disorder (MDD) (55). Results revealed that compared with the sham group (mimicking all attributes accept the intense heat), just one WBH therapy treatment showed significantly reduced depression scores maintained across the 6-week post-intervention study period.

WATER

We categorized this domain to encapsulate aspects pertaining to the influence of direct consumption of water, and the exposure to water, including the use of general hydrotherapy, balneotherapy (treatment of disease *via* bathing in natural mineral springs), and water-based physical activity (56).

Mammalian life requires water for existence, with the human body being composed of approximately 60% water (57). Aside from the importance of adequate hydration for the proper electrolyte balance, intracellular function, and extracellular communication, there may be mood and cognitive consequences of dehydration (58). In respect to mental health effects, a novel study assessing mild dehydration (produced by intermittent moderate exercise) was conducted on 25 healthy females. Participants undertook three 8-h, placebo-controlled experiments involving different hydration states (based on exercise or diuretic-induced states) (59). While most aspects of cognition were not affected, significant adverse effects of 1.36% dehydration showed a degradation in mood, increased perception of task difficulty, lower concentration, and more headache symptoms. This equates to a moderate level of dehydration (many studies will not push the body past 1.50% dehydration due to an increasing range of negative consequences).

The therapeutic application of water is evident in many cultures, especially in respect to natural mineral spa bathing (commonly in hot springs). One study (n = 237) comparing balneotherapy in spa resorts with paroxetine in treating generalized anxiety disorder showed a significant advantage of the spa treatment as assessed on anxiety scales, with remission and sustained response rates also significantly higher in those treated with balneotherapy (60). When compared to progressive muscle relaxation for stress-relief, short-term balneotherapy provided higher subjective ratings of relaxation with healthy participants (n = 49) and was similarly beneficial in decreasing salivary cortisol (61).

Balneotherapy has also been shown to improve quality of life and symptoms of chronic pain in fibromyalgia patients. A study conducted at the Dead Sea for 10 days (n = 48) demonstrated significant improvements on all well-being measures (62). Further evidence from Ozkurt et al. (63) supported these positive effects for fibromyalgia sufferers (n = 50), with their 2-week treatment producing significant improvements on all outcome measures, including pain, fibromyalgia impact, depression, and quality of life. In both studies, follow-up assessments showed physical improvements lasting 3 months on average, while psychological improvements were shorter-lasting, suggesting the benefits of regular balneotherapy in managing fibromyalgia. The classical use of contemporary steam rooms also provides an ambient therapeutic interface with both heat and water.

While in-depth exploration of water-based physical activities are outside the auspices of this review, a couple of novel applications of immersive water-based activities are worth noting. A recent study evaluated Deptherapy, a UK-based charity that provides a scuba diving intervention as support to military veterans who experienced life-changing injuries from combat (64). A total of 15 male veterans were assessed in an uncontrolled format both prospectively and retrospectively on a range of quantitative measures of mental well-being and functional ability outcomes. Participants reported enhancement on a range of psychosocial well-being measures. The researchers posit that scuba diving has the potential in part to benefit injured veterans due to the requirement of complete focus and the feeling of weightlessness when underwater. Another water-based application is in the use of "surf therapy," which has shown to improve participants' well-being (65, 66). It is however recognized that this offers a range of other ancillary benefits (beyond direct effects from the immersion in water), including increased mindfulness and atelic skill development, exposure to fresh air and sunlight, and general physical activity.

AIR

We categorized this domain to encapsulate aspects pertaining to the influence of direct exposure to fresh clean air, conscious and more effective breathing, and specific breathing exercises (such as utilized in yoga, known as *pranayama*). This may be achieved *via* regulated breathing-focused biofeedback techniques (67), which may reduce anxiety and perceived stress. For instance, regulation of natural breathing synchronizes electrical activity in human piriform (olfactory) cortex, as well as modulating limbic-related brain areas (which includes amygdala and hippocampus; key brain areas affecting anxiety/stress, and memory) (68).

One key environmental factor that is recognized to influence physical health involves the increased exposure to particulate air pollution, which is one common issue of modernity (69). This has been found to have a potential profound effect on the central nervous system. Exposure to air pollution, for example, has been found in a longitudinal study of 537 elderly Koreans to be associated with an increase in depressive symptoms (70). Additionally, evidence from a cross-sectional study indicates that secondhand cigarette smoke is positively associated with increased depressive symptoms in smoking-naive people (even after adjustment for a range of demographic factors and comorbidities) (71, 72).

Emerging preclinical evidence suggests that air pollution may induce oxidative stress, neuroinflammation, microglial activation, and cerebrovascular dysfunction, while potentially altering the blood–brain barrier (73). For example, a mouse model study investigated whether long-term (10 months) exposure to ambient fine airborne particulate matter compared to filtered air affected depression-related animal behavior and cognitive responses (74). The data revealed that mice exposed to long-term air pollution displayed more depressive-like responses and impairments in spatial learning and memory as compared with mice exposed to filtered air.

As well as the quality of the air that we breathe, the way that we breathe is also associated with our health and well-being. While functional and dysfunctional breathing are difficult to define, dysfunctional breathing, including restricted, shallow, rapid, or irregular breathing, is implicated in a range of physical and psychological health conditions (67). In particular, dysfunctional breathing is recognized as symptomatic of depression and anxiety, and there is a corresponding high prevalence of depression and anxiety among people with chronic breathing disorders (75).

Mindful breath awareness (MBA) and breath regulation techniques (BRTs) have been reported as the most commonly used mind–body therapy by adults with medical conditions in the United States (76) and the second most commonly used of all complementary health approaches (second only after all natural dietary supplements combined) (77). MBA and BRTs are commonly used as components of psychological and complementary treatments for mental health conditions, including cognitive behavior therapy (CBT), mindfulness-based cognitive therapy (MBCT), mindfulness-based stress reduction (MBSR), and mind–body practices in general, including yoga, taichi, qigong, relaxation training, and mindfulness and other forms of meditation (78). Each of these has been studied in clinical research and included in numerous reviews (78–82).

Clinical studies that have focused on BRTs as a primary intervention for general mental health are mostly yoga-based breathing exercises. MBA and BRTs are integral to several aspects of yoga practice. For example, yoga postures are ideally done with MBA and coordination of breath with movements; specific yoga BRTs (known as *pranayama*), relaxation, and meditation techniques often use the breath as a means to relax and focus the mind. Several clinical studies have found that yoga BRTs were effective in reducing severity of depressive symptoms (83–87). One RCT using a yoga BRT technique, known as Sudarshan Kriya Yoga (SKY), found that the technique was equally as effective as both electroconvulsive therapy (ECT) and a commonly prescribed pharmacological antidepressant (imipramine) for clinical depression over a 4-week period (85). Later studies using the same yoga BRT also found reductions in depressive symptoms among alcohol-dependent participants following a detox program (87) and reductions in posttraumatic stress (PTS) and depressive symptoms among survivors of the 2004 Southeast Asia Tsunami (84). More recent studies that incorporate MBA into multi-component yoga interventions have also found benefits for reducing symptoms of depression and anxiety and improving well-being (83, 86). Streeter and colleagues have also found preliminary evidence that suggests that breath-centered yoga practices increase gamma amino-butyric acid (GABA) levels in the brain, which is associated with improvements in depression (88).

Several researchers have postulated neuro-physiological models to explain the benefits of breath-centered yoga practices in diverse, frequently comorbid medical conditions, including mental health disorders, based on the concept and evidence that yoga practices reduce allostatic load in stress response systems and restore homeostasis and balance in the human system (88, 89). They hypothesize that breath-centered yoga-based practices 1) correct underactivity of the parasympathetic nervous system (PNS), in part through stimulation of the vagus nerves, the main peripheral pathway of the PNS; 2) increase low levels of GABA; and 3) reduce the allostatic load of stress. Depression, anxiety, PTS, and chronic pain exemplify medical and mental health conditions that are exacerbated by stress, have low heart rate variability (HRV) and impaired GABAergic activity, respond to pharmacologic agents that increase activity of the GABA system, and show symptom improvement in response to breath-centered yoga-based interventions (88, 89).

DISCUSSION

As detailed above, the "elements" in both a classical and a contemporary sense have effects on our mental health and are potentially modifiable aspects that can be harnessed as therapeutic interventions. The most robust interventional evidence currently available shows tentative support for several use of the elements *via* horticultural and nature-exposure therapy, green exercise/physical activity, sauna and heat therapy, balneotherapy, and breathing exercises. It should be noted that, in many cases, these interventions were not studied in definitive diagnosed psychiatric disorders and thus it is premature to consider these therapies to be gold standard treatments. Regardless, the evidence does reveal many positive general mental health benefits. The mechanisms of action underpinning these lifestyle medicine approaches are varied (due to the breadth of interventions covered). More attention is required to tease out the direct health effect of the elements, as many interventions will have other confounding aspects such as physical activity, mindfulness, or attention-based activity, they may also have a social interface component, and finally commonly will have a range of nature-based environmental influences (involving increased exposure to sunlight, fresh air, etc). As detailed above, known health effects for example include early morning light increasing serotonin and cortisol production, modulation of core temperature boosting circulation and the immune response, breathing regulation affecting a range of neurochemical effects and HRV and blood flow dynamics, and exposure to flora and fauna altering the microbiome.

While it is understood that this paper does not follow a strict reductive analysis of specific techniques for specified psychiatric disorders, it is intended to provide a paradigm to be able to expand a different way of thinking, particularly for the consideration of novel interventions that may work alongside conventional treatments to enhance mental health. It is clearly accepted that many of the interventions do not currently possess firm evidentiary support, and further research employing randomized and controlled designs (ideally within mixed-methods designs) is required. Promising areas of future inquiry concern further research into the impact of the elements on mental health, in particular interventions such as sauna and heat therapy, hydrotherapy, and nature-exposure therapies.

There are many potential benefits of "harnessing the four elements" for health purposes. This approach can be recognized as being considered part of the emerging field of "lifestyle medicine." Aside from providing the fundamentals of sustaining life, and the potential mental health benefits detailed above, there are a range of ancillary advantages. Such approaches may enhance social connectivity, improve physical health, may enhance brain health and cognition, and increase "self-efficacy" or mastery (90). These approaches are generally very low-cost, although choices may be limited in developing countries and those with overindustrialized, polluted environments. In respect to clinical considerations for more mainstream lifestyle medicine implementation, recent data from Sweden suggest that there are a range of barriers still persisting (91). Major factors for why lifestyle modifications are not being more commonly implemented in clinical practice include a lack of knowledge and roles, lack of organizational support and resources, a low perceived importance of these measures, and a deficit of time to provide the needed attention. Overcoming these barriers within the mental health sphere also presents with more challenges in respect to increased comorbidity, potential motivational issues, lower socioeconomic status in those with more severe mental illness, and a deficit in most jurisdictions of qualified clinical staff with lifestyle medicine-focused skills and training. While there is no easy solution at present, the increased academic emphasis on the emerging lifestyle medicine field should increase awareness and, with an evolving evidentiary base, be able to interface more profoundly with policy makers and clinical bodies.

One further "element" that may be considered within the elemental paradigm is the philosophical consideration of a fifth element, which has been termed as "void," "space," or "ether." This element is generally not present in the Hippocratic–Western framework, yet it is found in other traditional systems such as Ayurveda. A more abstract-related connection to this concept is that of our understanding of space and the quantum physics field. Quantum theorists postulate the importance of quantum physics for cognitive neuroscience and psychiatry, and suggest that the laws of quantum mechanics may have an influence on the dynamics of consciousness and the nature of mind (92). A further curious factor relating to space and mental health is a well-documented phenomenon known as the "overview effect," experienced by astronauts travelling into space (93, 94). Viewing the Earth from space has often prompted astronauts to report overwhelming emotion and feelings of identification with humankind and the planet as a whole.

Psychological constructs, such as awe and self-transcendence, appear to contribute to a psychological understanding of the experience of vast open spaces. While such experiences may be associated with well-being and increased altruism and other prosocial behavior, in some cases they can also be associated with increased fear and anxiety (94). There are many factors associated with mental health, open spaces, and space travel, and they warrant further investigation for mental health implications, including for the majority of us who do not leave the planet.

At the heart of this paper is encouragement for the psychiatric field (and the broader medical field) to consider going back to basics in terms of understanding the importance and the potential utilization of the elements for mental health. Of course, we are not diminishing the importance of pharmacotherapy and psychological techniques for psychiatric disorders. We are however saying that nature still holds a key to addressing many of the woes that currently plague society. We are becoming increasingly more socially isolated and hyperstimulated, and connecting more intimately to the biosphere and our fellow humans will always provide mental health sustenance.

AUTHOR CONTRIBUTIONS

JS: lead author and contributor to the earth section. MdM: contribution to section on air. FH: contribution to section on water, referencing, and editing. JT: contribution to section on fire.

REFERENCES

Logan AC, Selhub EM. Vis Medicatrix naturae: does nature "minister to the mind"? *Biopsychosoc Med* (2012) 6(1):11. doi: 10.1186/1751-0759-6-11

Hidaka B. Depression as a disease of modernity: explanations for increasing prevalence. *J Affect Disord* (2012) 140(3):205–14. doi: 10.1016/j.jad.2011.12.036

Roberts M. Modernity, mental illness and the crisis of meaning. *J Psychiatr Ment Health Nurs* (2007) 14(3):277–81. doi: 10.1111/j.1365-2850.2007.01074.x

Logan AC, Katzman MA, Balanzá-Martínez V. Natural environments, ancestral diets, and microbial ecology: is there a modern "paleo-defi t disorder"? Part I. *Physiol Anthropol* (2015) 34:1. doi: 10.1186/s40101-015-0041-y

Stelmack R, Stalikas A. Galen and the humour theory of temperament. *Pers Individ Dif* (1991) 12(3):255–63. doi: 10.1016/0191-8869(91)90111-N

Patwardhan B, Warude D, Pushpangadan P, Bhatt N. Ayurveda and traditional Chinese medicine: a comparative overview. *Evid Based Complement Alternat Med* (2005) 2(4):465–73. doi: 10.1093/ecam/neh140

Keniger L, Gaston K, Irvine K, Fuller R. What are the benefits of interacting with nature? *Int J Environ Res Public Health* (2013) 10:913–35. doi: 10.3390/ijerph10030913

Barton J, Rogerson M. The importance of greenspace for mental health. *BJPsych Int* (2017) 14(4):79–81. doi: 10.1192/S2056474000002051

Tasnim N, Abulizi N, Pither J, Hart MM, Gibson DL. Linking the gut microbial ecosystem with the environment: does gut health depend on where we live? *Front Microbiol* (2017) 8:1935. doi: 10.3389/fmicb.2017.01935

Aerts R, Honnay O, Van Nieuwenhuyse A. Biodiversity and human health: mechanisms and evidence of the positive health effects of diversity in nature and green spaces. *Br Med Bull* (2018) 127(1):5–22. doi: 10.1093/bmb/ldy021

Nan J, Ho R. Effects of clay art therapy on adults outpatients with major depressive disorder: a randomized controlled trial. *J Affect Disord* (2017) 217:237–45. doi: 10.1016/j.jad.2017.04.013

Dadvand P, Tischer C, Estarlich M, Llop S, Dalmau-Bueno A, López- Vicente M, et al. Lifelong residential exposure to green space and attention: a population-based prospective study. *Environ Health Perspect* (2017) 125(9):097016. doi: 10.1289/EHP694

Wahrborg P, Petersson I, Grahn P. Nature-assisted rehabilitation for reactions to severe stress and/or depression in a rehabilitation garden: long-term follow-up including comparisons with a matched population-based reference cohort. *J Rehabil Med* (2014) 46(3):271–6. doi: 10.2340/16501977-1259

Vujcic M, Tomicevic-Dubljevic J, Grbic M, Lecic-Tosevski D, Vukovic O, Toskovic O. Nature based solution for improving mental health and well-being in urban areas. *Environ Res* (2017) 158:385–92. doi: 10.1016/j. envres.2017.06.030

Detweiler MB, Self JA, Lane S, Spencer L, Lutgens B, Kim DY, et al. Horticultural therapy: a pilot study on modulating cortisol levels and indices of substance craving, posttraumatic stress disorder, depression, and quality of life in veterans. *Altern Ther Health Med* (2015) 21(4):36–41.

Gonzalez M, Hartig T, Patil GG, Martinsen EW, Kirkevold M. A prospective study of group cohesiveness in therapeutic horticulture for clinical depression. *Int J Ment Health Nurs* (2011) 20(2):119–29. doi: 10.1111/j.1447-0349.2010.00689.x

Tse M. Therapeutic effects of an indoor gardening programme for older people living in nursing homes. *J Clin Nurs* (2010) 19(7–8):949–58. doi: 10.1111/j.1365-2702.2009.02803.x

Van Den Berg A, Custers M. Gardening promotes neuroendocrine and affective restoration from stress. *J Health Psychol* (2011) 16(1):3–11. doi: 10.1177/1359105310365577

Barton J, Pretty J. What is the best dose of nature and green exercise for improving mental health? A multi-study analysis. *Environ Sci Technol* (2010) 44(10):3947–55. doi: 10.1021/es903183r

Annerstedt M, Wahrborg P. Nature-assisted therapy: systematic review of controlled and observational studies. *Scand J Public Health* (2011) 39(4):371–88. doi: 10.1177/1403494810396400

Thompson Coon J, Boddy K, Stein K, Whear R, Barton J, Depledge MH. Does participating in physical activity in outdoor natural environments have a greater effect on physical and mental wellbeing than physical activity indoors? A systematic review. *Environ Sci Technol* (2011) 45(5):1761–72. doi: 10.1021/es102947t

Calogiuri G, Evensen K, Weydahl A, Andersson K, Patil G, Ihlebæk C, et al. Green exercise as a workplace intervention to reduce job stress. Results from a pilot study. *Work* (2015) 53(1):99–111. doi: 10.3233/WOR-152219

Takayama N, Korpela K, Lee J, Morikawa T, Tsunetsugu Y, Park BJ, et al. Emotional, restorative and vitalizing effects of forest and urban environments at four sites in Japan. *Int J Environ Res Public Health* (2014) 11(7):7207–30. doi: 10.3390/ijerph110707207

Mao G, Lan XG, Cao YB, Chen ZM, He ZH, Lv YD, et al. Effects of short-term forest bathing on human health in a broad-leaved evergreen forest in Zhejiang Province, China. *Biomed Environ Sci* (2012) 25(3):317–24. doi: 10.3967/0895-3988.2012.03.010

Mao G, Cao Y, Wang B, Wang S, Chen Z, Wang J, et al. The salutary influence of forest bathing on elderly patients with chronic heart failure. *Int J Environ Res Public Health* (2017) 14(4):368. doi: 10.3390/ijerph14040368

Chun MH, Chang MC, Lee S-J. The effects of forest therapy on depression and anxiety in patients with chronic stroke. *Int J Neurosci* (2017) 127(3):199–203. doi: 10.3109/00207454.2016.1170015

Berget B, Braastad BO. Animal-assisted therapy with farm animals for persons with psychiatric disorders. *Ann Ist Super Sanita* (2011) 47(4):384–90. doi: 10.4415/ANN_11_04_10

Hahn IH, Grynderup MB, Dalsgaard SB, Thomsen JF, Hansen AM, Kaergaard A, et al. Does outdoor work during the winter season protect against depression and mood difficulties? *Scand J Work Environ Health* (2011) 37(5):446–9. doi: 10.1016/j.psychres.2008.10.025

Radua J, Pertusa A, Cardoner N. Climatic relationships with specifi clinical subtypes of depression. *Psychiatry Res* (2010) 175(3):217–20. doi: 10.1016/j.psychres.2008.10.025

Sanders KM, Stuart AL, Williamson EJ, Jacka FN, Dodd S, Nicholson G, et al. Annual high-dose vitamin D3 and mental well-being: randomised controlled trial. *Br J Psychiatry* (2011) 198(5):357–64. doi: 10.1192/bjp.bp.110.087544

Berk M, Sanders KM, Pasco JA, Jacka FN, Williams LJ, Hayles AL, et al. Vitamin D deficiency may play a role in depression. *Med Hypotheses* (2007) 69(6):1316–9. doi: 10.1016/j.mehy.2007.04.001

Berk M, Jacka F. Preventive strategies in depression: gathering evidence for risk factors and potential interventions. *Br J Psychiatry* (2012) 201:339–41. doi: 10.1192/bjp.bp.111.107797

Knippenberg S, Damoiseaux J, Bol Y, Hupperts R, Taylor BV, Ponsonby AL, et al. Higher levels of reported sun exposure, and not vitamin D status, are associated with less depressive symptoms and fatigue in multiple sclerosis. *Acta Neurol Scand* (2014) 129(2):123–31. doi: 10.1111/ane.12155

Thorn L, Hucklebridge F, Esgate A, Evans P, Clow A. The effect of dawn simulation on the cortisol response to awakening in healthy participants. *Psychoneuroendocrinology* (2004) 29(7):925–30. doi: 10.1016/j.psyneuen.2003.08.005

Ciarleglio CM, Resuehr HE, McMahon DG. Interactions of the serotonin and circadian systems: nature and nurture in rhythms and blues. *Neuroscience* (2011) 197:8–16. doi: 10.1016/j.neuroscience.2011.09.036

Lingjaerde O, Foreland AR, Dankertsen J. Dawn simulation vs. lightbox treatment in winter depression: a comparative study. *Acta Psychiatr Scand* (1998) 98(1):73–80. doi: 10.1111/j.1600-0447.1998.tb10045.x

Avery DH, Eder DN, Bolte MA, Hellekson CJ, Dunner DL, Vitiello MV, et al. Dawn simulation and bright light in the treatment of SAD: a controlled study. *Biol Psychiatry* (2001) 50(3):205–16. doi: 10.1016/S0006-3223(01)01200-8

Terman M, Terman JS. Controlled trial of naturalistic dawn simulation and negative air ionization for seasonal affective disorder. *Am J Psychiatry* (2006) 163(12):2126–33. doi: 10.1176/ajp.2006.163.12.2126

Tsonis J. Sauna studies as an academic field: a new agenda for international research. *Lit Aesth* (2016) 26:41–82. Retrieved from: https://openjournals.library.sydney.edu.au/index.php/LA/article/view/11424/10827.

Hussain J, Cohen M. Clinical effects of regular dry sauna bathing: a systematic review. *Evid Based Complement Alternat Med* (2018) 2018, Article ID 1857413, pp. 30. doi: 10.1155/2018/1857413

Hannuksela M, Ellahham S. Benefits and risks of sauna bathing. *Am J Med* (2001) 110:118–26. doi: 10.1016/S0002-9343(00)00671-9

Laukkanen T, Khan H, Zaccardi F, Laukkanen J. Association between sauna bathing and fatal cardiovascular and all-cause mortality events. *JAMA Intern Med* (2015) 175(4):542–8. doi: 10.1001/jamainternmed.2014.8187

Zaccardi F, Laukkanen T, Willeit P, Kunutsor S, Kauhanen J, Laukkanen J. Sauna bathing and incident hypertension: a prospective cohort study. *Am J Hypertens* (2017) 30(11):1120–5. doi: 10.1093/ajh/hpx102

Kunutsor S, Laukkanen T, Laukkanen J. Sauna bathing reduces the risk of respiratory diseases: a long-term prospective cohort study. *Eur J Epidemiol* (2017) 32:1107. doi: 10.1007/s10654-017-0311-6

Laukkanen T, Kunutsor S, Kauhanen J, Laukkanen J. Sauna bathing is inversely associated with dementia and Alzheimer's disease in middle-aged Finnish men. *Age Ageing* (2017a) 46(2):245–9. doi: 10.1093/ageing/afw212

Aaland M. *Sweat: the illustrated history and description of the Finnish sauna, Russian bania, Islamic hammam, Japanese mushi-buro, Mexican temescal, and American Indian & Eskimo sweat lodge.* Santa Barbara, CA: Capra Press (1978).

Buijze GA, Sierevelt IN, van der Heijden BC, Dijkgraaf MG, Frings-Dresen MH. The effect of cold showering on health and work: a randomized controlled trial. *PloS One* (2016) 11(9):e0161749. doi: 10.1371/journal.pone.0161749

Kauppinen K. Sauna, shower, and ice water immersion: physiological responses to brief exposures to heat, cool, and cold. Part III: body temperatures. *Arctic Med Res* (1989) 48:75–86.

Radtke T, Poerschke D, Wilhelm M, Trachsel L, Tschanz H, Matter F, et al. Acute effects of Finnish sauna and cold-water immersion on haemodynamic variables and autonomic nervous system activity in patients with heart failure. *Eur J Prev Cardiol* (2016) 23(6):593–601. doi: 10.1177/2047487315594506

Tsonis J. 'Another city, another sauna': travel as Saunatarian praxis. *Fieldw Rel* (2018) 13(1):81–106. doi: 10.1558/firn.36290

Laukkanen T, Laukkanen J, Kunutsor S. Sauna bathing and risk of psychotic disorders: a prospective cohort study. *Med Princip Pract* (2018) 27:562–9. doi: 10.1159/000493392

Kuusinen J, Heinonen M. Immediate aftereffects of the Finnish sauna on psychomotor performance and mood. *J App Psych* (1971) 56(4):336–40. doi: 10.1037/h0032942

Hayasakaa S, Nakamurab Y, Kajiic E, Ided M, Shibataa Y, Nodaa Y, et al. Effects of charcoal kiln saunas (jjimjilbang) on psychological states. *Comp Ther Clin Prac* (2008) 14:143–8. doi: 10.1016/j.ctcp.2007.12.004

Kanji G, Weatherall M, Peter R, Purdie G, Page R. Efficacy of regular sauna bathing for chronic tension-type headache: a randomized controlled study. *J Altern Complement Med* (2015) 21(2):103–9. doi: 10.1089/acm.2013.0466

Janssen C, Lowry C, Mehl M, Allen J, Kelly K, Gartner D, et al. Whole-body hyperthermia for the treatment of major depressive disorder: a randomized clinical trial. *JAMA Psychiatry* (2016) 73(8):789–95. doi: 10.1001/jamapsychiatry.2016.1031

Gascon M, Zijlema W, Vert C, White M, Nieuwenhuijsen M. Outdoor blue spaces, human health and well-being: a systematic review of quantitative studies. *Int J Hyg Environ Health* (2017) 220(8):1207–21. doi: 10.1016/j.ijheh.2017.08.004

Jéquier E, Constant F. Water as an essential nutrient: the physiological basis of hydration. *Eur J Clin Nutr* (2010) 64:115–23. doi: 10.1038/ejcn.2009.111

Masento NA, Golightly M, Field DT, Butler LT, van Reekum CM. Effects of hydration status on cognitive performance and mood. *Br J Nutr* (2014) 111(10):1841–52. doi: 10.1017/S0007114513004455

Armstrong LE, Ganio MS, Casa DJ, Lee EC, McDermott BP, Klau JF, et al. Mild dehydration affects mood in healthy young women. *J Nutr* (2012) 142(2):382–8. doi: 10.3945/jn.111.142000

Dubois O, Salamon R, Germain C, Poirier MF, Vaugeois C, Banwarth B, et al. Balneotherapy versus paroxetine in the treatment of generalized anxiety disorder. *Complement Ther Med* (2010) 18(1):1–7. doi: 10.1016/j.ctim.2009.11.003

Matzer F, Nagele E, Bahadori B, Dam K, Fazekas C. Stress-relieving effects of short-term balneotherapy - a randomized controlled pilot study in healthy adults. *Forsch Komplementmed* (2014) 21(2):105–10. doi: 10.1159/000360966

Neumann L, Sukenik S, Bolotin A, Abu-Shakra M, Amir M, Flusser D, et al. The effect of balneotherapy at the Dead Sea on the quality of life of patients with fibromyalgia syndrome. *Clin Rheumatol* (2001) 20(1):15–9. doi: 10.1007/s100670170097

Ozkurt S, Dönmez A, Karagülle M, Uzunoğlu E, Turan M, Erdoğan N. Balneotherapy in fibromyalgia: a single blind randomized controlled clinical study. *Rheumatol Int* (2012) 32(7):1949–54. doi: 10.1007/s00296-011-1888-9

Morgan A, Sinclair H, Tan A, Thomas E, Castle R. Can scuba diving offer therapeutic benefit to military veterans experiencing physical and psychological injuries as a result of combat? A service evaluation of Deptherapy UK. *Disabil Rehabil* (2018) 29:1–9. doi: 10.1080/09638288.2018.1480667

Caddick N, Smith B, Phoenix C. The effects of surfing and the natural environment on the well-being of combat veterans. *Qual Health Res* (2015) 25(1):76–86. doi: 10.1177/1049732314549477

Godfrey C, Devine-Wright H, Taylor J. The positive impact of structured surfing courses on the wellbeing of vulnerable young people. *Commun Pract* (2015) 88(1):26–9.

Courtney R, Greenwood K, Cohen M. Relationships between measures of dysfunctional breathing in a population with concerns about their breathing. *J Bodyw Mov Ther* (2011) 15:24–34. doi: 10.1016/j.jbmt.2010.06.004

Zelano C, Jiang H, Zhou G, Arora N, Schuele S, Rosenow J, et al. Nasal respiration entrains human limbic oscillations and modulates cognitive function. *J Neurosci* (2016) 36(49):12448–67. doi: 10.1523/JNEUROSCI.2586-16.2016

Anderson O, Thundiyil J, Stolbach A. Clearing the air: a review of the effects of particulate matter air pollution on human health. *J Med Toxicol* (2012) 8(2):166–75. doi: 10.1007/s13181-011-0203-1

Lim YH, Kim H, Kim JH, Bae S, Park HY, Hong YC. Air pollution and symptoms of depression in elderly adults. *Environ Health Perspect* (2012) 120(7):1023–8. doi: 10.1289/ehp.1104100

Bandiera FC, Arheart KL, Caban-Martinez AJ, Fleming LE, McCollister K, Dietz NA, et al. Secondhand smoke exposure and depressive symptoms. *Psychosom Med* (2010) 72(1):68–72. doi: 10.1097/PSY.0b013e3181c6c8b5

World Health Organization. *Protection from exposure to second-hand tobacco smoke: policy recommendations*. UCSF: Center for Tobacco Control Research and Education (2007). Retrieved from: https://escholarship.org/uc/ item/0nb6z24q.

Genc S, Zadeoglulari Z, Fuss SH, Genc K. The adverse effects of air pollution on the nervous system. *J Toxicol* (2012) 2012, Article ID 782462, pp. 23. doi: 10.1155/2012/782462

Fonken LK, Xu X, Weil ZM, Chen G, Sun Q, Rajagopalan S, et al. Air pollution impairs cognition, provokes depressive-like behaviors and alters hippocampal cytokine expression and morphology. *Mol Psychiatry* (2011) 16(10):987–95. doi: 10.1038/mp.2011.76

Kunik M, Roundy K, Veazey C, Souchek J, Richardson P, Wray N, et al. Surprisingly high prevalence of anxiety and depression in chronic breathing disorders. *Chest* (2005) 127(4):1205–11. doi: 10.1378/chest.127.4.1205

Bertischa S, Wee C, Phillips R, McCarthy E. Alternative mind–body therapies used by adults with medical conditions. *J Psychosom Res* (2009) 66(6):511–9. doi: 10.1016/j.jpsychores.2008.12.003

Clarke T, Black L, Stussman B, Barnes P, Nahin R. Trends in the use of complementary health approaches among adults: United States, 2002–2012. *Natl Health Stat Report* (2015) 10(79):1–16. Retrieved from: https://www. ncbi.nlm. nih.gov/pmc/articles/PMC4573565/.

Morgan A, Jorm A. Self-help interventions for depressive disorders and depressive symptoms: a systematic review. *Ann Gen Psychiatry* (2008) 7:13. doi: 10.1186/1744-859X-7-13

Cramer H, Lauche R, Langhorst J, Dobos G. Yoga for depression: a systematic review and meta-analysis. *Depress Anxiety* (2013) 30(11):1068–83. doi: 10.1002/da.22166

D'Silva S, Poscablo C, Habousha R, Kogan M, Kligler B. Mind-body medicine therapies for a range of depression severity: a systematic review. *Psychosomatics* (2012) 53:407–23. doi: 10.1016/j.psym.2012.04.006

Hofmann S, Sawyer A, Witt A, Oh D. The effect of mindfulness-based therapy on anxiety and depression: a meta-analytic review. *J Consult Clin Psychol* (2010) 78:169–83. doi: 10.1037/a0018555

Jorm A, Allen N, Morgan A, Ryan S, Purcell R. *A guide to what works for depression*. 2nd ed. Melbourne: Beyond Blue (2013). Retrieved from www.idfa. org.au/wp-content/uploads/2015/06/BB.WhatWorksForDepression.pdf.

de Manincor M, Bensoussan A, Smith CA, Barr K, Schweickle M, Donoghoe L, et al. Individualized yoga for reducing depression and anxiety, and improving well-being: a randomized controlled trial. *Depress Anxiety* (2016) 33(9):816–28. doi: 10.1002/da.22502

Descilo T, Vedamurtachar A, Gerbarg P, Nagaraja D, Gangadhar B, Damodaran B, et al. Effects of a yoga breath intervention alone and in combination with an exposure therapy for post-traumatic stress disorder and depression in survivors of the 2004 South-East Asia tsunami. *Acta Psychiatr Scand* (2010) 121(4):289–300. doi: 10.1111/j.1600-0447.2009.01466.x

Janakiramaiah N, Gangadhar BN, Naga Venkatesha Murthy PJ, Harish MG, Subbakrishna DK, Vedamurthachar A. Antidepressant efficacy of Sudarshan Kriya Yoga (SKY) in melancholia: a randomized comparison with electroconvulsive therapy (ECT) and imipramine. *J Affect Disord* (2000) 57(1–3):255–9. doi: 10.1016/S0165-0327(99)00079-8

Streeter C, Gerbarg P, Whitfield T, Owen L, Johnston J, Silveri M, et al. Treatment of major depressive disorder with iyengar yoga and coherent breathing: a randomized controlled dosing study. *J Altern Complement Med* (2017) 23:201–7. doi: 10.1089/acm.2016.0140

Vedamurthachar A, Janakiramaiah N, Hegde J, Shetty T, Subbakrishna D, Sureshbabu S, et al. Antidepressant efficacy and hormonal effects of Sudarshana Kriya Yoga (SKY) in alcohol dependent individuals. *J Affect Disord* (2006) 94:249–53. doi: 10.1016/j.jad.2006.04.025

Streeter C, Gerbarg P, Saper R, Ciraulo D, Brown R. Effects of yoga on the autonomic nervous system, gamma-aminobutyric-acid, and allostasis in epilepsy, depression, and post-traumatic stress disorder. *Med Hypotheses* (2012) 78:571–9. doi: 10.1016/j.mehy.2012.01.021

Brown R, Gerbarg P. Sudarshan kriya yogic breathing in the treatment of stress, anxiety, and depression: part I - neurophysiologic model. *J Altern Complement Med* (2005) 11(2):189–201. doi: 10.1089/acm.2005.11.189

Donnelley M. Functional mastery of health ownership: a model for optimum health. *Nurs Forum* (2018) 53(2):117–21. doi: 10.1111/nuf.12223

Kardakis T, Jerden L, Nystrom ME, Weinehall L, Johansson H. Implementation of clinical practice guidelines on lifestyle interventions in Swedish primary healthcare – a two-year follow up. *BMC Health Serv Res* (2018) 18:227. doi: 10.1186/s12913-018-3023-z

Tarlaci S. Why we need quantum physics for cognitive neuroscience and psychiatry. *Neuroquantology* (2010) 8:66–76. doi: 10.14704/nq.2010.8.1.271

White F. *The overview effect: space exploration and human evolution*. Reston VA, USA: American Institute of Aeronautics and Astronautics (1998). doi: 10.2514/4.103223

Yaden D, Iwry J, Slack K, Eichstaedt J, Zhao Y, Vallient G, et al. The overview effect: awe and self-transcendent experience in space flight. *Psychol Conscious* (2016) 3:1–11. doi: 10.1037/cns0000086

13

Physical Activity for Executive Function and Activities of Daily Living in AD Patients

Lin Zhu[1], Long Li[1]*, Lin Wang[2]*, Xiaohu Jin[2] and Huajiang Zhang[3]

[1] School of Physical Education, Soochow University, Suzhou, China, [2] Department of Physical Education, Wuhan University of Technology, Wuhan, China, [3] College of Physical Education, Hubei University of Arts and Science, Xiangyang, China

*Correspondence:
Long Li
lilong@suda.edu.cn
Lin Wang
wanglin123@126.com

Objectives: The present study aimed to systematically analyze the effects of physical activity on executive function, working memory, cognitive flexibility, and activities of daily living (ADLs) in Alzheimer's disease (AD) patients and to provide a scientific evidence-based exercise prescription.

Methods: Both Chinese and English databases (PubMed, Web of Science, the Cochrane Library, EMBASE, VIP Database for Chinese Technical Periodicals, China National Knowledge Infrastructure, and Wanfang) were used as sources of data to search for randomized controlled trials (RCTs) published between January 1980 and December 2019 relating to the effects of physical activity on executive function, working memory, cognitive flexibility, and ADL issues in AD patients. Sixteen eligible RCTs were ultimately included in the meta-analysis.

Results: Physical activity had significant benefits on executive function [standard mean difference (SMD) = 0.42, 95% confidence interval (CI) 0.22–0.62, $p < 0.05$], working memory (SMD = 0.28, 95% CI 0.11–0.45, $p < 0.05$), cognitive flexibility (SMD = 0.23, 95% CI −0.02 to 0.47, $p < 0.01$), and ADLs (SMD = 0.68, 95% CI 0.19–1.16, $p < 0.05$) among AD patients. Subgroup analysis indicated that, for executive function issues, more than 60 min per session for 16 weeks of moderate-to-high-intensity dual-task exercises or multimodal exercise had a greater effect on AD patients. For working memory and cognitive flexibility issues, 60–90 min of moderate-intensity dual-task exercises 1–4 times/week was more effective. For ADL issues, 30–90 min of multimodal exercise at 60–79% of maximal heart rate (MHR) 3–4 times/week had a greater effect on AD patients.

Conclusions: Physical activity was found to lead to significant improvements in executive function, working memory, cognitive flexibility, and ADLs in AD patients and can be used as an effective method for clinical exercise intervention in these patients. However, more objective, scientific, and effective RCTs are needed to confirm this conclusion.

Keywords: exercise prescription, ADL, executive function, AD, physical activity

INTRODUCTION

Alzheimer's disease (AD) is a common disorder of the nervous system, accounting for disease in 60–70% of patients with dementia (Reitz et al., 2011), causing severe clinical, social, and economic problems (Prince et al., 2013). Features of dementia include progressive cognitive decline, including loss of memory, language, or executive function, and subsequent decline of social function, for example, activities of daily living (ADLs) (Allal et al., 2015). The cognitive process of the frontal lobe may also change, which is characterized by decreased attention and executive function, as evidenced by deficits in problem solving, planning, and organizing behavior and ideas, abstraction, judgment, cognitive flexibility, decision making, working memory, and self-monitoring (Avilla and Miotto, 2002; Yaari and Bloom, 2007). By 2050, the number of people ≥60 years old will increase by 1.25 billion (Prince et al., 2013), and there will be an estimated 115.4 million people with dementia (Maffei et al., 2017). Drug therapy has been shown to be beneficial to the cognitive function and dependence in ADLs in AD patients (Tan et al., 2014), but it also has side effects.

Based on the above factors, alternative treatment options for AD are necessary to achieve better treatment results. Some research shows that approximately one-third of all AD cases may be due to potentially modifiable factors, such as lack of physical activity (Norton et al., 2014), which means that the disease can be prevented. Furthermore, some human and animal studies have shown that physical activity can promote the improvement of cerebrovascular function, perfusion, and brain neural plasticity, which can prevent the gradual loss of cognitive function or executive function related to diseases, such as aging and dementia (Davenport et al., 2012; Erickson et al., 2012). Furthermore, physical activity is considered to have a significant effect on executive function (Wilbur et al., 2012), as confirmed recently in a large experiment of moderate-intensity exercise in sedentary older adults: in the subgroup with the weakest cognitive ability, executive function was improved. In recent years, more and more studies have confirmed the positive effect of physical activity among AD patients. Meanwhile, executive function can directly affect the ADLs or continued independence (Royall et al., 2000; Bell-McGinty et al., 2002; Cahn-Weiner et al., 2002). Some studies provide support for the hypothesis that commonly used clinical trials of executive function significantly predict the ADLs (Bell-McGinty et al., 2002; Cahn-Weiner et al., 2002). As such, with a decrease in executive function, a breakdown in successful execution and completion of complex behavioral procedures is likely, especially in subsets of ADLs involving executive control (Bell-McGinty et al., 2002). However, some ADLs (e.g., ambulating, cooking, reading, leisure, housework, and managing finances) promote improved physical, cognitive, and executive functions (Bell-McGinty et al., 2002; Cahn-Weiner et al., 2002; Jekel et al., 2015). More and more studies have shown that physical activity has a significant impact on improving executive function and ADL issues in AD patients, thus improving their quality of life. In addition, the World Health Organization (WHO) recommends that people over the age of 65 should take at least 150 min of moderate-intensity aerobic exercise (such as brisk walking and jogging) every week, 75 min of high-intensity aerobic exercise every week, or a combination of the two supplemented by muscle-strengthening activities (such as resistance exercise and stretching exercise) on 2 or more days every week (World Health Organization Physical Activity Older Adults, 2017).

Recently, a great deal of research has been carried out to evaluate the impact of physical activity on executive function or ADL issues among AD patients. Because of the differences in the intervention samples, timing, frequency, intensity, and duration, the specific effects on executive function and ADL issues among AD patients could have been different. Therefore, the aim of our meta-analysis was to evaluate the impact of physical activity on executive function and ADL issues in AD patients. Moreover, executive function is a complex construct that includes different functions, such as cognitive flexibility inhibition and working memory. However, there are few studies on inhibitory functions in AD patients. Therefore, this study assessed the specific effects of physical activity on cognitive flexibility and working memory issues in AD patients. This study also explored the internal regulation mechanism of physical activity on the executive functions of AD patients to provide a corresponding exercise prescription.

METHODS

Search Strategy

Literature was identified using the following databases: PubMed, Web of Science, the Cochrane Library, EMBASE, VIP Database for Chinese Technical Periodicals, China National Knowledge Infrastructure, and Wanfang. These databases were searched to identify randomized controlled trials (RCTs) published in any language between January 1, 1980 and December 31, 2019. The search terms used included "exercise or physical activity or aerobic exercise or physical exercise or aerobic fitness or walking or cycling or strength training or balance training or flexibility training" with AD terms including "AD or Alzheimer's disease or Alzheimer" as well as "executive function or executive functions or ADL or activities of daily living."

Inclusion Criteria

The selection criteria were as follows: (1) RCTs investigating the impact of any type of physical activity as an additional intervention on executive function or ADLs; (2) sample population including a group of old people (aged ≥50 years) and participants diagnosed with Alzheimer's-type dementia of any severity, excluding diagnoses of other dementias or mild cognitive impairment (MCI); (3) interventions in an experimental group involving physical activity (e.g., aerobic exercise, aerobic fitness, walking, cycling, strength training, balance training, and flexibility training) compared with different types of control groups (e.g., usual care, no physical activity, and no-intervention control group); (4) outcome indicators including test data on executive function and ADLs; and (5) publication language of Chinese or English.

Exclusion Criteria

The exclusion criteria were as follows: (1) duplicated studies; (2) reviews, observational studies, abstract-only articles (without full-text article available), and non-RCT studies; and (3) studies with no data or unclear data reported for analysis.

Collection of Studies

Two investigators (LZ and LW) independently reviewed the titles and abstracts from the search results and screened out the full texts that might meet the criteria. If a study met the inclusion criteria, it received a full-text article evaluation. When there was any disagreement between the two reviewers, a third reviewer (LL) was invited to discuss with them and to verify the eligibility of the uncertain article. All eligible studies included information, such as author, publication year, country, sample size, sample population age, intervention methods, duration, measurement standards, experimental results, and dropouts.

Data Extraction

Detailed information included the first author, publication year, participant characteristics (sample size and age range/mean age), intervention design (frequency, duration of each intervention session, duration, and follow-up), outcome measure, statistical analyses, and results. Meanwhile, we also extracted quantitative data from the research results: mean and standard deviation (SD) of executive function and ADLs between physical activity and usual care, including its corresponding sample size.

Methodological Quality Assessment

Two authors used the modified the Physical Therapy Evidence Database (PEDro) scale (Zou et al., 2019) to independently perform methodological quality assessment of each eligible study. This assessment consisted of nine items (randomization, concealed allocation, similar baseline, blinding of assessors, ≤15% dropouts, intention-to-treat analysis, between-group comparison, point measure and measures of variability, and isolate exercise intervention), and higher scores indicate better quality of the method.

Statistical Analysis

Stata 14.0 (StataCorp, Texas, USA) was used to calculate effect sizes [standardized mean difference (SMD)] of physical activity

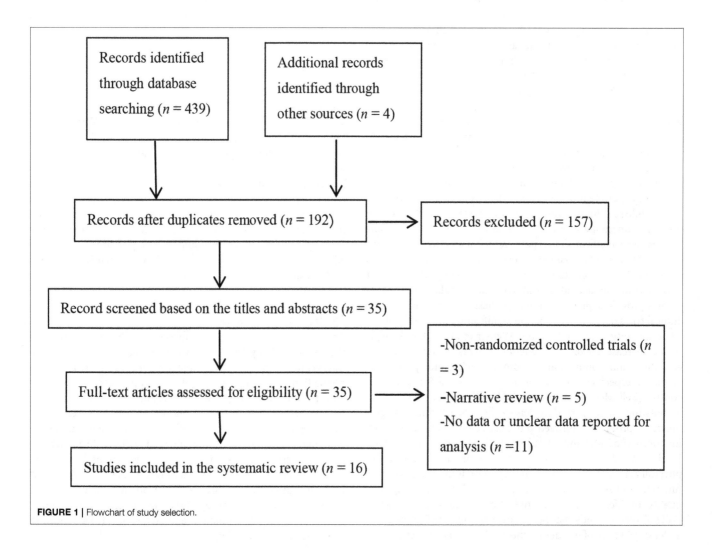

FIGURE 1 | Flowchart of study selection.

TABLE 1 | Summary characteristics of the included studies.

References	Country	Sample size (attrition rate)	Mean age or age range	Duration (W)	Experimental group intervention	Control group intervention	Outcome assessments	Follow-up
Morris et al. (2017)	US	76 (10.5%)	T = 74.4 (6.7) C = 71.4 (8.4)	26	AEx: 150 min/week of moderate-intensity aerobic exercise (cycling, walking, arm cranking on a specific ergometer)	ST: stretching and toning control program	EF	No
Fonte et al. (2019)	Italy	41 (0%)	T = 79 (9) C = 79 (7)	24	3 × 90 min/week moderate-intensity endurance and resistance training	Standard treatment	FAB/IADL	Yes
Ohman et al. (2016)	Helsinki	140 (21%)	T = 77.7 (5.4) C = 78.1 (5.3)	48	2 × 60 min/week executive function-related exercises, dual-task training, and balance, endurance, or aerobic exercises	Usual care	CDT/VF	No
Tootsa et al. (2017)	Sweden	186 (13.4%)	T = 84.4 (6.2) C = 85.9 (7.8)	16	3 × 45 min/week high-intensity functional exercise (HIFE) program (weight-bearing exercises, strength exercises, balance training)	Regular daily life	VF	No
Pedroso et al. (2017)	Brazil	42 (14.2%)	T = 77.6 (6.2) C = 79.2 (5.6)	12	3 × 60 min/week functional-task training: warm-up exercise period (walking, stretching exercises) + stimulated locomotion (walking up and down the stairs, zigzag jogging, etc.) + stimulate other activities of daily living (sitting down and getting up, moving objects)	Standard medical care	VF/DAFS-R	No
Holthoff et al. (2015)	Germany	30 (0%)	T = 72.4 (4.3) C = 70.6 (5.4)	12	3 × 30 min/week PA intervention program: motor-assisted or active resistance training of the legs on a movement trainer	Usual care	EF/ADCS-ADLs	Yes
Coelho et al. (2012)	Brazil	27 (0%)	T = 78 (7.3) C = 77.1 (7.4)	16	3 × 60 min/week multimodal exercise (strength/resistance exercises, agility, flexibility, strength, balance, and cognitive training)	Regular daily life	FAB/CDT	No
Silvaa et al. (2019)	Brazil	27 (0%)	T = 81.2 (8.8) C = 77.5 (8.0)	12	2 × 60 min/week multimodal training session (balance training, aerobic exercise, strength training)	Usual care	CDT/VF	No
Andrade et al. (2013)	Brazil	30 (0%)	T = 78.6 (7.1) C = 77.0 (6.3)	16	3 × 60 min/week multimodal exercise (warm-up, aerobic work, dual-task activities)	Usual care	EF/CDT	No
El-Kader and Al-Jiffr (2016)	Saudi Arabia	59 (32.2%)	T = 68.9 (5.7) C = 69.1 (6.1)	8	3 × 45 min/week aerobic exercise (warm-up, stretching exercises, aerobic exercise, cooling down [on treadmill with low speed and without inclination])	Usual treatment	SF-36PF	No
Rolland et al. (2017)	France	134 (17.9%)	T = 82.8 (7.8) C = 83.1 (7.0)	48	2 × 60 min/week aerobic, strength, flexibility, and balance training	Routine medical care	ADLs	No
Vreugdenhill et al. (2012)	Australia	40 (0%)	T = 73.5 (51–83) C = 74.7 (58–89)	16	7 × 30 min/week strength and balance training and brisk walking + usual treatment	Usual treatment	Barthel Index/IADL	Yes

(Continued)

TABLE 1 | Continued

References	Country	Sample size (attrition rate)	Mean age or age range	Duration (W)	Experimental group intervention	Control group intervention	Outcome assessments	Follow-up
Venturelli et al. (2011)	Italy	24 (14.3%)	T = 83 (6) C = 85 (5)	24	4 × 30 min/week moderate exercise (walking)	Routine care	Barthel Index	No
Vidoni et al. (2017)	Italy	65 (0%)	T = 74.1 (6.8) C = 71.1 (8.8)	26	AEx: 150 min/week of moderate-intensity aerobic exercise	ST: stretching and toning control program	BADL/IADL	No
Hoffmanna et al. (2016)	Denmark	200 (5%)	T = 69.8 (7.4) C = 71.3 (7.3)	16	3 × 30 min/week moderate-to-high-intensity aerobic exercise (ergometer bicycle, cross trainer, treadmill)	Usual treatment	SDMT/ADCS-ADLs	No
Chang et al. (2015)	China	60 (5%)	T = 70.7 (7.4) C = 70.2 (8.5)	16	3 × 60-90 min/week cycling or treadmill + routine medical care	Routine medical care	ADCS-ADLs	No

W, week; EF, executive function; AEx, aerobic exercise condition; ST, stretching and toning control condition; FAB, Frontal Assessment Battery; IADL, instrumental activity of daily living; CDT, clock-drawing test; VF, verbal fluency test; DAFS-R, Direct Assessment of Functional Status; ADCS-ADLs, Alzheimer's Disease Cooperative Study—Activities of Daily Living; SDMT, Symbol Digit Modalities Test; SF-36PF, SF-36: Physical Functioning; BADL, basic instrumental activities of daily living.

on executive function and ADLs. SMD was considered as small (0.2–0.49), moderate (0.5–0.79), or large (0.8). According to the intervention system review of the Cochrane Collaboration handbook, selection of fixed-effects or random-effects meta-analysis should be based on the actual effect of an intervention on outcome measures. Differences (standard mean difference, SMD) and 95% confidence intervals (95% CIs) were calculated. I^2 values of 25, 50, and 75% are considered to be low, medium, and high heterogeneity (Higgins et al., 2003). When the heterogeneity test $I^2 \geq 50\%$, a random-effects model was used for meta-analysis. In this study, regression analysis was used to study the degree of experimental heterogeneity. Subgroup analyses were performed according to categorical variables, including sample age, exercise intensity, frequency, duration, duration of each intervention session, and exercise type. Subgroup analysis was used to determine which subgroup was more effective for improving the executive function and ADLs among AD patients.

RESULTS

Study Selection

A total of 443 topic-related articles were identified from 7 databases and other resources (**Figure 1**). After removing duplicate articles, 192 articles remained. A total of 157 articles were deleted after titles and abstracts were screened for non-related articles ($n = 148$) and abstract-only articles ($n = 9$). The remaining 35 articles were further screened after reading the full-text articles. Nineteen studies were removed because they were non-RCTs ($n = 3$), reviews ($n = 5$), or had no or unclear outcome measures ($n = 11$). Finally, our meta-analysis included 16 eligible studies.

Characteristics of Eligible Studies

There were 16 eligible (Venturelli et al., 2011; Coelho et al., 2012; Vreugdenhill et al., 2012; Andrade et al., 2013; Chang et al., 2015; Holthoff et al., 2015; El-Kader and Al-Jiffr, 2016; Hoffmanna et al., 2016; Ohman et al., 2016; Morris et al., 2017; Pedroso et al., 2017; Rolland et al., 2017; Tootsa et al., 2017; Vidoni et al., 2017; Fonte et al., 2019; Silvaa et al., 2019) RCTs, as shown in **Table 1**. There were 1,181 participants in total; the smallest sample was 27 participants (Silvaa et al., 2019), and the largest sample was 200 participants (Holthoff et al., 2015). The age of the participants in the experiment ranged from 50 to 96 years old. The shortest experimental period was 8 weeks (El-Kader and Al-Jiffr, 2016), and the longest experimental period was 1 year (Rolland et al., 2017). The experimental group included various interventions, such as moderate-to-high-intensity physical activity, ergometer bicycle exercise, walking, cycling, strength training, balance training, and flexibility training. The control group was treated by usual care, standard treatment, routine medical care, etc. (**Table 1**).

Methodological Quality Assessment

The methodological quality score for all qualified studies was between 5 and 8 (**Table 2**). All studies were RCTs and had similar baseline characteristics, between-group comparisons, point measures, measures of variability description, and

TABLE 2 | Quality evaluation of eligible randomized controlled trials.

References	Item 1	Item 2	Item 3	Item 4	Item 5	Item 6	Item 7	Item 8	Item 9	Score
Morris et al. (2017)	1	0	1	0	1	0	1	1	1	6
Fonte et al. (2019)	1	1	1	1	1	0	1	1	1	8
Ohman et al. (2016)	1	0	1	0	0	0	1	1	1	5
Tootsa et al. (2017)	1	1	1	1	1	0	1	1	1	8
Pedroso et al. (2017)	1	0	1	0	1	0	1	1	1	6
Holthoff et al. (2015)	1	0	1	0	1	0	1	1	1	6
Coelho et al. (2012)	1	0	1	0	1	0	1	1	1	6
Silvaa et al. (2019)	1	0	1	0	1	0	1	1	1	6
Andrade et al. (2013)	1	0	1	0	1	0	1	1	1	6
El-Kader and Al-Jiffr (2016)	1	0	1	0	0	0	1	1	1	5
Rolland et al. (2017)	1	1	1	1	0	1	1	1	1	8
Vreugdenhill et al. (2012)	1	0	1	0	1	0	1	1	1	6
Venturelli et al. (2011)	1	1	1	1	0	0	1	1	1	8
Vidoni et al. (2017)	1	0	1	0	1	0	1	1	1	6
Hoffmanna et al. (2016)	1	0	1	0	1	0	1	1	1	6
Chang et al. (2015)	1	0	1	0	1	0	1	1	1	6

Item 1, randomization; Item 2, concealed allocation; Item 3, similar baseline; Item 4, blinding of assessors; Item 5, <15% dropouts; Item 6, intention-to-treat analysis; Item 7, between-group comparison; Item 8, point measure and measures of variability; Item 9, isolate exercise intervention; 1, explicitly described and present in details; 0, absent, inadequately described, or unclear.

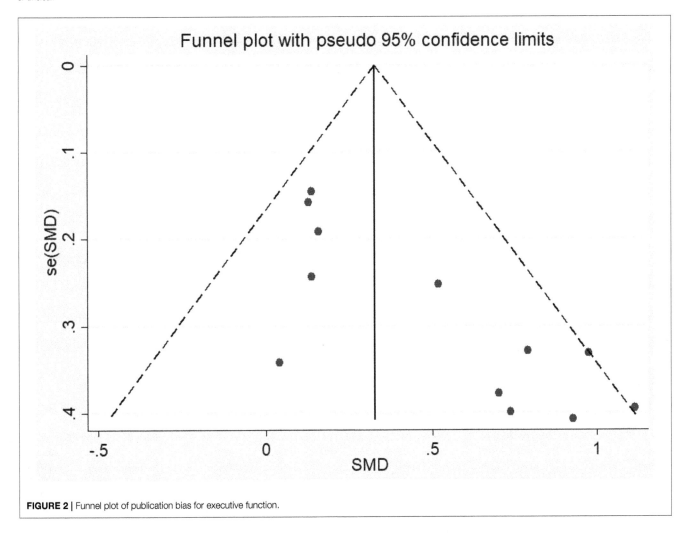

FIGURE 2 | Funnel plot of publication bias for executive function.

isolated exercise interventions. Only four studies had concealed allocations and blinding of assessors (Venturelli et al., 2011; Rolland et al., 2017; Tootsa et al., 2017; Fonte et al., 2019). The dropout rates in three of these studies were all higher than 15% (El-Kader and Al-Jiffr, 2016; Ohman et al., 2016; Rolland et al., 2017), and only one study used the intention-to-treat principle (Rolland et al., 2017).

Meta-Analysis of Outcome Indicators
Effect of Physical Activity on Executive Function Issues in AD Patients

Twelve articles (Coelho et al., 2012; Vreugdenhill et al., 2012; Andrade et al., 2013; Holthoff et al., 2015; Hoffmanna et al.,

2016; Ohman et al., 2016; Morris et al., 2017; Pedroso et al., 2017; Tootsa et al., 2017; Vidoni et al., 2017; Fonte et al., 2019; Silvaa et al., 2019) compared the effects of an intervention group and a control group on executive function before and after the experiment. An asymmetrical funnel plot was presented. The funnel plot shows that there were no outlier values (**Figure 2**). There was a moderate heterogeneity in the research literature (p = 0.047, I^2 = 44.8%), and a random-effects model was selected for the meta-analysis (**Figure 3**). The meta-analysis of 12 studies demonstrated that physical activity had significant effects on improving executive function in AD patients (SMD = 0.42, 95% CI 0.22–0.62, $p < 0.05$).

Covariates including age, intensity, frequency, time, and duration are likely to be the influencing factors for executive

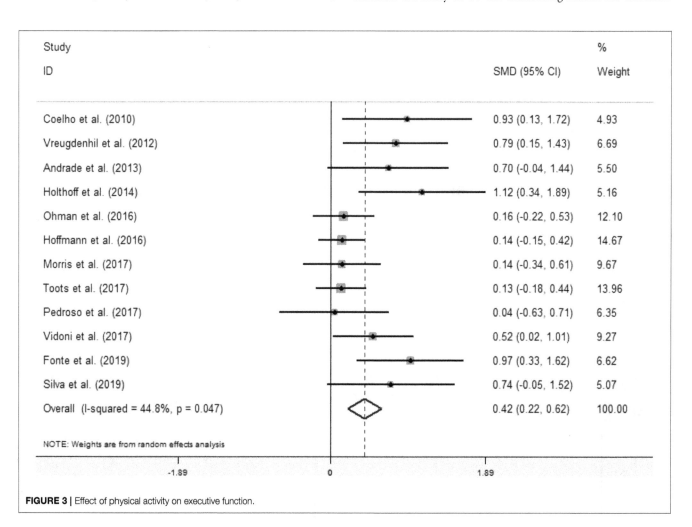

FIGURE 3 | Effect of physical activity on executive function.

TABLE 3 | Covariate regression analysis of executive function issues in AD patients.

_ES	Coef.	Std. err.	t	p > t	(95% CI)	
Age	0.0110741	0.0218454	0.51	0.63	−0.0423797	0.0645279
Intensity (%)	−0.0271544	0.0123192	−2.20	0.07	−0.0572985	0.0029897
Frequency (times/week)	0.1126148	0.0999144	1.13	0.303	−0.131867	0.3570966
Time (min)	0.0037139	0.0031768	1.17	0.287	−0.0040595	0.0114874
Duration (week)	−0.0245532	0.0129349	−1.9	0.106	−0.0562039	0.0070974
_cons	1.441027	1.818227	0.79	0.458	−3.008015	5.890069

TABLE 4 | Subgroup analysis of executive function issues in AD patients.

Group	Subgroup	N	SMD	95% CI	p	I^2
Age	65–75	5	0.44	0.109, 0.771	0.065	54.80%
	Older than 75	7	0.424	0.136, 0.713	0.086	45.80%
Intensity (%)	35–59	2	0.574	−0.356, 1.505	0.029	79.00%
	60–79	8	0.549	0.303, 0.794	0.293	17.40%
	80–89	2	0.134	−0.076, 0.343	0.968	0.00%
Frequency (times/week)	1–2 times/week	4	0.293	0.052, 0.534	0.403	0.00%
	3–4 times/week	7	0.473	0.155, 0.790	0.021	59.70%
	5–7 times/week	1	0.79	0.145, 1.435	—	—
Time (min)	30≤min<60	3	0.604	−0.023, 1.231	0.022	73.90%
	60≤min<90	7	0.424	0.136, 0.713	0.086	45.80%
	90≤min≤150	2	0.322	−0.049, 0.694	0.279	14.80%
Duration (week)	8–12 weeks	3	0.606	−0.033, 1.244	0.107	55.20%
	16 weeks	5	0.269	0.082, 0.692	0.047	44.80%
	24–48 weeks	4	0.387	0.051, 0.724	0.124	47.90%
Event	Single exercises	1	1.115	0.342, 1.888	—	—
	Dual-task exercises	3	0.492	−0.003, 0.988	0.144	48.3%
	Multimodal exercise	8	0.345	0.123, 0.567	0.111	40.1%

"—" heterogeneity test cannot be conducted due to the lack of literature.

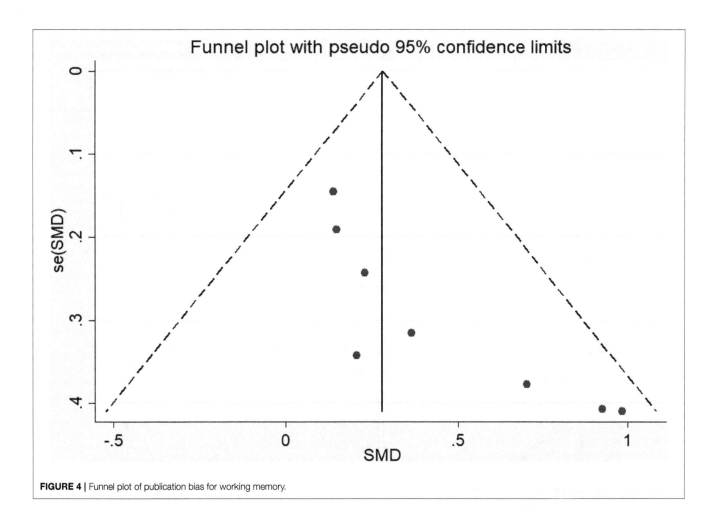

FIGURE 4 | Funnel plot of publication bias for working memory.

function issues in AD patients. The results of the regression of covariates for executive function issues in AD patients are presented in **Table 3**. For executive function, there were no significant effects of age (95% CI −0.0423797 to 0.0645279, $p = 0.63$), intensity (95% CI −0.0572985 to 0.0029897, $p = 0.07$), frequency (95% CI −0.131867 to 0.3570966, $p = 0.303$), time (95% CI −0.0040595 to 0.0114874, $p = 0.287$), or duration (95% CI −0.0562039 to 0.0070974, $p = 0.106$).

According to the sample population's age, exercise intensity, frequency, time, and duration, this study divided the research subjects into different subgroups, as shown in **Table 4**. The results from the subgroup analysis are as follows: (1) age: physical activity was beneficial for AD patients who were older than 75 years and had executive function issues. (2) Intensity: for executive function issues in AD patients, maintaining a 60–79 or an 80–89% maximal heart rate (MHR) during physical activity was more effective. (3) Frequency: the frequency of physical activity has a significant impact on the improvement of the executive function in AD patients, and the effect of 1–2 times/week was better than the effect of 3–4 or 5–7 times/week. (4) Time: a total of 60–150 min of physical activity per exercise session significantly improved executive function in AD patients. (5) Duration: an intervention duration of 16 or 24–48 weeks

showed a significant effect on executive function issues in AD patients. (6) Event: for executive function issues in AD patients, both dual-task exercises and multimodal exercise had significant effects.

Effect of Physical Activity on Working Memory Issues in AD Patients

Eight articles (Coelho et al., 2012; Andrade et al., 2013; Hoffmanna et al., 2016; Ohman et al., 2016; Morris et al., 2017; Pedroso et al., 2017; Fonte et al., 2019; Silvaa et al., 2019) evaluated the effects of physical activity on working memory issues in AD patients. An asymmetrical funnel plot was presented. The funnel plot shows that there were no outlier values (**Figure 4**). The heterogeneity test results of the included research literature were not significant ($p = 0.303$, $I^2 = 16.1\%$); thus, the fixed-effects model was used for meta-analysis (**Figure 5**). The meta-analysis of eight studies demonstrated that physical activity had significant effects on improving working memory in AD patients (SMD = 0.28, 95% CI 0.11–0.45, $p < 0.05$).

The results of the regression of covariates for cognitive flexibility issues in AD patients are presented in **Table 5**. For cognitive flexibility, there were no significant effects of age (95% CI −0.1637734 to 0.2960517, $p = 0.341$), intensity (95%

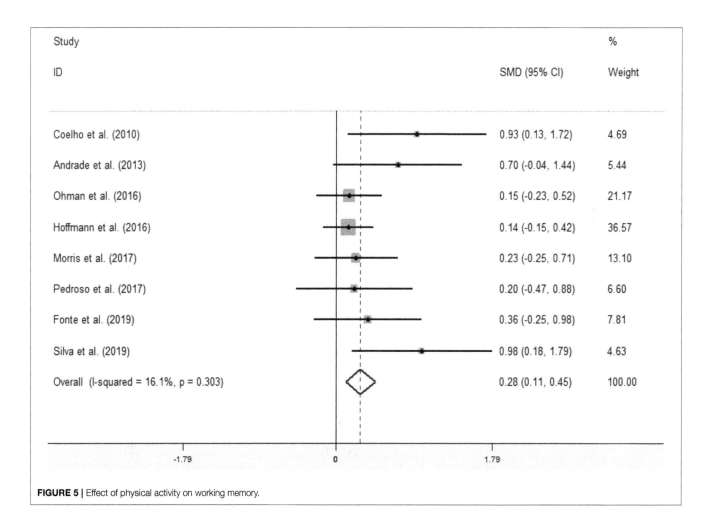

FIGURE 5 | Effect of physical activity on working memory.

TABLE 5 | Covariate regression analysis of working memory issues in AD patients.

_ES	Coef.	Std. err.	t	p > t	(95% CI)	
Age	0.0661391	0.0534351	1.24	0.341	−0.1637734	0.2960517
Intensity (%)	0.0060079	0.0481411	0.12	0.912	−0.2011265	0.2131423
Frequency (times/week)	−0.2336269	0.3742413	−0.62	0.596	−1.843857	1.376603
Time (min)	−0.0029123	0.0065205	−0.45	0.699	−0.0309679	0.0251433
Duration (week)	−0.0156879	0.0316051	−0.5	0.669	−0.1516738	0.1202981
_cons	−3.939082	7.507129	−0.52	0.652	−36.23965	28.36149

TABLE 6 | Subgroup analysis of working memory issues in AD patients.

Group	Subgroup	N	SMD	95% CI	p	I^2
Age	65–75	2	0.161	−0.084, 0.406	0.748	0.00%
	Older than 75	6	0.397	0.154, 0.641	0.265	22.40%
Intensity (%)	35–59	1	0.146	−0.229, 0.521	−	−
	60–79	5	0.408	0.126, 0.689	0.534	0.00%
	80–89	2	0.233	−0.036, 0.502	0.051	73.70%
Frequency (times/week)	1–2 times/week	3	0.274	−0.003, 90.550	0.174	42.70%
	3–4 times/week	5	0.284	0.064, 0.505	0.303	17.50%
Time (min)	30≤min<60	1	0.137	−0.148, 0.423	−	−
	60≤min<90	5	0.404	0.139, 0.668	0.169	37.80%
	90≤min≤150	2	0.279	−0.098, 0.657	0.734	0.00%
Duration (week)	8–12 weeks	2	0.526	0.011, 1.041	0.144	53.10%
	16 weeks	3	0.282	0.030, 0.535	0.303	16.10%
	24–48 weeks	3	0.212	−0.054, 0.478	0.837	0.00%
Event	Dual-task exercises	3	0.491	−0.014, 0.995	0.165	46.7%
	Multimodal exercise	5	0.396	0.012, 0.780	0.038	60.7%

CI −0.2011265 to 0.2131423, $p = 0.912$), frequency (95% CI −1.843857 to 1.376603, $p = 0.596$), time (95% CI −0.0309679 to 0.0251433, $p = 0.699$), or duration (95% CI −0.1516738 to 0.1202981, $p = 0.669$).

All eligible studies were analyzed in subgroups based on age, intensity, frequency, time, and duration, as shown in **Table 6**. The results from subgroup analysis are as follows: (1) age: physical activity was beneficial for AD patients aged 65–75 years with working memory issues. (2) Intensity: for working memory issues in AD patients, maintaining a 60–79% MHR during physical activity was more effective. (3) Frequency: the frequency of physical activity has a significant impact on the improvement of the working memory issues in AD patients, and the effect of 3–4 times/week was better than the effect of 1–2 times/week. (4) Time: a total of 60–150 min per exercise session significantly improved working memory in AD patients. (5) Duration: an intervention duration of 16 or 24–48 weeks showed a significant effect on working memory issues in AD patients. (6) Event: for working memory issues in AD patients, dual-task exercises had a significant effect.

Effect of Physical Activity on Cognitive Flexibility Issues in AD Patients

Nine articles (Vreugdenhill et al., 2012; Andrade et al., 2013; Holthoff et al., 2015; Hoffmanna et al., 2016; Ohman et al., 2016;

Pedroso et al., 2017; Tootsa et al., 2017; Vidoni et al., 2017; Silvaa et al., 2019) evaluated the effects of physical activity on cognitive flexibility issues in AD patients. An asymmetrical funnel plot was presented. According to the funnel plot, there were two outliers (**Figure 6**). There was a moderate heterogeneity in the research literature ($p = 0.025$, $I^2 = 54.5\%$), and the meta-analysis was performed using a random-effects models (**Figure 7**). **Figure 7** shows that the meta-analysis of nine studies demonstrated that physical activity had a significant effect on improving cognitive flexibility in AD patients (SMD = 0.23, 95% CI −0.02 to 0.47, $p < 0.01$).

The analysis of heterogeneity and sensitivity showed that there was considerable bias in the studies by Vreugdenhill et al. (2012) and Holthoff et al. (2015). Therefore, a meta-analysis of the remaining RCTs was performed after exclusion. The results showed that the heterogeneity was reduced ($I^2 = 7.4\%$, $p = 0.372$, SMD = 0.06, 95% CI −0.11, 0.23), and that the differences between groups were significant ($p < 0.01$).

The results of the regression of covariates for working memory issues in AD patients are presented in **Table 7**. For working memory, there were no significant effects of age (95% CI −0.2086577 to 0.2332289, $p = 0.608$), intensity (95% CI −0.2536149 to 0.2638656, $p = 0.843$), frequency (95% CI −5.644876 to 5.888054, $p = 0.833$), time (95% CI −0.0894664

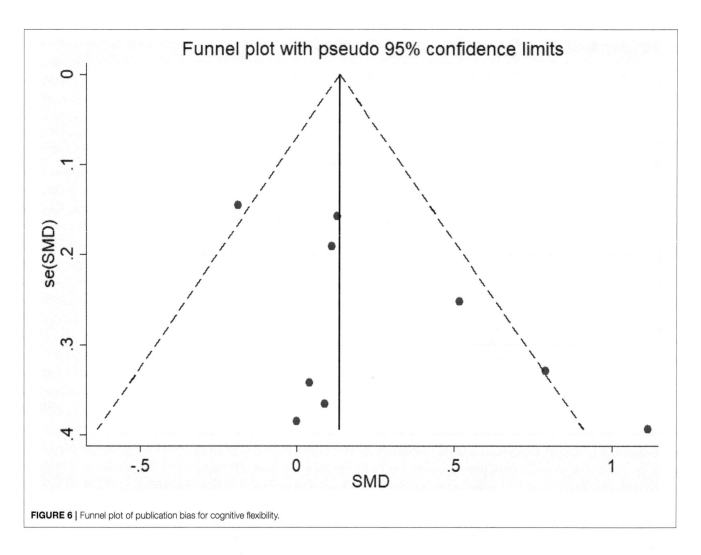

FIGURE 6 | Funnel plot of publication bias for cognitive flexibility.

to 0.1045166, $p = 0.505$), or duration (95% CI −0.2578807 to 0.2722502, $p = 0.789$).

The results from the subgroup analysis are as follows (**Table 8**): (1) age: physical activity was beneficial for cognitive flexibility issues in AD patients who were older than 75 years. (2) Intensity: for cognitive flexibility issues in AD patients, the effect of maintaining a 60–79 or 80–89% MHR was more effective. (3) Frequency: for cognitive flexibility issues in AD patients, the effect of performing physical activity 1–2 or 3–4 times/week was more effective. (4) Time: a total of 60–90 min per exercise session significantly improved cognitive flexibility in AD patients. (5) Duration: an intervention duration of 16 or 24–48 weeks showed a significant effect on cognitive flexibility issues in AD patients. (6) Event: for cognitive flexibility issues in AD patients, both dual-task exercises and multimodal exercise had significant effects.

Effect of Physical Activity on ADL Issues in AD Patients

Ten articles (Venturelli et al., 2011; Vreugdenhill et al., 2012; Chang et al., 2015; Holthoff et al., 2015; El-Kader and Al-Jiffr, 2016; Hoffmanna et al., 2016; Pedroso et al., 2017; Rolland

et al., 2017; Vidoni et al., 2017; Fonte et al., 2019) evaluated the effects of physical activity on ADL issues in AD patients. An asymmetrical funnel plot was presented. Funnel plot indicated that there were three outliers (**Figure 8**). Heterogeneity testing of the study literature showed high heterogeneity ($p < 0.000$, $I^2 = 86.4\%$), and a random-effects model was used for the meta-analysis (**Figure 9**). **Figure 9** shows that the meta-analysis of 10 studies demonstrated that physical activity had significant effects on improving ADLs in AD patients (SMD = 0.68, 95% CI 0.19–1.16, $p < 0.001$).

The analysis of heterogeneity and sensitivity showed that there was considerable bias in the studies by Venturelli et al. (2011), Holthoff et al. (2015), and El-Kader and Al-Jiffr (2016) thus, a meta-analysis of the remaining RCTs was performed after exclusion. The results showed that the heterogeneity was reduced ($I^2 = 45.1\%$, $p = 0.091$, SMD = 0.15, 95% CI −0.10, 0.39), and that the differences between groups were significant ($p < 0.001$).

The results of the regression of covariates for ADL issues in AD patients are presented in **Table 9**. For ADLs, there were no significant effects of age (95% CI −0.2683096 to 0.4846618, $p = 0.47$), intensity (95% CI −0.2702262 to 0.0794482, $p = 0.204$),

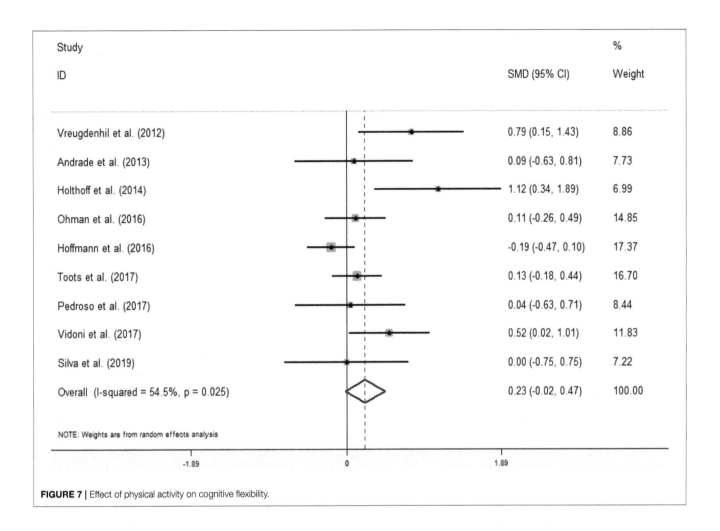

FIGURE 7 | Effect of physical activity on cognitive flexibility.

frequency (95% CI −1.392111 to 1.053637, $p = 0.72$), time (95% CI −0.0623979 to 0.035701, $p = 0.492$), or duration (95% CI −0.2969797 to 0.113052, $p = 0.281$).

The results from the subgroup analysis are as follows (**Table 10**): (1) age: physical activity was beneficial for ADL issues in AD patients who were older than 75 years. (2) Intensity: for ADL issues in AD patients, the effect of maintaining a 60–79% MHR was more effective. (3) Frequency: for ADL issues in AD patients, the effect of performing physical activity 3–4 times/week was more effective. (4) Time: a total of 30–60 or 60–90 min per exercise session significantly improved the ADL issues in AD patients. (5) Duration: for ADL issues in AD patients, the intervention duration was not important. (6) Event: for ADL issues in AD patients, multimodal exercise was significant.

DISCUSSION

The purpose of this systematic review and meta-analysis was to compile and analyze the literature pertaining to RCTs on physical activity (e.g., aerobic exercise, aerobic fitness, walking, cycling, strength training, balance training, and flexibility training) in relation to its influence on executive function, working memory, cognitive flexibility, and ADLs among AD patients to determine an optimal exercise prescription. The results suggest that physical activity can improve executive function, working memory, cognitive flexibility, and ADL issues in AD patients.

This systematic review investigated the influence of physical activity on executive function and ADL issues in AD patients. Research suggests that the effect size of executive function was 0.22–0.62 ($p < 0.05$), that of working memory was 0.11–0.45 ($p < 0.05$), that of cognitive flexibility was −0.02 to 0.47 ($p < 0.01$), and that of ADLs was 0.19–1.16 (p 0.001). Furthermore, significant heterogeneity may have been present in the study by Holthoff et al. (2015). In his study, physical activity was conducted on comfortable chairs to encourage patients to participate and prevent falls and other injuries. This method was different from those used in other studies and may be the cause of the heterogeneity.

The subgroup analysis showed that, for executive function issues, performing moderate-to-high-intensity dual-task exercises or multimodal exercise for more than 60 min per session for 16 weeks had a greater effect on AD patients. Regarding frequency, performing physical activity 1–2 times/week was

TABLE 7 | Covariate regression analysis of cognitive flexibility issues in AD patients.

_ES	Coef.	Std. err.	t	p > t	(95% CI)	
Age	0.0122856	0.0173886	0.71	0.608	−0.2086577	0.2332289
Intensity (%)	0.0051253	0.0203633	0.25	0.843	−0.2536149	0.2638656
Frequency (times/week)	0.121589	0.4538306	0.27	0.833	−5.644876	5.888054
Time (min)	0.0075251	0.0076334	0.99	0.505	−0.0894664	0.1045166
Duration (week)	0.0071848	0.0208611	0.34	0.789	−0.2578807	0.2722502
_cons	−2.169054	2.459361	0.88	0.540	−33.4182	29.08009

TABLE 8 | Subgroup analysis of cognitive flexibility issues in AD patients.

Group	Subgroup	N	SMD	95% CI	p	I^2
Age	65–75	2	−0.011	−0.258, 0.237	0.015	83.00%
	Older than 75	5	0.103	−0.104, 0.309	0.998	0.00%
Intensity (%)	35–59	1	0.112	−0.263, 0.487	–	–
	60–79	3	0.29	−0.058, 0.638	0.441	0.00%
	80–89	3	−0.039	−0.241, 0.163	0.336	8.30%
Frequency (times/week)	1–2 times/week	3	0.225	−0.053, 0.503	0.36	2.20%
	3–4 times/week	4	−0.025	−0.218, 0.168	0.506	0.00%
Time (min)	$30 \leq$ min <60	2	−0.042	−0.252, 0.168	0.141	53.90%
	$60 \leq$ min <90	4	0.082	−0.195, 0.359	0.994	0.00%
	$90 \leq$ min ≤ 150	1	0.518	0.024, 1.013	–	–
Duration (week)	8–12 weeks	2	0.424	−0.477, 0.525	0.174	56.80%
	16 weeks	3	−0.031	−0.233, 0.170	0.318	12.70%
	24–48 weeks	2	0.260	−0.039, 0.559	0.199	39.40%
Event	Dual-task exercises	2	0.107	−0.225, 0.440	0.960	0.00%
	Multimodal exercise	5	0.073	−0.175, 0.322	0.174	37.1%

found to be significant. In addition, for working memory and cognitive flexibility issues, performing 60–90 min of moderate-intensity dual-task exercises 1–4 times/week was more effective. The subgroup analysis indicated that, for ADL issues, maintaining a 60–79% MHR during multimodal exercise 3–4 times/week for 30–90 min each time had a greater effect on AD patients. In addition, in the subgroup analyses of executive function, working memory, cognitive flexibility, and ADL issues, maintaining a 35–59% MHR during physical activity did not show a strong effect compared with maintaining a 60–79 or an 80–89% MHR. Performing physical activity 1–4 times/week for 60–90 min per exercise session significantly improved executive function, working memory, cognitive flexibility, and ADL issues in AD patients. In addition, this meta-analysis provides evidence to support the inclusion of aerobic training and strength, flexibility, balance, and other physical activities to improve executive function and ADL issues in AD patients. For AD patients with executive function, working memory, cognitive flexibility, and ADL issues, both dual-task exercises and multimodal exercises had significant effects. Notably, for working memory and cognitive flexibility issues, dual-task exercises showed a strong influence compared with multimodal exercises. Coincidentally, our findings support the WHO recommendations (World Health Organization Physical Activity Older Adults, 2017). In addition, the characteristics of exercise intervention in the included studies support the frequency,

intensity, and time per session recommended by the WHO, but slightly lower than the WHO recommendations based on expert advice. Our meta-analysis showed that the current WHO recommendations can be considered an effective exercise prescription for AD patients; however, future studies are needed to determine which combinations of intervention methods, intensity, duration of each intervention session, frequency, and duration best improve executive function and ADL issues among older adults diagnosed with AD.

Systematic reviews showed that physical activity can improve the attention, cognitive function, executive function, and language of AD patients (Coelho et al., 2009; Farina et al., 2014). These authors agree that there is not enough theoretical support for the ideal intervention program, and that there is no consensus on the intensity, frequency, and duration of exercise. However, long-term physical activity stimulates growth factors, neurotransmitter synthesis, oxygenation, and plasticity to produce nerve and neuroprotective effects on the brain (Deslandes et al., 2009). The beneficial effects of physical activity on brain aging or dementia have not been well-documented (Herholz et al., 2013). However, animal studies have revealed that the activation of adult neurogenesis (Kempermann et al., 2010) or the increase in plasma levels of neuroplasticity-related brain-derived neurotrophic factors (Coelho et al., 2014) is related to physical activity. Furthermore, some mechanisms related to physical activity help to improve

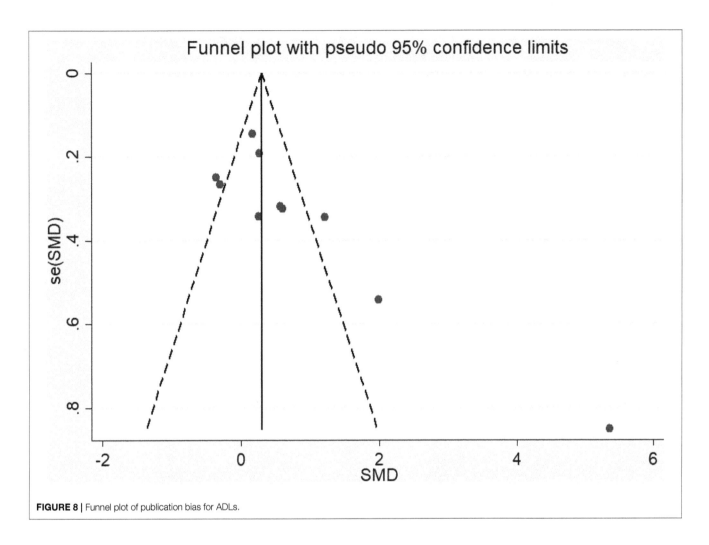

FIGURE 8 | Funnel plot of publication bias for ADLs.

cognitive function, such as improvement of the nervous system, including promoting the synthesis of neurotransmitters and improving cerebral blood flow (Eggermont et al., 2006; Lista and Sorrentin, 2009). Some studies have shown that physical activity can increase brain-derived neurotrophic factor and also have a positive impact on the brain neuroplasticity. Kramer and Erickson found that in rodents, physical activity induces increased levels of brain-derived neurotrophic factor in the frontal cortex, hippocampus, and cerebellum and promotes the formation of new capillaries in these areas (Kramer and Erickson, 2007). Some authors believe that physical activity improves cerebral circulation by increasing cerebral blood flow and oxygen supply (Hamer and Chid, 2009; Sofifi et al., 2011), while promoting cardiovascular and cerebrovascular health by lowering blood pressure and blood lipid levels. Physical activity also promotes inflammatory markers and can effectively enhance endothelial function (Kivipelto et al., 2005). Furthermore, physical activity can stimulate the proliferation of neurons in the hippocampus (Erickson et al., 2011). Therefore, the effect of physical activity on clinical performance in AD (e.g., cognitive and executive functions) may rely on improvement in brain functionality.

Previous studies have shown that physical activity can improve the cognitive and executive functions of the elderly with cognitive impairment (Scherder et al., 2005; Lautenschlager et al., 2008; Uffelen et al., 2008; Baker et al., 2010; Lam et al., 2011). The executive function is mainly responsible for the self-regulation of behavior and is the key cognitive resource, including the ability to initiate, plan, sequence, and monitor (Miyake and Friedma, 2012). In AD patients, executive dysfunction is a prominent clinical symptom that directly affects the patient's self-regulation of behavior and ADLs (Boyle et al., 2003; Razani et al., 2007).

The promoting effect of non-pharmacological treatment methods on the improvement of the condition of AD patients has been confirmed (Morley and Silve, 1995; Cohen-Mansfifield and Mintze, 2005). Interventions, such as physical activity, have been shown to improve cognitive function and executive function and are even effective for frail residents of nursing homes (Lazowski et al., 1999). At the same time, exercise intervention may produce effective protective mechanisms to prevent the decline in the ADLs. At present, it has been confirmed that suitable physical activities can inhibit the pathophysiological changes of AD by regulating the expression and hydrolysis of amyloid precursor protein, reducing the production of β

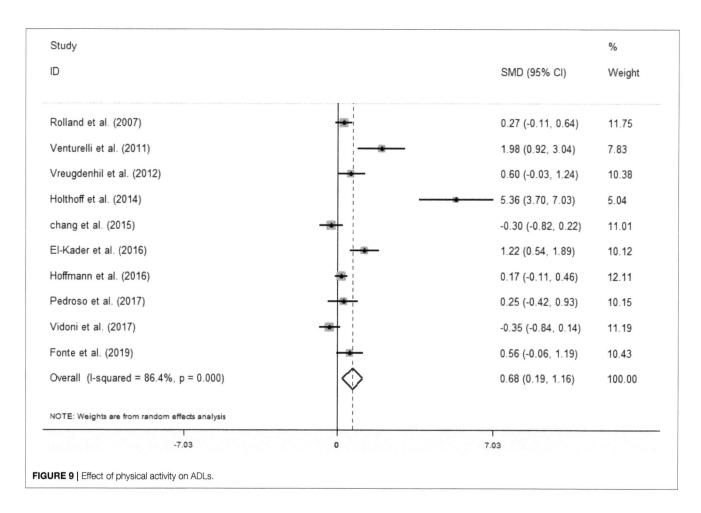

FIGURE 9 | Effect of physical activity on ADLs.

TABLE 9 | Covariate regression analysis of ADL issues in AD patients.

_ES	Coef.	Std. err.	t	p > t	(95% CI)	
Age	0.1081761	0.1355999	0.8	0.47	−0.2683096	0.4846618
Intensity (%)	−0.095389	0.0629716	−1.51	0.204	−0.2702262	0.0794482
Frequency (times/week)	−0.1692369	0.4404458	−0.38	0.72	−1.392111	1.053637
Time (min)	−0.0133484	0.0176663	−0.76	0.492	−0.0623979	0.035701
Duration (week)	−0.0919639	0.0738411	−1.25	0.281	−0.2969797	0.113052
_cons	2.195003	9.602787	0.23	0.83	−24.46661	28.85662

amyloid protein, and scavenging free radicals, among other actions (Radak et al., 2010; Foster et al., 2011). In addition, on the one hand, the decline of ADLs among AD patients is due to a decline in the cognitive level; on the other hand, it is closely related to the atrophy of muscles with the development of age and disease (Sakuma and Yamaguch, 2011). Physical activity is an important measure to combat skeletal muscle atrophy. It can increase the quality of skeletal muscle, output power of physical activity per unit time, and skeletal muscle endurance. According to the changes in muscle stimulation during physical activity, the number of activated transverse bridges can be increased, thereby enhancing muscle flexibility (Jin et al., 2020). Furthermore, the contraction ability of respiratory muscles is enhanced after exercise, which is conducive to the extension

of patient's trunk and limbs, and provides opportunities for improving limb coordination and strengthening exercise ability (Liu et al., 2018). Therefore, physical activity can improve ADLs in AD patients by increasing the quality of skeletal muscle, enhancing muscle activity, improving limb coordination, and exercise performance, etc.

In this review, one article showed that there was no significant effect of physical activity on executive function among AD patients. Specifically, Morris et al. (2017) showed that there was no significant difference in the improvement of executive function between the intervention group and the control group. Aerobic exercise interventions were used in this study, which are different from other interventions. This may be one of the reasons for the lack of a significant difference. However, aerobic

TABLE 10 | Subgroup analysis of ADL issues in AD patients.

Group	Subgroup	N	SMD	95% CI	p	I^2
Age	65–75	4	0.019	−0.358, 0.395	0.049	61.90%
	Older than 75	3	0.328	0.038, 0.618	0.708	0.00%
Intensity (%)	35–59	2	−0.02	−0.623, 0.582	0.05	73.90%
	60–79	4	0.255	−0.189, 0.699	0.096	52.70%
	80–89	1	0.172	−0.114, 0.458	–	–
Frequency (times/week)	1–2 times/week	2	−0.02	−0.623, 0.582	0.05	73.90%
	3–4 times/week	4	0.147	−0.158, 0.451	0.203	34.90%
	5–7 times/week	1	0.603	−0.031, 1.238	–	–
Time (min)	30≤ min <60	4	0.291	−0.087, 0.668	0.225	32.20%
	60≤ min <90	2	0.18	−0.159, 0.519	0.179	38.80%
	90≤ min ≤150	1	−0.349	−0.839, 0.141	–	–
Duration (week)	8–12 weeks	1	0.253	−0.42, 0.926	–	–
	16 weeks	3	0.137	−0.281, 0.554	0.091	58.30%
	24–48 weeks	3	0.142	−0.347, 0.632	0.049	66.80%
Event	Single exercises	1	−0.298	−0.821, 0.224	–	–
	Multimodal exercise	6	0.210	−0.033, 0.453	0.165	36.3%

"–" heterogeneity test cannot be conducted due to the lack of literature.

exercise interventions were also used in the study by Vidoni et al. (2017), and the results showed a significantly different effect on ADL issues in AD patients. This result suggests that aerobic exercise may be more effective in improving the quality and activity of skeletal muscle in AD patients. In general, more RCTs are required to demonstrate the effect of aerobic exercise on executive function and ADL issues in AD patients. In addition, other studies have shown that physical activity can improve executive function and ADL issues in AD patients. Therefore, physical activity is feasible and may provide an alternative or adjuvant treatment for patients with mild to moderate or even late AD and their family nurses.

LIMITATIONS

There are some limitations and deficiencies in this study. The authenticity and reliability of the results are affected by the course of disease and the frequency, time, intensity, and duration of the intervention in AD patients. There are certain differences in the quality of the eligible articles for our study: (1) only four studies showed their concealed allocation, which may be one of the reasons for the systematic bias of results (PEDro-scale, 2010). (2) Only four articles referred to blinding of assessors. (3) Most of the studies lacked a description of the course of the disease, which could have led to a lack of understanding of the effectiveness of physical activity on executive function and ADL issues in AD patients. (4) Most studies did not mention the severity of disease among patients with AD, which made it impossible to provide patients with more targeted exercise prescriptions. (5) Only two authors, Hoffmanna et al. (2016) and Silvaa et al. (2019), mentioned the effect of physical activity on inhibitory functions in AD patients. Studies on inhibitory executive functions among AD patients are scarce and were not included in the meta-analysis for the time being to avoid errors. Furthermore, the differences in

experimental intensity, time, frequency, duration, and outcome measure methods could have led to differences in outcomes and caused difficulty in explanations.

CONCLUSIONS

Research has proven that physical activity can effectively improve executive function, working memory, cognitive flexibility, and ADL issues in AD patients and may be an alternative or auxiliary treatment. In the future, it will necessary to provide more accurate neuropsychological evaluations of each executive function, working memory, cognitive flexibility, and ADL dimension and to grade the course of AD to obtain more accurate exercise prescriptions for physical activity interventions. In the absence of adverse reactions, medical profession could combine physical activity with daily medical treatment to optimize the treatment of executive function, working memory, cognitive flexibility, and performance of ADLs in AD patients. In addition, the conclusion of this study still needs to be confirmed by a high-quality large-sample RCT.

AUTHOR CONTRIBUTIONS

LW and LZ contributed to the idea and structural design plan for review. XJ and HZ applied the search strategy. LZ, LW, and LL applied the selection criteria to screen out qualified documents. LW and XJ completed the deviation risk assessment. LZ wrote the manuscript. LW, LL, and HZ edited the manuscript. All authors analyzed and interpreted the data. All authors have read the complete manuscript and reached a consensus on the manuscript version.

REFERENCES

Allal, G., Annweiler, C., Blumen, H. M., Callisaya, M. L., De-Cock, A. M., Kressig, R. W., et al. (2015). Gait phenotype from mild cognitive impairment to moderate dementia: results from the GOOD initiative. *Eur. J. Neurol.* 23, 527–541. doi: 10.1111/ene.12882

Andrade, L. P., Gobb, L. T. B., Coelh, F. G. M., and Christofolett, G. (2013). Benefits of multimodal exercise intervention for postural control and frontal cognitive functions in individuals with alzheimer's disease: a controlled trial. *JAGS* 61, 1919–1926. doi: 10.1111/jgs.12531

Avilla, R., and Miotto, E. (2002). Funcoes executivas no envelhecimento normal e na doenca de Alzheimer. *J. Bras. Psiquiatr.* 52, 53–63. Available online at: http://www.ipub.ufrj.br/#jbp.html

Baker, L. D., Fran, L. L., Foster-Schuber, K., Gree, P. S., Wilkinso, C. W., and McTierna, A. (2010). Effects of aerobic exercise on mild cognitive impairment: a controlled trial. *Arch. Neurol.* 67, 71–79. doi: 10.1001/archneurol.2009.307

Bell-McGinty, S., Podell, K., Franzen, M., Baird, A. D., and Williams, M. J. (2002). Standard measures of executive function in predicting instrumental activities of daily living in older adults. *Int. J. Geriatr. Psychiatry* 17, 828–834. doi: 10.1002/gps.646

Boyle, P. A., Mallo, P. F., Sallowa, S., Cahn-Weine, D. A., Cohe, R., and Cumming, J. L. (2003). Executive dysfunction and apathy predict functional impairment in alzheimer disease. *J. Geriatr. Psychiatry* 11, 214–221. doi: 10.1097/00019442-200303000-00012

Cahn-Weiner, D. A., Boyle, P. A., and Malloy, P. F. (2002). Tests of executive function predict instrumental activities of daily living in community-dwelling older individuals. *Appl. Neuropsychol.* 9, 187–191. doi: 10.1207/S15324826AN0903_8

Chang, C. H., Wan, W., Zh, Y., and Yan, S. Y. (2015). Study on the intervention of aerobic training on alzheimer's disease. *Chin. J. Rehabil. Med.* 11, 1131–1134. doi: 10.3969/j.issn.1001-1242.2015.11.007

Coelho, F., Vital, T. M., Stei, A. M., Arante, F. J., Rued, A. V., and Camarin, R. (2014). Acute aerobic exercise increases brain derived neurotrophic factor levels in elderly with alzheimer's disease. *J. Alz. Dis.* 39, 401–408. doi: 10.3233/JAD-131073

Coelho, F. G. M., Andrad, L. P., and Pedros, R. V. (2012). Multimodal exercise intervention improves frontal cognitive functions and gait in alzheimer's disease: a controlled trial. *Geriatr. Gerontol. Int.* 4, 1–6. doi: 10.1111/j.1447-0594.2012.00887.x

Coelho, F. G. M., Galduróz-Santos, R. F., Gobbi, S., and Stella, F. (2009). Atividade físicasistematizada e desempenho cognitivo com demência de alzheimer: uma revisão sistemática. *Revis. Brasileira Psiquiatria.* 31, 163–170. doi: 10.1590/S1516-44462009000200014

Cohen-Mansfifield, J., and Mintze, J. E. (2005). Time for change: the role of nonpharmacological interventions in treating behavior problems in nursing home residents with dementia. *Alzheimer Dis. Assoc. Disord.* 19, 37–40. doi: 10.1097/01.wad.0000155066.39184.61

Davenport, M. H., Hogan, D. B., Eskes, G. A., Longman, R. S., and Poulin, M. J. (2012). Cerebrovascular reserve: the link betweenfifit ness and cognitive function? *Exerc. Sport Sci. Rev.* 40, 153–158. doi: 10.1097/JES.0b013e3182553430

Deslandes, A., Moraes, H., Ferreira, C., Veiga, H., Silveira, H., Mouta, R., et al. (2009). Exercise and mental health: many reasons to move. *Neuropsychobiology* 59, 191–198. doi: 10.1159/000223730

Eggermont, L., Swaa, D., Luite, P., and Scherde, E. (2006). Exercise, cognition and alzheimer's disease: more is not necessarily better. *Neurosci. Biobehav. Rev.* 30, 562–575. doi: 10.1016/j.neubiorev.2005.10.004

El-Kader, S. M., and Al-Jiffr, O. H. (2016). Aerobic exercise improves quality of life, psychological well-being and systemic inflammation in subjects with alzheimer's disease. *Afr. Health Sci.* 16, 1045–1055. doi: 10.4314/ahs.v16i4.22

Erickson, K. I., Vos, M. W., and Prakas, R. S. (2011). Exercise training increases size of hippocampus and improves memory. *Proc. Natl. Acad. Sci. U.S.A.* 108, 3017–3022. doi: 10.1073/pnas.1015950108

Erickson, K. I., Weinstein, A. M., and Lopez, O. L. (2012). Physical activity, brain plasticity and alzheimer's disease. *Arch. Med. Res.* 43, 615–621. doi: 10.1016/j.arcmed.2012.09.008

Farina, F., Rusted, J., and Tabet, N. (2014). The effect of exercise interventions on cognitive outcome in alzheimer's disease: a systematic review. *Int. Psychogeriatr.* 26, 9–18. doi: 10.1017/S1041610213001385

Fonte, C., Smani, S., Pedrinoll, A., Munari, D., Gandolf, M., and Picell, A. (2019). Comparison between physical and cognitive treatment in patients with MCI and alzheimer's *disease. Aging* 5, 3138–3155. doi: 10.18632/aging.101970

Foster, P. P., Rosenblatt, K. P., and Kuljiš, R. O. (2011). Exercise-induced cognitive plasticity, implications for mild cognitive impairment and alzheimer's disease. *Front. Neurol.* 2:28. doi: 10.3389/fneur.2011.00028

Hamer, M., and Chid, Y. (2009). Physical activity and risk of neurodegenerative disease. *A systematic review of prospective evidence. Psychol. Med.* 39, 3–11. doi: 10.1017/S0033291708003681

Herholz, S. C., Herhol, R. S., and Herhol, K. (2013). Non-pharmacological interventions and neuroplasticity in early stage alzheimer's disease. *Expert Rev. Neurother.* 13, 1235–1245. doi: 10.1586/14737175.2013.845086

Higgins, J. P. T., Thompso, S. G., Deek, J. J., and Altma, D. G. (2003). Measuring inconsistency in metaanalyses. *BMJ Br. Med. J.* 327, 557–560. doi: 10.1136/bmj.327.7414.557

Hoffmanna, K., Sobolb, N. A., Frederiksena, K. S., Beyerb, N., Vogela, A., and Vestergaard, K. (2016). Moderate-to-high intensity physical exercise in patients with alzheimer's disease: a randomized controlled trial. *J. Alz. Dis.* 50, 443–453. doi: 10.3233/JAD-150817

Holthoff, V. A., Marschne, K., Schar, M., Stedin, J., and Meye, S. (2015). Effects of physical activity training in patients with alzheimer's dementia: results of a pilot RCT study. *PLoS ONE* 4:e0121478. doi: 10.1371/journal.pone.0121478

Jekel, K., Damian, M., and Wattmo, C. (2015). Mild cognitive impairment and defificits in instrumental activities of daily living: a systematic review. *Alzheimer Res. Ther.* 7:17. doi: 10.1186/s13195-015-0099-0

Jin, X. H., Wan, L., Li, S. J., Zh, L., Loprinz, D., and Fa, X. (2020). The impact of mind-body exercises on motor function, depressive symptoms, and quality of life in parkinso's disease: a systematic review and meta-analysis. *Int. J. Environ. Res. Public Health.* 17:31. doi: 10.3390/ijerph17010031

Kempermann, G., Fabe, K., Ehninge, D., Bab, H., Leal-Galici, P., and Garth, A. (2010). Why and how physical activity promotes experience-induced brain plasticity. *Front. Neurosci.* 4:189. doi: 10.3389/fnins.2010.00189

Kivipelto, M., Ngand, T., and Fratiglion, L. (2005). Obesity and vascular risk factors at midlife and the risk of dementia and alzheimers disease. *Arch. Neurol.* 62, 1556–60. doi: 10.1001/archneur.62.10.1556

Kramer, A. F., and Erickson, K. I. (2007). Capitalizing on cortical plasticity: infifluence of physical activity on cognition and brain function. *Trends Cogn. Sci.* 11, 342–348. doi: 10.1016/j.tics.2007.06.009

Lam, L. C., Cha, R. C., Won, B. M., Fun, A. W., Lu, V. W., and Ta, C. C. (2011). Interim follow-up of a randomized controlled trial comparing Chinese style mind body (Tai Chi) and stretching exercises on cognitive function in subjects at risk of progressive cognitive decline. *Int. J. Geriatr. Psychiatry* 26, 733–740. doi: 10.1002/gps.2602

Lautenschlager, N. T., Co, K. L., Flicke, L., Foste, J. K., Bockxmee, F. M., and Xia, J. (2008). Effect of physical activity on cognitive function in older adults at risk for alzheimer disease: a randomized trial. *J. Am. Med. Assoc.* 300, 1027–1037. doi: 10.1001/jama.300.9.1027

Lazowski, D. A., Ecclestone, N. A., and Myers, A. M. (1999). A randomized outcome evaluation of group exercise programs in long-term care institutions. *J. Gerontol. A Biol. Sci. Med. Sci.* 54A, M621–M628. doi: 10.1093/gerona/54.12.M621

Lista, I., and Sorrentin, G. (2009). Biological mechanisms of physical activity in preventing cognitive decline. *Cell. Mol. Neurobiol.* 30, 493–503. doi: 10.1007/s10571-009-9488-x

Liu, S. J., Ren, Z. B., Wang, L., Wei, G. X., and Zou, L. Y. (2018). Mind-body (Baduanjin) exercise prescription for chronic obstructive pulmonary disease: a systematic review with meta-analysis. *Int. J. Environ. Res. Public Health.* 15:1830. doi: 10.3390/ijerph15091830

Maffei, L., Picano, E., and Andreassi, M. G. (2017). Train the brain consortium. *Randomized trial on the effects of a combined physical/cognitive training in aged MCI subjects: the train the brain study. Sci. Rep.* 7:39471. doi: 10.1038/srep39471

Miyake, A., and Friedma, N. P. (2012). The nature and organization of individual differences in executive functions: four general conclusions. *Curr. Dir. Psychol. Sci.* 21, 8–14. doi: 10.1177/0963721411429458

Morley, J. E., and Silve, A. J. (1995). Nutritional issues in nursing home care. *Ann. Intern. Med.* 123, 850–859. doi: 10.7326/0003-4819-123-11-199512010-00008

Morris, J. K., Vidon, E. D., Johnson, D. K., Scive, A. V., Mahnke, J. D., Hone, R. A., et al. (2017). Aerobic exercise for alzheimer's disease: a randomized controlled pilot trial. *PLoS ONE* 2:e0170547. doi: 10.1371/journal.pone.0170547

Norton, S., Matthews, F. E., Barnes, D. E., Yaffe, K., and Brayne, C. (2014). Potential for primary prevention of alzheimer's disease: an analysis of population-based data. *Lancet Neurol.* 13, 788–794. doi: 10.1016/S1474-4422(14)70136-X

Ohman, H., Savikk, N., Strandber, T. E., Kautiaine, H., and Raivi, M. M. (2016). Effects of exercise on cognition: the finnish alzheimer disease exercise trial: a randomized, controlled trial. *JAGS* 64, 731–738. doi: 10.1111/jgs.14059

PEDro-scale (2010). Available online at: https://www.pedro.org.au/simplified-chinese/pedro-scale/ (accessed August 4, 2010).

Pedroso, R. V., Ayán, C., Frag, F. G., and Silv, T. M. V. (2017). Effects of functional-task training on older adults with alzheimer's disease. *J. Aging Phys. Act.* 26, 97–105. doi: 10.1123/japa.2016-0147

Prince, M., Bryce, R., Albanese, E., Wimo, A., Ribeiro, W., and Ferri, C. P. (2013). The global prevalence of dementia: a systematic review and metaanalysis. *Alzheimers Dement.* 9, 63–75.e2. doi: 10.1016/j.jalz.2012.11.007

Radak, Z., Hart, N., and Sarga, L. (2010). Exercise plays a preventive role against alzheimer's disease. *J. Alz. Dis.* 20, 777–783. doi: 10.3233/JAD-2010-091531

Razani, J., Casa, R., Won, J. T., Lu, P., Aless, C., and Josephso, K. (2007). Relationship between executive functioning and activities of daily living in patients with relatively mild dementia. *Appl. Neuropsychol.* 14, 208–214. doi: 10.1080/09084280701509125

Reitz, C., Brayne, C., and Mayeux, R. (2011). Epidemiology of alzheimer disease. *Nat. Rev. Neurol.* 7, 137–152. doi: 10.1038/nrneurol.2011.2

Rolland, Y., Pillar, F., Klapouszcza, A., and Reynis, E. (2017). Exercise program for nursing home residents with alzheimer's disease: a 1-year randomized, controlled *trial. J. Am. Geriatr. Soc.* 55, 158–165. doi: 10.1111/j.1532-5415.2007.01035.x

Royall, D. R., Chiodo, L. K., and Polk, M. J. (2000). Correlates of disability among elderly retirees with "subclinical" cognitive impairment. *J. Gerontol. A Biol. Sci. Med. Sci.* 55, M541–M546. doi: 10.1093/gerona/55.9.M541

Sakuma, K., and Yamaguch, A. (2011). The recent understanding of the neurotrophin's role in skeletal muscle adaptation. *J. Biomed. Biotechnol.* 2011:201696. doi: 10.1155/2011/201696

Scherder, E. J., Van-Paassche, J., Deije, J. B., Van Der Knokk, S., Orlebek, J. F. K., and Burger, I. (2005). Physical activity and executive functions in the elderly with mild cognitive impairment. *Aging Ment. Health* 9, 272–280. doi: 10.1080/13607860500089930

Silvaa, F. O., Ferreira, J. V., and Plácido, J. (2019). Three months of multimodal training contributes to mobility and executive function in elderly individuals with mild cognitive impairment, but not in those with alzheimer's disease: a randomized controlled *trial. Maturitas* 126, 28–33. doi: 10.1016/j.maturitas.2019.04.217

Sofifi, F., Valecch, D., and Bacc, D. (2011). Physical activity and risk of cognitive decline. *A meta-analysis of prospective studies. J. Intern. Med.* 269, 107–117. doi: 10.1111/j.1365-2796.2010.02281.x

Tan, C. C., Yu, J. T., Wang, H. F., Tan, M. S., Meng, X. F., Wang, C., et al. (2014). Effificacy and safety of donepezil, galantamine, rivastigmine, and memantine for the treatment of alzheimer's disease: a systematic review and meta-analysis. *J. Alzheimers Dis.* 41, 615–631. doi: 10.3233/JAD-132690

Tootsa, A., Littbran, H., Bostro, G., Hornste, C., and Holmberg, H. (2017). Effects of exercise on cognitive function in older people with dementia: a randomized controlled trial. *J. Alz. Dis.* 60, 323–332. doi: 10.3233/JAD-170014

Uffelen, J. G., Chinapa, M. J., Mechele, W., and Hopman-Roc, M. (2008). Walking or vitamin B for cognition in older adults with mild cognitive impairment? *A randomised controlled trial. Br. J. Sports Med.* 42, 344–351. doi: 10.1136/bjsm.2007.044735

Venturelli, M., Scarsin, R., and Schen, F. (2011). Six-month walking program changes cognitive and ADL performance in patients with Alzheimer. *J. Alzheimers Dis.* 26, 381–388. doi: 10.1177/1533317511418956

Vidoni, E. D., Perale, J., Alshehr, M., Gile, A. M., and Siengsuko, C. F. (2017). Aerobic exercise sustains performance of instrumental activities of daily living in early-stage alzheimer disease. *J. Geriatr. Phys. Ther.* 42, 1–6. doi: 10.1519/JPT.0000000000000172

Vreugdenhill, A., Cannel, J., Davie, A., and Raza, G. (2012). A community-based exercise programme to improve functional ability in people with alzheimer's disease: a randomized controlled trial. *Scand. J. Caring Sci.* 26, 12–19. doi: 10.1111/j.1471-6712.2011.00895.x

Wilbur, J., Marquez, D. X., Fogg, L., Wilson, R. S., Staffifileno, B. A., Hoyem, R. L., et al. (2012). The relationship between physical activity and cognition in older latinos. *J. Gerontol. B Psychol. Sci. Soc. Sci.* 67, 525–534. doi: 10.1093/geronb/gbr137

World Health Organization Physical Activity and Older Adults (2017). Available online at: http://www.who.int/dietphysicalactivity/factsheet_olderadults/en (accessed January 18, 2017).

Yaari, R., and Bloom, J. C. (2007). Alzheimer's disease. *Semin. Neurol.* 27, 32–41. doi: 10.1055/s-2006-956753

Zou, L. Y., Han, J., Li, X. C., Yeung, A., Hui, S. C., Tsang, W. N., et al. (2019). The effects of tai chi on lower limb proprioception in adults aged over 55: a systematic review and meta-analysis. *Arch. Phys. Med. Rehabil.* 100, 1102–1113. doi: 10.1016/j.apmr.2018.07.425

14

Depression in Somatic Disorders: Is there a Beneficial Effect of Exercise?

Astrid Roeh[1*], Sophie K. Kirchner[1], Berend Malchow[2], Isabel Maurus[1], Andrea Schmitt[1,3], Peter Falkai[1] and Alkomiet Hasan[1]

[1] Department of Psychiatry and Psychotherapy, University Hospital, Ludwig-Maximilians University Munich, Munich, Germany, [2] Department of Psychiatry and Psychotherapy, Universitätsklinikum Jena, Jena, Germany, [3] Laboratory of Neuroscience (LIM27), Institute of Psychiatry, University of São Paulo, São Paulo, Brazil

Correspondence:
Astrid Roeh
astrid.roeh@med.uni-muenchen.de

Background: The beneficial effects of exercise training on depressive symptoms are well-established. In the past years, more research attention has been drawn to the specific effects of exercise training on depressive symptoms in somatically ill patients. This reviews aims at providing a comprehensive overview of the current findings and evidence of exercise interventions in somatic disorders to improve depressive symptoms.

Methods: We systematically searched PubMed and Cochrane databases and extracted meta-analyses from somatically ill patients that underwent exercise interventions and provided information about the outcome of depressive symptoms.

Results: Of the 4123 detected publications, 39 were selected for final analysis. Various diseases were included (breast-cancer, prostate cancer, mixed-cancer, cardiovascular disease, coronary heart disease, hemodialysis, fibromyalgia syndrome, acute leukemia, other hematological malignancies, heart failure, HIV, multiple sclerosis, mixed neurological disorders, Parkinson's disease, stroke, ankylosing spondylitis, traumatic brain injury, lupus erythematodes). Most meta-analyses (33/39) found beneficial effects on depressive symptoms, but quality of the included studies as well as duration, intensity, frequency, and type of exercise varied widely.

Conclusion: Exercise training has the potential to improve depressive symptoms in patients with somatic disorders. For specific training recommendations, more high quality studies with structured exercise programs and better comparability are needed.

Keywords: depressive symptoms, training, aerobic, somatic disease, comorbidity

INTRODUCTION

Depression alone and comorbid with other chronic somatic diseases accounts for significant disease burden worldwide (1, 2). By 2030, depression is in addition to HIV/AIDS and ischemic heart disease assumed to be one of the three leading causes of burden of disease (3). Exercise therapy in depressive patients, as an independent intervention and as an adjunct intervention to antidepressant medication or psychotherapy, has been discussed to improve clinical outcomes in somatic diseases (4, 5). Compared to pharmacological treatment, the beneficial effects of exercise seem to be similar and are present at short-term and during follow-up periods of up to one year (6, 7). Especially for somatically unstable patient, this offers new treatment perspectives without the common side-effects of psychopharmacological medication. Usually both the depressive symptoms and the underlying somatic condition improve as a consequence of exercise therapy.

In a large World Health Survey of 245 404 participants from 60 countries, an average between 9.3 and 23.0% of participants with one or more chronic physical diseases had comorbid depressive symptoms (2). For numerous somatic diseases, an association with depression is well-established. For example, patients with multiple sclerosis (8), stroke (9), parkinson's disease (10), diabetes mellitus (11), breast cancer (12) or heart failure (13) have an elevated risk for developing a major depressive disorder (MDD). From a psychiatric perspective, it is important to note that a recently published study with 1,237,194 participants showed that individuals who exercised (various types of disciplines) had 1.49 (43.2%) fewer days of poor mental health in the past month than non-exercising individuals (14).

As the comorbid physical diseases often complicate the pharmacological treatment of depressive symptoms, further research approaches with a focus on alternative therapy options are urgently needed. Based on the beneficial effects of physical exercise in MDD (15), prior studies investigated the effects of exercise in patients with somatic disorders and comorbid depressive symptoms. A meta-analysis of different chronic illnesses including stroke, ischemic heart attack, fibromyalgia, dementia, and other psychiatric diseases, revealed a significant overall reduction of depressive symptoms. The majority of effects were derived from cardiovascular diseases, chronic pain and fibromyalgia (16). The results lead to the conclusion that physical exercise seems to have positive effects on depressive symptoms in patients with various somatic diseases without subdividing the different diseases with specific recommendations. However, a comprehensive overview of the available evidence of how exercise may improve depressive symptoms in patients with somatic diseases is lacking.

In this systematic meta-review, we will provide a detailed overview of recent meta-analyses evaluating different somatic diseases with comorbid depressive symptoms. The efficacy and the types and durations of exercise will be analyzed. Up to date, meta-analyses of specific diseases or disease groups (e.g., cardiovascular diseases) have been published as well as meta-analyses comprising different somatic diseases with an emphasis on cardiovascular diseases, fibromyalgia and pain (16). With our review, we aim to close this gap and point to limitations of prior studies as well as possible future research strategies.

METHODS

We systematically searched PubMed and Cochrane databases with all combinations of the following search terms: depressive disorder OR depression AND exercise, depressive disorder OR depression AND physical activity, depressive disorder OR depression AND endurance training, depressive disorder OR depression AND training, depressive disorder OR depression AND resistance training, depressive disorder OR depression AND aerobic, depression OR depressive disorder AND somatic AND exercise, depression OR depressive disorder AND physical illness. The database search was last updated on 31th July 2018. All citations were screened for relevance by title in a first step, by abstract in a second step and by full-text in a last step. In all included meta-analyses, the citations were screened manually for further relevant meta-analyses that may have not been detected by the systematic search. The systematic literature search and selection was performed by AR, the selection was afterwards reviewed independently by SK.

Both AR and SK retrieved the relevant information and the results were compared. In case of disagreement, a third author (AH) was consulted. Inclusion criteria were: meta-analysis investigating the effects of exercise on depressive symptoms in patients with comorbid physical illness based on interventional trials, published within the past 10 years. Exclusion criteria contained meta-analyses published earlier than within the past 10 years, systematic reviews without meta-analyses, meta-analyses in non-English language, meta-analyses only investigating depressive patients with no somatic comorbidities, lack of data post-intervention. No limitations were defined for the type or duration of exercise and the type of somatic illness.

RESULTS

Study Selection

The initial search without further restrictions resulted in 103,468 citations. After limiting the citations for the past 10 years, 60,430 citations remained. When only considering the meta-analyses, 4,123 citations remained and after eliminating duplicates, 981 citations were included for further analysis. The screening on title-level eliminated 869 citations (112 remaining), the screening on abstract-level another 63 citations (49 remaining). After full-text screening, 39 citations remained for final analysis (see **Figure 1**).

Study Characteristics

Table 1 provides an overview of the included somatic diseases. The duration of the single studies varied between three (46) to 52 (21) weeks, the intensity between one time (51) and seven times (37) per week and the duration of the sessions between 30 and 122 min (16). Adherence rate was solely reported in two meta-analyses (21, 22) and intensity of the training with heart rate controlled exertion in one meta-analysis (37). The interventions consisted of aerobic exercise, resistance training, balance training, yoga, moderate cycling, walking, nordic walking, running, swimming, tai chi chuan, qigong, Bobath exercises, jogging, calisthenics. Across all trials, the mean sample size was 658 with a minimum of 39 (28) and a maximum of 3.425 (36). Depressive symptoms were rated with different questionnaires (observer or self-assessment): BDI (Beck Depression Inventory), CDI (Children Depression Inventory), CES-D (Center for Epidemiological Studies Depression Scale), DASS (Depression Anxiety Stress Scales), GDS (Geriatric Depression Scale), HAD (Hospital Anxiety and Depression Scale), HAM-D (Hamilton Rating Scale for Depression), SCL-90 (Symptom Checklist-90), TAS (Toronto Attitude Scale), POMS (Profile of Mood States), SAS (Symptom Assessment Scale), CSDD (Cornell Scale for Depression in Dementia), IDS-SR (Inventory of Depressive Symptomatology Self Report), LPD (Levine-Pilowsky Depression Questionnaire), MADRS

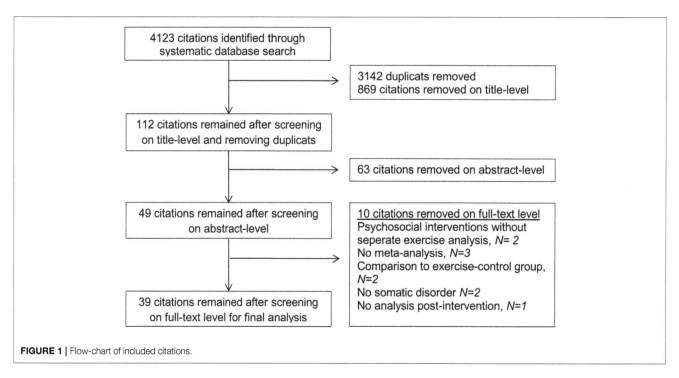

FIGURE 1 | Flow-chart of included citations.

TABLE 1 | Included somatic diseases.

Somatic disease in meta-analysis	No. of meta-analyses	References
Breast cancer	7	(17–23)
Mixed cancer types	7	(24–30)
Prostate cancer	3	(31–33)
Cardiovascular disease	1	(34)
Coronary Heart disease	1	(35)
Heart failure	2	(36, 37)
Intradialytic patients	2	(38, 39)
Hemodialysis patients	1	(40)
Fibromyalgia	2	(41, 42)
Ankylosing spondylitis	1	(43)
Lupus erythematodes	1	(44)
Acute leukemia	1	(45)
Hematological malignancies	1	(46)
HIV	1	(47)
Multiple sclerosis	3	(16, 48, 49)
Mixed neurological disorders	1	(50)
Parkinson disease	1	(51)
Stroke	2	(52, 53)
Traumatic brain injury	1	(54)
Total	39	

HIV, human immunodeficiency virus.

(Montgomery-Asberg Depression Rating Scale), MDI (Major Depression Inventory), POMS (Profile of Mood States), QOL (Quality of Life), DASS (Depression Anxiety Stress Scales), TAS (Toronto Attitude Scale), MAACL (Multiple Affect Adjective Checklist), HDCDS (Hare-Davis Cardiac Depression Scale),

SDS (Self-rating Depression Scale), BSI-18 (Brief Symptom Inventory). Thus, in the different meta-analyses, various different questionnaires were used, most often self-rating questionnaires: the BDI I/II in 26, the HADS in 18 and the CES-D in 17 meta-analyses. The majority of meta-analyses included more than three different questionnaires. As observer-rating scales, HAMD was used in four and MADRS in three meta-analyses.

Risk of Bias Within and Across Studies

Most meta-analyses (51) reported about different cancer-type patients followed by neurological disorders (7). For other diseases, such as HIV, only one meta-analysis could be identified. The variety of exercise modalities and the different durations of interventions lead to a reduced general transferability of the conclusions. Recommendations regarding effects of specific interventions on depressive symptoms in specific somatic conditions can hardly be drawn. None of the trials included in the respective meta-analyses could be declared double-blind as this is challenging to fulfill with exercise interventions. The application of various different rating-scales is another potential risk of bias. Moreover, most of the included studies in the respective meta-analyses did not define depressive symptoms as primary outcome parameter.

Results of Individual Studies

A detailed summary of the included studies with inclusion/exclusion criteria, study population, intervention summary and outcomes is provided in **Tables 2, 3**.

Exercise Interventions in Cancer Patients
Exercise interventions in breast cancer patients
Our search resulted in seven meta-analyses that met the inclusion criteria. The majority found positive effects of

TABLE 2 | Methods and Limitations of the included meta-analyses.

References	Included trials, sample size	Included population/inclusion criteria	Intervention	Rating Scales	Quality and possible moderators
Adamson et al. (50)	23 studies, N = 1.324 participants	1) Adults aged >18 years 2) Any diagnosed neurologic disorder (ad or dementia, migraine, ms, parkinson disease, spinal cord injury, and traumatic brain injury) Excluded: fibromyalgia, rheumatoid arthritis	Aerobic exercise, resistance training, balance training, yoga, and others involving a combination of these exercises. No limits concerning frequency, intensity, or duration of the exercise intervention.	BDI, BDI-II, CES-D, CSDD, GDS, HAD, IDS-SR, MADRS, LPD, MDI, POMS	123/26 studies evaluated depression. 13 of the 26 studies Received a score >6 on the PEDro scale. 3 trials identified depression as primary endpoint.
Bergenthal et al. (46)	3 RCTs, N = 249	1) RCTs comparing an aerobic physical exercise intervention, intending to improve the oxygen system, in addition to standard care with standard care 2) Only for adults suffering from hematological malignancies.	Studies that evaluated aerobic exercise (such as moderate cycling, walking, Nordic walking, running, swimming and other related forms of sport) or aerobic exercise in addition to strength training were included. Studies that investigated the effect of training programs that were composed of yoga, tai chi chuan, qigong or similar types of exercise were excluded. Duration of the intervention between 3 and 12 weeks with 3–5 sessions per week.	NR	3/9 studies could be included in the meta-analysis for depression (secondary endpoint). Low quality of evidence.
Brown et al. (24)	37 RCTs, N = 2.929	1) RCT comparing an exercise intervention with a control group 2) Report of depression outcomes 3) Adults diagnosed with any type of cancer, regardless of stage of diagnosis or type of treatment At baseline, the standardized metric of depressive symptoms was 34.2 and ranged from 3.49 to 81.5. 65% Breast Cancer, 5% Prostate cancer, 5% Leukemia, 5% Lymphoma, 20% diverse groups of cancer	Exercise interventions occurring in any setting, with or without supervision. Mean length of the exercise interventions was 13.2 weeks with an average of 3.0 sessions per week lasting 49.1 min/session.	CES-D, POMS, BDI, HAS, SAS	The mean PEDro score of the exercise interventions was 7.061 suggesting relatively high methodological quality.
Buffart et al. (25)	8 RCTs, N = 471	1) Design: RCT 2) Population: adults with any cancer diagnosis either during or post treatment 3) Intervention: yoga including physical postures (asanas) 4) Control group: non-exercise or wait-list 5) Outcome: physical and psychosocial outcomes Average age of the participants ranged from 44 to 63 years. 1 study with lymphoma patients, the rest with breast cancer patients.	All included a supervised yoga program with physical poses (yoga asanas), combined with breathing techniques (pranayama) and relaxation or meditation (savasana or dhanya). Median program duration was 7 weeks with a range of 6 weeks to 6 months. In general, the number of classes per week ranged from one to three, and home practice was encouraged in nine studies, supported by audio or videotapes. Session duration ranged from 30 to 120 min; three studies did not report the session duration.	HADS-D, BDI, CES-D, POMS	The median quality score was 67% (range: 22–89%). All but one study were of high quality. 8 of 16 studies evaluated depression.
Carayol et al. (17)	9 RCTs, N = 801	1) Participants were adult women diagnosed with breast cancer. 2) Presented a randomized, controlled experimental design 3) Included an intervention program involving physical activity (yoga-based interventions were included whereas relaxation-based were not) 4) Intervention program was scheduled during adjuvant cancer therapy (chemotherapy and/or radiotherapy), (v) assessed at least one psychological outcome among fatigue, anxiety, depression, and QoL 5) Provided pre and post-intervention data to calculate standardized mean differences(SMDs) The median age of included patients was 50.5 years old. All patients with breast cancer have been diagnosed with non-metastatic cancer and were undergoing adjuvant therapy, i.e., chemotherapy and/or radiotherapy during exercise intervention.	Exercise duration between 5 and 26 weeks, 2–6 sessions per week of 30–60 min. Interventions consisted of aerobic exercise and/or resistance training or Yoga.	CES-D, HADS-D, BDI, POMS	Regarding methodological quality, median score was 7, ranging from 2 to 9. 9/17 studies evaluated depression.

(Continued)

TABLE 2 | Continued

References	Included trials, sample size	Included population/inclusion criteria	Intervention	Rating Scales	Quality and possible moderators
Chung et al. (38)	4 RCTs, $N = 212$	1) This review included randomized controlled trials (RCTs) published in the English or Chinese language 2) participants aged >18 years diagnosed with end stage renal disease (ESRD) requiring maintenance hemodialysis (HD) as renal replacement therapy 3) participants undergoing HD for more than 3 months who received exercise training during HD sessions (intradialytic)	Exercise interventions included aerobic cycling alone, resistance training, cycling or resistance training and aerobic cycling combined with strength training or range of motion. Each exercise session lasted 10–90 min. The exercise program lasted between 8 and 48 weeks.	Zung Depression Scale, BDI	In over half of the studies, there was a low or unclear risk of detection bias. 4/17 studies evaluated depression.
Craft et al. (26)	14 RCTs, $N = 1,371$ participants	1) RCTs of adults diagnosed with cancer 2) Comparison of an exercise program with usual care 3) The exercise program was chronic in nature (i.e., at least 4 weeks in duration) 4) Reported depressive symptoms pre- and post-intervention 5) Utilized a depression inventory or a clinician interview to quantify depressive symptoms 6) published in English Average age of participants was 51.6 years. 9 (60%) breast cancer, 1 colorectal cancer, 1 lymphoma, 2 prostate cancer and 2 diverse groups of cancer	All studies included an aerobic exercise component, with several also including a strength training component.	CES-D, BDI, HADS, QOL	Only 1 trial identified depression as primary endpoint. 11 RCTs with PEDro "high" quality. Potential moderators: exercise location, Supervised and partially supervised exercise, exercise bout durations of >30 min.
Cramer et al. (19)	6 RCTs, $N = 161$	1) RCTs 2) Studies of adult (older than 18 years) patients with a history of breast cancer 3) Studies that compared yoga with no treatment or any active treatment 4) No restrictions were made regarding yoga tradition, length, frequency or duration of the program. Co-interventions were allowed. 5) Studies that assessed health-related quality of life or well-being and/or psychological health.	Yoga interventions were heterogeneous. Program length and intensity varied, ranging from daily interventions over 1 week to one intervention per week over 6 months.	CES-D, HADS, BDI	Generally, risk of selection bias was high. 6/10 studies evaluated depression.
Cramer et al. (18)	11 RCTs, $N = 496$ (7 RCTs yoga vs. No therapy) $+ N = 226$ (4 RCTs, yoga vs. Psychosocial intervention)	1) RCT 2) Compared yoga interventions vs. no therapy or vs. any other active therapy in women with a diagnosis of non-metastatic or metastatic breast cancer 3) Assessed at least one of the primary outcomes on patient-reported instruments, including health-related quality of life, depression, anxiety, fatigue or sleep disturbances	Of the 24 included studies: the duration of yoga programs ranged from 2 weeks to 6 months, with a median duration of 8 weeks; the frequency of yoga interventions ranged from one to 10 (median: two) weekly yoga sessions of 20 to 120 (median: 67.5) min in length.	HADS, BDI, CES-D, POMS	11/24 studies evaluated depression.
Dalgas et al. (48)	12 RCTs, $N = 476$	1) RCT design 2) Enrollment of participants with definite MS according to the McDonald criteria 3) Evaluate an exercise intervention that was compared with either non-training controls, active controls or another exercise intervention 4) Inclusion of a primary validated measure of depressive symptoms available in English	resistance training, endurance training, combined training (i.e., resistance training + endurance training) or as other exercise modalities	BDI, MDI, IDS-SR, HADS, POMS, CES-D	Only one of the RCT studies applied depressive symptoms As the primary outcome. Average PEDro score was 5.6 ± 1.3 points.
Eng and Reime (52)	13 RCTs, $N = 1,022$	1) Confirmed diagnosis of stroke by medical records, imaging, or clinical examination 2) Adult patients over 18 years of age 3) Intervention and control group treatments clearly defined 4) Baseline and follow-up of at least 4 weeks available for depressive symptoms The time since stroke ranged from 30 days to 6 years and the patients' age ranged from 21 to 93 years.	Progressive resistance training, functional, aerobic exercises, treadmill exercises, Bobath exercises, individualized exercises with education, community-based rehabilitation services including physical therapy and occupational therapy. Eleven of the 13 studies had a frequency of at least two sessions per week for a minimal duration of 4 weeks. The length of the intervention ranged from 4 weeks to 12 weeks.	HAD, GDS, BDI, CES-D	PEDro scale ranged from three to eight.

(Continued)

TABLE 2 | Continued

References	Included trials, sample size	Included population/inclusion criteria	Intervention	Rating Scales	Quality and possible moderators
Ensari et al. (49)	13 RCTs, N = 477	The mean baseline depressive symptoms of the study samples were below established thresholds for clinically relevant depressive symptoms in the majority of studies (12/13). 1) Studies that compared exercise training vs. no-treatment control Reliable and valid measures of depressive symptoms (e.g., HADs, CES-D) as an outcome assessment pre/post intervention in patients with MS 2) Only samples in 2 of the studies had mean scores above the threshold for moderate depressive symptomatology.	Aerobic and an-aerobic. 7 of the 13 studies had a frequency of at least 3 sessions per week.	BDI, IDS, MDI, HADS, CES-D, POMS	9 of the 13 studies received a score of 6 or higher on the PEDro scale. Exploratory analyses only identified depression symptom scale as a potential moderator variable (p = 0.04).
Fong et al. (27)	4 RCTs, N = 168 4 RCTs with different outcome measurements, N = 533	Adult patients (aged ≥18) Patients diagnosed with cancer 3) Patients who had completed their main treatment for cancer but might be still undergoing hormonal treatment 4) And assessed the effect of physical activity on health indicators ¾ included studies evaluated breast cancer, 1 endometrial cancer.	All 4 studies used aerobic exercise.	BDI, HADS, POMS	4/34 studies evaluated depression via BDI and were included in the meta-analysis. 2 studies used the HADS and 2 the POMS. No overall analysis was performed.
Furmaniak et al. (20)	5 RCTs, N = 674	1) RCTs of exercise training during adjuvant (including neoadjuvant) treatment (radiotherapy chemotherapy) for women with non-metastatic breast cancer 2) Exercise training during adjuvant (including neoadjuvant) treatment (radiotherapy, chemotherapy) for women with non-metastatic breast cancer. 3) Studies that assessed the effects of all forms of repeatedly performed aerobic or resistance exercise or both with program duration of at least 6 weeks	Aerobic or resistance training.	BDI, CES-D	Cochranes risk of bias tool. 1 study evaluated depression via HADS and was not included in the meta-analysis. 5/32 studies evaluated depression.
Gomes Neto et al. (39)	3 RCTs, N = 88	1) Studies that included hemodialysis patients randomized to two different intra-dialytic exercise training modalities or to a group of specific exercise modality and group of usual care without exercise training. 2) Studies that enrolled patients with cardiac or respiratory diseases were excluded	Combined aerobic and resistance training.	BDI	3/56 studies evaluated depression with the BDI.
Graven et al. (53)	54 RCTs, 10 with exercise and 2 for meta-analysis, N = 137	1) Patients with a primary diagnosis of cerebrovascular accident 2) Participants who were community-dwelling 3) RCTs 4) Trial outcomes that measured at least one of the domains of participation, the mood disorder of depression and HRQoL (using validated scales that are commonly applied) 5) Interventions conducted in the community setting by predominantly nursing or allied health practitioners 6) The availability of an English full text version	All the studies incorporated an experimental exercise regime that was of an intensity of two to three sessions per week over a 6–12-week duration (average 9.8 weeks).	CES-D, GDS-15	PEDro methodological rating of at least four points was an inclusion criterion.
Herring et al. (16)	14 RCTs, N = 624	1) English-language peer-reviewed publications 2) Adults aged >18 years with a formal diagnosis of MS 3) Randomized allocation to either an exercise intervention or a non-active control condition that lacked exercise training 4) A measure of depressive symptoms measured at baseline and at mid- and/or post-intervention The mean age was 44.0 years. The mean percentage of women was 75%. Mean reported disease duration was 9.8 years, and mean baseline Expanded Disability Status Scale (EDSS) score was 3.4.	Aerobic, Resistance Aerobic+, Resistance+, Yoga Exercise training consisted of three sessions per week, 51 min per session, and 11 weeks in duration. Based on reported methods, PwMS were prescribed 122 (SD = 38) min of exercise per week. The mean exercise training adherence rate was 85%.	BDI, CES-D, HADS-D, IDS-SR, POMS-D, MDI	Mean PEDro score was 5.86. Depressive symptoms were not the primary outcome in any of the included trials.

(Continued)

TABLE 2 | Continued

References	Included trials, sample size	Included population/inclusion criteria	Intervention	Rating Scales	Quality and possible moderators
Langhorst et al. (41)	6 RCTs, $N = 306$	1) RCTs 2) Studies with meditative movement therapies 3) Patients diagnosed with FMS on recognized criteria, of any age 4) Studies should assess at least one key domain of FMS (pain, sleep, fatigue), health-related quality of life (HRQOL) and depression	Tai Chi and/or Yoga, and/or Qi Gong. In the whole review (7 studies), the number of sessions was 12 (8–24). The total treatment time was 18 (6–48) h.	BDI, CES-D, CDI	Publication bias was assessed by Egger's intercept test and Begg's rank correlation test at the significance level $p < 0.05$. 6/7 studies evaluated depression.
Liang et al. (43)	3 RCTs/quasi-RCTs, $N = 121$	1) Adults diagnosed by a rheumatologist as having AS (ankylosing spondylitis) 2) Participants > 18 years 3) Quasi-randomized and randomized controlled trials (RCT), in which at least one of the groups received home-based exercise therapy	Home-based exercise program including muscle relaxation, flexibility exercises for cervical, thoracic and lumbar spine, range of motion exercises of coxofemoral joints, stretching exercises for the major muscle groups, muscular strengthening, straight posture, and respiratory exercises.	BDI	3/6 trials investigated depression. The research team performed an analysis of all included studies (6), using a funnel plot to determine publication bias in all the literature. The outcome from the funnel shows asymmetry, thereby indicating that publication bias possibly exists in the included studies.
Lin et al. (29)	8 RCTs, $N = 519$	1) Randomized control trial design 2) Examination of yoga or MBSR (mindfulness based stress reduction) on psychological health, quality of life, and physical health of cancer patients 6 studies assessed the effects of yoga for patients with breast cancer, 1 for patients with lymphoma, and 1 for mixed cancer population.	The style of yoga used and the duration and frequency of the yoga sessions varied among all studies. Intervention duration ranged from 6 to 24 weeks.	HADS, CES-D, POMS SCL-90-R	8/10 studies evaluated depressive symptoms. Of the 10 studies, the PEDro scores ranged from 4 to 7.
Lin et al. (28)	2 RCTs, $N = 39$	1) Randomized controlled trials (RCTs) published in a peer-reviewed journal 2) Patients of any age, diagnosed with any type of gynecological cancer (i.e., cancers of the vulva, vagina, cervix, uterus, ovary, fallopian tube and placenta), at any stage of their illness 3) studies including an intervention with any type of exercise component (i.e., aerobic training, muscle strengthening, stretching exercises or education regarding exercise) The mean age of the participants across all studies (7) ranged from 52.1 to 63.9 years.	The length of interventions ranged from 5 days to 6 months. Participants were coached to meet the physical activity guidelines of at least 30 min of physical activity on 5 days per week.	BDI, BDI-II	The mean PEDro score was 5.3 (standard deviation 1.5) out of 10 for the whole analysis (7 studies). 2 of the 7 studies assessed depressive symptoms.
Liu et al. (35)	2 RCTs/CCTs, $N = 84$	1) Patients with CHD (coronary heart disease), regardless of disease stage and severity. Eligible CHD diagnoses included myocardial infarction (MI), angina or a revascularization procedure (coronary artery bypass grafting or percutaneous coronary intervention) 2) Thai Chi intervention, no limits were imposed on type, duration, frequency, length or intensity of the Tai Chi intervention. 3) RCTs, non-randomized controlled clinical trials (CCTs) 4) Articles published in English or Chinese	Thai Chi groups, duration of 3 months and 2–5 sessions per week.	SDS	2/11 studies evaluated depressive symptoms. The two studies were rated as 'moderate' regarding global quality.
Newby et al. (31)	4 RCTs, $N = 466$	1) RCTs 2) Comparison of any intervention to treat depression in patients with prostate cancer 3) Entry criteria for depressive scores did not have to be severe enough to be considered a case of Diagnostic and Statistical Manual major depressive disorder (clinical depression)	For most studies, the intervention was 6–9 weeks. Precise exercise regimen was not stated.	CES-D, HADS, GDS, BDI	4/9 studies evaluated depression. Overall quality was fair (3 studies) to poor (1 study).

(Continued)

TABLE 2 | Continued

References	Included trials, sample size	Included population/inclusion criteria	Intervention	Rating Scales	Quality and possible moderators
O'Brien et al. (47)	2 RCTs, N = 65	1) RCTs with human participants who were HIV positive 2) adults 18 years of age or older 3) aerobic exercise intervention performed at least three times/week, at least 20 min per session for at least 4 weeks 4) a randomized controlled comparison group	Aerobic exercise was defined as a regimen containing aerobic interventions performed at least three times per week for at least 4 weeks. Aerobic interventions included but were not limited to walking, jogging, cycling, rowing, stair stepping, and swimming. Interventions may or may not have been supervised.	POMS	2/10 studies evaluated depression via POMS and were included in the meta-analysis.
O'Dwyer et al. (44)	3 RCTs, N = 75	1) Quasi-randomized and randomized controlled trials in SLE (systemic lupus erythematodes) comparing at least one exercise group to controls 2) Studies evaluating adults diagnosed with SLE by established criteria 3) studies with participants under 18 years of age were excluded 4) studies comparing exercise to no intervention controls, studies comparing different exercise or physical activity protocols (e.g., aerobic exercise vs. strengthening exercise), and studies comparing an exercise-based intervention to another treatment approach (e.g., relaxation)	Exercise-based interventions comprised one or more of the following components: range of motion (stretching), resistance training, or aerobic exercise. 3–6 weeks of duration and 2–3 sessions/week.	BDI	Overall risk of bias of these studies was unclear.
Patsou et al. (21)	14 RCTs, N = 1.701	1) Written in English 2) Published in 2011 and beyond 3) Participants were adult women diagnosed with breast cancer based on mammography and biopsy 4) Included an intervention program involving physical activity 5) Randomized controlled trial (experimental) design 5) Results for depression outcomes The median age of the included breast cancer survivors was 52 years. In all studies, women had been diagnosed with 0–IIIc stage breast cancer.	Aerobic, resistance, aerobic and resistance, yoga exercises The length of the interventions ranged from 6 to 52 weeks. The reported exercise frequency was 2–3 sessions per week for the majority of the studies, while duration varied from 30 to 90 min per session and weekly exercise duration ranged from 90 to 270 min. All studies had over 80% up to as high as 99% retention rates, while adherence rates, when reported, varied from 70 to 92.7%.	HADS, CES-D, BDI-II, POMS	The mean PEDro score of the studies was 6.1 ± 2, indicating High quality. Depression was the sole primary outcome measure in only one study, while in three more studies, depression was included either as primary or not as psychosocial/psychological outcome.
Perry et al. (54)	2 RCTs/7 non-RCTs, N = 188	1) Participants aged 18 or older and have sustained a TBI (traumatic brain injury) 2) Interventions must utilize physical exercise 3) Depression-related outcome measure	Eight out of the nine studies had an aerobic intervention including treadmill, exercise bike and swimming, one study used a walking intervention. The intervention length was between 8 and 12 weeks, apart from one study which had just two sessions, 1 week apart	BDI, HAM-D, POMS, BRUMS, CES-D, HADS	Majority of included trials was non-randomized, no PEDro scores provided.
Samartzis et al. (36)	9 RCTs (+ 4 RCTs with SSRI comparison), N = 3.425	1) An experimental CHF patient group, and a CHF patient group as controls that received standard care 2) Patients were randomly allocated 3) Both groups were evaluated for depression before and after the intervention, by using psychometric instruments 4) data were published	Home and hospital exercise training interventions.	HAM-D,BDI-II, BDI, MADRS, GDS, MAACL	No PEDro scores provided. A trend for superiority of hospital-based exercise training for depression was noted.
Singh et al. (22)	14 RCTs, N = 1005	1) RCTs in which at least 50% of the sample was diagnosed with Stage II+ breast cancer 2) Exercise trials 3) Trials were eligible regardless of the level of supervision provided, mode of intervention delivery, intervention duration or intensity. Median recruitment rate was 56% (1–96%), 15 withdrawal rate was 10% (0–41%) and adherence rate was 82% (44–99%).	Aerobic exercise, resistance exercise, combined,	POMS, HADS, CES-D, Greene Climacteric Scale, BDI, Functional Living Index of Cancer	14/61 trials evaluated depression. 38/61 trials were rated as "high quality" according to the PEDro score.

(Continued)

TABLE 2 | Continued

References	Included trials, sample size	Included population/inclusion criteria	Intervention	Rating Scales	Quality and possible moderators
Song et al. (51)	4 RCTs, N = 148	1) RCTs and prospective non-randomized controlled and observational studies published in English 2) Parkinson's disease was the primary disease and Tai Chi and/or Qigong were the primary interventions were included. 3) RCTs	3 studies used Thai Chi, 1 study used Qigong. The duration of interventions ranged from 7 to 16 weeks. Individual intervention sessions ranged from 45 to 90 min, and the frequency of classes varied between 1 and 3 times per week.	BDI, GDS, MADRS	5/21 studies (4 RCTs) evaluated depression.
Song et al. (40)	8 RCTs, N = 368	1) RCTs 2) patients with ESRD (end-stage renal disease) undergoing HD (hemodialysis) for more than 3 months 3) 18 years and older 4) exercise training compared to routine HD treatment or exercise training with pharmacological treatment compared to the same pharmacological treatment	Aerobic exercise, resistance training, flexibility training, Yoga, Pilates. The duration of one intervention and the total interventions ranged from 15 min to 90 min and 4 weeks to 48 weeks (12 months).	BDI, HADS, Zung Depression Scale	8/15 trials evaluated depression. Cochrane risk of bias tool was applied.
Sosa-Reina et al. (42)	11 RCTs, N = 641	1) RCTs comparing types of therapeutic exercise or comparing therapeutic exercise with a control group receiving another intervention or standard care 2) Studies with participants older than 18 years, diagnosed with FMS (fibromyalgia syndrome) in the absence of significant comorbidity 3) Studies using aerobic, strengthening, or stretching exercises or a combination of these were considered. Studies of exercise interventions based on activities such as yoga or tai-chi were excluded. Almost all the participants were women (97.90%). The average age of participants was 42.36 years.	Aerobic exercise, combined exercise, muscle strengthening, flexibility, stretching.	BDI, HAD, and VAS	11/14 studies evaluated depression. It was concluded that all the studies included in this meta-analysis exceeded minimum thresholds for methodological and scientific quality.
Tu et al. (37)	16 RCTs, N = 3.226	1) RCTs 2) Included patients (>18 years old) with either systolic HF or HF with a preserved EF of any etiology in the control and in the intervention group (diagnosis based on LVEF or clinical findings) 3) Patients received exercise training either alone or as part of a comprehensive cardiac rehabilitation program (i.e., included components such as psychological intervention or health education) 4) compared with a standard medical treatment or education placebo control group 5) reported the effect of exercise training on depression or depressive Symptoms The median age of the populations ranged between 54 and 81 years.	Walking, bicycle, treadmill, games, jogging, calisthenics, Tai Chi Chuan, and strength training. Frequency 2–7 days/week; duration 20–60 min per session; intensity 40–80% of maximum heart rate, 60–70% of maximal heart rate reserve, or maximum oxygen uptake; and overall length of the programme 6 weeks to 1.5 years.	BDI, CES-D, GDS, HADS, HAM-D, HDCDS	Jadad scale between 2 and 7. Antidepressant effect was not influenced by age, duration of the exercise intervention, or exercise setting, but rather by LVEF and the exercise mode; HF patients with LVEFs of <50%, as well as aerobic exercise intervention, demonstrated consistent benefits on depressive symptoms.
Vashistha et al. (32)	3 RCTs, N = NR	1) RCTs published in English 2) The population of interest was men with clinically diagnosed prostate cancer and participation in a prescribed exercise program 3) Acceptable exercise interventions included Pilates, yoga, mind-body stress reduction, tai chi, walking alone or in combination with cycling, cycling, resistance training, strength training, qigong, aerobic exercise, anaerobic exercise, and/or stretching. 4) Included studies had to contain one of the following primary outcome measures: cancer-specific QOL, overall QOL, fatigue, depression, and/or anxiety. No limit was placed on the duration of exercise intervention or length of follow-up.	Walking, stretching, and light resistance exercises, aerobic exercise, QiGong. Study duration varied from 4 weeks to 6 months (whole study, N = 13).	BSI-18	5/13 studies evaluated depression, 3 used the BSI-18 and were enrolled in the meta-analysis. Using the Cochrane Collaboration tool for risk of bias assessment for all 13 RCTs included in our systematic review, we found that 10 studies had high risk of bias, two had unclear risk of bias, and one had low risk of bias.

(Continued)

TABLE 2 | Continued

References	Included trials, sample size	Included population/inclusion criteria	Intervention	Rating Scales	Quality and possible moderators
Wang et al. (34)	4 RCTs, N = 245	1) Published RCTs 2) Patients with CVD including ischemic heart disease or coronary artery disease, cerebrovascular disease, diseases of the aorta and arteries, and peripheral vascular disease 3) Articles that compared an intervention group (e.g., tai chi, qigong, baduanjin) with a control group that performed other exercises (egg, strength exercises), that received usual care, or that did not undergo any intervention.	Thai Chi, aerobic exercise. Duration of the intervention between 5 and 12 weeks.	HAMD, POMS	4/35 studies evaluated depression. A low risk of incomplete outcome bias was reported in 31 articles (88.5%), whereas a low risk of selective reporting bias was reported in most articles (n = 28, 73.6%).
Wayne et al. (30)	7 RCTs, N = 783	1) Randomized controlled trials (RCTs), prospective non-randomized controlled studies, and prospective non-controlled studies published in English 2) cancer was the primary disease and Tai Chi and/or Qigong were the primary interventions Most studies evaluated breast cancer patients. Other cancers included ovary, lung, gastrointestinal and colorectal cancer.	Intervention duration between 6 and 12 weeks.	POMS, CES-D, BDI, HADS, BSI-18, DASS-21	7/15 studies evaluated depression. Quality of RCTs indicated an overall low to high risk of bias For the 7 RCTs.
Ying et al. (33)	2 RCTs, N = 124	1) All participants were adult men and the diagnoses of prostate cancer were based on pathology reports and staging studies 2) The participants all underwent ADT (androgen deprivation therapy) for at least 3 months 3) Lifestyle interventions contain dietary advices, aerobic and resistance exercises, and physical activity 4) The patients had minimum lifestyle intervention duration of 6 weeks Exclusion criteria: Men with diabetes, uncontrolled hypertension, cardiovascular disease and unstable bony metastases.	Aerobic and resistance exercise. Duration between 12 and 24 weeks.	NR	Jadad scores between 3 and 5. 2/11 RCTs evaluated depression.
Zhu et al. (23)	8 RCTs, N = 751	1) English language 2) Adopted a randomized controlled trial design, comparing exercise intervention group with control group (usual care, maintain current activity level, or waitlist) 3) Included adults diagnosed with breast cancer 4) Evaluated the effects of exercise in breast cancer patients.	The main types of exercise interventions reported in this meta-analysis were aerobic, resistance, and stretching exercises. Duration in the whole study (n = 33) between 5 weeks and 6 months.	NR	8/33 studies evaluated depression. Delphi criteria were used for assessment of quality, the studies were heterogenous in the level of quality.
Zhou et al. (45)	3 RCTs, N = 128	1) participants with a diagnosis of AL [either acute myelocytic leukemia (AML) or acute lymphoblastic leukemia (ALL)] undergoing induction therapy or post-remission therapy 2) Intervention: an exercise component, regardless of the type of exercise 3) Comparison intervention: standard care with no exercise intervention or instruction 4) Outcome measures including depression 5) Study design: a randomized controlled trial (RCT) or a quasi-experimental design trial	Aerobic exercise, mixed-modality exercise. Duration was reported for 2 of the studies with 3–12 weeks.	HADS	3/9 studies evaluated depression. Risk of bias was heterogenous.

BDI, Beck Depression Inventory; CDI, Children Depression Inventory; CES-D, Center for Epidemiological Studies Depression Scale; DASS, Depression Anxiety Stress Scales; GDS, Geriatric Depression Scale; HAD, Hospital Anxiety and Depression Scale; HAM-D, Hamilton Rating Scale for Depression; SCL-90, Symptom Checklist-90; TAS, Toronto Attitude Scale; POMS, Profile of Mood States; SAS, Symptom Assessment Scale; CSDD, Cornell Scale for Depression in Dementia; IDS-SR, Inventory of Depressive Symptomatology Self Report; LPD, Levine-Pilowsky Depression; MADRS, Montgomery-Asberg Depression Rating Scale; MDI, Major Depression Inventory; POMS, Profile of Mood States; QOL, Quality of Life; DASS, Depression Anxiety Stress Scales; TAS, Toronto Attitude Scale; MAACL, Multiple Affect Adjective Checklist; HDCDS, Hare-Davis Cardiac Depression Scale; SDS, Self-rating Depression Scale; BSI-18, Brief Symptom Inventory; BRUMS, Brunel Mood Scale; NR, not reported.

TABLE 3 | Outcomes of the included meta-analyses.

References	Results/Main Outcomes
Adamson et al. (50)	Results from the meta-analysis yielded a small but statistically significant effect of 0.28 for depression reduction overall (SE = 0.07; 95% CI: 0.15 to 0.41; p = 0.00). The effect of exercise on depression is slightly larger (0.36) in the MS studies compared with the other studies (0.20), but this difference was not statistically significant.
Bergenthal et al. (46)	The pooled result of three trials (N = 249) for depression shows a statistically significant benefit for the exercise arm (SMD = 0.25; 95% CI:−0.00 to 0.50; p = 0.05).
Brown et al. (24)	Exercise provided a small overall reduction in depressive symptoms compared to standard care among all types of cancer ds = −0.13, 95% CI: −0.26 to −0.01). Collectively, the 40 effect sizes lacked homogeneity I^2 = 55%, 95% CI: 35 to 68, p < 0.001. Subgroup analysis by cancer type revealed significant reductions in depressive symptoms among breast cancer survivors d = −0.17, 95% CI: −0.32 to −0.02, but no significant difference in depressive symptoms among prostate, leukemia, lymphoma, and colorectal cancer survivors.
Buffart et al. (25)	After excluding outliers, yoga resulted in significant large reductions in depression (d = −0.69; 95% CI: 1.02 to −0.37).
Carayol et al. (17)	Exercise resulted in an improvement of depressive symptoms (d = −0.275, 95% CI: −0.457 to −0.094, p = 0.003). I^2 = 39% (p = 0.09).
Chung et al. (38)	Exercise improved depressive symptoms (d = −1.233, SE = 0.482, 95% CI: −2.177 to −0.289, p = 0.010). Heterogeneity: χ^2 = 23.80,p < 0.001; I^2 = 87.40%
Craft et al. (26)	Mean ES of (−0.22, 95% CI: −0.43 to −0.009; p = 0.04) under a random effects model, when comparing exercise interventions to control groups.
Cramer et al. (19)	Evidence for large short-term effects were found for depression (SMD = −1.59, 95% CI: −2.68 to −0.51; p < 0.01). Heterogeneity: Chi² = 84.03, df = 5 (p < 0.00001); I^2 = 94% Long-term effects (2 studies, N = 43) of up to 24 weeks did not show significant results.
Cramer et al. (18)	Comparison of yoga vs. no therapy: Yoga did not appear to reduce depression (pooled SMD = −0.13, 95% CI −0.31 to 0.05; seven studies, 496 participants; low-quality evidence). Comparison of yoga vs. psychosocial/educational interventions provided moderate-quality evidence indicating that yoga can reduce depression (pooled SMD = −2.29, 95% CI: −3.97 to −0.61; 4 studies, 226 participants).
Dalgas et al. (48)	In summary the meta-analysis indicated a small beneficial effect of exercise on depressive symptoms in people with MS. The SMD across studies was(g = −0.37, 95% CI: −0.56 to −0.17).
Eng and Reime (52)	Overall, physical exercise resulted in less depressive symptoms over 13 studies involving 1022 patients (SMD = −0.13, 95% CI: −0.26 to −0.01, I^2 = 6%, p = 0.03) with low heterogeneity. Ten studies evaluated the effect on depressive symptoms after a period of time had elapsed following the exercise sessions (range from 10 weeks to 9 months). Physical exercise did not change depressive symptoms over these 10 follow-up studies involving 889 patients (SMD = −0.04, 95% CI: −0.17 to 0.09, I^2 = 1%, p = 0.53).
Ensari et al. (49)	The weighted mean ES was small, but statistically significant (g = 0.36, SE = 0.09, 95% CI: 0.18 to 0.54, Z = 3.92, p < 0.001), indicating the exercise training resulted in an improvement in depressive symptoms compared to control.
Fong et al. (27)	Measured by the Beck depression inventory, physical activity was associated with reduced depression (−4.1, 95% CI: −6.5 to −1.8; p < 0.01) in survivors of mixed types of cancer. Four other studies in the sample used the HADS (two) or POMS (two). The results for HADS were (−0.5, 95%CI: −2.8 to 1.7, p = 0.64 and for POMS −7.5, 95 CI:−16.0 to 1.0, p = 0.09).
Furmaniak et al. (20)	Exercise may lead to little or no improvement in depression (SMD = −0.15, 95% CI: −0.30 to 0.01, test for overall effect: Z = 1.86; p = 0.062). Heterogeneity: Tau² = 0.0; Chi² = 3.73, df = 5; p = 0.59; I^2 = 0.0%.
Gomes Neto et al. (39)	Exercise lead to a reduction in depression symptoms (−7.32; 95% CI: −9.31 to −5.33). Test for overall effect size Z = 7.21, p < 0.00001.
Graven et al. (53)	When the data from the two studies was pooled; (SMD = −2.03, 95% CI: −3.22 to −0.85) immediately after the intervention phase (note, different time points were used in the two studies for the follow-up assessment).
Herring et al. (16)	Exercise training significantly reduced depressive symptoms by a heterogeneous mean effect of 0.55 (95% CI: 0.31 to 0.78, p < 0.001). A significant improvement in fatigue (β = 0.37, Z = 2.21, p≤0.03) accounted for significant variation in the overall effect of exercise on depressive symptoms.
Langhorst et al. (41)	Meditative movement therapies improved depressive symptoms (SMD = −0.49, 95% CI: −0.76 to −0.22, p = 0.0004 Heterogeneity I^2 = 27%; Tau² = 0.03). 2 studies evaluated the follow-up (N = 132), with no significant improvement of depressive symptoms. In subgroup analyses, only Yoga yielded significant effects on depression at final treatment.
Liang et al. (43)	A statistically significant difference was observed (MD = −2.31, 95% CI: −3.33 to −1.30, p = 0.001), which indicated that home-based exercise interventionsreduced the depression scores, compared to the control groups. No significant heterogeneity between home-based exercise groups and control groups (p = 0.24, I^2 = 30%).
Lin et al. (29)	Improvement of depressive symptoms (−0.95, 95% CI: −1.55 to −0.36, test for overall effect: Z = 3.15, p = 0.002). Heterogeneity: τ^2 = 0.63, χ^2 = 66.81, df = 7, p < 0.00001); I^2 = 90%.
Lin et al. (28)	No significant effects were found for depression and health-related quality of life. (No SMD or CI provided)

(Continued)

TABLE 3 | Continued

References	Results/Main Outcomes
Liu et al. (35)	The Thai Chi group had a significantly lower level of depression (SMD 9.42, 95% CI: 13.59 to 5.26, $p < 0.001$, $I^2 = 81\%$, $N = 168$) compared with the non-active control groups.
Newby et al. (31)	Exercise interventions significantly reduced depressive symptoms (Point estimate -0.961, SE $= 0.319$, CI 95% -1.585 to -0.337, $Z = -3.017$, $p = 0.003$).
O'Brien et al. (47)	One meta-analysis was performed and demonstrated a significant improvement in the depression-dejection subscale of the Profile of Mood States Scale (POMS) by a reduction of 7.68 points for participants in the aerobic exercise intervention group compared with the non-exercising control group (95% CI: -13.47 to -1.90, $p = 0.009$, $I^2 = 94\%$, $p < 0.0001$).
O'Dwyer et al. (44)	A meta-analysis including three studies found significantly lower depression scores in the exercise groups compared to controls (SMD $= -0.40$ SD; 95% CI: -0.71 to -0.09, test for overall effect size $Z = 2.54$, $p = 0.01$).
Patsou et al. (21)	Reduction in depressive symptoms showed a small to moderate effect of depressive symptoms in favor of the exercise $g = -0.38$ (95% CI -0.89 to 0.13, $p = 0.14$).
	With regard to the type of the exercise intervention, aerobic interventions yielded a large and significant effect on depression at the last follow-up (3–6 months) measurement compared with the control groups ($g = -1.23$, 95% CI: -1.97 to -0.49, $p = 0.001$).
Perry et al. (54)	This represents a statistically significant, positive small to medium overall effect size of physical exercise to reduce depressive symptoms in people following TBI (SMC $= 0.48$, 95% CI $= 0.16$ to 0.81).
	Tests of heterogeneity were significant ($p < 0.01$), confirming that heterogeneity was present amongst the studies included in the analysis.
Samartzis et al. (36)	Interventions using exercise training appeared more effective compared to usual care (SMD $= 0.391$, 95% CI: 0.213 to 0.569). There was a trend for SSRI superiority compared to exercise training for improving depression ($Q = 3.257$, df $= 1$, $p = 0.071$).
Singh et al. (22)	Large effect in favor of exercise SMD $= 0.66$, 95%, CI: 0.52 to 0.80, $p < 0.01$, $I^2 = 90\%$; high heterogeneity.
	Intervention duration had an effect on depression ($\chi^2 = 7.93$, df $= 1$, $p < 0.01$), with interventions lasting longer than 12 weeks producing a large effect (SMD $= 0.84$, 95% CI: 0.65 to 1.03, $p < 0.01$) and interventions lasting 12 weeks or less having a moderate effect (SMD $= 0.44$, 95% CI: 0.23 to 0.65, $p < 0.01$).
Song et al. (51)	A fixed-effect model indicated that TCQ significantly reduced depression scores compared to control groups, with an overall medium effect size ($g = -0.457$, 95% CI: -0.795 to -0.118, $p = 0.008$). Q- value ($p = 0.739$) and I^2 (0%) indicated limited heterogeneity.
Song et al. (40)	Exercise training was able to reduce depression in HD patients (SMD $=-0.95$, 95% CI: -1.18 to -0.73; $Z = 8.33$, $p < 0.00001$).
Sosa-Reina et al. (42)	There is strong evidence from intention-to-treat and per protocol analysis that exercise reduces symptoms of depression (-0.40, 95% CI: -0.55 to -0.24; $p < 0.001$). Values of Cohen's g suggested that exercise had a small effect on symptoms of depression.
Tu et al. (37)	Strong evidence of a decrease in the symptoms of depression with exercise (SMD -0.38, 95% CI: -0.55 to -0.21, $p < 0.00001$) in 3–6 months follow-up.
Vashistha et al. (32)	The pooled data did not reveal a significant improvement in depression (-3.02, 95%CI: -7.83 to 1.79, test for overall effect: $Z = 1.23$, $p = 0.22$).
	Heterogeneity: Tau² $= 9.80$; Chi² $= 4.64$, df $= 1$, $p = 0.03$; $I^2 = 78\%$.
Wang et al. (34)	The HAMD scores of patients performing TCEs improved (MD -3.97, 95% CI: -5.05 to -2.89, $p < 0.001$; $I^2 = 0$, $p = 0.91$) compared with those of patients in the control group, based on a random-effects model.
	The POMS depression scale scores of the patients performing TCEs significantly improved (MD -3.02, 95% CI: -3.50 to -2.53, $p < 0.001$; $I^2 = 0\%$, $p = 0.76$) compared with those of patients in the control group, based on a random-effects model.
Wayne et al. (30)	The overall effect size based on a random-effects model favors TCQ on depression in cancer patients ($g = -0.27$, 95% CI: -0.44 to -0.11, $p = 0.001$). A subgroup meta-analysis limited to five RCTs using an active control group showed a statistically non-significant trend toward TCQ improving depression ($g = -0.22$, 95% CI:-0.47 to 0.02, $p = 0.080$). A subgroup meta-analysis limited to the three RCTs with a no-treatment control group showed a statistically positive effect of TCQ.
Ying et al. (33)	No obvious difference in mitigating depression (SMD $= -0.18$, 95% CI: -0.54 to 0.17, $p = 0.31$).
Zhu et al. (23)	Exercise intervention reduced depression, (SMD $= -2.08$, 95% CI: -3.36 to -0.80, $p = 0.001$, $I^2 = 2\%$, $p = 0.41$).
Zhou et al. (45)	Based on the data for depression, there were no significant differences in these parameters between the exercise and control groups (SMD $= -0.15$, 95% CI: -0.51 to 0.22, $p = 0.28$, p for heterogeneity $= 0.57$, $I^2 = 0\%$).

exercise on depressive symptoms in these cohorts (17, 21–23, 55). Different types of interventions were summarized (aerobic, resistance, aerobic and resistance, yoga exercises), with one meta-analysis providing more detailed information about differences between the exercise types: aerobic interventions yielded a large and significant effect on depression at the last follow-up measurement compared with the non-exercising control group (21). Another meta-analysis pointed toward the beneficial effects of an intervention duration of longer than 12 weeks (22).

One meta-analysis only showed little improvement in depression after exercise intervention (20). The two remaining meta-analyses with overlapping populations of Cramer et al.

(18, 19) were heterogeneous. In the 2012 analysis, large short-term effects were shown (19), in the 2017 analysis these results could not be reproduced (18).

Exercise interventions in mixed cancer-samples
Most of these meta-analyses included a majority of breast-cancer patients.

Yoga intervention Buffart et al. showed significant large reductions in depressive symptoms of yoga interventions, one of the included RCTs included lymphoma patients, the other 6 trials breast cancer (25). Lin et al. (29) summarized 6/8 RCTs with breast cancer and different forms of yoga interventions and showed that depressive symptoms improved significantly in the intervention groups (29).

In the cohort of Wayne et al. breast cancer was also the main disease. The overall effect size favored Thai Chi and QiGong interventions on depressive symptoms (30).

Aerobic or mixed intervention Brown et al. (24) (65% of patients with breast cancer) found a small overall reduction in depressive symptoms of aerobic and yoga interventions compared to standard care among all types of cancer. Subgroup analysis by cancer type revealed significant reductions in depressive symptoms among breast cancer survivors, but no significant difference in depressive symptoms among prostate, leukemia, lymphoma, and colorectal cancer survivors.

Another meta-analysis by Craft et al. revealed modest beneficial effects of exercise (26). Fong et al. evaluated 75% breast cancer patients and showed different outcomes with regard to different depression scales: measured by the BDI, physical activity (aerobic) was associated with reduced depression. Subgroups of four RCTs used the HAMD and POMS scales, the outcomes in this cohort were not significant (27).

In another meta-analysis by Lin et al. (28) with various gynecological cancer-types and various types of activity (i.e., aerobic training, muscle strengthening, stretching exercises or education regarding exercise) no statistically significant improvement could be shown. None of the included RCTs appeared in both analyses (28).

Exercise interventions in Patients with Prostate Cancer
Three meta-analyses were found eligible for this review with regard to prostate cancer. All of them included various types of exercise and one meta-analysis included lifestyle interventions consisting of exercise and other interventions (e.g., dietary advice) (33). The largest meta-analysis with four RCTs found significantly reduced depressive symptoms, while the two smaller ones with 3 RCTs and 2 RCTs found no statistically significant differences (31–33).

Exercise Interventions in Patients With Cardiovascular Disease and Coronary Heart Disease
For cardiovascular diseases, one meta-analysis could be included in our meta- review (34). 4 RCTs summarizing patients with ischemic heart disease or coronary artery disease, cerebrovascular disease, diseases of the aorta and arteries, and peripheral vascular disease compared Thai Chi, qigong, baduanjin interventions to control interventions (e.g., strength training or no intervention). Both outcome measures (HAMD and POMS) showed significant improvements in the intervention groups. One meta-analysis with 2 RCTs/CCTs analyzed the effects of 3-months of Thai Chi Interventions and found positive effects in the intervention group concerning the depressive symptoms (35).

Exercise Interventions in Patients With Heart Failure
The two included meta-analyses showed an improvement in depressive symptoms compared to standard care in large cohorts (36, 37).

Intradialytic Exercise Interventions and Exercise Interventions in Hemodialysis Patients
We could include two meta-analyses for the cohort of intradialytic exercise (38, 39). Exercise interventions included aerobic training, resistance training, or a combination with strength training or range of motion. Both publications showed significant improvements of depressive symptoms (38, 39).

One meta-analysis included intradialytic exercise patients and exercise interventions in hemodialysis patients on non-dialytic days (40). Beneficial effects of exercise were reported.

Exercise Interventions in Patients With Fibromyalgia, Ankylosing Spondylitis and Lupus Erythematodes (LE)
The two cited meta-analyses for fibromyalgia (41, 42) were able to present improved depressive symptoms. The interventions were heterogeneous with Tai Chi and/or Yoga, and/or Qi Gong (41) and aerobic exercise, combined exercise, muscle strengthening, flexibility, stretching (42).

Our search resulted in one meta-analysis that revealed a statistically significant beneficial effect of home-based stretching exercise in reducing depressive symptoms in patients with ankylosing spondylitis (43).

In a meta-analysis of patients with LE, significantly lower depression scores were found in the exercise groups (stretching or aerobic exercise) compared to controls (44).

Exercise Interventions in Patients With Acute Leukemia and Other Hematological Malignancies
Our systematic search resulted in two meta-analyses, one including solely acute leukemia (45) and one including various hematological malignancies (46). Zhou et al. found no significant differences between the exercise (aerobic exercise, mixed-modality exercise) and control groups, whereas Bergenthal showed a statistically significant benefit for the exercise group with aerobic exercise or combined aerobic/strength exercise in a larger cohort.

Exercise Interventions in Patients With HIV
We were able to identify one meta-analysis with a small sample size and various forms of exercise interventions (e.g., walking, jogging, cycling, rowing, stair stepping, and swimming). A significant improvement could be displayed in the depression-dejection sub scale of the POMS d (47).

Exercise Interventions in Patients With Neurological Diseases
Three meta-analyses revealed small but significantly positive effects of exercise on depressive symptoms in multiple sclerosis (16, 48, 49). Different forms of exercise were allowed (Aerobic, Resistance Aerobic+, Yoga).

In Parkinson's disease, exercise interventions (Tai Chi and/or Qigong) led to significantly improved depressive symptoms (51).

Overall, physical exercise resulted in less depressive symptoms in the two suitable meta-analyses of stroke patients (52, 53).

After 10 weeks of follow-up, this beneficial effect could not be maintained (52).

One meta-analysis included various neurological disorders and various exercise interventions. Depressive symptoms were significantly reduced. The effect of exercise on depression was slightly larger in the MS studies compared with the other studies. In addition to the above mentioned neurological disorders (with overlapping single studies), other diseases like Alzheimer's disease, were included (50).

Exercise Interventions in Patients With Traumatic Brain Injury

In one meta-analysis, two RCTs and seven non-RCTs were included and found statistically significant, positive effects of exercise on depressive symptoms (54).

DISCUSSION

We were able to include 39 meta-analyses confirming that the application of exercise as an add-on treatment in patients with somatic disorders is a frequently studied intervention. As stated above, different reasons for this observation can be discussed: the positive effects in depression alone (15), the principle lack of side-effects and the overall improvement of fitness and mortality. In our meta-review, most meta-analyses showed these (expected) beneficial effects of exercise on depressive symptoms (33/39). The six meta-analyses without these effects evaluated different exercise modalities in different types of diseases (18, 20, 28, 32, 33, 45). One of these meta-analyses provided data of breast cancer patients receiving yoga therapy and found no significant effect on depressive symptoms of yoga when comparing to no therapy, but did find significant improvements of depressive symptoms when comparing yoga to psychosocial intervention (7 and 4 included trials) (18). Another meta-analysis with breast-cancer patients found no significant results (20). The smallest of the included meta-analyses with 39 participants (2 trials) also evaluated depressive symptoms in any type of gynecological cancer and found no significant effects (28). Neither of the two meta-analyses with prostate cancer patients nor the meta-analyses with acute lymphoblastic leukemia (ALL) patients found significant reductions in depressive symptoms (32, 33, 45).

Five meta-analyses reported long-term effects with follow-up periods from 3 to 9 months of the exercise interventions (19, 21, 37, 41, 52). The results were heterogeneous with two meta-analyses showing no significant effects in a 3 to 9 months period (19, 52). One meta-analysis only found positive long-term effects during 3 to 6 months for one of the possible exercise interventions in subgroup analyses (41). The two remaining meta-analyses pointed to positive long-term effects in a 3–6 months period (21, 37). In all of these studies except one (37) the follow-up cohort was much smaller compared to the overall sample size. The small sample sizes on the one hand and the small number of meta-analyses in total restrict the generalizability of these results. Future studies should include a follow-up period of at least 3 months (preferably three and 3 months assessments) to accumulate data for meaningful statements.

Following the American College of Sports Medicine (ACSM) guidelines, healthy adults should engage in moderate aerobic exercise training for ≥ 30 min per day on ≥ 5 days per week, vigorous aerobic exercise training for ≥ 20 min per day on ≥ 3 days per week, or a combination of both moderate and vigorous aerobic training. On another 2–3 days, healthy adults should perform resistance exercises for each of the major muscle groups and flexibility exercises for each major muscle-tendon groups on ≥ 2 days per week (56). Future studies should lean on these recommendations to help homogenize the results.

In literature, many different rating scales (self- and observer-rating) have been introduced to assess depressive symptoms, reflecting the variety of questionnaires used in the original trials and the consecutive meta-analyses. For example, the practice guidelines for the treatment of depression in Germany (57) list nine possible questionnaires as valid tools. In specific somatic disorders, validation studies of the most often used scales were performed: HAMD for multiple sclerosis patient (58) and for stroke patients (59). BDI for cancer patients (60) and heart failure patients (61). In a mixed cancer population, a review recommended the CES-D as most precise instrument if depression is the sole focus (62). It has been stated that discrepancies between BDI and HAMD scores (self- and observer rating scales) could be due to different personality traits (e.g., high neuroticism is associated with higher BDI scores) and that therefore both should be regarded separately (63). To date, valid recommendations for all included somatic disorders or general recommendations for specific questionnaires to access depressive symptoms could not be identified. For future studies, similar outcome measured should be implemented to ensure comparability and both self- and observer rating scales should be combined.

The possible reasons for the varying observations regarding the different intervention types and the measuring time points could be the same reasons that complicate meta-analyses of the existing exercise trials. As stated above, in none of the meta-analyses, the included trials had matching exercise protocols regarding type, duration and frequency of the intervention. Most often no data was provided about the attendance rate of the participants and about the aerobic capacity before/after the intervention as a controlling variable. The quality of the trials ranged from very low to good quality (also with regard to the exercise-specific difficulty of blinding the intervention). In none of the meta-analyses the depressive symptoms after the exercise intervention were the primary endpoint in all of the included trials, so moreover the validity of the conclusions has to be discussed cautiously.

In summary, we were able to identify a large interest in this field of research for the above demonstrated reasons. In most of the meta-analyses, regardless of the underlying somatic disease, beneficial effects of exercise on depressive symptoms could be observed—keeping in mind that depressive symptoms were mainly secondary outcomes in the included studies. Some of the somatic diseases, especially cancer and in this field breast cancer, were overrepresented compared to others like heart failure.

More standardized trials with better comparability are required to draw specific conclusions about the recommended type and duration of exercise in different diseases. The current findings point to beneficial effects of various forms of exercise, but the implementation in guidelines and for example in therapy strategies that are supported more extensively is still difficult because of the lack of clarity of specific outcomes. Especially the diversity of outcome parameters impedes the comparability of interventions within and between somatic disorders. Moreover, most meta-analyses did not report types of other antidepressant interventions like medication or psychotherapy. Thus, it is difficult to answer the question whether exercise therapy is efficient as an add-on treatment to an ongoing pharmaco- or psychotherapy or whether it should be offered as a single intervention in patients with somatic disorders and depression. Finally, information is sparse regarding whether patients continue to exercise after the intervention (e.g., in sport clubs) or whether their overall activity level (e.g., measured by pedometers or more accurately by accelerometers) increases and how this is related to outcome.

CONCLUSION

In this meta-review, we provide an overview of existing evidence for the effects of exercise on depressive symptoms in various somatic disorders. The results are promising, but meaningful recommendations are lacking because of heterogeneous study protocols. For better comparability, we would recommend to implement the following standards in future studies: homogeneous outcome measures, one self-rating scale (e.g., BDI) and one observer-rating scale (e.g., HAMD or MADRS). Moreover, specific information of other antidepressant treatments (especially medication and psychotherapy) should be consistently reported. State and duration of the somatic disease should be provided. Future studies should lean on recommendation of the ACSM regarding type and intensity of the intervention (e.g., moderate aerobic exercise training for ≥ 30 min per day on ≥ 5 days per week or vigorous aerobic exercise training for ≥ 20 min per day on ≥ 3 days per week; on another 2–3 days, resistance exercises for each of the major muscle groups and flexibility exercises for each major muscle-tendon groups on ≥ 2 days per week) (56). For aerobic training, bicycle ergometers are a widely-used and practical possibility (also for e.g., patients with arthrosis). The duration of the intervention should last at least 12 weeks. Attendance rates, setting (e.g., group activity, with/without supervision) and training intensity should be monitored, preferably with spiroergometric examinations at the start and the end of the study. Follow-up examinations of 3 and 6 months should be performed, and also in this period, information about antidepressant medication should be provided. On these occasions, information about the overall fitness level (e.g., via pedometer/accelerometer measurements over at least 3 days or via activity questionnaires like IPAQ) should be documented.

AUTHOR CONTRIBUTIONS

AR and AH conceived the study. AR and SK performed the qualitative analyses. AR, SK, IM, and AH wrote the first draft. AS and PF supervised the project. BM provided methodological advice; and all authors were involved in the reviewing the manuscript and approved the final version of the manuscript.

REFERENCES

Luppa M, Heinrich S, Angermeyer MC, König H-H, Riedel-Heller SG. Cost- of-illness studies of depression: a systematic review. *J Affect Disord.* (2007) 98:29–43. doi: 10.1016/j.jad.2006.07.017

Moussavi S, Chatterji S, Verdes E, Tandon A, Patel V, Ustun B. Depression, chronic diseases, and decrements in health: Results from the World Health Surveys. *Lancet.* (2007) 370:851–8. doi: 10.1016/S0140-6736(07)61415-9

Mathers CD, Loncar D. Projections of global mortality and burden of disease from 2002 to 2030. *PLoS Med.* (2006) 3:e442. doi: 10.1371/journal.pmed.0030442

Kvam S, Kleppe CL, Nordhus IH, Hovland A. Exercise as a treatment for depression: a meta-analysis. *J Affect Disord.* (2016) 202:67–86. doi: 10.1016/j.jad.2016.03.063

Rethorst CD, Wipfli BM, Landers DM. The antidepressive effects of exercise: A meta-analysis of randomized trials. *Sports Med.* (2009) 39:491–511. doi: 10.2165/00007256-200939060-00004

Blumenthal JA, Babyak MA, Doraiswamy PM, Watkins L, Hoffman BM, Barbour KA, et al. Exercise and pharmacotherapy in the treatment of major depressive disorder. *Psychosom Med.* (2007) 69:587–96. doi: 10.1097/PSY.0b013e318148c19a

Hoffman BM, Babyak MA, Craighead WE, Sherwood A, Doraiswamy PM, Coons MJ, et al. Exercise and pharmacotherapy in patients with major depression: one-year follow-up of the SMILE study. *Psychosom Med.* (2011) 73:127–33. doi: 10.1097/PSY.0b013e31820433a5

Solaro C, Gamberini G, Masuccio FG. Depression in multiple sclerosis: epidemiology, aetiology, diagnosis and treatment. *CNS Drugs.* (2018) 32:117–33. doi: 10.1007/s40263-018-0489-5

Arwert HJ, Meesters JJL, Boiten J, Balk F, Wolterbeek R, Vliet Vlieland TPM. Post stroke depression, a long term problem for stroke survivors. *Am J Phys Med Rehabil.* (2018) 97:565–71. doi: 10.1097/PHM.0000000000 000918

Camargo CHF, Serpa RA, Jobbins VA, Berbetz FA, Sabatini JS. Differentiating between apathy and depression in patients with parkinson disease dementia. *Am J Alzheimer's Dis Other Dement.* (2018) 33:30–4. doi: 10.1177/1533317517728333

Eker S. Prevalence of depression symptoms in diabetes mellitus. *Open Access Maced J Med Sci.* (2018) 6:340–3. doi: 10.3889/oamjms.2018.085

Park EM, Gelber S, Rosenberg SM, Seah DSE, Schapira L, Come SE, et al. Anxiety and depression in young women with metastatic breast cancer: a cross-sectional study. (2018). *Psychosomatics* 59:251–8. doi: 10.1016/j.psym.2018.01.007

Gagin R, HaGani N, Shinan-Altman S, Roguin A. Coping with depression and anxiety among heart failure patients. *Harefuah.* (2018) 157:81–4.

Chekroud SR, Gueorguieva R, Zheutlin AB, Paulus M, Krumholz HM, Krystal JH, et al. Association between physical exercise and mental health in 1·2 million individuals in the USA between 2011 and 2015: A cross-sectional study. *Lancet Psychiatry.* (2018) 5:739–46. doi: 10.1016/S2215-0366(18)30227-X

Schuch FB, Vancampfort D, Richards J, Rosenbaum S, Ward PB, Stubbs B. Exercise as a treatment for depression: a meta-analysis adjusting for publication bias. *J Psychiatr Res.* (2016) 77:42–51. doi: 10.1016/j.jpsychires.2016.02.023

Herring MP, Puetz TW, O'Connor PJ, Dishman RK. Effect of exercise training on depressive symptoms among patients with a chronic illness: a systematic review and meta-analysis of randomized controlled trials. *Arch Intern Med.* (2012) 172:101–11. doi: 10.1001/archinternmed. 2011.696

Carayol M, Bernard P, Boiche J, Riou F, Mercier B, Cousson-Gelie F, et al. Psychological effect of exercise in women with breast cancer receiving adjuvant therapy: what is the optimal dose needed? *Ann Oncol.* (2013) 24:291–300. doi: 10.1093/annonc/mds342

Cramer H, Lauche R, Klose P, Lange S, Langhorst J, Dobos GJ. Yoga for improving health-related quality of life, mental health and cancer-related symptoms in women diagnosed with breast cancer. *Coch Database Syst Rev.* (2017) 1:CD010802. doi: 10.1002/14651858.CD010802.pub2

Cramer H, Lange S, Klose P, Paul A, Dobos G. Yoga for breast cancer patients and survivors: a systematic review and meta-analysis. *BMC Cancer.* (2012) 12:412. doi: 10.1186/1471-2407-12-412

Furmaniak AC, Menig M, Markes MH. Exercise for women receiving adjuvant therapy for breast cancer. *Cochr Database Syst Rev.* (2016) 9:CD005001. doi: 10.1002/14651858.CD005001.pub3

Patsou ED, Alexias GD, Anagnostopoulos FG, Karamouzis MV. Effects of physical activity on depressive symptoms during breast cancer survivorship: a meta-analysis of randomised control trials. *ESMO Open.* (2017) 2:e000271. doi: 10.1136/esmoopen-2017-000271

Singh B, Spence RR, Steele ML, Sandler CX, Peake JM, Hayes SC. A systematic review and meta-analysis of the safety, feasibility and effect of exercise in women with stage II+ breast cancer. *Arch Phys Med Rehabil.* (2018) 99:2621– 36. doi: 10.1016/j.apmr.2018.03.026

Zhu G, Zhang X, Wang Y, Xiong H, Zhao Y, Sun F. Effects of exercise intervention in breast cancer survivors: a meta-analysis of 33 randomized controlled trails. *OncoTargets Ther.* (2016) 9:2153–68. doi: 10.2147/OTT.S97864

Brown JC, Huedo-Medina TB, Pescatello LS, Ryan SM, Pescatello SM, Moker E, et al. The efficacy of exercise in reducing depressive symptoms among cancer survivors: a meta-analysis. *PLoS ONE.* (2012) 7:e30955. doi: 10.1371/journal.pone.0030955

Buffart L, van Uffelen M, Jannique GZ, Riphagen II, Brug J, van Mechelen W, Brown WJ, et al. Physical and psychosocial benefits of yoga in cancer patients and survivors, a systematic review and meta-analysis of randomized controlled trials. *BMC Cancer.* (2012) 12:559. doi: 10.1186/1471-2407-12-559

Craft LL, Vaniterson EH, Helenowski IB, Rademaker AW, Courneya KS. Exercise effects on depressive symptoms in cancer survivors: a systematic review and meta-analysis. *Cancer Epidemiol Biomarkers Prev.* (2012) 21:3–19. doi: 10.1158/1055-9965.EPI-11-0634

Fong DYT, Ho JWC, Hui BPH, Lee AM, Macfarlane DJ, Leung SSK, et al. Physical activity for cancer survivors: Meta-analysis of randomised controlled trials. *BMJ.* (2012) 344:e70. doi: 10.1136/bmj.e70

Lin K-Y, Frawley HC, Denehy L, Feil D, Granger CL. Exercise interventions for patients with gynaecological cancer: a systematic review and meta-analysis. *Physiotherapy.* (2016) 102:309–19. doi: 10.1016/j.physio.2016.02.006

Lin K-Y, Hu Y-T, Chang K-J, Lin H-F, Tsauo J-Y. Effects of yoga on psychological health, quality of life, and physical health of patients with cancer: a meta-analysis. *Evid Based Compl Altern Med.* (2011) 2011:659876. doi: 10.1155/2011/659876

Wayne PM, Lee MS, Novakowski J, Osypiuk K, Ligibel J, Carlson LE, et al. Tai Chi and Qigong for cancer-related symptoms and quality of life: a systematic review and meta-analysis. *J Cancer Surviv.* (2017). doi: 10.1007/s11764-017- 0665-5

Newby TA, Graff JN, Ganzini LK, McDonagh MS. Interventions that may reduce depressive symptoms among prostate cancer patients: a systematic review and meta-analysis. *Psychooncology.* (2015) 24:1686–93. doi: 10.1002/pon.3781

Vashistha V, Singh B, Kaur S, Prokop LJ, Kaushik D. The effects of exercise on fatigue, quality of life, and psychological function for men with prostate cancer: systematic review and meta-analyses. *Eur Urol Focus.* (2016) 2:284– 95. doi: 10.1016/j.euf.2016.02.011

Ying M, Zhao R, Jiang D, Gu S, Li M. Lifestyle interventions to alleviate side effects on prostate cancer patients receiving androgen deprivation therapy: a meta-analysis. *Jpn J Clin Oncol.* (2018) 48:827–34. doi: 10.1093/jjco/ hyy101

Wang X-Q, Pi Y-L, Chen P-J, Liu Y, Wang R, Li X, et al. Traditional chinese exercise for cardiovascular diseases: systematic review and meta-analysis of randomized controlled trials. *J Am Heart Assoc.* (2016) 5:e002562. doi: 10.1161/JAHA.115.002562

Liu T, Chan AW, Liu YH, Taylor-Piliae RE. Effects of Tai Chi-based cardiac rehabilitation on aerobic endurance, psychosocial well-being, and cardiovascular risk reduction among patients with coronary heart disease: a systematic review and meta-analysis. *Eur J Cardiovasc Nurs.* (2017). 17:368- 383 doi: 10.1177/1474515117749592

Samartzis L, Dimopoulos S, Tziongourou M, Koroboki E, Kyprianou T, Nanas S. SSRIs versus exercise training for depression in chronic heart failure: a meta-analysis of randomized controlled trials *Int J Cardiol.* (2013) 168:4956–8. doi: 10.1016/j.ijcard.2013.07.143.

Tu R-H, Zeng Z-Y, Zhong G-Q, Wu W-F, Lu Y-J, Bo Z-D, et al. Effects of exercise training on depression in patients with heart failure: a systematic review and meta-analysis of randomized controlled trials. *Eur J Heart Fail.* (2014)

16:749–57. doi: 10.1002/ejhf.101

Chung Y-C, Yeh M-L, Liu Y-M. Effects of intradialytic exercise on the physical function, depression and quality of life for haemodialysis patients: a systematic review and meta-analysis of randomised controlled trials. *J Clin Nurs.* (2017) 26:1801–13. doi: 10.1111/jocn.13514

Gomes Neto M, Lacerda FFR, de Lopes AA, Martinez BP, Saquetto MB. Intradialytic exercise training modalities on physical functioning and health-related quality of life in patients undergoing maintenance hemodialysis: Systematic review and meta-analysis. *Clin Rehabil.* (2018) 32:1189–202. doi: 10.1177/0269215518760380

Song Y-Y, Hu R-J, Diao Y-S, Chen L, Jiang X-L. Effects of exercise training on restless legs syndrome, depression, sleep quality, and fatigue among hemodialysis patients: a systematic review and meta-analysis. *J Pain Symptom Manage.* (2018) 55:1184–95. doi: 10.1016/j.jpainsymman.2017.12.472

Langhorst J, Klose P, Dobos GJ, Bernardy K, Hauser W. Efficacy and safety of meditative movement therapies in fibromyalgia syndrome: a systematic review and meta-analysis of randomized controlled trials. *Rheumatol Int.* (2013) 33:193–207. doi: 10.1007/s00296-012-2360-1

Sosa-Reina MD, Nunez-Nagy S, Gallego-Izquierdo T, Pecos-Martin D, Monserr at J, Alvarez-Mon M. Effectiveness of therapeutic exercise in fibromyalgia syndrome: a systematic review and meta-analysis of randomized clinical trials. *Biomed Res Int.* (2017) 2017:2356346. doi: 10. Z155/2017/2356346

Liang H, Zhang H, Ji H, Wang C. Effects of home-based exercise intervention on health-related quality of life for patients with ankylosing spondylitis: a meta-analysis. *Clin Rheumatol.* (2015) 34:1737–44. doi: 10.1007/s10067-015- 2913-2

O'Dwyer T, Durcan L, Wilson F. Exercise and physical activity in systemic lupus erythematosus: a systematic review with meta-analyses. *Semin Arthritis Rheum.* (2017) 47:204–15. doi: 10.1016/j.semarthrit.2017.04.003

Zhou Y, Zhu J, Gu Z, Yin X. Efficacy of exercise interventions in patients with acute leukemia: a meta-analysis. *PLoS ONE.* (2016) 11:e0159966. doi: 10.1371/journal.pone.0159966

Bergenthal N, Will A, Streckmann F, Wolkewitz K-D, Monsef I, Engert A, et al. Aerobic physical exercise for adult patients with haematological malignancies. *Cochr Database Syst Rev.* (2014) 11:CD009075. doi: 10.1002/14651858.CD009075.pub2

O'Brien KK, Tynan A-M, Nixon SA, Glazier RH. Effectiveness of aerobic exercise for adults living with HIV: systematic review and meta-analysis using the Cochrane Collaboration protocol. *BMC Infect Dis.* (2016) 16:182. doi: 10.1186/s12879-016-1478-2

Dalgas U, Stenager E, Sloth M. The effect of exercise on depressive symptoms in multiple sclerosis based on a meta-analysis and critical review of the literature. *Eur J Neurol.* (2015) 22:443. doi: 10.1111/ene. 12576

Ensari I, Motl RW, Pilutti LA. Exercise training improves depressive symptoms in people with multiple sclerosis: results of a meta-analysis. *J Psychosom Res.* (2014) 76:465–71. doi: 10.1016/j.jpsychores.2014. 03.014

Adamson BC, Ensari I, Motl RW. Effect of exercise on depressive symptoms in adults with neurologic disorders: a systematic review and meta-analysis. *Arch Phys Med Rehabil.* (2015) 96:1329–38. doi: 10.1016/j.apmr.2015.01.005

Song R, Grabowska W, Park M, Osypiuk K, Vergara-Diaz GP, Bonato P, et al. The impact of Tai Chi and Qigong mind-body exercises on motor and non-motor function and quality of life in Parkinson's disease: A systematic review and meta-analysis. *Parkinsonism Relat Disord.* (2017) 41:3–13. doi: 10.1016/j.parkreldis.2017.05.019

Eng JJ, Reime B. Exercise for depressive symptoms in stroke patients: a systematic review and meta-analysis. *Clin Rehabil.* (2014) 28:731–9. doi: 10.1177/0269215514523631

Graven C, Brock K, Hill K, Joubert L. Are rehabilitation and/or care co- ordination interventions delivered in the community effective in reducing depression, facilitating participation and improving quality of life after stroke? *Disabil Rehabil.* (2011) 33:1501–20. doi: 10.3109/09638288.2010. 542874

Perry DC, Sturm VE, Peterson MJ, Pieper CF, Bullock T, Boeve BF, et al. Association of traumatic brain injury with subsequent neurological and psychiatric disease: a meta-analysis. *J Neurosurg.* (2016) 124:511–26. doi: 10.3171/2015.2.JNS14503

Bae S-C, Gun SC, Mok CC, Khandker R, Nab HW, Koenig AS, et al. Improved health outcomes with etanercept versus usual DMARD therapy in an Asian population with established rheumatoid arthritis. *BMC Muscul Disord.* (2013) 14:13. doi: 10.1186/1471-2474-14-13

Garber CE, Blissmer B, Deschenes MR, Franklin BA, Lamonte MJ, Lee I-M, et al. American college of sports medicine position stand. Quantity and quality of exercise for developing and maintaining cardiorespiratory, musculoskeletal, and neuromotor fitness in apparently healthy adults: Guidance for prescribing exercise. *Med Sci Sports Exerc.* (2011) 43:1334–59. doi: 10.1249/MSS.0b013e318213fefb

AWMF. *S3-Leitlinie/Nationale VersorgungsLeitlinie Unipolare Depression: Langfassung.* 2nd ed. Berlin (2015).

Raimo S, Trojano L, Spitaleri D, Petretta V, Grossi D, Santangelo G. Psychometric properties of the Hamilton Depression Rating Scale in multiple sclerosis. *Qual Life Res.* (2015) 24:1973–80. doi: 10.1007/s11136-015-0940-8

Aben I, Verhey F, Lousberg R, Lodder J, Honig A. Validity of the beck depression inventory, hospital anxiety and depression scale, SCL- 90, and hamilton depression rating scale as screening instruments for depression in stroke patients. *Psychosomatics.* (2002) 43:386–93. doi: 10.1176/appi.psy.43.5.386

Mystakidou K, Tsilika E, Parpa E, Smyrniotis V, Galanos A, Vlahos L. Beck depression inventory: exploring its psychometric properties in a palliative care population of advanced cancer patients. *Eur J Cancer Care.* (2007) 16:244–50. doi: 10.1111/j.1365-2354.2006.00728.x

Lahlou-Laforêt K, Ledru F, Niarra R, Consoli SM. Validity of beck depression inventory for the assessment of depressive mood in chronic heart failure patients. *J Affect Disord.* (2015) 184:256–60. doi: 10.1016/j.jad.2015. 05.056

Luckett T, Butow PN, King MT, Oguchi M, Heading G, Hackl NA, et al. A review and recommendations for optimal outcome measures of anxiety, depression and general distress in studies evaluating psychosocial interventions for English-speaking adults with heterogeneous cancer diagnoses. *Supportive Care Cancer.* (2010) 18:1241–62. doi: 10.1007/s00520-010-0932-8

Schneibel R, Brakemeier E-L, Wilbertz G, Dykierek P, Zobel I, Schramm E. Sensitivity to detect change and the correlation of clinical factors with the hamilton depression rating scale and the beck depression inventory in depressed inpatients. *Psychiatry Res.* (2012) 198:62–7. doi: 10.1016/j.psychres.2011.11.014

15

A Perspective on Implementing Movement Sonification to Influence Movement (and Eventually Cognitive) Creativity

Luca Oppici[1,2]*, Emily Frith[3] and James Rudd[4]

[1]Psychology of Learning and Instruction, Department of Psychology, School of Science, Technische Universität Dresden, Dresden, Germany, [2]Centre for Tactile Internet with Human-in-the-Loop (CeTI), Technische Universität Dresden, Dresden, Germany, [3]Cognitive Neuroscience of Creativity Laboratory, Department of Psychology, Penn State University, State College, PA, United States, [4]Research Institute for Sport and Exercise Sciences, Liverpool John Moores University, Liverpool, United Kingdom

*Correspondence:
Luca Oppici
luca.oppici@tu-dresden.de

Creativity represents an important feature in a variety of daily-life and domain-specific contexts. Recent evidence indicates that physical movement serves as a key resource for exploring and generating task-relevant creative ideas, supporting the embodied perspective on creative cognition. An intuitive link between movement and creative cognition is movement creativity. The process of exploring the movement solutions an environment offers (i.e., affordances) and exploiting novel, functional, and creative movements may translate to and improve how individuals explore and generate novel ideas. Opening perception to the variety of affordances ("conventional" and novel) an environment offers drives creative movement. Teachers and coaches can promote this process by designing a learning environment that invites performers to consider and utilize novel movement solutions. In this article, we present a rationale for using movement sonification to promote creative movement. Movement sonification consists of mapping a movement parameter into sound, with a sound being triggered or changing according to how movement unfolds. We argue that movement sonification can facilitate the emergence of creative movement *via* enhancing perception of currently performed movements and invite performers to utilize novel affordances, and emphasizing information for regulating subsequent creative actions. We exemplify this concept in a creative dance intervention for children during physical education classes. In conclusion, we contend that learning to explore original dance sequences using movement sonification may provide a meaningful link between creative movement and creative cognition. Children may use their minds *and* bodies as tools for creative thinking and exploration, such as shaping letters with their bodies.

Keywords: creative cognition, embodied cognition, exercise-cognition, affordance, functional similarity, education, creative

INTRODUCTION

Creativity is a relatively new term with its genesis in the 20th century. In 1968, Wyrick was one of the first to explore an embodied approach to creativity research through emphasizing the importance of movement and its relationship with the environment (Wyrick, 1968). Creative cognition represents an important feature in a variety of daily-life and domain-specific contexts, and the embodied perspective on creative cognition contends that body movement plays a key and active role in the development of creative ideas. An intuitive link between body movement and creative cognition is creative movement. Creative movement is generally defined as a functional and original movement solution to achieve a task goal (Memmert and Perl, 2009; Hristovski et al., 2011), and could be instrumental for creative cognition given its prominence in the art and sport domains (e.g., dance). The process by which creative movement emerges may influence and enhance how creative ideas are generated. Importantly, broadening perception of what the task and environment offers and exploring different solutions to solve a motor task promotes creative movement and can eventually contribute to generating creative ideas. Here, we discuss how the strategy of sonifying a movement – movement sonification – can be used to promote creative movement. While this concept is not novel and sonification has been already used to promote creative movement, primarily in dance improvisation (e.g., Lem et al., 2010; Diniz et al., 2012; Rizzo et al., 2018; Dahlstedt and Dahlstedt, 2019; Erdem et al., 2019), we think that a clear rationale for its implementation in the context of movement creativity is lacking. We present our approach grounded in ecological psychology and discuss how movement sonification can invite performers to explore the variety of movement opportunities (i.e., affordances) the environment offers, thus promoting creativity. Importantly, we also highlight the potential implications that this approach and, more generally, creative movement can have on creative cognition.

CREATIVE COGNITION

Creative cognition is often understood as a collection of mental operations that promote the generation of novel and task- or context-relevant ideas (Sternberg and Lubart, 1999; Runco and Jaeger, 2012). Creative thinking is esteemed across many domains, including large-scale scientific achievement, technological innovation, and artistic expression (Cropley, 2006; Moran, 2010). However, small-scale creativity is also an important outlet for self-expression as individuals learn to initiate and pursue novel approaches to everyday problem-solving (Richards, 2010). Practicing everyday creative thinking may be particularly beneficial to the development of a cognitive skillset that lends itself to the fulfillment of creative thinking potential at more impactful levels. This is because, while ability, experience, and capacity indisputably influence the value of creative thoughts, the same cognitive processes are thought to contribute to the production of both seminal and everyday creative ideas (Runco, 2014).

Given the breadth and diversity of creative outcomes, our approach centers on highlighting the role of everyday creative thinking in context (Cropley, 2006; Amabile, 2018). Specifically, several foci of cognitive creativity research encompass strategies for increasing creative thinking in educational contexts (Craft, 2003; Beghetto and Kaufman, 2010; Moran, 2010; Pllana, 2019) by supporting holistic academic success, mental health and well-being, and reinforcing diversity and cross-cultural inclusivity (Lubart and Georgsdottir, 2004; Glaveanu et al., 2019). To this end, it is important to highlight that creative thinking is suggested to be less of an inflexible, enduring personality trait consigned to the minds of geniuses, and is considered more of an externally-modifiable faculty (Amabile, 2018). In other words, creative thinking is proposed to be shaped by both intrinsic factors, including task-relevant skills and motivation, as well as external circumstances, such as affordances and constraints within the task environment (Ward et al., 1999; Amabile, 2018). A context-centered perspective of creative cognition, therefore, permits a broader exploration of the value of everyday creative thinking as a conduit for the construction of meaning across the lifespan.

THE ROLE OF EMBODIMENT IN CREATIVE COGNITION

Understanding which mental and contextual factors may promote or inhibit creative thinking processes is integral to establishing models that adequately address creative cognition across domains (Ward et al., 1999). Embodied cognition frameworks interleave both mental and physical dynamics of problem-solving, contending that the mind, body, and environment shape the problem/task-goal space, and their interaction guides thought and action that are appropriate to solving the problem (Shapiro and Stolz, 2019). The body may support cognition by offering a means to manipulate and explore the problem-space and reduce cognitive load (Risko and Gilbert, 2016). For example, reading tilted words on a computer screen often requires physical movement (i.e., tilting the head) to accomplish this demanding task, rather than relying solely on mental rotation to match the tilted word stimuli with stored representations of normally-oriented text in semantic memory (Jolicoeur, 1988; Risko and Gilbert, 2016).

The role of movement for creative thinking may be particularly important from a developmental perspective, as a wealth of evidence suggests that early acquisition of motor skills is positively associated with cognitive developments, including memory, language, and problem-solving ability (see Frith et al., 2019). An important mechanism underlying the benefits of movement for cognition is functional similarity between task-relevant movement and cognitive process (Tversky, 2009). Functional similarity between mental and physical operations is thought to scaffold and offload cognition, meaning that the body is a conduit for meaningfully exploring and externalizing task-relevant solutions (both physical and mental). For example, Bara and Bonneton-Botté (2018) demonstrated that movement-based educational programs have the potential to support learning in early childhood compared to sedentary approaches.

In this study, kindergarteners were taught to (1) move their arms to draw letters in the air, and (2) walk along letter outlines drawn on the ground. This motor intervention was associated with higher letter recognition and handwriting quality compared to practicing visual recognition of letters and handwriting practice alone. Recent creativity work has also shown that moving *via* gesture (Kirk and Lewis, 2017), and matching (functionally similar) emotional states with physical exertion in dance (Hutton and Sundar, 2010) promoted divergent thinking performance. These findings offer additional credence to the purported role of functional similarity within the mind-body relationship. Taken together, physical movement may serve as a resource for exploring and generating creative ideas and solutions. It is therefore plausible that *creative* movement and *creative* thought processes share functional similarities which reinforce the utility of embodied cognition in this domain.

Practicing and discovering creative movements may further enhance how creative ideas are generated. Building on functional similarity, the process of exploring the movement solutions an environment offers and exploiting novel, functional movements may translate to and improve how individuals explore and generate novel ideas. Indeed, fluid, unstructured and unconstrained (in a way creative) movement has been suggested to serve as a pathway to fluid, distributed thought, which may parallel creative thought processes (Leung et al., 2012; Slepian and Ambady, 2012; Kuo and Yeh, 2016; Zhou et al., 2017). While the link between movement and cognitive creativity has not been thoroughly considered in the literature, in the embodied creativity domain, emphasis should be placed on designing a training environment that offers novel affordances and invites individuals to explore how they might effectively generate creative movement. Considering the prominence of creativity within various physical domains (e.g., dance and sport), we speculate that this approach may have a favorable impact on creative cognition as well.

CREATIVE MOVEMENT

Creative movement is generally defined as a functional and original movement solution to achieve a task goal (Memmert and Perl, 2009; Hristovski et al., 2011; Orth et al., 2017). From an ecological dynamics approach, movement emerges from a continuous, cyclical, and prospective coupling of perception, cognition, and action, situated in the dynamic performer-environment interaction (Gibson, 1979; Davids et al., 1994; Warren, 2006). Humans move to perceive what opportunities for action their environment offers (i.e., affordances), perceive affordances to (self) organize their movement, and, cyclically, movement reveals new (flow of) information that specifies affordances (Michaels and Beek, 1995; Chemero, 2003; Fajen, 2005; Bruineberg and Rietveld, 2014). Across an affordance landscape, some affordances stand out and invite performers to certain actions (Bruineberg and Rietveld, 2014; Rietveld and Kiverstein, 2014; van Dijk and Rietveld, 2016). For example, a variety of actions can be performed in a school gym, but a ball on the ground and a goal create intentionality for most

children to perform a kicking action. Creative movement however emerges overtime and from a transformational process, involving search, exploration and discovery of novel, and functionally efficient actions (Hristovski et al., 2009; for an example in dance improvisation, see Kimmel et al., 2018; Rudd et al., 2020). Hypothetically, humans have both opportunities and capacities to perform different creative movements to achieve the same or different goals. In fact, a rich landscape of affordances constantly surrounds a moving organism, offering a vast array of movement options (Bruineberg and Rietveld, 2014; Rietveld and Kiverstein, 2014), and the human body is a multi-stable, degenerate system that can flexibly switch between different movement patterns (Kelso, 2012; Seifert et al., 2013). The more enriched an environment and greater the action capabilities of an individual the higher the possibilities for innovation through interaction creating an abundance of movement options (Bruineberg and Rietveld, 2014; Rietveld and Kiverstein, 2014).

Supporting and teaching creativity to emerge is however a tricky affair as people, typically, are attracted to and utilize affordances to guide their movement that are commonly accepted in their society (Rietveld and Kiverstein, 2014; van Dijk and Rietveld, 2016). In other words, they follow the norm, do what is typically done, and act within their comfort zone. For example, if a teacher turns on the music during a physical education (PE) class and ask children to dance, anecdotally, they will all likely perform a handful of dance movements, which correspond to the current "hits," e.g., "the floss dance." Teaching creativity requires designing learning environments that offer a broad range of task-relevant affordances as well as a safe space to encourage an individual to continuously explore functional and novel movement solutions. For example, in teaching the high jump, the introduction of foam-safety mats allowed for safe exploration and practice of landing on the back, which promoted the emergence of a new creative and highly functional movement solution – the "Fosbury Flop." In this sense, teachers are considered environmental designers that can influence learners' intention and invite them to explore and discover a range of movement solutions. This safe and non-judgmental (i.e., no correct technique) exploration of an affordance landscape will see individuals experimenting and creating a wide range of movement solutions to the task (Rasmussen et al., 2017; Woods et al., 2020). Keeping with the dance example and pertinent to this paper, the teacher's instructions should frame a child's intentionality to be open to new dance movements, explore different movement sequences, and add variability into their movements with the music, and in doing so moving away from the floss dance. Common strategies currently used are instructions (e.g., "avoid imitating your peers" in a class setting) and manipulation of task and environmental constraints (e.g., rules and equipment; Hristovski et al., 2011, 2012; Torrents et al., 2015, 2016). In summary, creative movement emerges when a performer perceives and utilizes novel affordances, and a learning environment (including framing of individual's intentionality) that encourages perceptual-motor exploration promotes creativity. Here, we provide a theoretical rationale to promote the development of creative movement using movement sonification.

MOVEMENT SONIFICATION

Movement sonification may represent an innovative strategy to enrich a learning environment and promote the development of movement creativity. It consists of mapping a movement parameter into sound, and depending on how the specified movement parameter (s) change (s) a sound is triggered or changes characteristics, e.g., frequency and amplitude (Effenberg, 2005; Hermann et al., 2011; Dyer et al., 2017). For example, a sound tone is triggered when a joint angle exceeds a certain threshold (e.g., Boocock et al., 2019) or a music melody is progressively distorted in reference to the amplitude of a joint angle increase (e.g., Lorenzoni et al., 2019). Given the inherent tight link between movement and sound (Stanton and Spence, 2020), movement sonification has recently gained an increased interest in the motor learning and control field as a suitable strategy to deliver augmented feedback (Sigrist et al., 2013; Dyer et al., 2015). In fact, sonification of a movement parameter has been shown to enhance a multimodal perception of intrinsic feedback (e.g., proprioceptive information) and the dynamics of perception-action coupling (Dyer et al., 2017), typically resulting in improved motor learning and performance (for reviews, see Effenberg et al., 2016; Schaffert et al., 2019). Here, we discuss how movement sonification can also be used to influence movement creativity.

Movement sonification can be used to enhance how a performer perceives the (currently) utilized affordances, directing them to novel affordances, and promote a change in a learner's intentionality toward an exploration of a new, functional, and creative movement. Once a learner is aware of the currently used affordances and changes their intentionality toward trying out new movements, they start a movement exploration process that will promote the emergence of movement creativity. The exploration process will perturb the performer-environment dynamic (e.g., learner and music) and will shape new affordances for novel creative movement. A learner can spontaneously change their intention ("I hear the sound changing as I change my moves, I should experiment with these movements and sounds") or teacher's should educate the learner's attention toward the environmental shift caused by their movement, thus supporting the learner's knowledge of the environment (Gibson, 1979). Importantly, movement sonification *per se* does not shape novel affordances but invites learners to explore a broad range of new movements, which in turn will create new affordances. In short, the key component for movement creativity to emerge is a learner's exploration of movement options, and movement sonification can promote this process. These mechanisms are discussed hereafter, and their application is exemplified in a creative dance intervention for children during PE classes, which represents a suitable learning context for creative movement.

As previously mentioned, a critical component for creative movement to emerge is a learner's perceptual openness and attunement to the rich landscape of affordances surrounding them (Rietveld and Kiverstein, 2014). A performer should be aware of the currently used affordances and be invited to find new solutions. In this context, movement sonification can enhance one's awareness of the movement solutions they are currently adopting and support a change in their intentionality toward

trying different (functional) movements. Previous research has shown that sonification increased dancers' awareness of the "movement vocabulary" they were using and movement sequences they were performing and facilitated their exploration of novel movement patterns (Diniz et al., 2012; Françoise et al., 2014; Wood et al., 2017). With this, we are not suggesting that movement sonification should direct a performer's attentional focus to their movement (which has been shown to be detrimental for motor performance and learning; Wulf, 2013), but instead it should enhance a performer's perception of how they are currently using the variety of movement possibilities the environment is offering. In short, movement sonification will promote an enhanced performer's attunement to the dynamics of task-environment they are embedded in. Keeping with the previous dance example, if a PE teacher turns on music and asks their children to create dance moves, they likely will replicate current dance "hits" (i.e., a handful of movements). To encourage children to find new movement, some parameter of the music (such as frequency and tempo) can be mapped onto children's movement and change according to how they find new movements. An initial assessment of children's typical dance moves is needed to set a child's movement signature as reference, and a selected music parameter can change when child deviates from their movement signature. If necessary, to educate a child's attention toward knowledge of the environment, the teacher could briefly explain how a child's movement can change music, and invite their students to explore movements to manipulate and play with the speed and tempo of the music through their movements. This will enhance children's perception of their currently adopted movement (i.e., music does not change if they perform the usual movement) and invite them to try new movement (i.e., music changes).

Movement sonification is mapped within the coupling of perception and action, and represents an informational constraint that can facilitate releasing a movement's degrees of freedom (hence creativity, see Hristovski et al., 2011; Torrents et al., 2020). From the cyclical coupling of perception and action, action "creates" new information for further action, and sonification can amplify this newly "created" information and encourage learners to perceive and exploit this information. This can be particularly relevant for sequences of movements and movement improvisation (e.g., in dance), whereby each movement is regulated on the (information about) previous movement. In this sense, movement sonification facilitates a learner's perception of the "novel" affordances. Previous research in dance improvisation has shown that sonification enhanced participants' variety of novel movements relative to a no-sonification condition (Yamaguchi and Kadone, 2017) and supported the creation of Japanese dance sequences (Dahlstedt and Dahlstedt, 2019). Keeping with the dance example, the PE teacher can ask their children to create dance movement sequences, but this time there is not a predefined music and children's movement will create music. Each child's movement is mapped onto a different sound, and children are instructed to create music by combining different movements (for an example of this procedure, see Landry and Jeon, 2017). They are also encouraged to create different combination of sounds by creatively combining movements. By doing this, children have to continuously perceive each movement they perform and regulate the next movement accordingly. This approach will also promote exploration, movement fluency, and functionality, as the produced sound will encourage children to move fluently to "create" a nice and smooth music.

Movement sonification can also motivate performers to pursue new creative movement and increase enjoyment especially in children. Sonification will readily "tell" and reward a performer when a new movement is created and it will encourage children to explore movement in a fun and safe environment. They can play with their movement repertoire *via* the different sounds they can create. Another important aspect worth mentioning is that movement sonification puts performers in charge of the task they are performing. This can likely promote self-regulation (key in embodied cognition, Diamond, 2016; Diamond and Ling, 2020), especially in children, as they have to self-regulate their behavior to keep up with the task and keep the task engaging and fun. Movement sonification will "tell" them straight away if they are disengaging with the task. Lastly, movement sonification can be mapped on movement of each individual, even in a classroom setting, thus it can support the individuality and non-linearity of learning (Newell et al., 2001; Pacheco et al., 2019). The learning intervention will be individualized and will follow the non-linear movement improvement, aligning with the principles of nonlinear pedagogy (Chow et al., 2007, 2015).

Teachers and coaches play a pivotal role in guiding their students toward using sonification for creating original movement. As previously mentioned, they should oversee the creativity process and, if necessary, guide attention to specify knowledge of the environment (Gibson, 1979), this can be done through careful instructions, encouraging their students to explore different and novel movement possibilities. This needs to be done in conjunction with individualizing the movement parameter(s) to sonify. A variety of parameters can be sonified and various sonification techniques have been proposed in the literature (e.g., Hermann et al., 2011; Siegel, 2012). It is beyond the scope of this article to discuss this issue in detail, but we can say that the selection of parameter(s) to sonify is context specific and depends on the teacher's goal and possibilities (Landry et al., 2014). In a school PE context (as per our example), financial constraints and limited technological expertise may restrict sonification options. However, simple and relatively low-cost strategies can still be implemented. For example, accelerometers placed on pupils' joints (e.g., wrists and ankles) can sonify movement acceleration, difference in acceleration between body parts, or parts of the body involved in the movement (e.g., see Françoise et al., 2014; Yamaguchi and Kadone, 2017). In such a scenario, the teacher can invite students to explore different movement speed and fluency, and change how they activate the different body parts. Ultimately, schools should not bear the cost of developing a suitable strategy. We presented a principled approach that can underpin the design and development of sonification techniques

to influence movement creativity, and we hope that inter-disciplinary collaboration between universities and industry can support schools in the process, as advocated through a transdiscplinary approach by Vaughan et al. (2019).

CONCLUSION

In this article, we argue for an embodied approach to creativity that emphasizes the important relationship between movement and cognition in the development of creativity. The development of technologies such as sonification offers new opportunities for designing learning environments that promote creativity. We provided a rationale for using movement sonification to promote creative movement and exemplified its use in creative dance for children. Our approach allows to better understand the embodied nature of creativity as the sonification is "embodied in perception and action" providing a rich landscape for future research to explore creativity. The tasks that can be created can be cognitively challenging and involve a high degree of problem solving that may transfer to more divergent and creative thinking in the classroom.

We contend that learning to explore original dance sequences using movement sonification may provide a meaningful link between creative movement and creative cognition. This association is predicated, in part, on functional similarities between novel actions and thought, such that the process of learning how novel movement parameters map onto sound may facilitate perception-action coupling in novel contexts sharing similar features. In this vein, children may be more inclined to exploit environmental affordances in the classroom after experiencing the self-regulatory process of creating music through physical movement. This may mean that children become more likely to rely on their minds *and* bodies as tools for creative thinking and exploration, such as using their whole bodies to learn the shapes of letters and numbers or acting out scenes from history and science lessons as a strategy for learning new concepts. Future empirical work is necessary to investigate whether and how transfer may unfold from movement sonification to diverse creative problem-solving contexts.

AUTHOR CONTRIBUTIONS

All authors conceptualized, drafted, edited, reviewed, and approved the manuscript.

ACKNOWLEDGMENTS

LO is supported by the Excellence Strategy of the DFG (EXC 2050/1 – Project ID 390696704 – Cluster of Excellence "Centre for Tactile Internet with Human-in-the-Loop").

REFERENCES

Amabile, T. M. (2018). *Creativity in context: Update to the social psychology of creativity*. New York: Routledge.

Bara, F., and Bonneton-Bottè, N. (2018). Learning letters with the whole body: visuomotor versus visual teaching in kindergarten. *Percept. Mot. Skills* 125, 190–207. doi: 10.1177/0031512517742284

Beghetto, R. A., and Kaufman, J. C. (2010). *Nurturing creativity in the classroom*. New York: Cambridge University Press.

Boocock, M., Naudé, Y., Taylor, S., Kilby, J., and Mawston, G. (2019). Influencing lumbar posture through real-time biofeedback and its effects on the kinematics and kinetics of a repetitive lifting task. *Gait Posture* 73, 93–100. doi: 10.1016/j.gaitpost.2019.07.127

Bruineberg, J., and Rietveld, E. (2014). Self-organization, free energy minimization, and optimal grip on a field of affordances. *Front. Hum. Neurosci.* 8:599. doi: 10.3389/fnhum.2014.00599

Chemero, A. (2003). An outline of a theory of affordances. *Ecol. Psychol.* 15, 181–195. doi: 10.1207/S15326969ECO1502_5

Chow, J. Y., Davids, K., Button, C., and Renshaw, I. (Eds.) (2015). *Nonlinear pedagogy in skill acquisition: An introduction*. (London: Routledge).

Chow, J. Y., Davids, K., Renshaw, I., Button, C., Shuttleworth, R., and Araújo, D. (2007). The role of nonlinear pedagogy in physical education. *Rev. Educ. Res.* 77, 251–278. doi: 10.3102/003465430305615

Craft, A. (2003). The limits to creativity in education: dilemmas for the educator. *Br. J. Educ. Stud.* 51, 113–127. doi: 10.1111/1467-8527.t01-1-00229

Cropley, A. (2006). Creativity: a social approach. *Roeper Rev.* 28, 125–130. doi: 10.1080/02783190609554351

Dahlstedt, P., and Dahlstedt, A. S. (2019). "OtoKin: mapping for sound space exploration through dance improvisation" in Paper Presented at the International Conference on New Interfaces for Musical Expression; June 3–6, 2019; Brazil.

Davids, K., Handford, C., and Williams, M. (1994). The natural physical alternative to cognitive theories of motor behaviour: an invitation for interdisciplinary research in sports science? *J. Sports Sci.* 12, 495–528. doi: 10.1080/02640419408732202

Diamond, A. (2016). "Why improving and assessing executive functions early in life is critical" in *Executive function in preschool-age children: Integrating measurement, neurodevelopment, and translational research*. eds. J. A. Griffin, P. McCardle and L. S. Freund (Washington: American Psychological Association), 11–43.

Diamond, A., and Ling, D. S. (2020). "Review of the evidence on, and fundamental questions about, efforts to improve executive functions, including working memory" in *Cognitive and working memory training: Perspectives from psychology, neuroscience, and human development*. eds. J. M. Novick, M. F. Bunting, M. R. Dougherty and W. E. Randall (New York: Oxford University Press), 145–389.

Diniz, N., Coussement, P., Deweppe, A., Demey, M., and Leman, M. (2012). An embodied music cognition approach to multilevel interactive sonification. *J. Multimodal User In.* 5, 211–219. doi: 10.1007/s12193-011-0084-2

Dyer, J. F., Stapleton, P., and Rodger, M. W. M. (2015). Sonification as concurrent augmented feedback for motor skill learning and the importance of mapping design. *Open Psychol. J.* 8, 192–202. doi: 10.2174/1874350101508010192

Dyer, J. F., Stapleton, P., and Rodger, M. (2017). Mapping sonification for perception and action in motor skill learning. *Front. Neurosci.* 11:463. doi: 10.3389/fnins.2017.00463

Effenberg, A. O. (2005). Movement sonification: effects on perception and action. *IEEE MultiMedia* 12, 53–59. doi: 10.1109/MMUL.2005.31

Effenberg, A. O., Fehse, U., Schmitz, G., Krueger, B., and Mechling, H. (2016). Movement sonification: effects on motor learning beyond rhythmic adjustments. *Front. Neurosci.* 10:219. doi: 10.3389/fnins.2016.00219

Erdem, C., Schia, K. H., and Jensenius, A. R. (2019). "Vrengt: a shared body-machine instrument for music-dance performance" in Paper Presented at the International Conference on New Interfaces for Musical Expression; June 3–6, 2019; Brazil.

Fajen, B. R. (2005). Perceiving possibilities for action: on the necessity of calibration and perceptual learning for the visual guidance of action. *Perception* 34, 717–740. doi: 10.1068/p5405

Françoise, J., Fdili Alaoui, S., Schiphorst, T., and Bevilacqua, F. (2014). "Vocalizing dance movement for interactive sonification of laban effort factors" in Paper Presented at the Proceedings of the 2014 Conference on Designing Interactive Systems; June 21–25, 2014; Vancouver, BC, Canada.

Frith, E., Loprinzi, P. D., and Miller, S. E. (2019). Role of embodied movement in assessing creative behavior in early childhood: a focused review. *Percept. Mot. Skills* 126, 1058–1108. doi: 10.1177/0031512519868622

Gibson, J. J. (1979). *The ecological approach to visual perception*. Boston: Houghton Mifflin.

Glaveanu, V. P., Hanchett Hanson, M., Baer, J., Barbot, B., Clapp, E. P., Corazza, G. E., et al. (2019). Advancing creativity theory and research: a socio-cultural manifesto. *J. Creat. Behav.* 0, 1–5. doi: 10.1002/jocb.395

Hermann, T., Hunt, A., and Neuhoff, J. G. (Eds.) (2011). *The sonification handbook*. (Berlin, Germany: Logos Publishing House).

Hristovski, R., Davids, K., and Araujo, D. (2009). "Information for regulating action in sport: metastability and emergence of tactical solutions under ecological constraints" in *Perspectives on cognition and action in sport*. eds. D. Araujo, H. Ripoll and M. Raab (Hauppauge, NY: Nova Science Publishers), 43–57.

Hristovski, R., Davids, K., Araujo, D., and Passos, P. (2011). Constraints-induced emergence of functional novelty in complex neurobiological systems: a basis for creativity in sport. *Nonlinear Dynamics Psychol. Life Sci.* 15, 175–206.

Hristovski, R., Davids, K., Passos, P., and Araujo, D. (2012). Sport performance as a domain of creative problem solving for self-organizing performer-environment systems. *Open Sports Sci. J.* 5, 26–35. doi: 10.2174/1875399X01205010026

Hutton, E., and Sundar, S. S. (2010). Can video games enhance creativity? Effects of emotion generated by dance dance revolution. *Creat. Res. J.* 22, 294–303. doi: 10.1080/10400419.2010.503540

Jolicoeur, P. (1988). Mental rotation and the identification of disoriented objects. *Can. J. Psychol.* 42, 461–478. doi: 10.1037/h0084200

Kelso, J. A. S. (2012). Multistability and metastability: understanding dynamic coordination in the brain. *Philos. Trans. R. Soc. Lond. Ser. B Biol. Sci.* 367, 906–918. doi: 10.1098/rstb.2011.0351

Kimmel, M., Hristova, D., and Kussmaul, K. (2018). Sources of embodied creativity: interactivity and ideation in contact improvisation. *Behav. Sci.* 8:52. doi: 10.3390/bs8060052

Kirk, E., and Lewis, C. (2017). Gesture facilitates children's creative thinking. *Psychol. Sci.* 28, 225–232. doi: 10.1177/0956797616679183

Kuo, C. Y., and Yeh, Y. Y. (2016). Sensorimotor-conceptual integration in free walking enhances divergent thinking for young and older adults. *Front. Psychol.* 7:1580. doi: 10.3389/fpsyg.2016.01580

Landry, S., and Jeon, M. (2017). "Participatory design research methodologies: a case study in dancer sonification" in Paper Presented at the 23rd International Conference on Auditory Display; June 19–23, 2017; Pennsylvania, US.

Landry, S., Ryan, J. D., and Jeon, M. (2014). "Design issues and considerations for dance-based sonification" in Paper Presented at the 20th International Conference on Auditory Display. June 22–25, 2017. New York, USA.

Lem, A., Paine, G., and Drummond, J. (2010). "A dynamic sonification device in improvisational music therapy" in Paper Presented at the 4th International Technology, Education and Development Conference; March 8–10, 2010; Spain.

Leung, A. K. Y., Kim, S., Polman, E., Ong, L., and Qiu, L. (2012). Embodied metaphors and creative "acts". *Psychol. Sci.* 23, 502–509. doi: 10.1177/0956797611429801

Lorenzoni, V., Staley, J., Marchant, T., Onderdijk, K. E., Maes, P. J., and Leman, M. (2019). The sonic instructor: a music-based biofeedback system for improving weightlifting technique. *PLoS One* 14:e0220915. doi: 10.1371/journal.pone.0220915

Lubart, T. I., and Georgsdottir, A. (2004). "Creativity: developmental and cross-cultural issues" in *Creativity: When east meets west*. eds. S. Lau, A. N. N. Hui and G. Y. C. Ng (River Edge, NJ: World Scientific Publishing Company), 23–54.

Memmert, D., and Perl, J. (2009). Analysis and simulation of creativity learning by means of artificial neural networks. *Hum. Mov. Sci.* 28, 263–282. doi: 10.1016/j.humov.2008.07.006

Michaels, C., and Beek, P. (1995). The state of ecological psychology. *Ecol. Psychol.* 7, 259–278. doi: 10.1207/s15326969eco0704_2

Moran, S. (2010). "The roles of creativity in society" in *The Cambridge handbook of creativity*. eds. J. C. Kaufman and R. J. Sternberg (New York, NY: Cambridge University Press), 74–90.

Newell, K. M., Liu, Y., and Mayer-Kress, G. (2001). Time scales in motor learning and development. *Psychol. Rev.* 108, 57–82. doi: 10.1037/0033-295X.108.1.57

Orth, D., van der Kamp, J., Memmert, D., and Savelsbergh, G. J. P. (2017). Creative motor actions as emerging from movement variability. *Front. Psychol.* 8:1903. doi: 10.3389/fpsyg.2017.01903

Pacheco, M. M., Lafe, C. W., and Newell, K. M. (2019). Search strategies in the perceptual-motor workspace and the acquisition of coordination, control, and skill. *Front. Psychol.* 10:1874. doi: 10.3389/fpsyg.2019.01874

Pllana, D. (2019). Creativity in modern education. *World J. Educ.* 9, 136–140. doi: 10.5430/wje.v9n2p136

Rasmussen, L. J. T., Østergaard, L. D., and Glăveanu, V. P. (2017). Creativity as a developmental resource in sport training activities. *Sport Educ. Soc.* 24, 491–506. doi: 10.1080/13573322.2017.1403895

Richards, R. (2010). "Everyday creativity" in *The Cambridge handbook of creativity.* eds. J. C. Kaufman and R. J. Sternberg (New York, NY: Cambridge University Press), 189–215.

Rietveld, E., and Kiverstein, J. (2014). A rich landscape of affordances. *Ecol. Psychol.* 26, 325–352. doi: 10.1080/10407413.2014.958035

Risko, E. F., and Gilbert, S. J. (2016). Cognitive offloading. *Trends Cogn. Sci.* 20, 676–688. doi: 10.1016/j.tics.2016.07.002

Rizzo, A., El Raheb, K., Cisneros, R. E. K., Whatley, S., Zanoni, M., Camurri, A., et al. (2018). "WhoLoDancE: whole-body interaction learning for dance education" in Paper Presented at the EUROMED International Conference on Digital Heritage; October 29 – November 3, 2018; Cyprus.

Rudd, J. R., Pesce, C., Strafford, B. W., and Davids, K. (2020). Physical literacy, a journey of individual enrichment: an ecological dynamics rationale for enhancing performance and physical activity in all. *Front. Psychol.* 11:1904. doi: 10.3389/fpsyg.2020.01904

Runco, M. A. (2014). "Big C, little c" creativity as a false dichotomy: reality is not categorical. *Creat. Res. J.* 26, 131–132. doi: 10.1080/10400419.2014.873676

Runco, M. A., and Jaeger, G. J. (2012). The standard definition of creativity. *Creat. Res. J.* 24, 92–96. doi: 10.1080/10400419.2012.650092

Schaffert, N., Janzen, T. B., Mattes, K., and Thaut, M. H. (2019). A review on the relationship between sound and movement in sports and rehabilitation. *Front. Psychol.* 10:244. doi: 10.3389/fpsyg.2019.00244

Seifert, L., Button, C., and Davids, K. (2013). Key properties of expert movement systems in sport: an ecological dynamics perspective. *Sports Med.* 43, 167–178. doi: 10.1007/s40279-012-0011-z

Shapiro, L., and Stolz, S. A. (2019). Embodied cognition and its significance for education. *Theory Res. Educ.* 17, 19–39. doi: 10.1177/1477878518822149

Siegel, W. (2012). "Dancing the music: interactive dance and music" in *The Oxford handbook of computer music.* ed. R. T. Dean (Oxford, UK: Oxford University Press).

Sigrist, R., Rauter, G., Riener, R., and Wolf, P. (2013). Augmented visual, auditory, haptic, and multimodal feedback in motor learning: a review. *Psychon. Bull. Rev.* 20, 21–53. doi: 10.3758/s13423-012-0333-8

Slepian, M. L., and Ambady, N. (2012). Fluid movement and creativity. *J. Exp. Psychol. Gen.* 141, 625–629. doi: 10.1037/a0027395

Stanton, T. R., and Spence, C. (2020). The influence of auditory cues on bodily and movement perception. *Front. Psychol.* 10:3001. doi: 10.3389/fpsyg.2019.03001

Sternberg, R. J., and Lubart, T. I. (1999). "The concept of creativity: prospects and paradigms" in *Handbook of creativity.* ed. R. J. Sternberg (New York, NY: Cambridge University Press), 3–15.

Torrents, C., Balagué, N., Ric, Á., and Hristovski, R. (2020). The motor creativity paradox: constraining to release degrees of freedom. *Psychol. Aesthet. Creat. Arts.* doi: 10.1037/aca0000291 [Epub ahead of print]

Torrents, C., Ric, Á., and Hristovski, R. (2015). Creativity and emergence of specific dance movements using instructional constraints. *Psychol. Aesthet. Creat. Arts* 9, 65–74. doi: 10.1037/a0038706

Torrents, C., Ric, A., Hristovski, R., Torres-Ronda, L., Vicente, E., and Sampaio, J. (2016). Emergence of exploratory, technical and tactical behavior in small-sided soccer games when manipulating the number of teammates and opponents. *PLoS One* 11:e0168866. doi: 10.1371/journal.pone.0168866

Tversky, B. (2009). "Spatial cognition: embodied and situated" in *Cambridge handbook of situated cognition.* eds. P. Robbins and M. Aydede (Cambridge: Cambridge University Press), 201–216.

van Dijk, L., and Rietveld, E. (2016). Foregrounding sociomaterial practice in our understanding of affordances: the skilled intentionality framework. *Front. Psychol.* 7:1969. doi: 10.3389/fpsyg.2016.01969

Vaughan, J., Mallett, C. J., Davids, K., Potrac, P., and Lopez-Felip, M. A. (2019). Developing creativity to enhance human potential in sport: a wicked transdisciplinary challenge. *Front. Psychol.* 10:2090. doi: 10.3389/fpsyg.2019.02090

Ward, T. B., Smith, S. M., and Finke, R. A. (1999). "Creative cognition" in *Handbook of creativity.* ed. R. J. Sternberg (New York, NY: Cambridge University Press), 189–212.

Warren, W. H. (2006). The dynamics of perception and action. *Psychol. Rev.* 113, 358–389. doi: 10.1037/0033-295X.113.2.358

Wood, K., Cisneros, R. E., and Whatley, S. (2017). Motion capturing emotions. *Open Cult. Stud.* 1, 504–513. doi: 10.1515/culture-2017-0047

Woods, C. T., McKeown, I., Rothwell, M., Araujo, D., Robertson, S., and Davids, K. (2020). Sport practitioners as sport ecology designers: how ecological dynamics has progressively changed perceptions of skill 'acquisition' in the sporting habitat. *Front. Psychol.* 11:654. doi: 10.3389/fpsyg.2020.00654

Wulf, G. (2013). Attentional focus and motor learning: a review of 15 years. *Int. Rev. Sport Exerc. Psychol.* 6, 77–104. doi: 10.1080/1750984X.2012.723728

Wyrick, W. (1968). The development of a test of motor creativity. *Restor. Q.* 39, 756–765. doi: 10.1080/10671188.1968.10616608

Yamaguchi, T., and Kadone, H. (2017). Bodily expression support for creative dance education by grasping-type musical interface with embedded motion and grasp sensors. *Sensors* 17:1171. doi: 10.3390/s17051171

Zhou, Y., Zhang, Y., Hommel, B., and Zhang, H. (2017). The impact of bodily states on divergent thinking: evidence for a control-depletion account. *Front. Psychol.* 8:1546. doi: 10.3389/fpsyg.2017.01546

16

Why do People with Schizophrenia Exercise? A Mixed Methods Analysis among Community Dwelling Regular Exercisers

Patrick A. Ho [1]*, Danielle N. Dahle [2] and Douglas L. Noordsy [3]*

[1] Department of Psychiatry, Geisel School of Medicine Dartmouth, Hanover, NH, United States, [2] Harvard Medical School, Division of Psychotic Disorders, McLean Hospital, Belmont, MA, United States, [3] Department of Psychiatry and Behavioral Sciences, Stanford University School of Medicine, Stanford University, Stanford, CA, United States

*Correspondence:
Patrick A. Ho
patrick.a.ho@hitchcock.org
Douglas L. Noordsy
dnoordsy@stanford.edu

Individuals with schizophrenia have reduced rates of physical activity, yet substantial proportions do engage in independent and regular exercise. Previous studies have shown improvement in symptoms and cognitive function in response to supervised exercise programs in people with schizophrenia. There is little data on motivations of individuals who exercise independently, or their chosen type, duration, or setting of exercise. This study explores motivational parameters and subjective experiences associated with sustained, independent exercise in outpatients with a diagnosis of schizophrenia or schizoaffective disorder. Participants completed a semi-structured interview and then were given a prospective survey containing visual analog scales of symptom severity and the Subjective Exercise Experiences Scales to complete immediately before and after three sessions of exercise. Results from the semi-structured interview were analyzed by modified content analysis. The most important reason for exercise was self-image, followed closely by psychological and physical health. Among psychological effects, participants reported exercise was most helpful for mood and cognitive symptoms. The prospective ratings demonstrated 10–15% average improvements in global well-being, energy, and negative, cognitive and mood symptoms, with almost no change in psychosis, after individual exercise sessions. This suggests that non-psychotic parameters are more susceptible to inter-session decay of exercise effects, which may reinforce continued exercise participation.

Keywords: schizophrenia, exercise, lifestyle psychiatry, psychiatry, community dwelling adults with schizophrenia, qualitative analysis

INTRODUCTION

The benefits of exercise are well-established and include not only weight loss and improved cardiovascular fitness, but also a reduction in risk of early mortality and cognitive decline (1, 2). Exercise also has the potential to prevent or delay the onset of several mental health disorders (3, 4). More recent studies have shown that exercise can have therapeutic effects for patients with psychiatric disorders and can specifically help to control and reduce the symptoms of schizophrenia (4, 5). Randomized controlled trials (RCTs) have identified that exercise significantly improves negative symptoms (such as social withdrawal, anergia, or apathy) but few studies have shown an improvement in positive symptoms (most notably delusions or hallucinations) of schizophrenia (6–8). A recent review of 10 RCTs found significant improvement in global cognition among those receiving an exercise intervention, with medium to large effect sizes for improvements in working memory, social cognition and attention (9). Recent designs have turned toward combining exercise with cognitive rehabilitation in an attempt to magnify effects (10). Some studies have identified release of neurotrophic factors, changes in regional or global brain volume and even preservation of telomere length and integrity as possible biological underpinnings of these benefits (11).

As noted by Farholm and Sorenson, physical activity may be quite challenging for those with severe mental illness due to several barriers such as medication side effects, symptoms of mental illness, lack of support and even motivation (12). While many studies have addressed the other barriers, relatively few studies address motivation. A recent systematic review and meta-analysis of patients with any severe mental illnesses (such as schizophrenia, schizoaffective disorder, bipolar disorder, major depressive disorder, etc.) found that 91% of the participants were motivated to exercise to "improve health" with the most common response being "losing weight." "Improving mood" and "reducing stress" were other common responses. These same patients also identified many barriers to participating in physical activity (13). When the motivations for exercise of people suffering specifically from "early psychosis" were examined, improving health also stood out as the main motivator for exercise. Interestingly, this subpopulation did not identify weight loss as the top motivator for exercise, as "increasing fitness/energy" was the top response followed by "taking your mind off things" and "being more confident in a gym." The author points out that weight loss may not be a realistic goal in the short term, and it is encouraging that there are other more important motivators for physical activity (14).

Existing study designs have typically evaluated the addition of a time-limited exercise regimen to the routines of patients with schizophrenia who live a sedentary lifestyle. A recent meta-analysis by Vancampfort found that half of patients with severe mental illness do not get more than 150 min of moderate aerobic exercise per week (15). Conversely, this analysis indicates that there is a substantial subset of patients with severe mental illness who do exercise regularly. To our knowledge, no research has been conducted on the subset of patients with schizophrenia who have independently and spontaneously incorporated exercise into their lifestyles.

There are several advantages of exercise over other modes of therapy. First, exercise can lead to improvement in both the individual's physical and mental health. Second, exercise is the only available intervention in schizophrenia, a disorder associated with atrophic brain changes, which has clear and sustained neurotrophic effects (16). Additionally it is available to individuals who are apprehensive about taking medications or have contraindications to medications. It requires no equipment or access to a provider. It can be done at any time convenient to the individual and can be varied to meet the individual's specific needs or tastes. It requires only time, and can provide structured activity to a daily schedule. Finally it can be used as an adjunctive therapy that may allow the individual to minimize the use of other modes of therapy such as medications or to combat side effects associated with anti-psychotic medications such as weight gain (17).

There is currently very little evidence to guide clinicians in methods to support individuals with schizophrenia engaging in regular exercise (18). Furthermore, most studies lack data on the subjective experience of participants or how an individual's motivation to exercise can be sustained beyond the end of the study intervention. This study used a semi-structured interview to explore factors motivating sustained, independent exercise in a population of individuals with a diagnosis of schizophrenia spectrum disorder and prospectively evaluated the mental health effects of individual sessions of exercise in these individuals.

METHODS

The project received approval from the university institutional review board. The investigators identified eligible participants from throughout the clinical care sites of a medical center in rural New Hampshire and Vermont. Participants were drawn from the authors' usual care clinics for people with schizophrenia spectrum disorders including a residential treatment program and a community mental health center. Encouragement of a healthy lifestyle was routinely incorporated into care, but treatment was otherwise typical for patients with schizophrenia. Inclusion criteria for participating were being of age 18 years or older, with a diagnosis of schizophrenia, schizoaffective, or schizophreniform disorder, and exercising spontaneously for at least 30 min, three times a week, for at least a month. Participants could have co-morbid diagnoses, such as depression or substance use disorder. Participants were taking a range of commonly prescribed antipsychotic medications including risperidone, clozapine, olanzapine, and aripiprazole. Few were taking first generation agents. Exclusion criteria were irregular exercise or physical activity that did not meet definition of exercise (e.g., hyperactivity that is not planned or purposeful or whose objective is not improving physical fitness *per se*) and inability to read or write in English.

Informed consent was obtained from all potential participants prior to screening with the modified SCID. Once an eligible diagnosis was confirmed, participants completed a semi-structured interview following a template with one of the investigators (DND or DLN). The interview included demographic information, as well as, open-ended questions regarding the reasons for exercise, whether exercise helped manage symptoms, what participants do to motivate themselves to exercise, and information on exercise type, frequency, duration, and interruptions. The investigators then reviewed the instructions for participant self-rating before and after three future sessions of exercise. After reviewing how to complete the scales, participants were given 3 sets of pre- and post-exercise scales with a stamped envelope and offered a $10 gift card to return the study materials to investigators once completed. Laboratory and medication data were collected by chart review using the most recent available results.

In order to assess each patient's experience with exercise, we selected the Subjective Exercise Experience Scale (19) (SEES), a 12-item self-report scale assessing three general categories of subjective responses to exercise stimuli: positive well-being (e.g., great), psychological distress (e.g., miserable), and fatigue (e.g., tired). For each item on the SEES, participants rate how strongly they are experiencing each feeling state along a 7-point Likert scale, ranging from 1 (not at all) to 7 (very much so). The SEES has been shown to have high internal consistency across a variety of populations.

Given the lack of an existing psychosis self-report scale, we also created a simple scale using a visual analog format to capture each participant's experience of well-being and symptoms in their natural exercise environment, which we named the Noordsy-Dahle Subjective Experience Scale (NDSE). The NDSE asked participants to rate the present status of their symptoms and wellbeing on a 10 cm line. The NDSE was constructed with 2 items each for psychosis (hallucinations, delusions), negative symptoms (motivation, social interest), mood (depression, anxiety) and cognition (clarity of thought, concentration). Global well-being was measured with the well-validated Lehman Quality of Life (QOL) scale (20), and an additional item rating energy, a dimension identified by many patients as central to their well-being (21). A detailed description of each item was provided, as well as, anchors at each end of the visual analog line. For psychosis and mood items, 0 corresponded to "none," and 10 to "extreme." For motivation, social interest, cognition and energy items, 0 was low and 10 was high. On the global QOL item, 0 corresponded to "delighted," and 10 to "terrible." Mean pre-workout scores on the NDSE were calculated for each item to provide a reference baseline.

The data collected from the semi-structured interview was analyzed by modified content analysis. Participant answers were categorized using a priori categories included in the interview template (available on request) but were also searched for any emerging themes that were not hypothesized prior to the interview. Responses were coded and collated by theme and frequencies calculated. The data collected on the NDSE was converted into numerical values by measuring the point marked by the participant from 0 to 10 cm along the visual analog line. These values and the numerical values from the SEES were used to calculate the change from pre- to post-exercise for each item in each episode of exercise rated and then the mean change in each item across all exercise sessions was calculated.

RESULTS

Twenty-three participants were enrolled in the study and completed the semi-structured interview. Participants had a mean age of 37.6 years (standard deviation 13.5 years, range 18–67 years). Seventy percent were male, 30% were female and there was an average duration of illness of 15.4 years. Fourteen participants (61%) returned the pre-post NDSE and SEES ratings for three exercise episodes, resulting in 42 ratings of response to exercise.

TABLE 1 | Study participant characteristics.

Variable	N = 23	%
Completion of scales	14	60.8
Male	16	69.5
Diagnosis		
Schizophrenia	10	43.5
Schizoaffective	13	56.5
Schizophreniform	0	0
Antipsychotic Use		
Participants on 1	13	56.5
Participants on >1	10	43.5
Co-morbidities		
Diabetes	3	13
Hypertension	5	21.7
Hyperlipidemia	5	21.7
Tobacco use	3	13
Health parameters	**Mean**	
BMI	28.9 kg/m^2	
Total cholesterol	176.3 mg/dL	
HDL	57 mg/dL	
LDL	91.2 mg/dL	
Triglycerides	142.1 mg/dL	
Blood glucose	102 mg/dL	
Systolic BP	122 mmHg	
Diastolic BP	80 mmHg	
Heart rate	87 BPM	

Demographic, metabolic, and treatment characteristics are presented in **Table 1**. 56.5% of the participants were diagnosed with schizoaffective disorder and 43.5% with schizophrenia. 56.5% of the participants were taking one antipsychotic medication at the time of the study, and 43.5% were prescribed more than one. Thirteen percent of the study participants used tobacco products during the study, 13% carried a diagnosis of diabetes, 22% had hyperlipidemia, and 22% had hypertension. Mean BMI was 28.9 kg/m^2 (overweight) and most recent mean serum glucose was 102 mg/dL (borderline high). However, mean blood pressure, pulse and lipid values were all in normal range.

In terms of medication treatment, 13 patients (56.5%) were on one antipsychotic medication while the other 10 (43.5%) were taking two antipsychotic medications during the study. The most common antipsychotic medications were clozapine (12 participants taking), olanzapine (5 participants taking), and aripiprazole (5 participants taking). Other participants were taking risperidone, quetiapine, paliperidone, lurasidone, and haloperidol. Finally, 2 participants were taking long acting injectable versions of antipsychotic medications: one on olanzapine and the other on paliperidone. Information on dosage was not collected. Mean pre-workout NDSE ratings ranged between 1.6 and 2.7 on psychosis and mood symptoms; 5.4–6.7 on motivation, social interest, cognition and energy items, and 3.7 on global QOL (**Table 2**).

Participants reported an average of 4.2 exercise sessions a week with 43.5% working out for more than 60 min. Most participants

TABLE 2 | NDSE mean pre-workout baseline scores.

NDSE item	Mean pre-workout score (cm)	Standard deviation
Global QOL	3.7	2.2
Anxiety	2.2	2
Depression	2.7	2.6
Energy	5.4	2.1
Hallucinations	1.6	2.5
Delusions	1.9	2.6
Motivation	5.9	2.5
Clarity of thought	6.7	2.4
Concentration	6.4	2.5
Social interest	5.7	2.8

TABLE 3 | Semi-structured interview participant responses.

Topic	Responses	Participants (%)
Who do you exercise for?	Myself	91
	Others	9.1
Why do you exercise?	Self-image[a]	69.6
	Psychological health	69.6
	Physical health	69.6
	Socialization	13
	Energy	13
What improves with exercise?	Depression	56.5
	Cognitive slowing	56.5
	Anxiety	43.5
	Amotivation	26.1
	Mindfulness	17.4
	Disorganization	11.5
	Hallucinations	8.7
	Paranoia	8.7
If you do not feel like exercising, what helps?	Reminding self of benefits	30.4
	Accountability partner	26
	Reminding self of goals	17.4
	Watch TV/YouTube	13
	Nothing	13
Exercise pattern throughout life	Started young with substantial interruptions[b]	61
	Regular since childhood	34.8
	Started as adult	4.3
If there was a substantial interruption, what motivated you to re-start?	Encouraged by doctor	35.3
	Did not feel as good	23.5
	Encouraged by family/friend	23.5
	Health reasons	11.8
Current types of exercise	Running/walking	91.3
	Weight Lifting	73.9
	Cycling	52.2
	Swimming	47.8
	Elliptical/Stair-climber	34.7
	Aerobics class, Pilates, dance	21.7
	Skiing/Snowboarding	21.7
	Organized sports	13
	Hiking	13
Duration of exercise (minutes)	30–44	30.4
	45–60	17.4
	More than 60	43.5
Who do you exercise with?	No one (workout alone)	63.5
	With one or more people	36.4

[a] Participants ranked this as the most important reason when asked to rank choices if multiple answers were given.
[b] The most common reason for an interruption was acute exacerbation of mental illness.

(63.5%) reported working out alone. Running, weight lifting, cycling and swimming were the most popular types of exercise, with smaller proportions engaging in more diverse forms of exercise.

Participants overwhelmingly reported (91%) that the reason that they exercise is for "myself" rather than for others. Most participants (61%) had learned to exercise early in life but noted at least one period of significant disruption, usually due to an exacerbation of their mental illness. The encouragement of a doctor was helpful in re-starting exercise for 35.5% of participants. Almost seventy percent (69.6%) of participants ranked the number one reason for exercising as "self-image." The same percentage of participants also reported psychological and physical health as very important reasons to exercise when allowed to choose more than one reason for why he or she exercised (**Table 3**).

On the SEES, study participants rated 0.6–0.2 point mean increases in feeling "Great," "Exhausted," "Positive," "Terrific," and "Strong" in response to exercise sessions (**Figure 2**). In addition, they rated 0.4–0.2 point mean reductions in feeling "Awful," "Crummy," and "Discouraged" (22).

A majority of participants (56.5%) identified depression and cognitive slowing to be improved by exercise and 43.5% reported that exercise improved their anxiety in the semi-structured interview. This is in contrast to 8.7% of participants who identified exercise as improving psychotic symptoms such as hallucinations or paranoia. This was consistent with the prospective NDSE ratings that showed 7–11% average decreases in anxiety and depression and 10–11% average increases in clarity of thought and concentration with almost no change on average in hallucinations and delusions in response to individual exercise sessions (**Figure 1**) (22). NDSE ratings also showed participants rated 9–15% average increases in global QOL, energy, motivation, and social interest with each exercise session (22).

DISCUSSION

Evidence pertaining to the effects of exercise in individuals with schizophrenia-spectrum disorders is growing. Typical designs, however, evaluate the effect of a time-limited exercise intervention on individuals who are sedentary at baseline. This study examined factors motivating and sustaining exercise in a unique population of individuals with schizophrenia-spectrum disorders who were already independently and regularly exercising. This study also examined whether self-reported retrospective mental health effects of exercise were

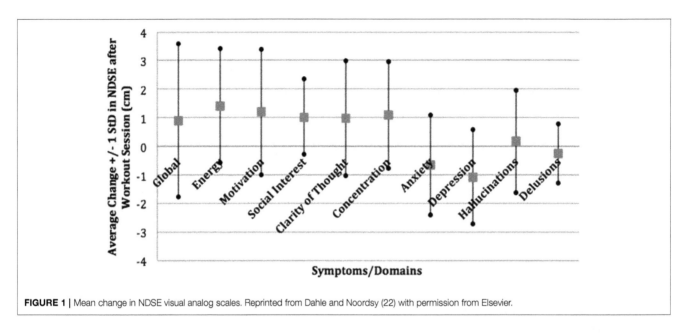

FIGURE 1 | Mean change in NDSE visual analog scales. Reprinted from Dahle and Noordsy (22) with permission from Elsevier.

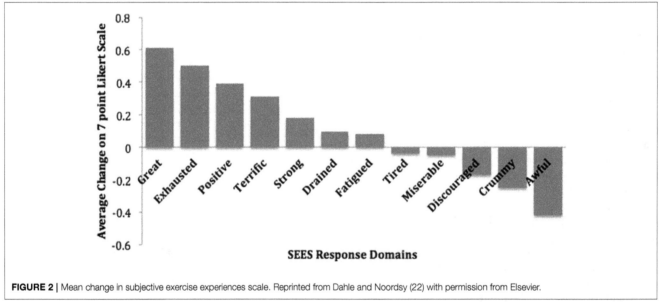

FIGURE 2 | Mean change in subjective exercise experiences scale. Reprinted from Dahle and Noordsy (22) with permission from Elsevier.

consistent with prospective ratings at the time of actual exercise sessions.

A recent systematic review found that people with schizophrenia engage in "significantly less" exercise than controls without schizophrenia, with about half of people with schizophrenia meeting a recommended 150 min of moderate physical activity per week (23). Our selected sample engaged in at least 90 min of exercise per week and reported an average of 4.2 sessions of running, weight lifting, cycling, swimming and other forms of exercise per week, with a majority reporting more than 45 min and nearly half reporting more than 60 min of exercise per session. Taken together, these findings indicate that while people with schizophrenia can stereotypically be considered inactive, some individuals engage in types and durations of

exercise that would be considered exceptional in the general population.

Our study showed that individuals with schizophrenia-spectrum disorders were most commonly motivated to exercise for "self-image" or, as one participant stated, "to look good in jeans." This is noteworthy, as overemphasis by the medical community on the physical and mental health benefits when attempting to motivate patients to add a routine of physical exercise may be misguided. This motivation is consistent with past research on motivation for exercise in other populations. As noted by Brudzynski and Ebben in a study of body image and exercise in a midwestern university population, "appearance, was identified as the most common contributor to individual exercise behaviors" (24). While the patients in our study did identify physical and mental health reasons as motivators for exercising, these were neither the primary nor the most important reasons. Furthermore, the finding that most of this unique population developed regular exercise habits during youth suggests the importance of culture and community in shaping healthy habits that can be sustained despite a diagnosis of major mental illness. It also shows the important role that physicians can play in encouraging patients to resume regular exercise after a disruption due to an acute exacerbation of their illness.

Our finding that people with schizophrenia report improved global well-being, depression, anxiety, energy, motivation, and cognition is consistent with prior research on mental health effects of exercise across multiple populations (25). Effects on subjective energy are mixed and may represent differences in impact on physical and mental energy. The finding of improved mood, negative, and cognitive symptoms with limited impact on positive symptoms is consistent specifically with prior research among people with schizophrenia (26). Although the effects were subjective and modest, these findings were consistent across both semi-structured interviews and structured prospective ratings.

Our sample reported low mean levels of psychosis and mood symptoms, moderate levels of motivation, social interest, cognition and energy and slightly favorable QOL immediately prior to their naturalistic exercise sessions. While population norms have not been established for the NDSE and there was substantial variability, these ratings suggest that our study participants were not highly symptomatic prior to exercise. This could mean that independent exercise represents a marker of high functioning, or be due to accrued benefits of their exercise activity. It is also possible that participants chose to exercise at times when they were less symptomatic or experienced anticipatory improvement in symptoms and well-being prior to exercising.

We found modest changes on the SEES and NDSE ratings of mental health parameters from immediately before to immediately after individual sessions of exercise. It is logical that single session effects would be smaller than cumulative effects over months of exercise. Given that respondents engaged in 30–60 + min of exercise per session, these effects are occurring quite rapidly. Participants were selected for sustained exercise, so they have likely accrued gains in their mental health prior to participation. These measures are targeting the time-limited effects of exercise that fade prior to the next exercise session. Therefore, the semi-structured interview provides evidence on the global effects of sustained exercise over individuals' moderate to long-term awareness, while the SEES and NDSE ratings hone in on the immediate reinforcing effects of individual exercise sessions. This suggests that benefits of exercise in non-psychotic symptom domains are subject to decay in the 1–2 day period between exercise sessions.

A meaningful subset of participants did report improvement in symptoms of psychosis in response to exercise in the interview, which was not reflected in the mean NDSE ratings. This suggests that the impact of exercise on the subjective experience of psychosis may be more gradual and sustained. It is also possible that the subset that reported improvement in psychosis were less likely to return completed NDSE ratings, or that low baseline levels of psychotic symptoms created floor effects.

The biological effects of vigorous sustained physical activity or exercise on the human body are numerous and include cardiovascular, pulmonary, metabolic, musculoskeletal, and immunologic regulation, as well as, changes in brain functioning and anatomy (27). In people with psychiatric disorders, no single mechanism has been found to account for the diverse range of health effects of exercise. Several have been suggested: (1). biochemical changes such as increased levels of neurotransmitters (e.g., endorphins or serotonin) or altered stress reactivity (hypothalamus-pituitary-adrenal axis), (2). physiological changes such as improved cardiovascular function or thermogenesis, and (3). psychological changes such as social support, sense of autonomy, experience of mastery, enhanced body image, self-efficacy, and improved coping skills (e.g., use of distraction) (25, 28, 29). One mechanism that has been proposed for people with schizophrenia is exercise-induced neurogenesis and synaptic proliferation. A study by Pajonk et al. found exercise-induced increases in hippocampal volume and decreases in positive and negative symptoms within 3 months, and another by Scheewe et al. found increases in gray matter volume and cortical thickness by 6 months (16, 30). While there is some evidence to suggest that neurogenic effects may develop relatively quickly in response to exercise, meaningful effects on mental and physical health will likely require sustained lifestyle changes (13).

Our study was limited by several factors. Our study relied on self-report and the use of less structured probes for the interview portion of the assessment. Interviewers may have elicited responses that participants might not have offered spontaneously. Validated measures of negative symptoms rely heavily on rater observation and it is not clear that people can accurately self-report this construct. Our study population was small, and recruited from a rural sample of patients. Although this convenience sample may not be representative of people with schizophrenia in other settings, all patients from the authors' usual care clinics who met criteria and consented to participate within the recruitment window were included. Another limitation is that the NDSE is not yet validated (a validation study is underway). Our participants, however, found the NDSE easy to use and demonstrated an expected degree of responsiveness to individual exercise sessions. Their responses on the NDSE closely paralleled their responses on the well-established SEES.

CONCLUSIONS

To our knowledge, this is the first study to examine a cohort of active and community dwelling individuals diagnosed with schizophrenia in order to describe their exercise patterns and subjective experiences. The granular detail on effects of individual exercise sessions provides a unique view into the experience of exercise for people living with schizophrenia. Our findings establish that some individuals with schizophrenia engage in regular physical exercise that stem from earlier life activities. These individuals identify primary motivations similar to those of people who do not have schizophrenia.

Duration and frequency of exercise rival those of community amateur athletes, and mean metabolic parameters are largely healthy despite BMI in overweight range. Individual sessions of exercise are rapidly reinforced by improvements in several areas including well-being, energy, and non-psychotic symptoms.

ETHICS STATEMENT

This study was carried out in accordance with the recommendations of the institutional review board of

Dartmouth-Hitchcock Medical Center with written informed consent from all subjects. All subjects gave written informed consent in accordance with the Declaration of Helsinki. The protocol was approved by the institutional review board of Dartmouth-Hitchcock Medical Center.

AUTHOR CONTRIBUTIONS

DD and DN contributed to study design and implementation. All authors contributed to manuscript preparation and approved the final draft.

REFERENCES

Correll CU, Solmi M, Veronese N, Bortolato B, Rosson S, Santonastaso P, et al. Prevalence, incidence and mortality from cardiovascular disease in patients with pooled and specific severe mental illness: a large-scale meta- analysis of 3,211,768 patients and 113,383,368 controls. World Psychiatry (2017) 16:163–80. doi: 10.1002/wps.20420

Gurusamy J, Gandhi S, Damodharan D, Ganesan V, Palaniappan M. Exercise, diet and educational interventions for metabolic syndrome in persons with schizophrenia: a systematic review. Asian J Psychiatr. (2018) 36:73–85. doi: 10.1016/j.ajp.2018.06.018

Ashdown-Franks G, Williams J, Vancampfort D, Firth J, Schuch F, Hubbard K, et al. Is it possible for people with severe mental illness to sit less and move more? A systematic review of interventions to increase physical activity or reduce sedentary behaviour. Schizophr Res. (2018). doi: 10.1016/j.schres.2018.06.058

Noordsy DL (ed). Lifestyle Psychiatry: Using Exercise, Diet and Mindfulness to Manage Psychiatric Disorders. Washington, DC: American Psychiatric Publishing.

Rimes RR, de Souza Moura AM, Lamego MK, de Sa Filho AS, Manochio J, Paes F, et al. Effects of exercise on physical and mental health, and cognitive and brain functions in schizophrenia: clinical and experimental evidence. CNS Neurol Disord Drug Targets (2015) 14:1244–54. doi: 10.2174/1871527315666151111130659

Gorczynski P, Faulkner G. Exercise therapy for schizophrenia. Schizophr Bull. (2010) 36:665–6. doi: 10.1093/schbul/sbq049

Wang PW, Lin HC, Su CY, Chen MD, Lin KC, Ko CH, et al. Effect of aerobic exercise on improving symptoms of individuals with schizophrenia: a single blinded randomized control study. Front Psychiatry (2018) 9:167. doi: 10.3389/fpsyt.2018.00167

Silva BA, Cassilhas RC, Attux C, Cordeiro Q, Gadelha AL, Telles BA, et al. A 20-week program of resistance or concurrent exercise improves symptoms of schizophrenia: results of a blind, randomized controlled trial. Rev Bras Psiquiatr. (2015) 37:271–9. doi: 10.1590/1516-4446-201 4-1595

Firth J, Stubbs B, Rosenbaum S, Vancampfort D, Malchow B, Schuch F, et al. Aerobic exercise improves cognitive functioning in people with schizophrenia: a systematic review and meta-analysis. Schizophr Bull. (2017) 43:546–56. doi: 10.1093/schbul/sbw115

Nuechterlein KH, Ventura J, McEwen SC, Gretchen-Doorly D, Vinogradov S, Subotnik KL. Enhancing cognitive training through aerobic exercise after a first schizophrenia episode: theoretical conception and pilot study. Schizophr Bull. (2016) 42(Suppl. 1):S44–52. doi: 10.1093/schbul/ sbw007

Archer T, Kostrzewa RM. Physical exercise alleviates health defects, symptoms, and biomarkers in schizophrenia spectrum disorder. Neurotox Res. (2015) 28:268–80. doi: 10.1007/s12640-015- 9543-y

Farholm A, Sorensen M. Motivation for physical activity and exercise in severe mental illness: a systematic review of cross-sectional studies. Int J Ment Health Nurs. (2016) 25:116–26. doi: 10.1111/inm.12217

Firth J, Rosenbaum S, Stubbs B, Gorczynski P, Yung AR, Vancampfort D. Motivating factors and barriers towards exercise in severe mental illness: a systematic review and meta-analysis. Psychol Med. (2016) 46:2869–81. doi: 10.1017/S0033291716001732

Firth J, Rosenbaum S, Stubbs B, Vancampfort D, Carney R, Yung AR. Preferences and motivations for exercise in early psychosis. Acta Psychiatr Scand. (2016) 134:83–4. doi: 10.1111/acps.12562

Vancampfort D, Firth J, Schuch FB, Rosenbaum S, Mugisha J, Hallgren M, et al. Sedentary behavior and physical activity levels in people with schizophrenia, bipolar disorder and major depressive disorder: a global systematic review and meta-analysis. World Psychiatry (2017) 16:308–15. doi: 10.1002/wps.20458

Pajonk FG, Wobrock T, Gruber O, Scherk H, Berner D, Kaizl I, et al. Hippocampal plasticity in response to exercise in schizophrenia. Arch Gen Psychiatry (2010) 67:133–43. doi: 10.1001/archgenpsychiatry.2009.193

Holley J, Crone D, Tyson P, Lovell G. The effects of physical activity on psychological well-being for those with schizophrenia: a systematic review. Br J Clin Psychol. (2011) 50:84–105. doi: 10.1348/014466510X496220

Beebe LH, Smith K, Burk R, McIntyre K, Dessieux O, Tavakoli A, et al. Effect of a motivational intervention on exercise behavior in persons with schizophrenia spectrum disorders. Commun Ment Health J. (2011) 47:628–36. doi: 10.1007/s10597-010-9363-8

MeAuley E, Courneya KS. The subjective exercise experiences scale (SEES): Development and preliminary validation. J Sport Exerc Psychol. (1994) 16:163–77. doi: 10.1123/jsep.16.2.163

Lehman AF. A quality of life interview for the chronically mentally ill. Eval Program Plann. (1988) 11:51–62. doi: 10.1016/0149-7189(88)90033-X

Ryan RM, Frederick C. On energy, personality, and health: Subjective vitality as a dynamic reflection of well-being. J Pers. (1997) 65:529–65.

Dahle D, Noordsy DL. Factors motivating spontaneous exercise in individuals with schizophrenia-spectrum disorders. Schizophr Res. (2018) 199:436–7. doi: 10.1016/j.schres.2018.03.022

Stubbs B, Firth J, Berry A, Schuch FB, Rosenbaum S, Gaughran F, et al. How much physical activity do people with schizophrenia engage in? A systematic review, comparative meta-analysis and meta-regression. Schizophr Res. (2016) 176:431–40. doi: 10.1016/j.schres.2016.05.017

Brudzynski LR, Ebben W. Body image as a motivator and barrier to exercise participation. Int J Exerc Sci. (2010) 3:3.

Knochel C, Oertel-Knochel V, O'Dwyer L, Prvulovic D, Alves G, Kollmann B, et al. Cognitive and behavioural effects of physical exercise in psychiatric patients. Prog Neurobiol. (2012) 96:46–68. doi: 10.1016/j.pneurobio.2011.11.007

Noordsy DL, Burgess JD, Hardy KV, Yudofsky LM, Ballon JS. Therapeutic potential of physical exercise in early psychosis. Am J Psychiatry (2018) 175:209–14. doi: 10.1176/appi.ajp.2017.170 60716

Firth J, Cotter J, Carney R, Yung AR. The pro-cognitive mechanisms of physical exercise in people with schizophrenia. Br J Pharmacol. (2017) 174:3161–72. doi: 10.1111/bph.13772

Wolff E, Gaudlitz K, von Lindenberger BL, Plag J, Heinz A, Strohle A. Exercise and physical activity in mental disorders. Eur Arch Psychiatry Clin Neurosci. (2011) 261(Suppl. 2):S186–91. doi: 10.1007/s00406-011- 0254-y

Oertel-Knochel V, Mehler P, Thiel C, Steinbrecher K, Malchow B, Tesky V, et al. Effects of aerobic exercise on cognitive performance and individual psychopathology in depressive and schizophrenia patients. Eur Arch Psychiatry Clin Neurosci. (2014) 264:589–604. doi: 10.1007/s00406-014-0485-9

Scheewe TW, van Haren NE, Sarkisyan G, Schnack HG, Brouwer RM, de Glint M, et al. Exercise therapy, cardiorespiratory fitness and their effect on brain volumes: a randomised controlled trial in patients with schizophrenia and healthy controls. Eur Neuropsychopharmacol. (2013) 23:675–85. doi: 10.1016/j.euroneuro.2012.08.008

17

Cardiorespiratory Fitness, Age and Multiple Aspects of Executive Function among Preadolescent Children

Zhuxuan Zhan[1,2], Jingyi Ai[3], Feifei Ren[4,5], Lin Li[1,2]*, Chien-Heng Chu[3]* and Yu-Kai Chang[3,6]*

[1]*Key Laboratory of Adolescent Health Assessment and Exercise Intervention of Ministry of Education, East China Normal University, Shanghai, China,* [2]*College of Physical Education and Health, East China Normal University, Shanghai, China,* [3]*Department of Physical Education, National Taiwan Normal University, Taipei, Taiwan,* [4]*Graduate Institute of Athletics and Coaching Science, National Taiwan Sport University, Taoyuan, Taiwan,* [5]*Department of Physical Education, Beijing Language and Culture University, Beijing, China,* [6]*Institute for Research Excellence in Learning Science, National Taiwan Normal University, Taipei, Taiwan*

Correspondence:
Lin Li
lilin.xtt@163.com
Chien-Heng Chu
cchu042@yahoo.com
Yu-Kai Chang
yukaichangnew@gmail.com

Cardiorespiratory fitness (CRF) and age have been positively associated with children's executive function; however, few studies have simultaneously assessed the associations between both variables and different aspects of executive function among preadolescent children. Therefore, the purpose of the current study was to evaluate the simultaneous influence of CRF and age on three aspects of executive function. Preadolescent children's ($n = 338$) CRF levels were estimated based on the Progressive Aerobic Cardiovascular Endurance Run (PACER) test and then grouped into two age groups (Young Group: 9–10 years old and Old Group: 11–12 years old). Hierarchical multiple regression analyses were conducted for the 2-back task, the Flanker task, and the Local-Global task to assess the influence of CRF and age on working memory, inhibitory control, and shifting, respectively. Preadolescent children with greater CRF levels were associated with higher response accuracy during the 2-back task and shorter response time across congruent and incongruent conditions of the Flanker task, whereas older children showed generally superior cognitive performance. Notably, only the Old Group's CRF was positively correlated with the accuracy in the switching condition of the Local-Global task. These findings suggest that CRF or age was generally associated with better performances in working memory and inhibitory control aspects of executive function. Furthermore, the positive influence of CRF on shifting may be modulated by developed cortical maturation.

Keywords: executive function, working memory, inhibitory control, shifting, maturation, Progressive Aerobic Cardiovascular Endurance Run, cardiorespiratory fitness

INTRODUCTION

Cardiorespiratory fitness (CRF), the direct indicator of individuals' cardiovascular and respiratory systems' overall capacity to perform physical activities, plays a critical role regarding physiological and psychological health. A higher CRF level has been linked to a lower metabolic syndrome risk and a cardiovascular disease risk (Twisk et al., 2000; Padilla-Moledo et al., 2012), increased volumes of certain cortical regions [e.g., the gray matter volume of the hippocampus and the basal ganglia (Chaddock et al., 2010a,b)], and lower risks of depression and anxiety (Biddle and Asare, 2011). The beneficial effects associated with higher CRF levels have been extended to academic performance in preadolescent school-aged children (Donnelly et al., 2016; Ruiz-Ariza et al., 2017; Chu et al., 2019). These improvements are possibly caused by CRF-related enhanced executive function, which is one of the foundations of academic performance (Hillman et al., 2009, 2014; Pontifex et al., 2011; Voss et al., 2011; Scudder et al., 2016; DiPietro et al., 2019).

Executive function is a top-down and meta-cognitive function required for conducting complex and goal-oriented operations. It consists of three distinct aspects: working memory, inhibitory control, and shifting (Miyake et al., 2000). Working memory, also known as updating, has been defined as the capacity of temporarily retaining relevant information and enables individuals to manipulate or further process this information (Miyake et al., 2000; Baddeley, 2012). Inhibitory control, also known as inhibition, refers to an individual's ability to deliberately control, inhibit, or override a prepotent response or the ability to ignore irrelevant information or interferences in the environment and focus on relevant information. Shifting, also known as cognitive flexibility, represents the switching of attention or response strategies between mental sets according to the task demands (Miyake et al., 2000). These three aspects of executive function are highly important to preadolescent children's learning and academic achievement (Kao et al., 2017a; Lippi et al., 2020).

A few studies have explored the associations between CRF and these three aspects of executive function separately (Tomporowski et al., 2015). Specifically, children with higher CRF assessed by the field-based CRF assessment [e.g., Progressive Aerobic Cardiovascular Endurance Run (PACER)] were associated with a superior performance on working memory capacity (Scudder et al., 2014, 2016). Cross-sectional research using the laboratory-based CRF assessment also revealed similar positive links between maximal oxygen consumption (VO_{2max}) and working memory capacity (Kamijo et al., 2011; Drollette et al., 2016; Kao et al., 2017b). Similarly, cross-sectional studies utilizing either field-based (e.g., PACER) or laboratory-based (e.g., VO_{2max}) CRF assessments to explore the associations between CRF and inhibitory control have revealed positive associations between CRF levels and task performance [e.g., shorter response times (Scudder et al., 2014; Drollette et al., 2016; Song et al., 2017) or higher response accuracy (Hillman et al., 2009; Pontifex et al., 2011; Scudder et al., 2014)], especially during the task condition requiring a more substantial amount of inhibitory control. Finally, similar findings of the beneficial effects of CRF on the shifting aspects of executive function have also been documented (Ishihara et al., 2018; Westfall et al., 2018).

Although relatively consistent evidence suggests a positive association between CRF and executive function, several potential limitations should be noted. First, prior studies examining the relationships between CRF and executive functions of children mainly used combined data across different age groups (e.g., aged 10–18 years) (Hillman et al., 2006; Themanson et al., 2006; Scudder et al., 2014; Kao et al., 2017b). Importantly, the cortical maturation trajectory of different parts of the brain

are not uniform and, consequently, the development trajectory of various aspects of executive function might differ from each other during early childhood (Best and Miller, 2010; Diamond, 2013). It is plausible that the capability of completing the cognitive tasks increases while the structural and functional development continuously progresses throughout adolescence into early adulthood in which the associations between CRF and executive function might be altered in different age groups of preadolescent children. Due to the complex laboratory-based CRF assessment and neuro-electrical equipment, the sample sizes in prior research were relatively small and less representative (Scudder et al., 2014). Finally, relatively few studies have simultaneously compared the various aspects of executive function among preadolescent school-aged children.

Accordingly, the current research aims to examine how CRF and age influence the three aspects of executive function – working memory, inhibitory control, and shifting – in a large sample of preadolescent school-aged children. It was hypothesized that the children with higher levels of CRF or at older ages might be associated with superior executive function as reflected in better cognitive task performance, and then the interactions between CRF and age would be observed.

MATERIALS AND METHODS

Participants
For this study, 377 school-aged preadolescent children were initially recruited. Eligible participants were screened by having to meet the following inclusion criteria: (1) age between 9 and 12 years old; (2) no history of psychiatric or neurological disease; (3) the anxiety scores assessed by the Chinese version of Self-Rating Anxiety Scale (Zung, 1971) were less than 50; (4) the depression scores assessed by the Chinese version of Children's Depression Inventory (Yu and Li, 2000) were less than 19; (5) the scores of the modified Chinese version of Raven's Standard Progressive Matrices were above the moderate levels; and (6) no history of cardiovascular disease.

Only those who completed the CRF and executive function assessments were included in the final analytical study. Three hundred thirty-eight children were finally recruited and grouped into the Young Group (9–10 years) and the Old Group (11–12 years) (**Table 1**).

The study was approved by the Institutional Review Board of East China Normal University, China. The written informed consent was obtained from children and their legal guardians before the children participated in the experiment.

CRF Assessment
In the current study, the PACER test, a multistage 20-m shuttle run test, was utilized to assess children's CRF performance. The PACER test is considered valid for accurately measuring CRF for wide age ranges of participants, and it has been utilized in several prior studies that examined the association between CRF and cognitive and academic performance (Scudder et al., 2014, 2016). The test-retest reliability ($r = 0.72$–0.89) and validity ($r = 0.51$–0.84) of the PACER have been well documented previously (Leger et al., 1988; Mahoney, 1992; Yu and Fang, 2002).

TABLE 1 | Preadolescents' demographic and cognitive-related characteristics of the Young and the Old Groups (mean ± SD).

Variables	Young Group	Old Group
No. of participants (% male)	150 (62.7%)	188 (64.9%)
Mean age (years)	9.49 ± 0.50	11.37 ± 0.48
Height (m)	1.37 ± 0.07	1.48 ± 0.08*
Weight (kg)	30.07 ± 5.70	36.88 ± 7.99*
BMI (kg.m^{-2})	16.02 ± 2.10	16.73 ± 2.47*
Estimated VO$_{2max}$ (ml.kg^{-1}.min^{-1})	49.77 ± 3.48	46.71 ± 3.76*
Anxiety score	37 ± 6.36	42 ± 6.31
Depression score	12.35 ± 4.48	11.64 ± 4.58
Raven's Standard Progressive Matrices score	53.7 ± 9.7	55.53 ± 3.63
2-back task		
RT (ms)	1190.08 ± 242.9	1081.41 ± 230.09*
Accuracy	0.70 ± 0.17	0.79 ± 0.17*
Flanker task		
Congruent RT (ms)	486.43 ± 108.71	463.37 ± 106.29
Congruent accuracy	0.69 ± 0.19	0.70 ± 0.19
Incongruent RT (ms)	503.47 ± 118.1	470. 67 ± 115.64*
Incongruent accuracy	0.65 ± 0.19	0.67 ± 0.19
Local-Global task		
Non-switching RT (ms)	901.65 ± 293.26	836.14 ± 242.53*
Non-switching accuracy	0.90 ± 0.15	0.91 ± 0.14
Switching RT (ms)	1100.84 ± 332.42	1050.04 ± 275.63
Switching accuracy	0.86 ± 0.14	0.86 ± 0.14

VO$_{2max}$, maximal oxygen consumption; RT, response time. *$p \leq 0.05$.

The PACER test was administered during participants' second visits by the trained physical education teachers following the standardized protocol (Welk and Meredith, 2008). Briefly, participants were instructed to perform a 5-min standardized warm-up, following run back and forth from one maker to another marker spaced 20-m apart while keeping pace with the prerecorded cadence. The frequency of beat increases 0.5 km/h every minute, with an initial speed of 8.5 km/h. Participants were encouraged to keep up with the beat for as long as possible. The test was terminated if the given participant failed to traverse the 20-m distance between the markers within the designated time twice or was no longer able to maintain the pace and voluntarily stopped. The higher the number of laps a participant completed, the higher the CRF level they had.

Based on the number of the laps a child completed, the index of CRF (i.e., the estimated VO$_{2max}$) was calculated using the following equation (Leger et al., 1988):

VO$_{2max}$ (ml.kg^{-1}.min^{-1}) = 31.025 + 3.238 × speed (speed corresponding to the final stage in km.h^{-1}) − 3.248 × age (years) + 0.1536 × age × speed

2-Back Task

The working memory aspect of executive function was assessed by the 2-back task that was programmed and ran using the E-prime software (v. 2.0, Psychology Software Tools, Inc.). The 2-back task is a modified N-back task, which has been a widely utilized paradigm to assess the capacity of working memory (Scudder et al., 2016; Ishihara et al., 2017). The 2-back task consisted of a sequence of white numeric digits (1–9), each measuring 1.5 cm × 1.5 cm. The stimulus was presented focally against a black background with a duration of 2,000 ms and a fixed intertrial interval of 3,000 ms. The task was composed

of two blocks of 25 trials each, with 60 s of rest between the blocks. The total duration of the tasks summed to about 7 min. The participants were instructed to press the #1 key on the numeric keypad if the current stimulus (trial n) was matched to the stimulus two trials earlier (trial $n-2$); otherwise, they were instructed to press the #2 key. Trials of 50% probability as represented required the participants to press the #1 key as the correct response. The primary behavioral indices were the response times of the correct responses and response accuracy.

Flanker Task

The inhibitory aspect of executive function was assessed by the modified Flanker task (Eriksen and Eriksen, 1974; Pindus et al., 2019) that was programmed and ran using the E-prime software. Each trial of the Flanker task consisted of a row of five parallel white arrows presented in the center of a 14″ LCD screen against a black background. The target arrow was posited in the middle, and two distractive arrows were on each side of the target arrow (flankers). Each trial appeared for 200 ms and then followed by a randomly selected various intertrial interval of 1,250–1,500 ms.

The Flanker task consisted of two types of trials: (1) the congruent trials (50%), in which the directions of all the arrows were the same (e.g., < < < < < or > > > > >) and (2) the incongruent trials (50%), in which the target arrow was pointed in the opposite direction from the flankers (e.g., < < > < < or > > < > >). The trials were separated into two blocks of 75 trials each, with 60 s of rest between the blocks. The overall number of congruent and incongruent trials were equal across the two blocks (50% of trials were congruent). The participants were instructed to press either the #1 or #2 key on the numeric keypad corresponding to the direction of the target arrow (left or right, respectively), as fast and accurately as possible.

If the participants responded within 200 ms, the stimuli disappeared, and the screen remained black for the rest of the 200 ms period. The response times of correct responses and response accuracy for congruent and incongruent conditions were recorded and assessed as the primary behavioral indices.

Local-Global Task

The shifting aspect of executive function was assessed by the modified Local-Global task (Ishihara et al., 2018) that was programmed and ran using the E-prime software. The Navon-like global/local figures (Navon, 1977) were utilized during the task as the stimuli was made of two target numeric digits (i.e., the numeric digit 1, and 2) and two neutral distractors (i.e., the numeric digit 3 and 4). The large global numeric digits (global level) consist of copies of small local numeric digits (local level), and all of the numeric digits were presented equally at the global and local levels. For instance, 25% of the global numeric digits were the target numeric digit 1, which might be composed of one of the local distractor numeric digits. Similarly, 25% of the local numeric digits were the target numeric digit 1, which could be organized to form the global distractor numeric digits.

The switching condition (i.e., the target numeric digits were switched from local to global levels or vice versa) consisted of 46.8% of the trials. On the other hand, the repetitive non-switching condition (i.e., the current target numeric digit and the previous target were at the same level; e.g., a target "global" numeric digit 2 followed by a target "global" numeric digit 1) accounted for 53.2% of the trials. Two blocks of 36 trials each were presented, with 60 s of rest between the blocks. The stimuli presented focally on a 14″ LCD screen would disappear soon after the participants made their responses, and the next stimulus appeared immediately. Participants were instructed to press the #1 key or the #2 key on the numeric keypad when they identified the presence of target stimuli (the numeric digit 1 or the numeric digit 2, respectively) at either the global level or the local level. The stimuli remained on the screen until a response was made. The response time for a correct response and the accuracy of the switching and repetitive non-swathing conditions were the main behavioral indices.

Procedures

Each eligible child participated for 3 separate days to complete the study. On their first visit, the children and their legal guardians completed the written informational concerns in a quiet indoor space. Additionally, their basic demographic data (e.g., gender, age, height, and weight) were collected or assessed. On their second visit, their CRF was assessed by the PACER test. On their third visit, three computer-based cognitive tasks were completed in a fixed order that lasted for an hour, with short breaks between cognitive tasks. The order of tests was as follows: the 2-back task, the Flanker task, and the Local-Global task. Before starting the formal cognitive tasks, the participants received detailed instructions regarding each cognitive task and have achieved at least 80% accuracy of the practice trials. Given the large number of children recruited for the current study, the primary researchers conducted the experiment during both morning and afternoon hours.

Statistical Analysis of Data

Descriptive statistics were calculated to summarize the baseline characteristics of the participants. A series of independent t-test were further conducted by assessing the differences between the demographic and cognitive-related data by age group.

Separate 2-step linear hierarchical regression analyses were performed for two indices from the 2-back task (correct target response time/accuracy), and four indices from the Flanker task (correct congruent response time/accuracy and correct incongruent response time/accuracy), and four indices from the Local-Global task (correct switching response time/accuracy and correct non-switching response time/accuracy).

To examine the contributions of CRF, age, and their interactions on the three aspects of executive function, the variables were entered into the regression model in the following order: (1) CRF estimated from PACER laps, age group (coded as 0 for the Young Group and 1 for the Old Group), and body mass index (BMI) (Step 1) and (Step 2) the interactions between CRF and the age group (Step 2). If a significant interaction between CRF and an age group was detected, a simple slope analysis (Aiken et al., 1991) was performed to examine the main effects of CRF on the Young Group and the Old Group. The multiple regression coefficients squared R^2 for the overall model (R^2), the stepwise changes in R^2 (ΔR^2),

and the standardized regression weight (β) for each predictor variable were reported. A significance level of $p < 0.05$ was set.

All statistical analyses were conducted using the SPSS® 21 statistical package (IBM Corporation, Armonk, NY, USA).

RESULTS

Participants Characteristics

Independent t-test of the demographic data revealed that the participants in the Old Group were taller, heavier, and had larger BMI values than the participants in the Young Group ($ps < 0.05$). The Old Group also had lower estimated VO_{2max} values than the Young Group ($p < 0.05$). None of the other demographic variables were significantly different between the two groups (all $ps > 0.05$) (**Table 1**).

Independent t-test of the cognitive-related measures revealed that the Old Group had shorter response times and higher accuracy in the 2-back task, shorter response times in the incongruent Flanker task condition, and shorter response times in the non-switching Local-Global task condition than the Young Group ($ps < 0.05$). None of the other cognitive-related measures were significantly different between the two groups (all $ps > 0.05$).

CRF, Age, and 2-Back Task

Regarding the response time, the regression analysis revealed a significant overall model effect of Step 1 ($\Delta R^2 = 0.06$, $p < 0.01$), with a significant negative effect for age ($\beta = -0.25$, $p < 0.01$) (**Table 2**). The overall model effect of Step 2 was not significant ($p = 0.79$); however, a significant negative effect for age ($\beta = -0.26$, $p < 0.01$) was observed.

Regarding the response accuracy, the overall model effect of Step 1 was significant ($\Delta R^2 = 0.07$, $p < 0.01$), with a significant positive effect for CRF ($\beta = 0.13$, $p = 0.04$) and for age ($\beta = 0.29$, $p < 0.01$). The overall model effect of Step 2 was not significant ($p = 0.12$); however, a significant positive effect for age ($\beta = 0.28$, $p < 0.01$) was observed.

CRF, Age, and Flanker Task

Regarding the response time of the congruent condition, the overall model effect of Step 1 was significant ($\Delta R^2 = 0.03$, $p < 0.01$), with significant negative effects for CRF ($\beta = -0.16$, $p < 0.01$) and for age ($\beta = -0.16$, $p < 0.01$) (**Table 2**). The overall model effect of Step 2 was not significant ($p = 0.23$); however, a significant positive effect for age ($\beta = -0.15$, $p = 0.01$) was observed. Regarding the response accuracy of the congruent condition, neither the overall model effects of Step 1 and Step 2 nor other variables (CRF, age group, and BMI) were significant (all $ps > 0.05$).

Regarding the response time of the incongruent condition, the overall model effect of Step 1 was significant ($\Delta R^2 = 0.04$, $p < 0.01$), with significant negative effects for CRF ($\beta = -0.13$, $p = 0.03$) and age ($\beta = -0.17$, $p < 0.01$). The overall model effect of Step 2 was not significant ($p = 0.22$); however, a significant negative effect for age ($\beta = -0.16$, $p = 0.01$) was observed. Regarding the response accuracy of the incongruent condition, neither the overall model effects of Step 1 and Step 2 nor other variables (CRF, age group, and BMI) were significant (all $ps > 0.05$).

TABLE 2 | Regression analysis for the associations between cardiorespiratory fitness, age, the 2-back task, and the Flanker task.

Model and variable	2-back task		Flanker task			
			Congruent		Incongruent	
	ΔR^2	β	ΔR^2	β	ΔR^2	β
Response time						
Step 1	0.06**		0.03**		0.04**	
CRF		−0.06		−0.16**		−0.13*
Age		−0.25**		−0.16**		−0.17**
BMI		0.03		−0.08		−0.10
Step 2	<0.001		0.004		0.004	
CRF		−0.08		−0.08		−0.04
Age		−0.26**		−0.15**		−0.16**
BMI		0.04		−0.09		−0.11
CRF × Age		0.02		−0.10		−0.11
Accuracy						
Step 1	0.07**		0.002		0.003	
CRF		0.13*		0.02		0.01
Age		0.29**		0.03		0.06
BMI		0.03		0.03		0.01
Step 2	0.01		0.002		0.001	
CRF		0.02		0.08		0.05
Age		0.28**		0.04		0.06
BMI		0.03		0.03		0.01
CRF × Age		0.13		−0.07		−0.05

BMI, body mass index; CRF, cardiorespiratory fitness. $*p \leq 0.05$; $**p \leq 0.01$.

TABLE 3 | Regression analysis for the associations between cardiorespiratory fitness, age and Local-Global task.

Model and variable	Non-switching		Switching	
	ΔR^2	β	ΔR^2	β
Response time				
Step 1	0.02		0.01	
CRF		−0.07		0.01
Age		−0.15**		−0.09
BMI		0.02		0.04
Step 2	0.001		0.003	
CRF		−0.12		0.07
Age		−0.16**		−0.08
BMI		0.02		0.04
CRF × Age		0.06		−0.09
Accuracy				
Step 1	0.002		0.01	
CRF		0.01		0.08
Age		0.01		0.02
BMI		0.05		0.04
Step 2	0.003		0.01*	
CRF		−0.06		−0.07
Age		−0.001		0.01
BMI		0.05		0.05
CRF × Age		0.09		0.19*

BMI, body mass index; CRF, cardiorespiratory fitness. $*p \leq 0.05$; $**p \leq 0.01$.

CRF, Age, and Local-Global Task

Regarding the response time of the non-switching condition, the overall model effect of Step 1 was not significant ($\Delta R^2 = 0.02$, $p = 0.07$); however, a significant negative effect for age ($\beta = −0.15$, $p < 0.01$) was observed (**Table 3**). The overall model effect of Step 2 was not significant ($p = 0.51$); however, a significant negative effect for age ($\beta = −0.16$, $p < 0.01$) was observed.

Regarding the response accuracy of the non-switching condition, neither the overall model effects of Step 1 and Step 2 nor the effects of the variables (CRF, age group, and BMI) were significant (all $ps > 0.05$).

Regarding the response time of the switching condition, neither the overall model effects of Step 1 and Step 2 nor the effects of the variables (CRF, age group, and BMI) were significant (all $ps > 0.05$). Regarding the response accuracy of the switching, neither the overall model effects of Step 1 nor the effects of the variables (CRF, age group, and BMI) were significant (all $ps > 0.05$). However, the overall model effect of Step 2 was significant ($\Delta R^2 = 0.01$, $p = 0.03$), with a significant positive effect for the interaction of CRF and age ($\beta = 0.19$, $p = 0.03$). Further decomposition of the interaction by the single slope analysis for each age group was carried out to test the significance of predicting the accuracy of CRF. The results revealed that CRF levels significantly associated with the higher switching accuracy among older children ($p = 0.02$), but the association was not observed in younger children (see **Figure 1**).

DISCUSSION

The current study was among the first large-sample investigations designed to better understand how CRF and age were associated with three aspects of executive function by using the 2-back task, the Flanker task, and the Local-Global task. The primary results revealed that CRF and age were positively associated with the performance of the 2-back task and the Flanker task. The interactions of CRF and age on the Local-Global task indicated the positive association between CRF and the performance of the switching condition in older preadolescents.

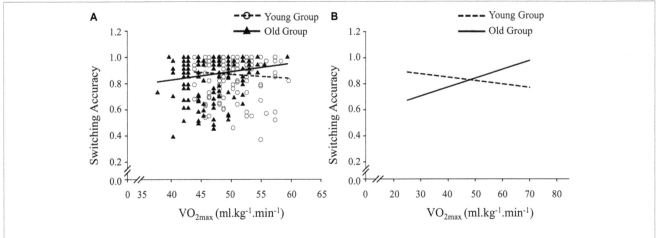

FIGURE 1 | Scatterplots of the relationships between cardiorespiratory fitness (i.e., VO_{2max}) and switching accuracy of the Local-Global task. **(A)** Raw data and **(B)** data that adjusted within the regression model.

The findings of CRF being positively associated with higher accuracy in the 2-back task suggest that CRF is linked to working memory. Similar findings were also observed in CRF and working memory assessed by different tasks. Scudder et al. (2014) reported that young children who completed more laps were associated with superior working memory (response accuracy and working memory d' scores) assessed using the field-based CRF (PACER test) and the spatial N-back paradigm. Laboratory-based assessed CRF (VO_{2max}) has also revealed increased response accuracy and working memory d' scores via N-back task (Drollette et al., 2016; Kao et al., 2017b). The subsequent 3-year longitudinal study further indicated that the positive correlations between increased CRF and enhanced working memory performance (the 2-back condition of the N-back task) were more potent at the more cognitively demanding task condition (Scudder et al., 2016). These studies that utilized different approaches to assess CRF and working memory provide a strong argument for the positive linkage between CRF and working memory from convergent perspectives.

The current study observed the association between CRF and inhibitory control aspect of executive function, regardless of the conditions of the Flanker task, being broadly consonant with prior research. In other words, children who completed a higher number of PACER laps were associated with better performance (i.e., shorter response times) in both congruent and incongruent conditions of the Flanker task relative to those completed few laps, suggesting a generally beneficial effect of CRF on inhibitory control among preadolescents (Scudder et al., 2014, 2016; Kao et al., 2017a; Raine et al., 2018; Westfall et al., 2018). Similar results showing an association between CRF levels and cognitive performance, regardless of the demands placed on executive function (including the differing demands of the congruent and incongruent conditions of the Flanker task), were also observed in elementary school children (Hillman et al., 2014; Scudder et al., 2014, 2016) and adolescents (Westfall et al., 2018). Collectively, the general improvements associated with CRF and inhibitory control-related tasks could be observed from preadolescent to adolescent children.

Along with CRF, our study also observed positive associations with age and working memory as well as age and inhibitory control, which are in line with prior developmental literature that the performance of working memory and inhibitory control continuously improved throughout childhood until the age of 15 years. The older children demonstrated superior working memory performance assessed by the N-back task and inhibitory control performance assessed by the Flanker task and evidenced by shorter response times or higher response accuracy (Best and Miller, 2010). Notably, a shorter response time without any of the negative impacts on the response accuracy for the Older Group suggests that age-induced increased performance does not result from the speed-accuracy trade off. In line with studies associated with CRF, these studies reflect a strong linkage between age and two types of executive function: working memory and inhibitory control. Our study has extended the existing knowledge by examining CRF and age simultaneously in preadolescent children.

The current findings have further demonstrated that age might moderate the correlation between CRF and shifting performance. Specifically, the positive relationship was only evident for older but not for younger preadolescent children during the more difficult parts of the task that require the upregulation of shifting ability. Our results have extended the previous research showing that 6–12-year-old children with a higher CRF were associated with shorter response times during the switching condition of the shifting paradigm (Ishihara et al., 2018) and have demonstrated that age might modulate the effects of CRF on shifting. The improvement of shifting ability (e.g., decreasing switching cost) usually continues into early adolescence following the inhibition and working memory processes (Huizinga et al., 2006; Best and Miller, 2010). A positive correlation between CRF levels in older adults and the performance of the task-switching paradigm (higher response accuracy for repeated and switching trials), which was mediated by the caudate nucleus volumes at the dorsal region (Verstynen et al., 2012), was observed. Thus, it is plausible that the limited beneficial effects of CRF on younger preadolescents were due to their lower levels of cortical maturation. Collectively, current findings have filled the gap of a lack of data concerning shifting and CRF in different ages of preadolescents (Verburgh et al., 2014) and have provided direct evidence of the performances on field tests of CRF and the shifting aspect of executive function.

To the best of our knowledge, this study was the first to investigate the CRF and working memory, inhibitory control, and shifting aspects of executive function simultaneously in a large sample of preadolescents from two age groups, thus making it possible to explore the associations between CRF, age, and more than one aspect of executive function in preadolescents. Despite the exciting findings from the current study, several limitations should be acknowledged. First, the CRF in the current study was assessed through the field-based PACER method. Although the maximum oxygen consumption (VO_{2max}) has been considered as the gold standard for CRF assessment, the requirement of sophisticated equipment and the relatively high cost limited the application in the settings such as school and populational-based studies (Castro-Pinero et al., 2010). Second, the order of conducting the cognitive tasks was not counterbalanced across groups and individuals, and the fixed order might influence the results of current findings. Lastly, since the current study was cross-sectional, the directions of the associations between CRF levels, ages, and cognitive performance could not be determined. Future research would benefit from utilizing longitudinal observational or randomized control interventional approaches so that the influence of the changes in CRF on various aspects of executive function among preadolescent children over time could be elucidated, and the associated causality could be more clearly established.

In conclusion, children with higher levels of CRF or older children were generally associated with better working memory, inhibitory control, and shifting aspects of executive function. Notably, the interaction of CRF and age on shifting further suggests the role of developed cortical maturation in the relationship between CRF and executive function.

ETHICS STATEMENT

The studies involving human participants were reviewed and approved by Institutional Review Board of East China Normal University, China. Written informed consent to participate in this study was provided by the participants' legal guardian/next of kin.

AUTHOR CONTRIBUTIONS

Conceptualization: ZZ, C-HC, JA, FR, LL, and Y-KC. Methodology: LL, FR, and Y-KC. Formal analysis: ZZ, LL, and Y-KC. Investigation: ZZ, JA, and LL. Data curation: ZZ, FR, and JA. Writing – original draft preparation: ZZ, C-HC, JA, and Y-KC. Writing – review and editing: all authors. Visualization: ZZ and JA.

REFERENCES

Aiken, L. S., West, S. G., and Reno, R. R. (1991). *Multiple regression: Testing and interpreting interactions.* Sage.

Baddeley, A. (2012). Working memory: theories, models, and controversies. *Annu. Rev. Psychol.* 63, 1–29. doi: 10.1146/annurev-psych-120710-100422

Best, J. R., and Miller, P. H. (2010). A developmental perspective on executive function. *Child Dev.* 81, 1641–1660. doi: 10.1111/j.1467-8624.2010.01499.x

Biddle, S. J., and Asare, M. (2011). Physical activity and mental health in children and adolescents: a review of reviews. *Br. J. Sports Med.* 45, 886–895. doi: 10.1136/bjsports-2011-090185

Castro-Pinero, J., Artero, E. G., Espana-Romero, V., Ortega, F. B., Sjostrom, M., Suni, J., et al. (2010). Criterion-related validity of field-based fitness tests in youth: a systematic review. *Br. J. Sports Med.* 44, 934–943. doi: 10.1136/bjsm.2009.058321

Chaddock, L., Erickson, K. I., Prakash, R. S., Kim, J. S., Voss, M. W., Vanpatter, M., et al. (2010a). A neuroimaging investigation of the association between aerobic fitness, hippocampal volume, and memory performance in preadolescent children. *Brain Res.* 1358, 172–183. doi: 10.1016/j.brainres.2010.08.049

Chaddock, L., Erickson, K. I., Prakash, R. S., Vanpatter, M., Voss, M. W., Pontifex, M. B., et al. (2010b). Basal ganglia volume is associated with aerobic fitness in preadolescent children. *Dev. Neurosci.* 32, 249–256. doi: 10.1159/000316648

Chu, C. H., Chen, F. T., Pontifex, M. B., Sun, Y., and Chang, Y. K. (2019). Health-related physical fitness, academic achievement, and neuroelectric measures in children and adolescents. *Int. J. Sport Exerc. Psychol.* 17, 117–132. doi: 10.1080/1612197X.2016.1223420

Diamond, A. (2013). Executive functions. *Annu. Rev. Psychol.* 64, 135–168. doi: 10.1146/annurev-psych-113011-143750

Dipietro, L., Buchner, D. M., Marquez, D. X., Pate, R. R., Pescatello, L. S., and Whitt-Glover, M. C. (2019). New scientific basis for the 2018 U.S. Physical Activity Guidelines. *J. Sport Health Sci.* 8, 197–200. doi: 10.1016/j.jshs.2019.03.007

Donnelly, J. E., Hillman, C. H., Castelli, D., Etnier, J. L., Lee, S., Tomporowski, P., et al. (2016). Physical activity, fitness, cognitive function, and academic achievement in children: a systematic review. *Med. Sci. Sports Exerc.* 48, 1197–1222. doi: 10.1249/MSS.0000000000000966

Drollette, E. S., Scudder, M. R., Raine, L. B., Davis Moore, R., Pontifex, M. B., Erickson, K. I., et al. (2016). The sexual dimorphic association of cardiorespiratory fitness to working memory in children. *Dev. Sci.* 19, 90–108. doi: 10.1111/desc.12291

Eriksen, B. A., and Eriksen, C. W. (1974). Effects of noise letters upon the identification of a target letter in a nonsearch task. *Percept. Psychophys.* 16, 143–149. doi: 10.3758/BF03203267

Hillman, C. H., Buck, S. M., Themanson, J. R., Pontifex, M. B., and Castelli, D. M. (2009). Aerobic fitness and cognitive development: event-related brain potential and task performance indices of executive control in preadolescent children. *Dev. Psychol.* 45, 114–129. doi: 10.1037/a0014437

Hillman, C. H., Kramer, A. F., Belopolsky, A. V., and Smith, D. P. (2006). A cross-sectional examination of age and physical activity on performance and event-related brain potentials in a task switching paradigm. *Int. J. Psychophysiol.* 59, 30–39. doi: 10.1016/j.ijpsycho.2005.04.009

Hillman, C. H., Pontifex, M. B., Castelli, D. M., Khan, N. A., Raine, L. B., Scudder, M. R., et al. (2014). Effects of the FITKids randomized controlled trial on executive control and brain function. *Pediatrics* 134, e1063–e1071. doi: 10.1542/peds.2013-3219

Huizinga, M., Dolan, C. V., and Van Der Molen, M. W. (2006). Age-related change in executive function: developmental trends and a latent variable analysis. *Neuropsychologia* 44, 2017–2036. doi: 10.1016/j.neuropsychologia.2006.01.010

Ishihara, T., Sugasawa, S., Matsuda, Y., and Mizuno, M. (2017). Improved executive functions in 6–12-year-old children following cognitively engaging tennis lessons. *J. Sports Sci.* 35, 2014–2020. doi: 10.1080/02640414.2016.1250939

Ishihara, T., Sugasawa, S., Matsuda, Y., and Mizuno, M. (2018). Relationship between sports experience and executive function in 6–12-year-old children: independence from physical fitness and moderation by gender. *Dev. Sci.* 21:e12555. doi: 10.1111/desc.12555

Kamijo, K., Pontifex, M. B., O'leary, K. C., Scudder, M. R., Wu, C. T., Castelli, D. M., et al. (2011). The effects of an afterschool physical activity program on working memory in preadolescent children. *Dev. Sci.* 14, 1046–1058. doi: 10.1111/j.1467-7687.2011.01054.x

Kao, S. C., Drollette, E. S., Scudder, M. R., Raine, L. B., Westfall, D. R., Pontifex, M. B., et al. (2017a). Aerobic fitness is associated with cognitive control strategy in preadolescent children. *J. Mot. Behav.* 49, 150–162. doi: 10.1080/00222895.2016.1161594

Kao, S. C., Westfall, D. R., Parks, A. C., Pontifex, M. B., and Hillman, C. H. (2017b). Muscular and aerobic fitness, working memory, and academic achievement in children. *Med. Sci. Sports Exerc.* 49, 500–508. doi: 10.1249/MSS.0000000000001132

Leger, L. A., Mercier, D., Gadoury, C., and Lambert, J. (1988). The multistage 20 metre shuttle run test for aerobic fitness. *J. Sports Sci.* 6, 93–101. doi: 10.1080/02640418808729800

Lippi, G., Mattiuzzi, C., and Sanchis-Gomar, F. (2020). Updated overview on interplay between physical exercise, neurotrophins, and cognitive function in humans. *J. Sport Health Sci.* 9, 74–81. doi: 10.1016/j.jshs.2019.07.012

Mahoney, C. (1992). 20-MST and PWC170 validity in non-Caucasian children in the UK. *Br. J. Sports Med.* 26, 45–47. doi: 10.1136/bjsm.26.1.45

Miyake, A., Friedman, N. P., Emerson, M. J., Witzki, A. H., Howerter, A., and Wager, T. D. (2000). The unity and diversity of executive functions and their contributions to complex "frontal lobe" tasks: a latent variable analysis. *Cogn. Psychol.* 41, 49–100. doi: 10.1006/cogp.1999.0734

Navon, D. (1977). Forest before trees: the precedence of global features in visual perception. *Cogn. Psychol.* 9, 353–383. doi: 10.1016/0010-0285(77)90012-3

Padilla-Moledo, C., Castro-Pinero, J., Ortega, F. B., Mora, J., Marquez, S., Sjostrom, M., et al. (2012). Positive health, cardiorespiratory fitness and fatness in children and adolescents. *Eur. J. Pub. Health* 22, 52–56. doi: 10.1093/eurpub/ckr005

Pindus, D. M., Drollette, E. S., Raine, L. B., Kao, S. C., Khan, N., Westfall, D. R., et al. (2019). Moving fast, thinking fast: the relations of physical activity levels and bouts to neuroelectric indices of inhibitory control in preadolescents. *J. Sport Health Sci.* 8, 301–314. doi: 10.1016/j.jshs.2019.02.003

Pontifex, M. B., Raine, L. B., Johnson, C. R., Chaddock, L., Voss, M. W., Cohen, N. J., et al. (2011). Cardiorespiratory fitness and the flexible modulation of cognitive control in preadolescent children. *J. Cogn. Neurosci.* 23, 1332–1345. doi: 10.1162/jocn.2010.21528

Raine, L. B., Kao, S. C., Pindus, D., Westfall, D. R., Shigeta, T. T., Logan, N. E., et al. (2018). A large-scale reanalysis of childhood fitness and inhibitory control. *J. Cogn. Enhanc.* 2, 170–192. doi: 10.1007/s41465-018-0070-7

Ruiz-Ariza, A., Grao-Cruces, A., De Loureiro, N. E. M., and Martínez-López, E. J. (2017). Influence of physical fitness on cognitive and academic performance in adolescents: a systematic review from 2005–2015. *Int. Rev. Sport Exerc. Psychol.* 10, 108–133. doi: 10.1080/1750984X.2016.1184699

Scudder, M. R., Drollette, E. S., Szabo-Reed, A. N., Lambourne, K., Fenton, C. I., Donnelly, J. E., et al. (2016). Tracking the relationship between children's aerobic fitness and cognitive control. *Health Psychol.* 35, 967–978. doi: 10.1037/hea0000343

Scudder, M. R., Lambourne, K., Drollette, E. S., Herrmann, S. D., Washburn, R. A., Donnelly, J. E., et al. (2014). Aerobic capacity and cognitive control in elementary school-age children. *Med. Sci. Sports Exerc.* 46, 1025–1035. doi: 10.1249/MSS.0000000000000199

Song, T. F., Chen, F. T., Chu, C. H., Chi, L., Liu, S., and Chang, Y. K. (2017). Obesity and cardiovascular fitness associated with inhibition of executive function: an ERP study. *J. Phys. Educ.* 50, 43–56. doi: 10.3966/102472972017035001004

Themanson, J. R., Hillman, C. H., and Curtin, J. J. (2006). Age and physical activity influences on action monitoring during task switching. *Neurobiol. Aging* 27, 1335–1345. doi: 10.1016/j.neurobiolaging.2005.07.002

Tomporowski, P. D., Mccullick, B., Pendleton, D. M., and Pesce, C. (2015). Exercise and children's cognition: the role of exercise characteristics and a place for metacognition. *J. Sport Health Sci.* 4, 47–55. doi: 10.1016/j.jshs.2014.09.003

Twisk, J. W., Kemper, H. C., and Van Mechelen, W. (2000). Tracking of activity and fitness and the relationship with cardiovascular disease risk factors. *Med. Sci. Sports Exerc.* 32, 1455–1461. doi: 10.1097/00005768-200008000-00014

Verburgh, L., Konigs, M., Scherder, E. J., and Oosterlaan, J. (2014). Physical exercise and executive functions in preadolescent children, adolescents and young adults: a meta-analysis. *Br. J. Sports Med.* 48, 973–979. doi: 10.1136/bjsports-2012-091441

Verstynen, T. F., Lynch, B., Miller, D. L., Voss, M. W., Prakash, R. S., Chaddock, L., et al. (2012). Caudate nucleus volume mediates the link between cardiorespiratory fitness and cognitive flexibility in older adults. *J. Aging Res.* 2012:939285. doi: 10.1155/2012/939285

Voss, M. W., Chaddock, L., Kim, J. S., Vanpatter, M., Pontifex, M. B., Raine, L. B., et al. (2011). Aerobic fitness is associated with greater efficiency of the network underlying cognitive control in preadolescent children. *Neuroscience* 199, 166–176. doi: 10.1016/j.neuroscience.2011.10.009

Welk, G. J., and Meredith, M. D. (2008). *Fitnessgram®/Activitygram® reference guide*. Dallas, TX: The Cooper Institute.

Westfall, D. R., Gejl, A. K., Tarp, J., Wedderkopp, N., Kramer, A. F., Hillman, C. H., et al. (2018). Associations between aerobic fitness and cognitive control in adolescents. *Front. Psychol.* 9:1298. doi: 10.3389/fpsyg.2018.01298

Yu, C. H., and Fang, C. L. (2002). Relationship between PACER test and maximal oxygen uptake. *J. Phys. Educ.*, 33–42.

Yu, D., and Li, X. (2000). Preliminary use of the children's depression inventory in China. *Chin. Ment. Health J.* 14, 225–227.

Zung, W. W. (1971). A rating instrument for anxiety disorders. *Psychosomatics* 12, 371–379. doi: 10.1016/S0033-3182(71)71479-0

The Experience of Sleep Problems and their Treatment in Young People at Ultra-High Risk of Psychosis

Felicity Waite [1,2,3]*, Jonathan Bradley [1,2,3], Eleanor Chadwick [1], Sarah Reeve [1], Jessica C. Bird [1,3] and Daniel Freeman [1,2,3]

[1] Department of Psychiatry, University of Oxford, Oxford, United Kingdom, [2] Sleep and Circadian Neuroscience Institute, University of Oxford, Oxford, United Kingdom, [3] Oxford Health NHS Foundation Trust, Oxford, United Kingdom

*Correspondence:
Felicity Waite
felicity.waite@psych.ox.ac.uk

We view sleep disruption as a contributory causal factor in the development of psychotic experiences. Clinical trials indicate that psychological interventions targeting insomnia result in improvements in both sleep and psychotic experiences. The aim of this study was to gain the perspective of young people at ultra-high risk of psychosis on their sleep problems and associated psychological treatment. Interviews were conducted with 11 patients, aged 15–22 years, at ultra-high risk of psychosis who had received a psychological sleep intervention. Responses were analyzed using thematic analysis. Disrupted sleep timing and a lack of routine were the characteristic hallmarks of participants' sleep problems. Sleep disturbance, psychological wellbeing, and functioning had a reciprocal relationship. There were negative expectations prior to therapy, however meaningful improvements occurred in sleep, mood, and functioning. The active implementation of therapy techniques was highlighted as important. These findings indicate that the treatment of sleep problems is highly valued and has a meaningful impact on wellbeing in young people at ultra-high risk of psychosis.

Keywords: at-risk-mental-state, ARMS, CBT, intervention, qualitative, schizophrenia

INTRODUCTION

Sleep disturbance has been identified as a potential causal factor in a range of severe mental health problems (1), including psychotic experiences (2, 3). In adolescents, sleep disruption and psychotic experiences overlap in genetic and environmental causes (4). Sleep problems are common during adolescence and have a significant impact on functioning (5, 6). In young people at high risk of serious mental health problems, sleep disturbance and circadian rhythm disruption are associated with poor outcomes and persistence of psychotic experiences (7–9). A consensus is emerging that "early treatment of sleep problems might reduce the risk of developing mental health problems and can be considered a helpful preventive strategy" (10). Sleep problems are important to be treated in their own right but also, if successfully reduced, have the potential for broad health benefits.

Cognitive Behavioral Therapy for insomnia (CBTi) has demonstrated treatment effects in adults and is the recommended first line treatment in clinical guidance (11). Importantly, improving sleep has been shown to result in additional benefits on mental health outcomes including anxiety, depression, psychotic experiences, and psychological wellbeing (12–14). However, CBTi has not been adequately tested in young people, either for its effects on sleep disturbance or potential wider effects on mental health outcomes.

Our group have conducted the first investigation of psychological interventions to treat sleep problems in young people at ultra-high risk of psychosis (15). In this case series, we found that the intervention was acceptable and may be associated with clinical benefits: following treatment, we found improvements in sleep, negative affect, and psychotic experiences. The effect sizes were large and the changes were maintained at the 1 month follow up.

Throughout the treatment development process, it is essential to incorporate the patient perspective on the phenomenology of the problem and the experience of receiving treatment. Previous qualitative studies have explored sleep problems in the absence of other mental health problems (16), or specifically in patients with sleep disturbance in the context of severe and enduring psychosis (17, 18). However, these accounts do not explore the specific developmental context of adolescence and early adulthood nor the novel target of addressing sleep as a preventative intervention for those at risk of serious mental health problems. The aim of the current study is to explore the experience of sleep problems and their treatment in young people at ultra-high risk of psychosis.

MATERIALS AND METHODS

Participants

Eleven patients, assessed as meeting criteria for ultra-high risk of psychosis based on attenuated psychosis [see (19) for full criteria] on the Comprehensive Assessment of At-Risk Mental States (CAARMS), took part in this qualitative study. All patients had recently received an adapted cognitive-behavioral intervention for sleep disturbance as part of a feasibility case series (15). Patients were identified based on their participation in the feasibility case series. All 11 patients approached consented to participate in the study. Participants were aged 15–22 years (mean = 18.27, $SD = 1.95$). Participants were employed full time ($n = 2$), part time ($n = 2$), or in education at school ($n = 4$) or university/higher education institution ($n = 3$). See **Table 1** for clinical and demographic details.

Intervention

The intervention is designed for young people to precisely target the key mechanisms which underpin sleep disturbance. It utilizes CBTi techniques, strategies to reduce hyperarousal, and circadian entrainment. The intervention is manualized in a modular format. All patients received 5 core modules:

(1) Psychoeducation, assessment, formulation, and goal setting,
(2) Establishing the environmental and lifestyle context for sleep (sleep hygiene),
(3) Stimulus control (re-associating bed with sleep) and strategies to reduce hyperarousal,
(4) Circadian entrainment (to regulate the timing of sleep by setting the sleep window, boosting zeitgebers for example meal and activity times, and increasing daytime activity),
(5) Relapse prevention.

Additional modules (addressing nightmares, voices, and motivation) were delivered according to the individualized

formulation of the young person's sleep problems. Further details of the intervention are reported by (15).

Procedure

Ethical approval for this study was obtained from an NHS research ethics committee. The interviews were conducted at participants' homes or at their local clinic. The interviews were conducted and audio-recorded by EC, a research worker, and transcribed verbatim. The mean duration of the interviews was 23 min ($SD = 10.8$) with a range of 10–47 min.

Semi-structured Interview

A semi-structured interview was developed by FW and JB. It focused on participants' experience of sleep problems and their treatment. The interview schedule was used flexibly, with additional verbal and non-verbal cues given to encourage elaboration. The participants' own vocabulary was used in relation to psychotic-like experiences. The interview schedule included four core questions: (1) "Can you tell me a bit about how things are for you at the moment?" (2) "Have there been any changes?" (3) "What was it like for you taking part in this therapy?" (4) "Is there anything that we haven't asked that you feel may have been important to your experience?" All participants focused their answers on sleep and its improvement therefore additional targeted prompts were not necessary.

Analysis

Thematic analysis is a widely used method for organizing, encoding, and identifying patterns within qualitative data. Analysis of this data set was carried out following the guidance provided by Braun and Clarke (22). First, the transcripts were read whilst listening to the corresponding audiotape to ensure accuracy and familiarity with the data set. Initial codes were then applied manually to segments of data and collated. Candidate themes were identified by organizing codes manually into theme-piles and a draft thematic map was created. Candidate themes were reviewed and data extracts within the themes were checked to ensure coherence within the theme and, if necessary, themes were adjusted. A candidate thematic map was developed and reviewed to ensure it represented the data set. The map was adjusted where necessary to better fit the data set. Finally, the accepted themes were refined and a thematic map finalized for the report (see **Figure 1**). Initial codes and candidate themes were developed by JB. SR and JCB (who were independent of the therapy and interviews) then joined JB in reviewing and refining the themes through an iterative process until a consensus was reached on the final thematic map.

RESULTS

Three main themes were developed, each with sub-themes. The finalized thematic map is shown in **Figure 1**. The first theme centered on the experience of sleep problems; the second and third themes related to the experience and utility of the intervention.

TABLE 1 | Demographic and clinical details of the participants, including data from baseline assessment.

Participant number	Gender	Ethnicity	Number of treatment sessions	Insomnia (ISI)	Wellbeing (WEMSBS)	Unusual thought content (CAARMS)[a]	Non-bizarre ideas (CAARMS)[a]	Perceptual abnormalities (CAARMS)[a]
1	Female	White	7	18	33	No	Yes	Yes
2	Male	Asian	8	18	26	Yes	Yes	Yes
3	Female	White	7	18	30	Yes	Yes	Yes
4	Male	White	8	16	36	Yes	Yes	Yes
5	Male	White	8	20	21	No	No	Yes
6	Male	White	7	14	43	Yes	No	Yes
7	Female	White	8	14	38	Yes	No	Yes
8	Female	White	7	19	38	Yes	No	No
9	Female	White	8	18	41	No	Yes	Yes
10	Male	White	8	15	49	Yes	Yes	Yes
11	Female	White	8	19	34	No	No	Yes

Insomnia Severity Index (20); WEMWBS, Warwick and Edinburgh Mental Wellbeing Scale (21); CAARMS, Comprehensive Assessment of At Risk Mental States (19); [a] Score of 3+ on CAARMS subscale.

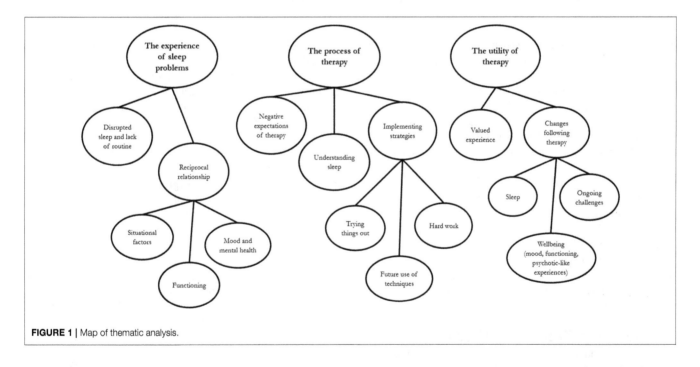

FIGURE 1 | Map of thematic analysis.

Theme 1: The Experience of Sleep Problems

Participants described a strong connection between disrupted sleep timing, lack of routine, and sleep problems. A reciprocal relationship between sleep disturbance, mental health problems, and daily functioning was also described.

"It Was a Lot of Just Feeling Tired at the Wrong Time" (P2) – Disrupted Sleep Timing and Lack of Routine

Participants frequently described their sleep problems as being characterized by delayed sleep phase and lack of routine: "I could be like staying up to about two, three o'clock in the morning and then going to sleep, and then I'd be napping for like an hour

or two during the day, and then staying up all night because I'd slept during the day" (P1). Circadian rhythm disruption included day-night reversal: "I was staying up until about like four in the morning, awake, and then I'd sleep until about three in the afternoon" (P7); "basically, I was nocturnal" (P5). This delayed sleep phase was reinforced by occupation in other activities at night: "when I went to bed, I'd sit there for ages, just on my phone or listening to music or something, without trying to sleep" (P6); "I'm ready to clock off, but my brain's not, and then I'm thinking through things" (P10); "I used to use my bed for work and things like that" (P11). Others identified a general lack of structure or predictability to their sleep patterns: "I just wouldn't really have a lot of structure to, kind of like, my sleeping pattern" (P9); "I never went to bed at the same time. I'd always be varying times, so that… Sometimes, it was even 3 or 4 h' difference" (P2).

"It Makes Everything a Lot Worse" (P2) – The Reciprocal Relationship

A complex interrelationship between sleep problems, mood, and functioning was described: "I would just sleep through the day and that like put a massive strain on like my social aspect and mood and my mental health, and I just think that it just turned my life like the other way around, so I would be up at night and then, because I was up at night, I wouldn't be up in the day and I wouldn't go out and see people because I was sleeping, and it was just… I just think it was very unhealthy" (P7). It was noted that poor sleep lowered mood, whether directly due to symptoms of insomnia, "not being able to get to sleep, not being able to stay asleep, and then being too tired during the day to actually do anything, which was really, really affecting my mood" (P3), or because of the social and functional consequences "It wasn't good for like my mental state, just like being by myself like not really talking to anyone" (P7). Others identified effects on anxiety, "it will pick up when I'm tired" (P11) or irritability "I'd just want to go home [and want to] go to sleep, and then, during the night, [I'd get] grouchy because I'd be like "I've got to go to sleep and I can't!'" (P1). Participants also noticed the reverse effect, where low mood or anxiety disrupted sleep: "I'm generally feeling quite low, so that very much affects my sleep" (P2); "I'm thinking about so much that I can't relax, and that will last for like a good hour or so every night" (P10). Participants described the reciprocal relationship between sleep disruption and everyday functioning: "I just would have been in bed, doing nothing, nothing like proactive or anything" (P7); "The more I get up in the night, the more I will just stay in bed for longer" (P1).

Other situational factors were identified in the onset or maintenance of sleep problems: "when I started, I wasn't sure whether we were moving out of the area, we were staying, we were kind of up in arms and everything" (P11); "like you have hormone cycles that affect your sleep as well" (P3); "I'm traveling 3 h a day by bus and things like that, which is always quite grueling" (P10).

Theme 2: The Process of Therapy

A theme was identified on the process of treating sleep problems. There were negative expectations of the therapy and its potential efficacy. Participants described two phases of therapy: understanding sleep and enacting strategies to improve it.

"I Didn't Think It Would Work at First" (P8) – Negative Expectations

There were a range of negative expectations regarding therapy. These included concerns about the potential efficacy of the treatment especially in the limited timeframe of the intervention, "when I started it, I was like no one can do this in 10 weeks" (P11); "I just thought…I'd give it a go and it probably wouldn't work" (P8). Particular intervention techniques also raised doubts: "some people [I'd heard in class], they were just like, oh, just sleep late, just, you know, like hot chocolate, or just count some sheep, and I was like, "Oh, it's just going to be that all over again!"

(P1); "little methods, such as like writing things down, and how actually when you think about that, that seems like it's not really going to do anything" (P2). There were negative expectations of the specific treatment model, "I never wanted to go through CBT, ever" (P11), and the style of therapy, "my worry was it was just going to be like some depressing…fest [laughing]" (P10). For some, there were concerns about judgment from the therapist: "I was scared that I was going to kind of be judged for like my sleep and stuff" (P9).

"I Learnt a Lot About Sleep" (P6) – Understanding Sleep

Participants' described the impact of monitoring sleep: "it sort of opened…well, not opened my eyes as such, but gave me a wider understanding of what actually affects my sleep" (P4); "with the sleep diaries, you thought more about your sleep and when you were sleeping" (P1); "I'd thought that maybe I wasn't getting enough sleep and I was tired during the day, but I didn't really think much more than that" (P6). For some participants, this revealed the scale of the sleep problem: "I didn't really realize how bad my sleep was" (P6); "I never would have imagined myself realizing how bad my sleep routine was" (P11). This detailed assessment allowed participants to gain awareness and knowledge regarding their sleep: "I learnt quite a lot, and it was just kind of… some obvious stuff, but it was said kind of in a way that I hadn't thought about before and I hadn't thought like how it was really affecting my sleep" (P9).

"I've Got a Repertoire of Skills Now" (P5) – Implementing Strategies

In developing a set of strategies to improve their sleep, participants identified a process of "trying things out": "I can just go, "Right, let's try this." If it doesn't work, I can try this. That works a bit. I can try this. That works even more" (P5); "It was just see what ones you can do, see what ones' work" (P9). This process included providing feedback on the strategy and then amending it or working on an alternative: "So, [my therapist] would give me a technique and then I'd come back and say 'This worked for me; this didn't work for me,' and then we could kind of work around that" (P3); "all the other things that we'd done before I felt they hadn't worked as much, and then we did the wind-down routine and it really helped" (P6).

Making changes to overcome sleep problems was challenging: "there's some days where I just want to like not move and just stay in my bed and just not do anything. It's hard to try and change that, to try and get myself motivated" (P7). Others identified specific strategies they found hard to implement: "the one thing I struggled with was kicking the laptop out my room, stop eating chocolate before bed, the amount of caffeine and things like that" (P11); "[my therapist] said if I get into bed and I don't fall asleep within 15 min, like to get back up again, like things like that, because once I'm in bed, I just don't really want to get back out of it [laughing]" (P8). For some, it was maintenance rather than implementation of strategies that was the challenge: "every time that I try to implement some of those strategies, there is a definite benefit, but it's quite difficult to maintain" (P10). However, implementation became easier over time: "it got easier, because I got used to what I was doing" (P8); "I've tried my best to sort of keep some of the routines... to where I don't even really think about them now" (P10).

A number of participants also talked about continuing to use strategies after completing therapy. Some were still actively using techniques and working toward their sleep goals: "I'm still doing the sleep plan" (P4); "I'm using a lot of the techniques that I was given through this" (P10); "I've been using the quarter-hour rule" (P9). Others reflected that they knew they could draw on the techniques if they needed to in the future and that the manual may be helpful for this: "if you begin to lose your sleep again, it's nice to be able to read back and remind yourself of what you did the last time" (P1); "if I sort of felt like I was having sleep problems again, I can go back to this and go, well, here's things I can use" (P5).

Theme 3: The Utility of Therapy

Participants gave extensive feedback on the intervention and its outcomes. The reciprocal relationship between sleep disturbance, mental health problems, and daily functioning identified within the earlier theme was reinforced by participants' observations of the benefits when their sleep improved.

"I've Quite Enjoyed the Therapy I've Had" (P1) – Valued Experience

The majority of participants gave positive feedback on the overall experience of the intervention. "it was very good, very interesting as well" (P4); "I thought it was really, really helpful" (P3). The specific style of treatment sessions, for example home visits, contact between sessions and active engagement were noted as important: "if I was struggling during the week, I could just email and say, "Having a tough day–any advice?" sort of thing. That was really helpful" (P3); "you guys are going sort of fairly... above and beyond sort of... even coming to my house" (P10); "It was kind of very friendly. It wasn't like scary" (P9). The collaborative approach to setting the focus of the session was valued: "[my therapist] was very happy to work through any other problems that I was having at the same time" (P3); "It is based, like, what you do during the day, diet, social life, like taking all that into account along with your sleep" (P1).

Limitations of the intervention were identified. This includes the treatment outcomes: "they don't solve the situation, too much, but it does still help" (P10); "I would say just the stuff about the nightmares. For some, it does work, but for others, it doesn't, which I can understand but I would like to try and find something that would work for all of them [nightmares]" (P4). There were contrasting responses to the booklets used in therapy: "the booklet things, did confuse me a bit" (P8), "the booklets were a little over-simplified" (P3). Some elements of the intervention delivered as standard in every session (the sleep diary, insomnia questionnaire, and session summary) were described as "repetitive" (P3 and P5) or "tedious" (P9).

"Everything has Kind of all Eased up at the Same Time" (P11) – Changes Following Therapy

Participants described improvements in their sleep following the intervention. Specific changes included: realigning circadian rhythm: "I do sleep now [laughing], at like the proper time" (P7), enhancing sleep quality: "waking up no more than twice during the night and not feeling concerned when I wake up" (P3), improving sleep onset latency and total sleep time: "I've been falling asleep quicker and spending more time asleep" (P4). Participants highlighted the importance of their sleep: "If I get a decent night's sleep, I'm not tired during the day" (P11); "I had originally thought it was more down to stuff during the day, like how much energy you had used on this activity or this activity or, again, what you're eating, but I didn't realize how much was down to sleep" (P10). Participants described issues related to their sleep which they would need to continue addressing such as increasing total sleep time "I'd say it's enough sleep, compared to where it was. It's still not a great amount" (P11) or hypnogogic/hypnopompic experiences "There was one thing that's still quite an issue [my therapist] called it hypnogogic experiences" (P10).

A number of participants directly linked improvements in their sleep to changes in mental health outcomes. The impact of improving sleep on mood and anxiety was reported: "I suffer from depression so it's not going to be high all the time, but because it's so highly linked with sleep, when I sleep better, I tend to have a better day" (P3); "the depression has been the big step. It's really eased. It's nowhere near where it used to be" (P11); "I find it also has helped my anxiety a lot. I'm able to cope with situations a lot better and kind of stay in control, which I think has come from me gaining control of my sleep a bit" (P9). Of particular relevance to a group at ultra-high risk of psychosis, improvements in sleep were also tentatively linked to improvements in sub-threshold psychotic symptoms: "since I've been sleeping better, my, visual things have like stopped" (P8); "I used to hear things quite a lot, like walking down the street, and that's subsided, almost entirely. I don't know whether that's a consequence of the work I've been doing with the psychologist [from the clinical team] or the sleep intervention or like a combination" (P3).

Mirroring the theme of the reciprocal relationship between sleep problems and broader difficulties, one participant summarized the wide effects of improving sleep: "the stuff that I normally wouldn't have done because I was physically just too tired, I find I can now have the energy to do that, those things, which makes me feel happy because I'm getting stuff done and I'm not getting stressed out at the fact that I haven't done the things that I wanted to do. It makes me feel happier" (P9). These concurrent changes in energy, mood, and functioning were noted both by individuals and their social networks: "my boyfriend in particular and then a couple of my friends, they've noticed how much more energy I have and how I've been contributing more in conversations" (P3).

DISCUSSION

To our knowledge, this is the first study to report the experience of sleep problems and their treatment in young people at ultra-high risk of psychosis. Participants gave vivid accounts about the importance of good sleep for mental health and day-to-day functioning. The experience of a delayed sleep phase, characteristic of the changes in sleep architecture in adolescence, was clearly described by participants. A lack of routine was identified as a key feature of sleep problems and thus a target for treatment.

A link between poor sleep, mood, sub-threshold psychotic experiences, and functioning was described. This is consistent with findings from a qualitative study of insomnia in adolescents with depression in which the negative impact of sleep disturbance on functioning was highlighted (23). The description of the reciprocal nature of sleep disturbance and mental health problems is aligned with accounts from patients with severe and enduring psychotic experiences (18). This supports theoretical models of sleep disruption as a causal factor in mental health problems (1). Importantly, in the current study, improvements in sleep were linked with improvements in mood, functioning, and psychological wellbeing.

Despite high treatment uptake rates there were negative expectations of therapy prior to taking part. It may be the case that some participants viewed their sleep problems as so intractable as to be untreatable – this attitude has been reported in patients with sleep problems in the context of established psychosis (17). Faulkner and Bee found that patients had pessimistic or neutral views on the likely effectiveness of "talking therapy" as an intervention for sleep problems, although individual components (e.g., stimulus control, increasing daytime activity) were seen as far more likely to be effective. What was notable, in the current study, was the spirit of experimentation, a willingness to try the intervention in spite of doubts about its efficacy. "Willingness to change" has been identified as a theme in other qualitative accounts of young people with sleep problems (24). It is unclear whether this disparity between expectation and engagement is specific to this age group (that is, whether adolescents are more willing to try strategies than other age groups) or whether it merely reflects the attitudes of those who express interest in research and so might be more willing to try the intervention in spite of reservations. Nevertheless, this finding may have specific implications for how this therapy may best be advertised and delivered in this group.

Two distinct phases of treatment were described: improving understanding of sleep and taking action to improve sleep. Prior to implementing new techniques, participants described the process of improving their understanding of sleep. Increasing knowledge of both good-quality and poor-quality sleep has been highlighted as an important target for identifying and treating sleep problems in adolescents (25). The current study indicates that young people at ultra-high risk of psychosis are keen to learn about sleep and value this information. In particular, participants described monitoring sleep as a route to increasing understanding. However, a limitation of the feasibility case series was the low rates of sleep diary completion (15). This reluctance to complete sleep diaries is consistent with findings from other studies, for example adolescents with depression identified sleep diaries as a barrier to treatment, regardless of the mode of delivery (23). Future research will need to addresses these discrepancies between desire to increase knowledge and the current tools for

monitoring sleep to ensure treatment is both engaging and effective.

Previous research has described how young people at ultra-high risk of psychosis have concerns regarding discussing unusual experiences and thus delayed help seeking (26). It is possible that sleep problems carry less stigma than other mental health problems. In the current study, participants described gaining control of sleep as a route to increasing control of their mental health and overall wellbeing. This may indicate that sleep problems could be an accessible first treatment target. This is an important consideration in the context of the current clinical guidance to improve timely access to services for early psychosis (27).

There were limitations to the present study. This was a selected sample in the context of a feasibility case series. Therefore, there is potential bias in their experiences. For example, themes identified on the experience of sleep problems may reflect the content of the intervention. The most likely bias is in the enthusiasm for the intervention. However, the findings of the present study fit both with the established evidence base in adults that psychological treatments for sleep problems are effective and the emerging literature indicating wider benefits to mental health. Clearly the findings of this small qualitative study are not generalizable. For example, the current study is not intended to reflect the experiences of sleep problems in early adolescence: given the changing developmental markers in sleep architecture, social demands, and cognitive development the current findings are limited to the late adolescent period (the peak age of onset for psychotic experiences). However, the aim of this study was to use first person accounts to inform theoretical and clinical developments. We believe the findings presented provide a resource to achieve this aim.

CONCLUSION

This study highlights the importance of addressing sleep problems in young people at ultra-high risk of psychosis, and provides insight on the motivations and reservations they have toward treatment. A number of key themes emerged related to treatment: negative expectations prior to treatment, two phases of therapy (understanding and action), and the importance of treatment style. These can be used to further develop the treatment and to optimize engagement. The findings support the promise of sleep interventions in young people, as reported in the feasibility study (15). Namely that, following therapy, participants reported improvements in their sleep, psychological wellbeing, and everyday functioning. The findings suggest that sleep interventions in this group should be given higher clinical and research priority.

ETHICS STATEMENT

This study was carried out in accordance with the recommendations of the Ethical Principles of Psychologists and Code of Conduct (28). All subjects gave written informed consent in accordance with the Declaration of Helsinki. The protocol was approved by the National Health Service South Central–Oxford A Research Ethics Committee (15/SC/0378).

AUTHOR CONTRIBUTIONS

FW and JB developed the interview for data collection. JB and EC recruited participants for the study. JB provided the intervention. FW provided clinical supervision. EC conducted the interviews for data collection. JB, SR, and JCB conducted the analysis. DF and FW provided overall supervision. FW took the main responsibility for drafting of the manuscript. All authors contributed to manuscript revision, read and approved the submitted version.

ACKNOWLEDGMENTS

We are very grateful to the patients who participated in the interviews.

REFERENCES

Harvey AG. A transdiagnostic approach to treating sleep disturbance in psychiatric disorders. *Cogn Behav Ther.* (2009) 38(Suppl. 1):35–42. doi: 10.1080/16506070903033825

Reeve S, Sheaves B, Freeman D. The role of sleep dysfunction in the occurrence of delusions and hallucinations: a systematic review. *Clin Psychol Rev.* (2015) 42:96–115. doi: 10.1016/j.cpr.2015. 09.001

Sheaves B, Bebbington PE, Goodwin GM, Harrison PJ, Espie CA, Foster RG, et al. Insomnia and hallucinations in the general population: findings from the 2000 and 2007 British Psychiatric Morbidity Surveys. *Psychiatry Res.* (2016) 241:141–46. doi: 10.1016/j.psychres.2016. 03.055

Taylor MJ, Gregory AM, Freeman D, Ronald A. Do sleep disturbances and psychotic-like experiences in adolescence share genetic and environmental influences? *J Abnorm Psychol.* (2015) 124:674–84. doi: 10.1037/abn00 00057

Johnson EO, Roth T, Schultz L, Breslau N. Epidemiology of DSM- IV insomnia in adolescence: lifetime prevalence, chronicity, and an emergent gender difference. *Pediatrics* (2006) 117:e247. doi: 10.1542/peds.200 4-2629

Shochat T, Cohen-Zion M, Tzischinsky O. Functional consequences of inadequate sleep in adolescents: a systematic review. *Sleep Med Rev.* (2014) 18:75–87. doi: 10.1016/j.smrv.2013.03.005

Lunsford-Avery JR, Orr JM, Gupta T, Pelletier-Baldelli A, Dean DJ, Smith Watts AK, et al. Sleep dysfunction and thalamic abnormalities in adolescents at ultra high-risk for psychosis. *Schizophr Res.* (2013) 151:148–53. doi: 10.1016/j.schres.2013. 09.015

Lunsford-Avery JR, Gonçalves Bda SB, Brietzke E, Bressan RA, Gadelha A, Auerbach RP, et al. Adolescents at clinical-high risk for psychosis: circadian rhythm disturbances predict worsened prognosis at 1-year follow-up. *Schizophr Res.* (2017) 189:37–42. doi: 10.1016/j.schres.2017. 01.051

Poe SL, Brucato G, Bruno N, Arndt LY, Ben-David S, Gill KE, et al. Sleep disturbances in individuals at clinical high risk for psychosis. *Psychiatry Res.* (2017) 249:240–3. doi: 10.1016/j.psychres.2016. 12.029

Blake MJ, Sheeber LB, Youssef GJ, Raniti MB, Allen NB. Systematic review and meta-analysis of adolescent cognitive–behavioral sleep interventions. *Clin Child Fam Psychol Rev.* (2017) 20:227–49. doi: 10.1007/s10567-017- 0234-5

National Institute for Health and Care Excellence. *Managing Long Term Insomnia (>4 weeks): NICE Clinical Knowledge Summary* (2015).

Freeman D, Waite F, Startup H, Myers E, Lister R, McInerney J, et al. Efficacy of cognitive behavioural therapy for sleep improvement in patients with persistent delusions and hallucinations (BEST): a prospective, assessor-blind, randomised controlled pilot trial. *Lancet Psychiatry* (2015) 2:975–83. doi: 10.1016/S2215-0366(15) 00314-4

Freeman D, Sheaves B, Goodwin GM, Yu LM, Nickless A, Harrison PJ, et al. The effects of improving sleep on mental health (OASIS): a randomised controlled trial with mediation analysis. *Lancet Psychiatry* (2017) 4:749–58. doi: 10.1016/ S2215-0366(17)30328-0

Sheaves B, Freeman D, Isham L, McInerney J, Nickless A, Yu LM, et al. Stabilising sleep for patients admitted at acute crisis to a psychiatric hospital (OWLS): an assessor-blind, pilot randomised controlled trial. *Psychol Med.* (2017) 48:1–11. doi: 10.1017/S00332917170 03191

Bradley J, Freeman D, Chadwick E, Harvey AG, Mullins B, Johns L, et al. Treating sleep problems in young people at ultra-high risk of psychosis: a feasibility case series. *Behav Cogn Psychother.* (2018) 46:276–91. doi: 10.1017/ S1352465817000601

Cheung JMY, Bartlett DJ, Armour CL, Saini B. The insomnia patient perspective, a narrative review. *Behav Sleep Med.* (2013) 11:369–89. doi: 10.1080/15402002.2012.694382

Faulkner S, Bee P. Experiences, perspectives and priorities of people with schizophrenia spectrum disorders regarding sleep disturbance and its treatment: a qualitative study. *BMC Psychiatry* (2017) 17:1–17. doi: 10.1186/s12888-017-1329-8

Waite F, Evans N, Myers E, Startup H, Lister R, Harvey AG, et al. The patient experience of sleep problems and their treatment in the context of current delusions and hallucinations. *Psychol Psychother Theory Res Pract.* (2016) 89:181–93. doi: 10.1111/papt. 12073

Yung AR, Yuen HP, McGorry PD, Phillips LJ, Kelly D, Dell'Olio M, et al. Mapping the onset of psychosis: the comprehensive assessment of at-risk mental states. *Aust N Z J Psychiatry* (2005) 39:964–71. doi: 10.1111/j.1440-1614.2005.01714.x

Bastien CH, Vallières A, Morin CM. Validation of the insomnia severity index as an outcome measure for insomnia research. *Sleep Med.* (2001) 2:297–307. doi: 10.1016/S1389-9457(00)00065-4

Tennant R, Hiller L, Fishwick R, Platt S, Joseph S, Weich S, et al. The Warwick-Edinburgh Mental Well-being Scale (WEMWBS): development and UK validation. Health Qual Life Outcomes (2007) 5:63. doi: 10.1186/1477-7525-5-63

Braun V, Clarke V. Using thematic analysis in psychology. *Qual Res Psychol.* (2006) 3:77–101. doi: 10.1191/1478088706q p063oa

Conroy DA, Czopp AM, Dore-Stites D, Dopp RR, Armitage R, Hoban TF, et al. A pilot study on adolescents with depression and insomnia: qualitative findings from focus groups. *Behav Sleep Med.* (2017) 15:22–38. doi: 10.1080/15402002.2015.10 65412

Paterson JL, Reynolds AC, Duncan M, Vandelanotte C, Ferguson SA. Barriers and enablers to modifying sleep behavior in adolescents and young adults: a qualitative investigation. *Behav Sleep Med.* (2017) doi: 10.1080/15402002.2016.1266489. [Epub ahead of print].

Orzech KM. A qualitative exploration of adolescent perceptions of healthy sleep in Tucson, Arizona, USA. *Soc Sci Med.* (2013) 79:109–16. doi: 10.1016/j. socscimed.2012.05.001

Byrne R, Morrison AP. Young people at risk of psychosis: a user- led exploration of interpersonal relationships and communication of psychological difficulties. *Early Interv Psychiatry* (2010) 4:162–8. doi: 10.1111/j.1751-7893.2010.00171.x

NHS England the National Collaborating Centre for Mental Health and National Institute for Health and Care Excellence. *Implementing the Early Intervention in Psychosis Access and Waiting Time Standard: Guidance* (2016). p. 57.

American Psychological Association (APA). *Ethical Principles of Psychologists and Code of Conduct (Including 2010 and 2016 Amendments)*. Washington, DC: APA (2017).

19

Dual-Task Interference in a Simulated Driving Environment: Serial or Parallel Processing?

Mojtaba Abbas-Zadeh[1]*, Gholam-Ali Hossein-Zadeh[1,2] and Maryam Vaziri-Pashkam[3]

[1]School of Cognitive Sciences, Institute for Research in Fundamental Sciences (IPM), Tehran, Iran, [2]School of Electrical and Computer Engineering, College of Engineering, University of Tehran, Tehran, Iran, [3]Laboratory of Brain and Cognition, National Institute of Mental Health, Bethesda, MD, United States

*Correspondence:
Mojtaba Abbas-Zadeh
mabbaszadeh@ipm.ir

When humans are required to perform two or more tasks concurrently, their performance declines as the tasks get closer together in time. Here, we investigated the mechanisms of this cognitive performance decline using a dual-task paradigm in a simulated driving environment, and using drift-diffusion modeling, examined if the two tasks are processed in a serial or a parallel manner. Participants performed a lane change task, along with an image discrimination task. We systematically varied the time difference between the onset of the two tasks (Stimulus Onset Asynchrony, SOA) and measured its effect on the amount of dual-task interference. Results showed that the reaction times (RTs) of the two tasks in the dual-task condition were higher than those in the single-task condition. SOA influenced the RTs of both tasks when they were presented second and the RTs of the image discrimination task when it was presented first. Results of drift-diffusion modeling indicated that dual-task performance affects both the rate of evidence accumulation and the delays outside the evidence accumulation period. These results suggest that a hybrid model containing features of both parallel and serial processing best accounts for the results. Next, manipulating the predictability of the order of the two tasks, we showed that in unpredictable conditions, the order of the response to the two tasks changes, causing attenuation in the effect of SOA. Together, our findings suggest higher-level executive functions are involved in managing the resources and controlling the processing of the tasks during dual-task performance in naturalistic settings.

Keywords: dual-task interference, driving, drift diffusion model, task order predictability, dual-task theories

INTRODUCTION

Humans have limited cognitive capacity. They can only attend to a few items in the scene (Pylyshyn and Storm, 1988; Huang et al., 2007), maintain and manipulate a few items in working memory (Kane and Engle, 2000; Engle, 2002), have limits in the amount of information they can store in short and long term memory (Anderson et al., 1996), and their performance is hindered when they are asked to handle multiple demands in close temporal proximity (Pashler, 1994a). One of the manifestations of this limited capacity is dual-task interference. When performing two tasks concurrently, reaction times increase and accuracies decrease as the two tasks get close together in time (Pashler and Johnston, 1989). During driving, this phenomenon manifests itself in performance declines when drivers attempt to drive and perform a secondary task simultaneously (Horrey and Wickens, 2004; Blanco et al., 2006; Strayer et al., 2017). Despite the importance of dual-task interference in everyday tasks such as driving and its potentially fatal consequences (Bakhit et al., 2018), most studies of dual-task interference have used artificial paradigms to investigate the underlying mechanisms of dual-task interference (Sigman and Dehaene, 2005, 2008; Miller et al., 2009). In this study, taking the artificial designs one step closer to the natural task of driving, we aim to examine the underlying mechanisms of dual-task interference in a simulated driving environment.

To systematically investigate dual-task interference in artificial tasks (Pashler and Johnston, 1989; Pashler, 1994a), the time interval between the onsets of the first and the second stimulus (henceforth referred to as the Stimulus Onset Asynchrony or SOA) has been varied. It has been shown that when the SOA decreases, the RTs increase and the accuracies decrease. This performance decline as a function of SOA has been used as a measure of dual-task interference. A couple of studies using a simulated driving environment have shown similar effects of SOA on dual-task interference (Levy et al., 2006; Hibberd et al., 2013). These studies provide evidence for dual-task interference in driving, but they do not shed light on its underlying mechanisms.

Several theories have been proposed to explain the dual-task interference; the two most influential of them are the "bottleneck theory" and the "central capacity sharing theory." According to the bottleneck theory, dual-task interference appears when the two tasks rely on the same processor. In this theory, this processor at any time can only be occupied by one of the two tasks (Pashler, 1994a). When the first task is being processed, the second task must wait for the first one to be finished so that the processor is released. Dividing each task into three stages of (1) perceptual, (2) response selection or decision, and (3) motor execution, the bottleneck theory proposes that the stimulus perception and the motor execution stages could be performed in parallel, while the decision stage is the bottleneck that could only process the two tasks in a serial manner (McCann and Johnston, 1992; Sigman and Dehaene, 2008). Many studies have proposed evidence in favor of the bottleneck theory (Pashler and Johnston, 1989; Pashler, 1994b; Ruthruff et al., 2001; Sigman and Dehaene, 2005). This theory predicts that the dual-task interference only affects the RT of the second task and has no effect on the response of the first task because the first task is processed by the decision stage first and postpones the processing of the second task (Pashler, 1994a).

On the other hand, the central capacity-sharing theory suggests that the limitation in the processing capacity is the main reason for dual-task interference. Unlike the bottleneck theory that assumes serial processing of the two tasks, this theory suggests that in the dual-task conditions, all three stages of perceptual, decision, and motor execution could process the two tasks in parallel (Posner and Boies, 1971; Kahneman, 1973; McLeod, 1977; Duncan, 1980). In this theory, only the decision process is limited in capacity, while there are no resource limitations for the perceptual and motor execution stages (Tombu and Jolicoeur, 2003). This theory predicts that dual-task interference affects the RT of both the first and the second tasks and that the size of this reaction time change depends on the size of the sharing portion. Several studies have provided evidence in favor of the capacity sharing theory. Some have observed a robust effect of dual-task interference on the RT of both the first and the second tasks (Carrier and Pashler, 1995; Tombu and Jolicoeur, 2002; Oriet et al., 2005; Sigman and Dehaene, 2006; Zylberberg et al., 2012).

Recently, Zylberberg et al. (2012) proposed a hybrid model for dual-task processing. They suggested that the decision stage of the two tasks is processed in parallel, while there exists a bottleneck in mapping the decision to the motor responses (**Figure 1D**). Zylberberg et al. (2012) used drift diffusion model (DDM) in a dual-task paradigm and showed that the drift rate and the post-decision time increase for the second task during dual-task interference. To do this, they used two simple artificial tasks. Currently, it is not clear whether these findings in artificial tasks could be generalized to real-world tasks such as driving. In the current study, we aimed to extend these findings to a naturalistic setting and investigate the nature of dual-task interference in our simulated driving environment. To do this, we explored the effect of SOA on driving performance and used a DDM to investigate if the driving and the secondary task are performed serially (as proposed by the central bottleneck theory) or in parallel (as proposed by the capacity sharing theory) or if a hybrid model best accounts for the results (as proposed by the Zylberberg et al., 2012).

A DDM could be used as a framework to model the different processing stages of two-choice tasks (Ratcliff, 1978, 2015; Ratcliff and Rouder, 1998). This model assumes that during a two-choice decision task, evidence accumulates gradually to reach one of two decision thresholds corresponding to the two choices. The perceptual, motor, and other non-decision related stages of task processing are modeled as the non-decision time in the DDM (henceforth referred to as non-decision time; **Figure 1**). The predictions of the bottleneck and the capacity sharing theories can be restated within the framework of the DDM. The bottleneck theory assumes that the decision stage of the two tasks is processed separately and sequentially and that at shorter SOAs, the processing of the decision stage of the second task is delayed until the decision stage of the first task is completed (**Figure 1B**). In other words, this theory predicts that the rate of evidence accumulation (drift rate) for the two tasks is constant across SOAs, while there is a delay before the start of evidence accumulation for the second task that translates to increased non-decision time at shorter SOAs. On the other hand, the capacity sharing theory suggests that the decision process for the two tasks are performed concurrently, and the resources for decision making are shared between the two tasks (**Figure 1C**). Therefore, this theory predicts a decrease in the rate of evidence accumulation of the two tasks at shorter SOAs and a constant non-decision time across SOAs. A hybrid account will have signatures of both bottleneck and capacity sharing theories, showing a decrease in the rate of evidence accumulation as well as an increased non-decision time.

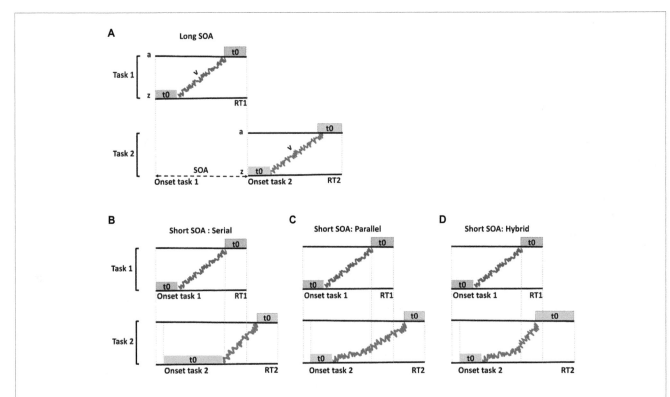

FIGURE 1 | A schematic of drift-diffusion modeling based on the predictions of the bottleneck, capacity sharing theories and a recent hybrid model proposed by Zylbelberg et al. (2012). V denotes the noisy evidence accumulation process (drift rate) in the decision stage of the two tasks, $t0$ denotes the non-decision time and a and z denote the decision threshold and the initial state of the decision processes, respectively. Here, only one threshold is shown, but there are two decision thresholds in the drift-diffusion model corresponding to the two alternatives of the two-choice tasks. **(A)** The processing stages of Task 1 (top) and Task 2 (bottom) in the long SOA condition. In the long SOA, the two tasks are processed independently, and there is no interference between the two tasks. **(B)** The processing stages of task 1 and task 2 in the short SOA based on the predictions of the bottleneck theory that suggests the evidence accumulation for Task 2 does not begin until that for Task 1 is complete. **(C)** The processing stages of Task 1 and Task 2 in the short SOA condition based on the predictions of the capacity sharing theory that suggests that the evidence accumulation for the two tasks happens simultaneously and in parallel but at slower rates compared to the long SOA conditions. **(D)** The processing stages of Task 1 and Task 2 in the short SOA condition based on the predictions of the hybrid model that suggests that the evidence accumulation for the two tasks happens simultaneously and in parallel but at slower rates and, in addition, a delay exists in the mapping of the decision to motor response in the short compared to the long SOA conditions.

Evidence for or against dual-task theories is mostly gathered through simple tasks. Typical examples include visual discrimination tasks (e.g., object, color, and orientation discrimination) or tone discrimination tasks (e.g., high pitch vs. low pitch). The predictions of these theories have not been sufficiently tested in more naturalistic, real-world conditions. Several differences exist between artificial tasks and real-world tasks such as driving. Examples of these include: (1) in the real-world driving situations, people often need to perform two or more motor movements sequentially to complete each driving task. For example, when the driver decides to turn right/left, he/she should rotate the wheel to turn the car to the correct location, and after a certain amount of time, turn the wheel in the opposite direction to straighten the car. This constraint may increase the demands of the driving task compared to other artificial tasks that usually require a single motor movement. (2) In the real-world driving events, time is a critical factor, and slow RTs might cause accidents. Most driving tasks have an intrinsic time limitation, while most artificial tasks do not put any constraints on the participant's response times. This intrinsic time limitation may alter behavior

in a natural setting compared to an artificial one. (3) In artificial dual-task experiments, none of the two tasks are intrinsically more important than the other one. In a dual-task paradigm, the main task is often the driving task, and the secondary task has less priority. This priority may also affect behavior in a dual-task paradigm. (4) The driving environment is a continuous environment that includes distracting elements in the scene, including the road and roadside elements, the movement in the scene caused by the interaction of the participant with the car, the car dashboard, odometer, and other car elements. These elements could alter behavior by either distracting the participants or facilitating the responses by providing an immersive experience. Most artificial tasks are discrete and contain isolated stimuli and a display that is not contingent upon the participants' responses. Considering these factors, in the current study, we designed a dual-task paradigm in a simulated driving environment to get one step closer to the real-world dual-task conditions. Although we are aware our paradigm does not replicate real-world driving, we think it has some of the main parameters of a lane change task in a driving situation. The first goal of this study is to measure the effect of SOA on the amount of dual-task interference in this paradigm and to examine the validity of dual-task theories in more naturalistic settings.

In most dual-task studies, the order of the presentation of the tasks has been kept fixed and predictable, and participants were explicitly instructed to perform the two tasks according to the order of the presentation. In contrast, task order is often random and unpredictable in real-world situations. One open question is whether the order of the response to the two tasks during driving is specified based on a first-come, first-served basis in which the order of the presentation determines the order of response, or a higher-order control mechanism determines this order.

In dual-task studies with simple designs (Sigman and Dehaene, 2005) in which the presentation order of the tasks is kept constant, and participants are often instructed to respond to the two tasks based on the presentation order, the first-come, first-served principle usually applies. However, recent studies which have made the order of the presentation of the two tasks unpredictable and have imposed no constraints for responding to the tasks according to the presentation order, support a higher-order control mechanism for managing the timing of the response to the two tasks (Sigman and Dehaene, 2006; Szameitat et al., 2006; Huestegge and Koch, 2010; Fernández et al., 2011; Leonhard, 2011). These studies have shown that increasing the perceptual difficulty of one of the tasks, such as degrading the stimulus, causes that task to be performed second (Sigman and Dehaene, 2006; Strobach et al., 2018; but see also Leonhard, 2011 for evidence on the contrary). Similarly, an increase in the difficulty of the decision (Fernández et al., 2011) or motor execution stages (Ruiz Fernández et al., 2013), causes participants to respond to that task later. These studies suggest that participants optimize the response order to decrease the total reaction time in dual-task conditions (Miller et al., 2009). All these studies have used simple artificial tasks rather than real-world naturalistic ones. It is still an open question if a higher-order control mechanism contributes to the response order in a naturalistic setting, such as a simulated driving environment. The second goal of this study was to measure the effect of task order predictability (OP) on the responses of the two tasks and the parameters of the DDM in naturalistic settings.

In sum, we aimed to investigate the underlying mechanism of dual-task interference in a simulated driving environment using drift-diffusion modeling. The paradigm consisted of a lane change task and an image discrimination task. We investigated the effect of SOA and the predictability of the order of the two tasks on the amount of dual-task interference. Using a DDM, we investigated whether the two tasks are processed in parallel or serially and how the predictability of the order of the two tasks influenced their processing. If the decision stages of the two tasks are processed serially, as predicted by the bottleneck theory, we expect the drift rate of the second task to be independent of SOA, and the non-decision time of the second task to be dependent on SOA. In contrast, if the decision stages of the two tasks are processed in parallel according to the predictions of the capacity sharing theory, we expect the drift rate of the second task to change and the non-decision time of the second task to not change across SOAs. Finally, if the decision stages of two tasks are processed in parallel, but there is some bottleneck in the process, as predicted by the hybrid model, we expect the drift rate and non-decision time of the second task to be dependent on SOA. These results will shed light on the underlying mechanisms of dual-task interference in more naturalistic settings.

MATERIALS AND METHODS

Participants
Twenty healthy, right-handed adults (11 females), aged 20–30, participated in the study. All participants had normal or corrected to normal vision. Additionally, all participants were not expert video game players, as defined by having less than 2 h of video-game usage per month in the past 2 years. All participants gave informed consent and were compensated for their participation.

Stimuli and Procedure
The dual-task paradigm consisted of a lane change driving task and an image discrimination task. The driving environment was designed in the Unity 3D game engine. Participants sat at a distance of 50 cm from a 22″ LG monitor with a refresh rate of 60 Hz and a resolution of 1,920 × 1,080 and responded to the tasks using a computer keyboard.

The driving environment consisted of a three-lane, desert road, without left/right turns or inclining/declining hills. Driving stimuli, composed of two rows of traffic cones (three cones in each row; **Figure 2A**), were presented on the two sides of one of the lanes in each trial, and the participants had to immediately redirect the car to the lane with the cones and pass through the cones. The space between the two rows of cones was such that the car could easily pass through them without collision. The cones were always presented in the lanes immediately to the left or immediately to the right of the car's lane so that the participants had to change only one lane per trial. The lane change was done gradually: the participant had to hold the corresponding key to direct the car in between the two rows of cones, and then release the key when the car was situated correctly. Any early or late key press or release would cause a collision with the cones and a performance loss in that trial. The fixation cross was jittered for 100 ms to provide online feedback in case of a collision with the traffic cones. The participants were instructed not to change lane before the cones appeared. Trials in which participants changed lane before the presentation of the cones were considered false and removed from the analysis. Using this method, we could divide a continuous driving task into individual trials with predetermined onset and ends. At the beginning of the block, participants speeded up to 80 km/h using the "up" arrow key with the middle finger of the right hand. During the block, the speed was kept constant, and the lane change was performed by pressing the right and left arrow with the middle and index fingers of their right hand, respectively. For the image discrimination task, a single image of either a scene

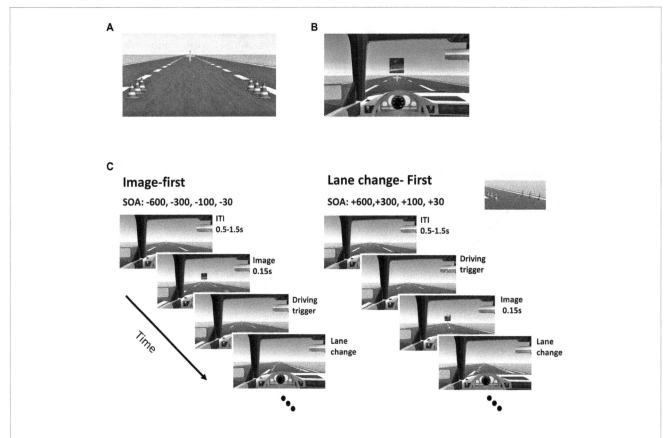

FIGURE 2 | Dual-task paradigm. **(A)** A sample display showing the driving stimulus consisting of two rows of traffic cones in the middle driving lane. The cones were randomly presented in each lane, and participants had to drive through them without collision. **(B)** A sample display showing an image discrimination presented above the fixation point. Participants determined if the image was a face or a scene. **(C)** The sequence of events for a sample trial in which the image task was presented first (left), and another in which the driving task was presented first (right). The inter-trial interval (ITI) varied between 0.5 and 1.5 s. The image lasted for 150 ms, and the cones were presented 30, 100, 300, or 600 before or after the image. Participants had to perform a lane change immediately after the appearance of the cones, and an image discrimination task immediately after the presentation of the image.

or a face was presented for 150 milliseconds centered at 2° eccentricity above the fixation cross (**Figure 2B**). The size of the image was 2.5° of visual angle. Participants pressed the "*x*" and "*z*" keys on the computer keyboard with the middle and index fingers of their left hand to determine whether the image was a face or a scene, respectively. The images were pseudo-randomly selected from a set of 864 images of scenes and 435 images of faces. We selected only natural scenes and neutral faces. If participants responded incorrectly, the green fixation cross turned red, and if they responded late, it turned orange for 100 ms. The length of each trial was 3 s, and the inter-trial interval varied randomly from 0.5 to 1.5 s. For the first trial in each block, the onset of the trial was set to 2 s after the beginning of the block. The end of the trial was set to when the rear end of the car reached the end of the set of traffic cones.

The experiment consisted of two different conditions: (1) "Predictable" task order condition, and (2) "Unpredictable" task order condition. In two experimental conditions, the two tasks were presented with eight possible SOAs (−600, −300, −100, −30, +30, +100, +300 and +600 ms). In the negative SOAs, the image discrimination was presented first (image-first,

Figure 2C), and in the positive SOAs, the lane change was presented first (lane change-first, **Figure 2C**). In the Predictable conditions, the order of the presentation was fixed, so that in two of the four blocks, the driving task was presented first, and in the other two, the image discrimination task was presented first. In the Unpredictable condition, the order of the presentation of the two tasks was not predictable in each trial. Trials with driving as the first task were interleaved with trials with the image discrimination as the first task. Before the start of each block, participants were informed about the type of the block.

In addition to the dual-task conditions, participants performed two single-task conditions: (1) single driving task and (2) single image discrimination task. In the single-task conditions, both the lane change and image stimuli were presented, but the participant only responded to one of them, ignoring the other. In the single image discrimination condition, the driving was on autopilot, and participants only responded to the images. In the single lane change condition, participants performed the lane change task and ignored the images.

Participants were told to focus on the fixation cross at the center of the page and respond to each task as fast as possible.

At the end of each block, participants were informed about their performance on each task as well as their total performance. The performance in the driving task was calculated as the percentage of trials in which the participant passed through the cones without collision. The performance in the image discrimination task was calculated as the percentage of correct identifications.

Participants completed four blocks of 64 trials for each dual-task condition and two blocks of 32 trials for each single-task condition. There was a 1-min interval between blocks and a 5-min break after finishing all the blocks in each condition. The order of the blocks was counterbalanced across participants.

Before performing the main experiment, all participants performed a block of 20 trials for every single-task. If their accuracy was 80% or higher, they proceeded to the main experimental blocks. Otherwise, they repeated blocks of 40 trials for each task until they reached 80% accuracy. After the single-task training, participants performed the dual-task training block. The dual-task training was similar to the single-task training block, with the difference that if after 20 trials, the dual-task performance did not reach the 75% threshold, the training was repeated with blocks of 50 trials.

Drift Diffusion Model Fitting

To investigate if the two tasks were processed serially, or in parallel we used a DDM in which each trial was modeled as a combination of a non-decision time and a decision time consisting of a random drift towards decision bound (**Figure 1**). Model parameters consisted of: (1) parameter z denoting the starting point of the decision process, (2) parameter a denoting the decision threshold, (3) parameter v representing the speed of information accumulation or drift rate, and (4) parameter $t0$ denoting the non-decision time pertaining to the combination of all other times in the trial excluding the drift-diffusion time. The DDM was implemented in the current study, by fitting the parameters z, a, v, and $t0$. We modified the DDM, so that z and a were independent of SOA, and v and $t0$ were dependent on SOA. Therefore, in the modified DDM, four values were fit for the parameter v and four values for the parameter $t0$ corresponding to the four SOAs, one value for the parameter a and one value for the parameter z across all SOAs.

We used the Fast-dm package, developed by Voss and Voss (2007), for model fitting. Fast-dm is a package for fast drift-diffusion modeling. This package uses a partial differential equation method and a simplex routine to obtain the parameters of the DDM, and uses the calculated cumulative density function (CDF) of the predicted RTs to estimate the goodness of fit using a Kolmogorov-Smirnov (KS) function (Voss and Voss, 2008; Voss et al., 2015). The DDM was fit separately for each task (lane change/image discrimination task) and each participant. We also calculated R^2 values as an additional measure to examine the goodness of fit of the model.

Data Analysis

Only the correct trials were used for the RT analysis. In the dual-task conditions, if the response to both tasks was correct, that trial was included in the analysis. The trials in which the

reaction time to each of the tasks was <200 ms and >1,500 ms were excluded from the analysis (3.48% of the trials). To quantify the effect of SOA on RTs and DDM parameters, one-way repeated-measures ANOVAs were used and to quantify the effect of SOA and task conditions on RTs, accuracies, and DDM parameters, two-way repeated-measures ANOVAs were used. A Greenhouse-Geisser correction was performed when sphericity had been violated. To compare the threshold, slope, and shift of the logistic regression function between the two task conditions, a paired t-test was used. We also performed three-way repeated measure ANOVAs with task condition, task order and SOA as three factors. The details of the statistical results are placed in **Supplementary Tables S1–S3**. In addition, we used t-test to statistically compare RTs, accuracies and DDM parameters between task conditions (dual vs. single/predictable vs. unpredictable) for each SOA. The details of the statistical tests for this analysis are placed in **Supplementary Tables S7–S9**. False Discovery Rate correction (Benjamini and Hochberg, 1995) was applied in all cases that multiple comparisons were performed.

We used a logistic regression model to examine the effect of SOA and OP on the order of the response of the two tasks. The probability that the lane change response was initiated before the image discrimination response was determined by the following formula:

$$\text{Logit } [P] = \beta_0 + \beta_1 C$$

where P stands for the probability that the lane change task was responded to first and C stands for SOAs. Parameters β_0 and β_1 were calculated for each participant. The model was fit separately on the data from the two dual-task conditions. A maximum likelihood estimation procedure was used for curve fitting.

RESULTS

Effect of Dual-Task Interference on RTs

We first focused our analysis on the dual-task condition with the predictable task order and compared it with the single-task conditions (**Figure 3**). We ran four two-way repeated-measures ANOVAs with task condition (dual/single), and SOA as factors separately for the lane change and the image discrimination and the lane change-first and image-first task orders. **Table 1** contains the details of the statistical results. Results showed a significant main effect of task condition with longer RTs in the dual- compared to the single-task condition in all cases [$Fs(1,19) > 6.21$, $ps < 0.023$, $\eta_p^2 > 0.24$]. The effect of SOA was significant in all cases [$Fs(3,57) > 6.5$, $ps < 0.006$, $\eta_p^2 > 0.25$] except for the lane change RTs in the lane change-first task order [$F(1.49, 26.84) = 2.55$, $p = 0.099$, $\eta_p^2 = 0.11$]. The interaction between task condition and SOA was also significant in all cases [$Fs(1,57) > 3.05$, $ps < 0.041$, $\eta_p^2 > 0.13$]. Further comparisons looking at the effect of SOA on RTs in the dual-task condition using one-way repeated-measures ANOVAs showed a significant effect of SOA on the RTs in all cases [$Fs(3,57) > 3.95$, $ps < 0.015$, $\eta_p^2 > 0.17$] except for the lane change when it was presented first [$F(1.6, 28.95) = 2.55$, $p = 0.49$, $\eta_p^2 = 0.02$]. Consistent with previous studies of

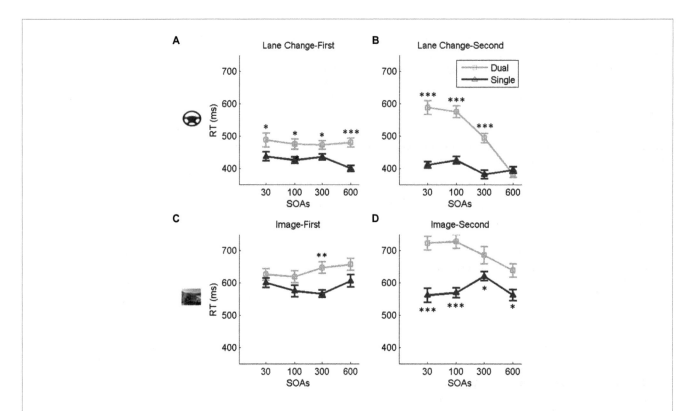

FIGURE 3 | Effect of task condition (dual vs. single) and SOA on RTs. **(A,B)** These panels indicate the RTs for the lane change in the lane change-first and lane change-second task orders, respectively, for the single-task (red) and the dual-task (blue) conditions. **(C,D)** These panels show the image discrimination RTs in the single (red) and the dual (blue) task conditions for the image-first and the image-second task orders, respectively. In all panels, errorbars show standard errors of mean and stars show a significant difference between task conditions for each SOA (* < 0.05, ** < 0.01, and *** < 0.001).

TABLE 1 | Results of two-way repeated-measure ANOVAs for the effect of task condition (dual vs. single), SOA, the interaction between the two on RTs, and SOA in dual shows the results of one-way repeated-measures ANOVAs for the effect of SOA on RTs separately in the dual-task condition.

		Lane change-first	Lane change-second	Image-first	Image-second
Task condition (dual vs. single)	F	10.19	43.10	6.22	23.20
	df	1, 19	1, 19	1, 19	1, 19
	p	**0.005**	**0.002**	**0.022**	**<0.0001**
	η_p^2	0.349	0.694	0.247	0.550
SOA	F	2.55	101.60	7.29	6.56
	df	1.49, 26*	3, 57	3, 57	1.8, 39*
	p	0.099	**0.0002**	**0.0002**	**0.005**
	η_p^2	0.119	0.843	0.277	0.257
Task condition × SOA	F	3.05	48.24	3.24	6.99
	df	3, 54	1.57, 29*	3, 57	3, 57
	p	**0.036**	**0.002**	**0.041**	**0.002**
	η_p^2	0.138	0.717	0.146	0.269
SOA in dual	F	0.657	103.7	7.10	8.35
	df	1.60, 28*	1.43, 27*	3, 57	1.61, 31*
	p	0.491	**0.002**	**0.002**	**0.002**
	η_p^2	0.023	0.845	0.272	0.305

All p-values were corrected for multiple comparisons, and Greenhouse-Geisser correction was done when necessary (indicated by a star). The significant p-values were shown in bold.

dual-task interference (Pashler and Johnston, 1989; Tombu and Jolicoeur, 2002; Sigman and Dehaene, 2005), when the image discrimination or the lane change tasks were presented second, the RTs increased at shorter SOAs. Interestingly, when the image discrimination was presented first, decreasing SOAs had an opposite effect, with shorter SOAs showing faster RTs.

These results have not been observed in previous dual-task studies and might be driven by participant's urge to finish the image discrimination task sooner in order to reduce the interference on driving.

Further analysis showed that the image discrimination RTs were generally longer than the lane change task RTs

(**Supplementary Figure S3**), but the magnitude of the dual-task effect was not different between the tasks (for more details see **Supplementary Table S6**). We also investigated if the image type (scenes vs. faces) affected RTs. Results showed no significant difference between scene image RTs and face image RTs [$t(159) = 1.13$, $p = 0.11$]. Also, the lance change RTs did not change in trials in which the image was a scene compared to those in which it was a face [$t(159) = 1.57$, $p = 0.118$].

We also calculated the accuracy of participants in single- and dual-task conditions. Results showed that the accuracies were above 95 and 90% for all conditions of the lane change task and the image discrimination task, respectively (**Supplementary Figures S1, S2**).

In sum, our results show a clear effect of SOA on driving and image discrimination RTs. The presence of these strong effects allows us to use SOA as a factor for drift-diffusion modeling in the next section to investigate the nature of dual-task interference in our simulated driving set up.

Drift-Diffusion Modeling of the Effect of Dual-Task Interference on RTs

Drift diffusion modeling was used to investigate if a change in SOA affects the drift rate, non-decision time, or both. The model could account for most of the variance in the data (R^2: Lane change-first 0.78 ± 0.03, Lane change-second 0.94 ± 0.02, Image-first 0.71 ± 0.04, and Image-second 0.84 ± 0.03), and the distribution of the RTs

from the model fit was not significantly different from the original data in all subjects and all conditions ($ps > 0.1$).

Next, we investigated the effect of SOA on the two model parameters v and $t0$, corresponding to the drift rate and non-decision times. Serial processing of the two tasks would lead to an increase in the $t0$ for the second task, while parallel processing of the two tasks would decrease the v for the second task at shorter SOAs. Results showed that when either of the two tasks was presented second, v decreased and $t0$ increased at shorter SOAs [$Fs(3,57) > 6.66$, $ps < 0.003$, $\eta_p^2 > 0.29$; **Figures 4B,D,F,H**]. No significant change in v or $t0$ was observed when driving was presented first ($p > 0.05$; **Figures 4A,E**) and a decrease in both $t0$ and v was observed at shorter SOAs when the image discrimination was presented first [$Fs(3,57) > 3.94$, $ps < 0.023$, $\eta_p^2 > 0.17$; **Figures 4C,G**]. The details of statistical tests are shown in **Table 2**. These results suggest that the two tasks are neither processed in a strictly parallel nor a strictly serial manner, as a change in the non-decision time is always accompanied by a change in the drift rate.

Effect of Task OP on RTs

To investigate the effect of task OP on the RTs during dual-task performance, we compared the main dual-task condition in which the task orders were predictable (i.e., the two task orders were presented in separate blocks) to a condition in which the task orders were unpredictable and varied randomly from trial to trial within a block. We ran four two-way

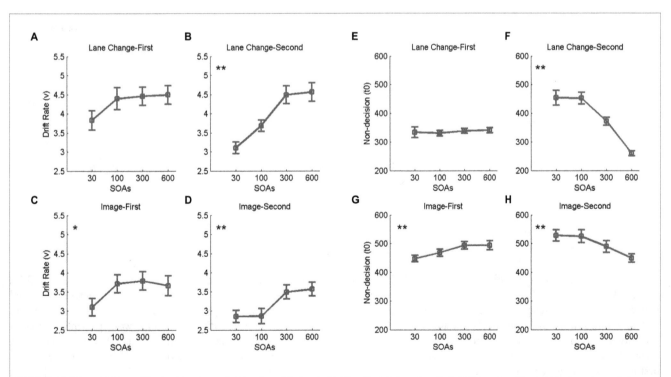

FIGURE 4 | Effect of SOA on drift rates (v) and non-decision times (t0). Panels **(A–D)** on the left show the effect of SOA on the drift rate (v) for lane change in the lane change-first **(A)** and lane change-second **(B)** conditions and that for the image discrimination in the image-first **(C)**, and image-second **(D)** conditions. Panels **(E–H)** on the right show the effect of SOA on non-decision time (t0) for lane change task in the lane change-first **(E)** and lane change-second **(F)** conditions and that for the image discrimination task in the image-first **(G)** and image-second **(H)** conditions. In all panels, errorbars show standard errors of mean and stars show a significant effect of SOA (* < 0.05 and ** < 0.01).

TABLE 2 | One-way repeated-measures ANOVAs for the effect of SOA on v and $t0$.

		Lane change-first		Lane change-second		Image-first		Image-second	
		v	$t0$	v	$t0$	v	$t0$	v	$t0$
SOA	F	1.59	3.46	15.03	64.42	3.95	7.96	6.67	12.20
	df	1.87, 35.53*	1.60, 30.43*	3, 57	1.59, 30.37*	3, 57	1.35, 25.80*	3, 57	1.86, 35.36*
	p	0.217	0.663	**0.002**	**0.001**	**0.022**	**0.006**	**0.002**	**0.001**
	η_p^2	0.078	0.018	0.442	0.772	0.172	0.295	0.296	0.391

All p-values were corrected for multiple comparisons and Greenhouse-Geisser correction was done when necessary (indicated by a star). The significant p-values are shown in bold.

TABLE 3 | Results of two-way repeated-measures ANOVAs for the effect of OP and SOA on RTs and one-way repeated-measures ANOVAs for effect SOA on RTs in the unpredictable condition.

		Lane change-first	Lane change-second	Image-first	Image-second
Task condition (predictable	F	10.21	11.81	3.53	4.29
vs. unpredictable)	df	1, 19	1, 19	1, 19	1, 19
	p	**0.005**	**0.012**	0.076	0.069
	η_p^2	0.350	0.383	0.157	0.184
SOA	F	2.83	88.89	3.35	7.55
	df	1.48, 28*	1.51, 28*	3, 57	1.65, 31*
	p	0.089	**0.0004**	**0.050**	**0.006**
	η_p^2	0.130	0.824	0.150	0.285
Task condition × SOA	F	5.02	7.06	3.37	3.07
	df	3, 57	3, 57	3, 57	1.83, 34*
	p	**0.003**	**0.004**	**0.041**	0.057
	η_p^2	0.215	0.271	0.151	0.139

All p-values were corrected for multiple comparison and Greenhouse-Geisser correction was done when necessary (indicated by a star). The significant p-values are shown in bold.

TABLE 4 | Results of two-way repeated-measures ANOVAs for the effect of OP and SOA on v and $t0$.

		Lane change-first		Lane change-second		Image-first		Image-second	
		v	$t0$	v	$t0$	v	$t0$	v	$t0$
OP	F	4.02	3.06	0.283	11.27	0.891	0.019	0.002	5.07
	df	1, 19	1, 19	1, 19	1, 19	1, 19	1, 19	1, 19	1, 19
	p	0.236	0.128	0.801	**0.012**	0.714	0.893	0.968	0.052
	η_p^2	0.175	0.139	0.015	0.372	0.045	0.001	0.001	0.211
SOA	F	2.10	1.33	28.02	43.23	7.23	9.03	3.45	5.93
	df	1.74, 33*	1.44, 27*	3, 57	1.40, 26*	3, 57	1.73, 32*	3, 57	1.93, 36*
	p	0.143	0.319	**0.002**	**0.002**	**0.002**	**0.002**	**0.036**	**0.008**
	η_p^2	0.100	0.056	0.596	0.695	0.276	0.322	0.157	0.238
OP × SOA	F	1.78	3.21	1.37	10.91	2.16	1.84	3.50	1.62
	df	3, 57	1.87, 35*	2.09, 39*	3, 57	3, 57	2.07, 39*	3, 57	2.19, 41*
	p	0.188	0.110	0.188	**0.003**	0.188	0.208	0.112	0.208
	η_p^2	0.086	0.145	0.084	0.365	0.100	0.089	0.156	0.079

All p-values were corrected for multiple comparisons and Greenhouse-Geisser correction was done when necessary (indicated by a star). The significant p-values are shown in bold.

repeated-measures ANOVAs with task condition (predictable/unpredictable) and SOA as the two factors, separately for the lane change and the image discrimination, and the lane change-first and image-first task orders. The details of the statistical tests are summarized in **Table 3**. The effects of OP, SOA, and their interaction on RTs were significant in both lane change-first and lane change-second conditions [$Fs > 5.03$, $ps < 0.013$, $\eta_p^2 > 0.21$; **Figures 5A,B**] except for the effect SOA on the lane change-first that was marginally significant [$F(1.48,28) = 2.83$, $p = 0.089$, $\eta_p^2 = 0.13$]. When the image discrimination was presented first (**Figure 5C**), OP had a marginally significant

effect on mean image discrimination RTs [$F(1,19) = 3.54$, $ps = 0.076$, $\eta_p^2 = 0.15$], and the interaction between OP and SOA was significant [$F(3,57) = 3.37$, $ps < 0.041$, $\eta_p^2 > 0.15$]. When the image discrimination was presented second (**Figure 5D**), the effect of OP on RTs [$F(1,19) = 4.29$, $ps = 0.069$, $\eta_p^2 = 0.18$], and the interaction between OP and SOA on RTs [$F(3,57) = 3.07$, $ps = 0.057$, $\eta_p^2 = 0.13$] were marginally significant.

Furthermore, we investigated the effect of SOA separately in the unpredictable conditions using one-way repeated-measures ANOVAs (note that the effects for the predictable condition

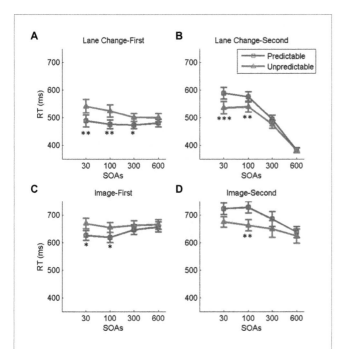

FIGURE 5 | Effect of OP and SOA on RTs. The two top panels show the RTs for the lane change in the lane change-first **(A)** and lane change-second **(B)** task orders for the predictable (blue) and the unpredictable (red) task order conditions. The two bottom panels show the RTs for the image discrimination task in the image-first **(C)** and image-second **(D)** task orders for the predictable (blue) and the unpredictable (red) task order conditions In all panels, error bars show standard errors of mean and stars show a significant difference between task conditions for each SOA (* < 0.05, ** < 0.01, and *** < 0.005).

are already reported in the previous section). The results showed a significant effect of SOA on the RTs in all cases $[Fs(3,57) > 3.75, ps < 0.015, \eta_p^2 > 0.16]$ except for when the image discrimination was presented first $[Fs(3,57) = 0.62, ps < 0.52, \eta_p^2 > 0.03]$.

In general, these results demonstrate that OP increases the mean RT of the first task and decreases the mean RT of the second task with the changes more pronounced when the tasks get closer together in time. These results show that unpredictability of the task order attenuates the effect of SOA on RTs for all cases except the lane change-first RTs. We next investigated the possible origin of this attenuation effect.

Effect of Task OP on the Response Order

To investigate the effect of SOA and OP on the order of the response to the two tasks, we calculated the probability that the lane change task was responded to first in each SOA and for each subject (**Figure 6A**) and fit a logistic regression model to these probability values. The model was fit separately for each of the two dual-task conditions, and an intercept (β_0 in the logistic model described in the methods) and a slope (β_1 in the logistic model) was calculated for each condition and each participant. We also calculated the SOA value in which the probability of responding to the lane change task first was 50% (T50). Then, to quantify the effect of OP on the response order, the model outputs and the T50 value across the two

experimental conditions were submitted to a paired t-test. OP had no significant effect on the shift (β_1) of the logistic function $[t(1,19) = 0.323\ p = 0.75;$ **Figure 6B**]. The slope of the logistic function (β_1) was significantly influenced by OP $[t(1,19) = 3.08, p = 0.006]$. Negative T50 values in both conditions show that participants had a general bias to respond to the lane change task first (**Figure 6C**) but this bias was the same across the two conditions $[t(1, 19) = 0.317, p = 0.75]$. At SOA = 0, in more than 60% of trials lane change was responded to first. In sum, these results showed that OP changes the response order to the two tasks and has no effect on the bias in favor of the lane change task.

Drift-Diffusion Modeling of the Effect of Task OP on RTs

Drift Diffusion Model (DDM) was fit to the data from the predictable and unpredictable task order conditions, separately, and output model parameters were compared for the two conditions. The results of model fitting on the unpredictable task order condition showed that the model could account for most of the variance in the data (R^2: lane change-first 0.70 ± 0.04, lane change-second 0.96 ± 0.01, image-first 0.75 ± 0.03 and image-second 0.82 ± 0.03) and the distribution of the RTs from the model fit was not significantly different from that of the original data in all subjects and all conditions ($ps > 0.09$). We ran two-way repeated-measures ANOVAs to investigate the effect of task condition (Predictable vs. Unpredictable) and SOA on the two parameters $t0$ and v, separately for the two task orders, and the lane change and the image discrimination tasks. The details of the statistical test are shown in **Table 4**. The effect of OP on v was not significant in all cases ($ps > 0.05$; **Figures 7A–D**). This effect on $t0$ was only significant in the lane change-second $[F(1,19) = 11.27, p = 0.012, \eta_p^2 = 0.37;$ **Figure 7F**] and marginally significant for image-second conditions $[F(1,19) = 5.07, p = 0.052, \eta_p^2 = 0.21;$ **Figure 7H**] and was not significant in the lane change-first and image-first conditions ($ps > 0.05$; **Figures 7E,G**). SOA had a significant effect on v and $t0$ in all conditions $[F(3,57) > 3.54, p < 0.02, \eta_p^2 > 0.15]$, except when the lane change task was presented first ($p > 0.05$; **Figure 7A**). The interaction of OP and SOA on $t0$ was only significant for lane change-second conditions $[F(3,57) = 10.91, p = 0.003, \eta_p^2 = 0.36;$ **Figure 7F**]. These results show that when either the image discrimination or the lane change tasks were presented second, unpredictability changed the non-decision time of the tasks. Note that the analysis of the response order showed that in the unpredictable condition, the second task was more likely to be responded to first. The changes in the order of response could be tightly related to the decrease in the non-decision time of the second task.

DISCUSSION

The purpose of this study was to investigate the underlying mechanisms of dual-task interference in a simulated lane change environment. We used a systematically controlled dual-task

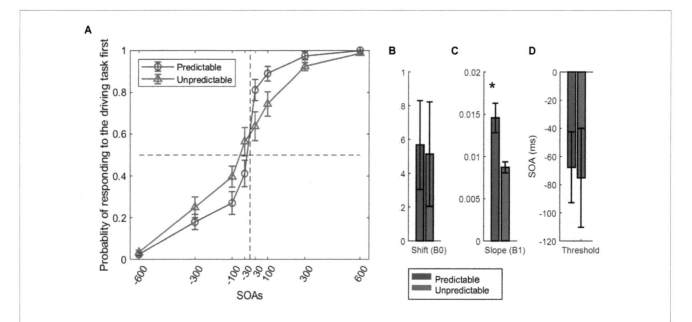

FIGURE 6 | Effect of OP on the response order. Predictable and Unpredictable conditions are shown in blue and red colors, respectively. **(A)** The probability of first responding to the lane change task plotted for the two task conditions. The curves are fit to the average data using a logistic regression function. **(B)** The shift of the logistic regression function (β_0), **(C)** the slope of the logistic function (β_1), and **(D)** The T50 (the SOA in which participants responded to the lane change task first with 50% probability), for the predictable (blue) and unpredictable (red) conditions. The shift did not differ between the two conditions, but the slope was shallower in the unpredictable condition ($p < 0.006$). There was a general bias for responding to the lane change task first in both conditions. In all panels, error bars show standard errors of mean. The star shows a significant difference between task conditions ($* < 0.05$).

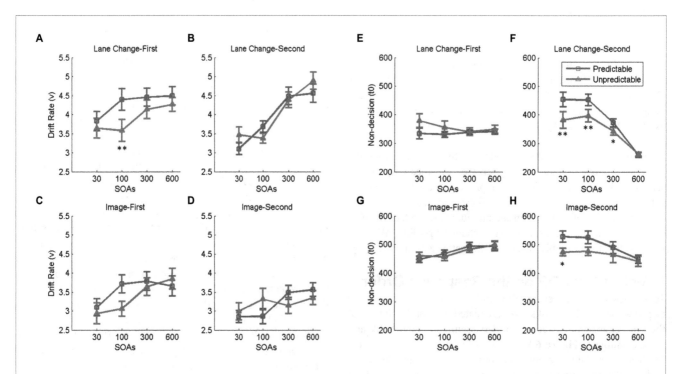

FIGURE 7 | Effect of OP and SOA on drift rates (v) and non-decision times ($t0$). Blue lines and red lines show the predictable and unpredictable task orders, respectively. Panels **(A–D)** on the left show the effect of OP and SOA on the drift rate (v) for lane change in the lane change-first **(A)** and lane change-second **(B)** conditions and that for the image discrimination in the image-first **(C)** and image-second **(D)** conditions. Panels **(E–H)** on the right show the effect of OP and SOA on non-decision time ($t0$) for lane change in the lane change-first **(E)** and lane change-second **(F)** conditions and that for the image discrimination task in the image-first **(G)** and image-second **(H)** conditions. In all panels, errorbars show standard errors of mean and stars show a significant difference between task conditions for each SOA ($* < 0.05$ and $** < 0.01$).

paradigm in which an image task was presented at set times before or after the lane change task. We investigated the effect of dual-task, SOA, and unpredictability of task order on subjects' performance and modeled the results using a DDM. Results showed strong dual-task effects on both tasks with stronger effects at shorter SOAs for the second tasks. DDM showed a change in both the drift rate and non-decision times, suggesting that a hybrid model containing features of both serial and parallel processing best accounts for the results. Unpredictability of the task order attenuated the effect of SOA by changing the order of the response to the two tasks. This effect induced a change in the non-decision time of the second task in the DDM.

The observation of a strong dual-task effect on both image discrimination and lane change RTs when they were presented second is compatible with the predictions of both capacity sharing and bottleneck theories. But our behavioral results are not fully compatible with either of the two theories. We observed a clear dual-task effect comparing the RTs of the single-task with the dual-task conditions when the tasks were presented first with longer RTs for the single-compared to the dual-task condition, and a decrease of RT at shorter SOAs for the image task. The bottleneck theory predicts no change in the RT in the single-compared to the dual-task, and the capacity sharing theory predicts an RT effect that increases at shorter SOAs. Our observations are different from those reported by Levy et al. (2006) and Hibberd et al. (2013) who only observed a dual-task effect for the second task in a simulated driving environment. In these two studies, for the driving task, participants performed a car following in which they pressed the brake pedal when the color of the brake light changed. In our study, for performing the driving, participants had to press a key, hold it, and tune the location of the car to avoid the collision. The more continuous and multi-step nature of the response in our study might have increased the time pressure and demands of the driving task, imposing a priority for processing it. This increased priority, in turn, may have caused the participant to not invest all their resources on the image task when they knew that a driving trigger may be presented soon. The increased priority may have also caused participants to try to respond to the first-presented image task faster at shorter SOAs to release resources for the driving task. These effects clearly suggest a more complex management of resources than what is suggested by the bottleneck or capacity sharing theories.

Results of our DDM analysis further confirm that neither the bottleneck theory with its prediction of a strictly serial processing of tasks nor the capacity sharing theory with predictions of a fully parallel processing can account for our results. This is because both the drift rate and the non-decision times of the second tasks are found to be modulated across SOAs. This result suggests some degree of capacity sharing for the processing of the two tasks. In addition, they suggest some delay in the processing of the second task due to a potential bottleneck. In other words, our results suggest that the best model to account for dual-task interference in driving is a hybrid model combining the two extremes suggested by capacity sharing and bottleneck theories. Zylberberg et al. (2012) modeled RT of the second task with a term for accumulation

time that includes the time from stimulus onset to end of the decision process and a term for the post-accumulation time that includes the time from the end of the decision process to the motor response. Their results showed that both accumulation and post-accumulation times increase in short compared to the long SOA conditions. These results are compatible with a hybrid model as they show that the dual-task interference decreases the efficacy of evidence accumulation without halting it and causes a delay in mapping the decision to motor response. In line with Zylberberg et al. (2012), the result of the current study demonstrates that the decision stage of the second task is processed in parallel with the decision stage of the first task, and there is also some bottleneck in processing the second task. In our DDM modeling, it is not possible to determine if the bottleneck is before or after the evidence accumulation stage. It is plausible that the mapping of the decision to the motor output happens in a serial manner, and this imposes a bottleneck on the production of the response, but proof of this point requires further studies.

Results of our task order predictability manipulation suggest the involvement of an active higher order control mechanism for scheduling the tasks (De Jong, 1995; Luria and Meiran, 2003; Sigman and Dehaene, 2006; Szameitat et al., 2006; Fernández et al., 2011; Leonhard, 2011; Ruiz Fernández et al., 2013) as opposed to passive scheduling of the tasks on a first-come first-served basis (Pashler, 1994b; Bunge et al., 2000; Jiang, 2004). A passive scheduling account would predict no effect of task order predictability on response orders while in our experiment, task order predictability changed the order of the response to the two tasks causing the RTs for the first task to increase and those for the second task to decrease. Our results do not fully replicate previous studies of task order predictability in simple artificial dual-tasks (Sigman and Dehaene, 2006; Töllner et al., 2012). These studies report an increase in RT for both the first and second tasks. However, unlike our paradigm these studies have instructed the participants to respond to the stimuli according to the presentation order. Imposing this artificial response order may have increased the dual-task costs leading to longer RTs (Strobach et al., 2018). Our paradigm is closer to naturalistic settings in which the secondary task can happen at any time relative to the driving event and are more applicable to natural settings.

Another feature of our data also favors an active account of task scheduling. Participants had an overall bias to respond to the lane change task first. Order predictability had no effect on this average bias. This bias might be due to the context of the lane change task and the intrinsic time pressure for responding to the lane change task in order to avoid collision with the cone obstacles. It may also be related to the differences in the difficulties between the image and lane change tasks. Miller et al. (2009) have suggested an RT optimization model for scheduling of tasks in dual-task paradigm. This model suggests that the participants' aim in a dual-task paradigm is to decrease the total RT (RT of the first task + RT of the second task). Therefore, they tend to respond to the easy task sooner than the difficult one. In other words, the duration of the components of the two tasks determines which task is responded to first (see Sigman and Dehaene, 2006 and Fernández et al., 2011 and Ruiz Fernández et al., 2013 for evidence in favor of this model). It is hard to evaluate if our results favor this model or not. In our paradigm, the decision time and non-decision times of the images task were slightly longer, while the motor stage of the lane change task was likely more difficult as it involved a series of motor movements. It is hard to speculate about the effect of each of these stages on the decision for task order without further experiments manipulating each stage in isolation. Regardless of the underlying reason, the prioritization of the lane change task over the image task shows that the order of the presentation of the tasks does not dictate the order of the processing.

Studies of working memory have categorized executive functions into distinct components (Jonides et al., 2008; Nee et al., 2013). These include shifting attention between items in working memory, updating the actively maintained items, and preventing interference from outside distractors and internal intrusions (Courtney et al., 2007; Bledowski et al., 2009; Nee et al., 2013). We did not have an explicit working memory task, but our behavioral and modeling results, in line with previous findings (De Jong, 1995; Meyer and Kieras, 1997; Szameitat et al., 2002; Piai and Roelofs, 2013) suggest that similar executive functions may be at play in our dual-task paradigm to coordinate which task should be prioritized and processed first, to divide the resources during the evidence accumulation of the two tasks, and to maintain the information of one task during the (possibly post-accumulation) bottleneck until the process of the other task is completed. Based on our results, we can speculate that resources are divided between tasks with a general preference for the first task and an additional preference for the lane change task. The information is then updated and maintained for the two tasks during the evidence accumulation and response selection phases, with the first task imposing constraints and interfering with the process of the second task.

We have used the broad term of interference for the phenomenon of performance decline and changes in the parameter of DDM in our dual-task paradigm. This term has been used in the literature to describe multiple distinct phenomena (Pashler, 1994a; Luck, 1998; Marois and Ivanoff, 2005; Johnston and McCann, 2006; Tombu et al., 2011), including performance declines due to internal processes and those related to distractions from external stimuli. In a dual-task paradigm, when the first task is being processed, the presence of the stimulus of the second task could serve as an external distractor. Once the process of the second task starts, the information from the second task is no longer an external distractor. The effect of this external distraction can be observed in our control single-task conditions, as in this condition, the stimuli for the ignored task are still present. Small modulations in the RTs in the single-task condition are possibly related to external distraction from the ignored task. The dual-task effect, however, is much stronger than this small modulation. This dual-task effect, observed especially in the second task, is due to proactive interference (Jonides and Nee, 2006) from the internal processing of the first task

imposing a reduction in the drift-diffusion rates of the second task. Other than this interference, task shifting may play some roles in our increased RTs. As discussed above, the changes in the non-decision time could be related to the shift between the two tasks during the post-accumulation phase (Zylberberg et al., 2012).

Our simulated driving paradigm was close to a real-life driving task in some respects such as having a continuous driving scene with a multi-lane road and a car dashboard and requiring a two-step response (pressing and releasing the button at prompt times) with an intrinsic time pressure for the driving task. But our paradigm also kept the driving task and driving environment as simple as possible to control the main experiment variables systematically. Participants drove at a constant speed in a high-way desert with no hill or turn, and other cars in our paradigm. The display was viewed on a 2D computer screen as opposed to a 3D environment. The responses were collected using button presses. Participants were only focused on the lane change in the driving task as opposed to real-world settings in which the driver has to control the brake, gas pedal, and steering wheel at the same time. Lastly, our image discrimination task was not a natural secondary task (although one could argue that many real-world tasks such as identifying images on traffic signs or billboards or determining if an item by the roadside is a human or an inanimate object involve similar mechanisms as our image discrimination task). These factors limit the generalizability of our task to a real-world driving scenario. Future studies with even more realistic driving simulators could determine if our results can be translated to real-world driving.

Another factor worth considering in future studies is the gaze behavior of participants during dual-task interference. In our experiment, we asked participants to fixate on a fixation point at the center of the screen close to the focus of the radial optical flow pattern, which is the natural position of the gaze during driving (Lappe et al., 2000). As such it is likely that our participants have kept their eyes on the fixation point. However, since we did not have eye tracking in our experiment, we cannot be certain about the gaze behavior of our participants. Future studies could shed light on the gaze behavior and its potential effects on dual-task interference in a driving task.

To sum up, here, for the first time, we used a simulated driving environment and a DDM to explore the processing of two tasks in a naturalistic dual-task setting. Our finding revealed that performing a secondary task while driving deteriorates the driving performance, whether presented before or after the driving task. Further investigations showed this effect might be caused by slower parallel processing of the driving task in the presence of a secondary task with some delays in the process, suggesting that a hybrid model best accounts for the results. Our results could be applicable for optimizing the design of driving assistance systems such as road signs, alarm systems, and other driver interfaces to reduce accidents. They could also inform precautionary measures aimed at reducing accidents in clinical populations with impaired executive control and should be considered in future neuroscience studies aiming to explore the neural underpinnings of dual-task interference in natural settings.

ETHICS STATEMENT

The studies involving human participants were reviewed and approved by the ethics committee of Iran University of Medical Sciences (ethics code: IR.IUMS.REC.1396.0435). The patients/participants provided their written informed consent to participate in this study.

AUTHOR CONTRIBUTIONS

MAZ: Conceptualization, methodology, investigation, formal analysis, and writing of the original draft. GHZ: Supervision and writing - review and editing. MVP: Supervision, conceptualization, methodology, and writing - review and editing. All authors contributed to the article and approved the submitted version.

ACKNOWLEDGMENTS

We thank Mahdi Shafiei for his assistance in developing the simulated driving environment and Sajjad Zabbah for his assistance in drift diffusion modeling. This research was supported in part by the Intramural Research Program of the NIH, National Institute of Mental Health (ZIA MH002035-39). The collection and analysis of the data was performed entirely at IPM. This manuscript has been released as a pre-print at bioRxiv (Abbas-Zadeh et al., 2019).

REFERENCES

Abbas-Zadeh, M., Hossein-Zadeh, G. -A., and Vaziri-Pashkam, M. (2019). Dual-task interference in a simulated driving environment: serial or parallel processing? *bioRxiv*, 853119. doi:10.1101/853119 [Preprint]

Anderson, J. R., Reder, L. M., and Lebiere, C. (1996). Working memory: activation limitations on retrieval. *Cogn. Psychol.* 30, 221–256. doi: 10.1006/cogp.1996.0007

Bakhit, P. R., Guo, B., and Ishak, S. (2018). Crash and near-crash risk assessment of distracted driving and engagement in secondary tasks: a naturalistic driving study. *Transp. Res. Rec.* 2672, 245–254. doi: 10.1177/0361198118772703

Benjamini, Y., and Hochberg, Y. (1995). Controlling the false discovery rate: a practical and powerful approach to multiple testing. *J. R. Stat. Soc. Ser. B Methodol.* 57, 289–300. doi: 10.2307/2346101

Blanco, M., Biever, W. J., Gallagher, J. P., and Dingus, T. A. (2006). The impact of secondary task cognitive processing demand on driving performance. *Accid. Anal. Prev.* 38, 895–906. doi: 10.1016/j.aap.2006.02.015

Bledowski, C., Rahm, B., and Rowe, J. B. (2009). What "works" in working memory? Separate systems for selection and updating of critical information. *J. Neurosci.* 29, 13735–13741. doi: 10.1523/JNEUROSCI.2547-09.2009

Bunge, S. A., Klingberg, T., Jacobsen, R. B., and Gabrieli, J. D. (2000). A resource model of the neural basis of executive working memory. *Proc. Natl. Acad. Sci.* 97, 3573–3578. doi: 10.1073/pnas.050583797

Carrier, L. M., and Pashler, H. (1995). Attentional limits in memory retrieval. *J. Exp. Psychol. Learn. Mem. Cogn.* 21, 1339–1348. doi: 10.1037//0278-7393.21.5.1339

Courtney, S. M., Roth, J. K., and Sala, J. B. (2007). "A hierarchical biased-competition model of domain-dependent working memory maintenance and executive control" in *Working memory: Behavioural and neural correlates*. 369–384.

De Jong, R. (1995). The role of preparation in overlapping-task performance. *Q. J. Exp. Psychol.* 48, 2–25. doi: 10.1080/14640749508401372

Duncan, J. (1980). The locus of interference in the perception of simultaneous stimuli. *Psychol. Rev.* 87, 272–300. doi: 10.1037/0033-295X.87.3.272

Engle, R. W. (2002). Working memory capacity as executive attention. *Curr. Dir. Psychol. Sci.* 11, 19–23. doi: 10.1111/1467-8721.00160

Fernández, S. R., Leonhard, T., Rolke, B., and Ulrich, R. (2011). Processing two tasks with varying task order: central stage duration influences central processing order. *Acta Psychol.* 137, 10–17. doi: 10.1016/j.actpsy.2011.01.016

Hibberd, D. L., Jamson, S. L., and Carsten, O. M. (2013). Mitigating the effects of in-vehicle distractions through use of the psychological refractory period paradigm. *Accid. Anal. Prev.* 50, 1096–1103. doi: 10.1016/j.aap.2012.08.016

Horrey, W. J., and Wickens, C. D. (2004). Driving and side task performance: the effects of display clutter, separation, and modality. *Hum. Factors* 46, 611–624. doi: 10.1518/hfes.46.4.611.56805

Huang, L., Treisman, A., and Pashler, H. (2007). Characterizing the limits of human visual awareness. *Science* 317, 823–825. doi: 10.1126/science.1143515

Huestegge, L., and Koch, I. (2010). Crossmodal action selection: evidence from dual-task compatibility. *Mem. Cogn.* 38, 493–501. doi: 10.3758/MC.38.4.493

Jiang, Y. (2004). Resolving dual-task interference: an fMRI study. *NeuroImage* 22, 748–754. doi: 10.1016/j.neuroimage.2004.01.043

Johnston, J. C., and McCann, R. S. (2006). On the locus of dual-task interference: is there a bottleneck at the stimulus classification stage? *Q. J. Exp. Psychol.* 59, 694–719. doi: 10.1080/02724980543000015

Jonides, J., Lewis, R. L., Nee, D. E., Lustig, C. A., Berman, M. G., and Moore, K. S. (2008). The mind and brain of short-term memory. *Annu. Rev. Psychol.* 59, 193–224. doi: 10.1146/annurev.psych.59.103006.093615

Jonides, J., and Nee, D. E. (2006). Brain mechanisms of proactive interference in working memory. *Neuroscience* 139, 181–193. doi: 10.1016/j.neuroscience.2005.06.042

Kahneman, D. (1973). Attention and effort. *Vol. 1063*. Citeseer.

Kane, M. J., and Engle, R. W. (2000). Working-memory capacity, proactive interference, and divided attention: limits on long-term memory retrieval. *J. Exp. Psychol. Learn. Mem. Cogn.* 26, 336–358. doi: 10.1037//0278-7393.26.2.336

Lappe, M., Grigo, A., Bremmer, F., Frenz, H., Bertin, R. J., and Israël, I. (2000). "Perception of heading and driving distance from optic flow." in *Proceedings of the Driving simulator conference*; September 2000.

Leonhard, T. (2011). Determinants of central processing order in psychological refractory period paradigms: central arrival times, detection times, or preparation? *Q. J. Exp. Psychol.* 64, 2012–2043. doi: 10.1080/17470218.2011.573567

Levy, J., Pashler, H., and Boer, E. (2006). Central interference in driving: is there any stopping the psychological refractory period? *Psychol. Sci.* 17, 228–235. doi: 10.1111/j.1467-9280.2006.01690.x

Luck, S. J. (1998). Sources of dual-task interference: evidence from human electrophysiology. *Psychol. Sci.* 9, 223–227. doi: 10.1111/1467-9280.00043

Luria, R., and Meiran, N. (2003). Online order control in the psychological refractory period paradigm. *J. Exp. Psychol. Hum. Percept. Perform.* 29, 556–574. doi: 10.1037/0096-1523.29.3.556

Marois, R., and Ivanoff, J. (2005). Capacity limits of information processing in the brain. *Trends Cogn. Sci.* 9, 296–305. doi: 10.1016/j.tics.2005.04.010

McCann, R. S., and Johnston, J. C. (1992). Locus of the single-channel bottleneck in dual-task interference. *J. Exp. Psychol. Hum. Percept. Perform.* 18:471. doi: 10.1037/0096-1523.18.2.471

McLeod, P. (1977). A dual task response modality effect: support for multiprocessor models of attention. *Q. J. Exp. Psychol.* 29, 651–667. doi: 10.1080/14640747708400639

Meyer, D. E., and Kieras, D. E. (1997). A computational theory of executive cognitive processes and multiple-task performance: part I. Basic mechanisms. *Psychol. Rev.* 104, 3–65. doi: 10.1037/0033-295x.104.1.3

Miller, J., Ulrich, R., and Rolke, B. (2009). On the optimality of serial and parallel processing in the psychological refractory period paradigm: effects of the distribution of stimulus onset asynchronies. *Cogn. Psychol.* 58, 273–310. doi: 10.1016/j.cogpsych.2006.08.003

Nee, D. E., Brown, J. W., Askren, M. K., Berman, M. G., Demiralp, E., Krawitz, A., et al. (2013). A meta-analysis of executive components of working memory. *Cereb. Cortex* 23, 264–282. doi: 10.1093/cercor/bhs007

Oriet, C., Tombu, M., and Jolicoeur, P. (2005). Symbolic distance affects two processing loci in the number comparison task. *Mem. Cogn.* 33, 913–926. doi: 10.3758/bf03193085

Pashler, H. (1994a). Dual-task interference in simple tasks: data and theory. *Psychol. Bull.* 116, 220–244. doi: 10.1037/0033-2909.116.2.220

Pashler, H. (1994b). Graded capacity-sharing in dual-task interference? *J. Exp. Psychol. Hum. Percept. Perform.* 20, 330–342. doi: 10.1037//0096-1523.20.2.330

Pashler, H., and Johnston, J. C. (1989). Chronometric evidence for central postponement in temporally overlapping tasks. *Q. J. Exp. Psychol.* 41, 19–45. doi: 10.1080/14640748908402351

Piai, V., and Roelofs, A. (2013). Working memory capacity and dual-task interference in picture naming. *Acta Psychol.* 142, 332–342. doi: 10.1016/j.actpsy.2013.01.006

Posner, M. I., and Boies, S. J. (1971). Components of attention. *Psychol. Rev.* 78, 391–408. doi: 10.1037/h0031333

Pylyshyn, Z. W., and Storm, R. W. (1988). Tracking multiple independent targets: evidence for a parallel tracking mechanism. *Spat. Vis.* 3, 179–197. doi: 10.1163/156856888X00122

Ratcliff, R. (1978). A theory of memory retrieval. *Psychol. Rev.* 85, 59–108. doi: 10.1037/0033-295X.85.2.59

Ratcliff, R. (2015). Modeling one-choice and two-choice driving tasks. *Atten. Percept. Psychophys.* 77, 2134–2144. doi: 10.3758/s13414-015-0911-8

Ratcliff, R., and Rouder, J. N. (1998). Modeling response times for two-choice decisions. *Psychol. Sci.* 9, 347–356. doi: 10.1111/1467-9280.00067

Ruiz Fernández, S., Leonhard, T., Lachmair, M., Ulrich, R., and Rolke, B. (2013). Processing order in dual-tasks when the duration of motor responses varies. *Universitas Psychologica* 12, 1439–1452. doi: 10.11144/Javeriana.UPSY12-5.podt

Ruthruff, E., Pashler, H. E., and Klaassen, A. (2001). Processing bottlenecks in dual-task performance: structural limitation or strategic postponement? *Psychon. Bull. Rev.* 8, 73–80. doi: 10.3758/BF03196141

Sigman, M., and Dehaene, S. (2005). Parsing a cognitive task: a characterization of the mind's bottleneck. *PLoS Biol.* 3:e37. doi: 10.1371/journal.pbio.0030037

Sigman, M., and Dehaene, S. (2006). Dynamics of the central bottleneck: dual-task and task uncertainty. *PLoS Biol.* 4:e220. doi: 10.1371/journal.pbio.0040220

Sigman, M., and Dehaene, S. (2008). Brain mechanisms of serial and parallel processing during dual-task performance. *J. Neurosci.* 28, 7585–7598. doi: 10.1523/JNEUROSCI.0948-08.2008

Strayer, D. L., Cooper, J. M., Turrill, J., Coleman, J. R., and Hopman, R. J. (2017). The smartphone and the driver's cognitive workload: a comparison of apple, Google, and Microsoft's intelligent personal assistants. *Can. J. Exp. Psychol.* 71, 93–110. doi: 10.1037/cep0000104

Strobach, T., Hendrich, E., Kübler, S., Müller, H., and Schubert, T. (2018). Processing order in dual-task situations: the "first-come, first-served" principle

and the impact of task order instructions. *Atten. Percept. Psychophys.* 80, 1785–1803. doi: 10.3758/s13414-018-1541-8

Szameitat, A. J., Lepsien, J., Von Cramon, D. Y., Sterr, A., and Schubert, T. (2006). Task-order coordination in dual-task performance and the lateral prefrontal cortex: an event-related fMRI study. *Psychol. Res.* 70, 541–552. doi: 10.1007/s00426-005-0015-5

Szameitat, A. J., Schubert, T., Müller, K., and Von Cramon, D. Y. (2002). Localization of executive functions in dual-task performance with fMRI. *J. Cogn. Neurosci.* 14, 1184–1199. doi: 10.1162/0898929027608 07195

Töllner, T., Strobach, T., Schubert, T., and Mueller, H. J. (2012). The effect of task order predictability in audio-visual dual task performance: just a central capacity limitation? *Front. Integr. Neurosci.* 6:75. doi: 10.3389/fnint.2012. 00075

Tombu, M. N., Asplund, C. L., Dux, P. E., Godwin, D., Martin, J. W., and Marois, R. (2011). A unified attentional bottleneck in the human brain. *Proc. Natl. Acad. Sci.* 108, 13426–13431. doi: 10.1073/pnas.1103583108

Tombu, M., and Jolicoeur, P. (2002). All-or-none bottleneck versus capacity sharing accounts of the psychological refractory period phenomenon. *Psychol. Res.* 66, 274–286. doi: 10.1007/s00426-002-0101-x

Tombu, M., and Jolicoeur, P. (2003). A central capacity sharing model of dual-task performance. *J. Exp. Psychol. Hum. Percept. Perform.* 29, 3–18. doi: 10.1037//0096-1523.29.1.3

Voss, A., and Voss, J. (2007). Fast-dm: a free program for efficient diffusion model analysis. *Behav. Res. Methods* 39, 767–775. doi: 10.3758/bf031 92967

Voss, A., and Voss, J. (2008). A fast numerical algorithm for the estimation of diffusion model parameters. *J. Math. Psychol.* 52, 1–9. doi: 10.1016/j. jmp.2007.09.005

Voss, A., Voss, J., and Lerche, V. (2015). Assessing cognitive processes with diffusion model analyses: a tutorial based on fast-dm-30. *Front. Psychol.* 6:336. doi: 10.3389/fpsyg.2015.00336

Zylberberg, A., Ouellette, B., Sigman, M., and Roelfsema, P. R. (2012). Decision making during the psychological refractory period. *Curr. Biol.* 22, 1795–1799. doi: 10.1016/j.cub.2012.07.043

20

Lifestyle Modifications for Migraine Management

Mendinatou Agbetou [1,2†] and Thierry Adoukonou [1,2,3†]*

[1] Department of Neurology, University of Parakou, Parakou, Benin, [2] Clinic of Neurology, Teaching Hospital of Parakou, Parakou, Benin, [3] Inserm U1094, IRD U270, Univ. Limoges, CHU Limoges, EpiMaCT - Epidemiology of Chronic Diseases in Tropical Zone, Institute of Epidemiology and Tropical Neurology, OmegaHealth, Limoges, France

Correspondence:
Thierry Adoukonou
adoukonouthierry@yahoo.fr

[†] *These authors have contributed equally to this work*

Migraine is a disabling disease that inflicts a heavy burden on individuals who suffer from it. Significant advances are being made in understanding the pathophysiology and treatment of the disease. The role of lifestyle modifications has become increasingly predominant. We reviewed the current and available data on the role of a healthy lifestyle in the management of migraine. Physical activity, management of obesity, a healthy diet, and a better lifestyle, such as adequate sleep and avoidance of drug abuse, significantly contribute to reducing the frequency and severity of attacks. It is important to consider these factors in the overall management strategies for migraine sufferers.

Keywords: migraine, lifestyle modification, physical activity, obesity, diet

INTRODUCTION

The Global Burden of Disease study in 2016 identified migraine as the second leading cause of years lived with disability (1) with an age-standardized disability-adjusted life years rate of 596.8 per 100,000 (2). The number of productive days at work was reduced by half or more as headache was significantly higher in occurrence in migraine sufferers (3). The direct and indirect costs and their impact on family, social, and professional life are also high (4, 5). The estimated cost of productivity loss associated with presenteeism (absenteeism) due to migraine was calculated at 21.3 billion US$/year in some studies (3). Episodic migraine can progress to chronic migraine, and about 3% of patients with episodic migraine report a very severe headache-related disability, as defined by the Migraine Disability Assessment Scale (6). Approximately 25% of individuals with chronic migraine have headache-related disability (6). Many risk factors contribute to chronicity and increase in episodic migraine frequency (7), some of which are modifiable, such as overuse of acute migraine medication, obesity, metabolic syndrome, depression, and stressful life events (8, 9). These risk factors may serve as targets for future preventive interventions. Even if the results are not unanimous, several publications have confirmed the effectiveness of reducing the burden of migraine with changes in the lifestyles of migraine sufferers (10). Migraine preventive therapy helps reduce the frequency of migraine attacks, days with migraine and headache, severity of symptoms, frequency of acute migraine therapy, and migraine-related disability (11). Here, we review the role of lifestyle changes and their benefits in managing migraine.

METHODS

This was a general mini-review and not a systematic review. For this general mini-review, the research was conducted in three electronic databases (PubMed, ISI Web of Science, and Google scholar). The keywords used were migraine, lifestyle, alcohol, obesity, overweight, caffeine, physical activity, smoking, diet, hydration, depression, insomnia, and drug abuse. Only articles published between January 2000 and May 2021 in French or English were included. We also used other articles from gray literature.

MIGRAINE AND LIFESTYLE MANAGEMENT

In addition to migraine attack trigger identification and avoidance, avoidance of risk factors for developing more frequent migraine attacks through a change in lifestyle is an important part of preventive measures for migraine (**Figure 1**). It has no side effects and is indicated for all migraine sufferers at a low cost with little risk to the patient (12). The acronym SEED, which means Sleep, Exercise, Eat, and Diary, was proposed in a recent update to summarize the lifestyle changes needed to improve migraine (10). Non-pharmacological treatments have been shown to be effective in controlling migraine (13, 14). Regular lifestyle behavior helps to control chronic migraine as patients without regular lifestyle behaviors are more likely to have chronic migraine than episodic migraine (12).

Physical Activity

Obesity, defined as a body mass index (BMI) [weight (kg)/height2 (m2)] $\geq$ 30, is associated with an increased frequency and severity of attacks among patients with episodic migraine (15). The interrelationships between migraine frequency and obesity are not well-known, but a bidirectional link between the two conditions has been noted (16). Migraine is significantly associated with obesity and being overweight, whereas the clinical features of migraine are not associated with BMI (15). Meta-analysis of the available observational studies suggested an association between migraine and obesity that is likely mediated by sex and migraine frequency (17, 18). In addition, BMI category has a consistent and increasing relationship with transformed migraine prevalence (16), and chronic migraine was associated with insulin resistance status, particularly when it is combined with obesity (8). In obese migraine patients, hypothalamic deregulation leads to alterations in peptides, neurotransmitters, and adipocytokines involved in energy homeostasis and regulation of feeding, especially via the orexinergic system (19, 20). Serotonin or orexins A or B can influence food intake, along with the feeling of satiety and modulation of nociceptive messages. Another hypothesis highlights the possible role of increased intracranial pressure found in a proportion of obese patients and some migraine patients (21). Pro-inflammatory mediators, including IL-1, IL-6, tumor necrosis factor-α, and calcitonin gene-related peptide (CGRP), play an important role in the pathophysiological mechanisms of these two conditions (22, 23). Likewise, an inflammatory state, induced by leptin and adiponectin secreted by adipose tissue, exists in obesity, and actively contributes to increasing migraine frequency or migraine transformation (24). Overactivation of the reward circuitry in obesity can lead to food addiction and/or excessive eating behaviors (25). In addition, one of the side effects of some migraine medications is weight gain (26).

Low levels of physical activity are associated with an increased migraine frequency (27). Therefore, weight loss may be proposed to reduce headache frequency and severity (28). Several strategies can be used to achieve this goal, including behavioral weight loss, pharmacotherapy, and bariatric surgery. However, weight loss is the recommended first-line treatment (29). Behavioral therapy in diet and physical activity interventions are more widely available and are recommended as primary intervention strategies. Outside of migraine attacks, internet-based resources, physical groups, or individual activities encourage physical activity in migraine sufferers (27). Approximately 150–300 min of moderate-intensity aerobic exercise per week (30) and increased lifestyle activities, such as walking the dog, parking farther away, or taking the stairs are encouraged. An aerobic exercise program that included relaxation had a similar effect to topiramate in reducing migraine pain intensity and frequency (31). Moreover, activities such as walking, jogging, cross-training, and cycling also have beneficial effects when completed for 30–60 min, 3–5 times a week. Physical activity has a positive cross-sectional effect on most of the modifiable risk factors of migraine and can improve the patients' quality of life (32, 33). Apart from weight loss, stress reduction, decreased anxiety, depressed mood, and depression, physical activity improves sleep efficiency and sleep quality, thereby inducing deep sleep, reducing daytime sleepiness, and decreasing the frequency of medication use to aid sleep (30).

Diet

Diet is an important lifestyle aspect. However, there is no specific diet for migraine sufferers. For individuals who are obese, a weight-loss diet is recommended. The total daily caloric intake of between 1,200 and 1,500 calories for women and 1,500 to 1,800 calories for men can be adjusted to induce weight loss (29). Several diets can improve migraine symptoms such as the following: elimination diets, diets high in certain nutrients, and epigenetic diets. Diet strategies, such as low fat, low carbohydrate, and high protein diet, can result in weight loss and similar cardiovascular benefits (29). Elimination diets require the identification of provocative dietary ingredients and their subsequent elimination (34). One example is the gluten-free diet among patients with celiac disease, which decreases headache or migraine frequency from 51.6 to 100% (35). Other elimination diets, such as immunoglobulin G-elimination, antihistamine, tyramine-free, and low-fat diets have contradictory results and might cause malnutrition in cases of total avoidance (36–38). Moreover, low-glycemic index diets showed improvement in migraine frequency in a diet group and in a control group of patients who took a standard migraine-preventive medication (39). On the other hand, diets high in certain food or ingredient ratios can also provide satisfactory results. Diets containing high levels of omega-3 fatty acids and low levels of omega-6 fatty acids reduce the duration and frequency of migraine (40, 41). Ketogenic diet in overweight individuals, low-sodium diet in pre-hypertensive patients or the elderly population, and a high-sodium diet among young women without hypertension and with a low-to-normal BMI or who have postural tachycardia syndrome may be beneficial (42,

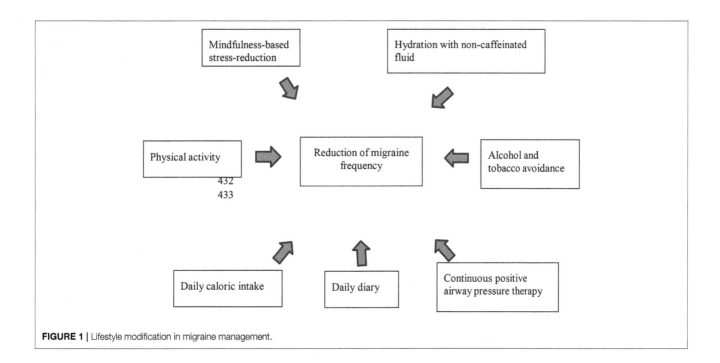

FIGURE 1 | Lifestyle modification in migraine management.

43). Neuroprotection, improvement in mitochondrial function, compensation for serotonergic dysfunction, decrement in CGRP levels, and suppression of neuroinflammation are the main mechanisms of action of these diets (42, 43). An epigenetic diet that can target DNA methylation, such as a folate-rich diet (44), modified Atkins, and Mediterranean diet, has also been reported (41). Some studies have demonstrated that migraine is more common when meals are skipped, particularly breakfast (45, 46). Thus, the standard advice for migraine sufferers is to take meals at regular intervals. In all cases, an appropriate diet selected by physicians and dietitians is recommended to ensure the psychosocial well-being of migraine sufferers.

Alcohol and Smoking

Alcohol is a trigger for migraine attacks in 75% of patients (47) through an inflammatory pathophysiologic mechanism (48). Other mechanisms may be involved, including vasodilatory effects, dehydration, toxicity, histamine, tyramine, sulfites, flavonoids, and 5-HT release (48). At this step, red wine is most indexed. However, all forms of alcohol may be trigger factors (49).

The pathogenesis of smoking or the use of nicotine in migraine onset is controversial and their action is direct on the central nervous system (50). Migraine attacks can be triggered by smoking (51). Particularly, if the total number of cigarettes smoked exceeds 5/day, it could subjectively precipitate a migraine attack (52). Among former smokers, smoking cessation is recommended (50).

Hydration

Headache is associated with fluid restriction and dehydration (53). A decrease in blood volume would result in poor oxygenation of the brain (54). Increased hydration status in migraine leads to a balanced plasma osmolality and ion concentrations and can improve migraine (55). The recommended amount of water intake is not well-known. In some studies, it varies from 1.8 to 4 L per day (56, 57). According to the Institute of Medicine, daily water intake is a function of age and gender and median total water intake for adults ranges from 2.7 to 3.7 L with extremes of 1.4 to 6.2, or 9–13 cups per day (58).

Caffeine and Migraine

Caffeine is an adenosine receptor antagonist with reversible effects on migraine. Its regular use is a risk factor for more frequent headaches. In addition, caffeine withdrawal can also induce headaches (59–61). There is a dose-dependent risk of headache, with a prevalence of 6.3 (62) to 14.5% (63).

Therefore, limiting caffeine consumption per day or discontinuation of caffeine consumption has been suggested.

Psychiatric Comorbidity

A stressful lifestyle is linked to both the onset of migraine attacks and weight gain. Anxiety and depression are psychiatric comorbidities and risk factors for migraine, with higher odds of anxiety than depression (64). Depression is a significant predictor of chronic migraine onset (OR = 1.65, 95% CI 1.12–2.45) with a depression-dose effect (9). They share a bidirectional relationship where major depression increases the risk of migraine and migraine increases the risk for major depression (65). Cognitive-behavioral therapy in individualized sessions or group sessions, either in person or online, improves mental status, impacts weight loss, and decreases migraine symptoms (66). Mindfulness-based stress-reduction programs can reduce pain intensity, headache frequency, and disability and improve self-efficacy and quality of life by encouraging pain acceptance (67, 68). In addition, relaxation techniques are used in migraine management, leading to progressive muscle relaxation and adequate deep breathing techniques (69). All these methods can be combined to reduce the morbidity of migraine.

Sleep Comorbidities

Lower quality of life, increased stress levels, and psychiatric comorbidities have been highlighted among migraine sufferers with sleep disorders (70). In addition, the risk of developing migraine in adults with sleep-related breathing disorders has increased (71). Poor sleep is a migraine trigger in which sleep apnea and insomnia are associated with migraine burden—symptoms that must be screened (72). Other common sleep disorders include short sleep duration, snoring, sleep-related breathing disorders, and restless leg syndrome (71, 73, 74). Insomnia prevalence among subjects with probable migraine is higher than in non-headache controls with a headache frequency. Similarly, Headache Impact Test-6 scores were also significantly higher in migraine sufferers with insomnia than in those without insomnia (75). Sleep is an effective treatment for migraine attacks (11) and there is a sleep hygiene benefit in chronic migraine, including keeping the bedroom quiet, dark, and cool; keeping the bed for sleep only; avoiding phones, tablets, or television in the bedroom; and having a regular bedtime (76, 77).

Insomnia can be managed by sleep and restriction of naps (78), while continuous positive airway pressure therapy for sleep apnea reduces the frequency of migraine (79).

Diary and Migraine Applications and Devices

A regular electronic diary of attacks is considered superior to a paper diary (80). Currently, there is a quartet of cellphone medication adherence apps (81). These can track triggers, duration, frequency, topography, type, and associated signs to better characterize migraine. Many apps and devices integrated into smartphones are currently available and provide an electronic daily diary for headaches (82), leading to better management of migraine and better adherence to treatment (83). In addition, thanks to the applications, patients stay connected with a community of other patients suffering from migraine, thereby improving their stress and low mood (84).

Drug overuse is a major risk factor for migraine chronicity and an increase in headache frequency (24). A daily headache diary can help the evaluation for acute migraine medication use and allow management or discontinuation of such drugs.

CONCLUSION

Migraine triggers are numerous. Lifestyle modifications and avoidance of triggers are essential in reducing the frequency and severity of migraine attacks. Managing obesity, alcohol, and tobacco consumption discontinuation, regular physical activity, sufficient hydration, and a healthy lifestyle are highly accessible and cost-efficient interventions for any patient with migraine. Nevertheless, large cohort follow-up studies on this population are warranted to obtain more information on environmental and lifestyle factors.

AUTHOR CONTRIBUTIONS

MA was involved in acquisition of data and drafted the manuscript for intellectual content. TA was involved in design and conceptualization of the study and final approval of the version to be published.

REFERENCES

Vos T, Abajobir AA, Abate KH, Abbafati C, Abbas KM, Abd-Allah F, et al. Global, regional, and national incidence, prevalence, and years lived with disability for 328 diseases and injuries for 195 countries, 1990–2016: a systematic analysis for the Global Burden of Disease Study 2016. *Lancet.* (2017) 390:1211–59.

Kyu HH, Abate D, Abate KH, Abay SM, Abbafati C, Abbasi N, et al. Global, regional, and national disability-adjusted life-years (DALYs) for 359 diseases and injuries and healthy life expectancy (HALE) for 195 countries and territories, 1990–2017: a systematic analysis for the Global Burden of Disease Study 2017. *Lancet.* (2018) 392:1859–922.

Shimizu T, Sakai F, Miyake H, Sone T, Sato M, Tanabe S, et al. Disability, quality of life, productivity impairment and employer costs of migraine in the workplace. *J Headache Pain.* (2021) 22:29. doi: 10.1186/s10194-021-01243-5

Stokes M, Becker WJ, Lipton RB, Sullivan SD, Wilcox TK, Wells L, et al. Cost of health care among patients with chronic and episodic migraine in canada and the usa: results from the international burden of migraine study (IBMS): July/August 2011. *Headache J Head Face Pain.* (2011) 51:1058– 77. doi: 10.1111/j.1526-4610.2011.01945.x

Munakata J, Hazard E, Serrano D, Klingman D, Rupnow MFT, Tierce J, et al. Economic burden of transformed migraine: results from the american migraine prevalence and prevention (AMPP) Study. *Headache J Head Face Pain.* (2009) 49:498–508. doi: 10.1111/j.1526-4610.2009.01369.x

Buse DC, Manack AN, Fanning KM, Serrano D, Reed ML, Turkel CC, et al. Chronic migraine prevalence, disability, and sociodemographic factors: results from the american migraine prevalence and prevention study. *Headache J Head Face Pain.* (2012) 52:1456–70. doi: 10.1111/j.1526-4610.2012.02223.x

Scher IA, Stewart FW, Ricci AJ, Lipton BR. Factors associated with the onset and remission of chronic daily headache in a population-based study. *Pain.* (2003) 106:81–9. doi: 10.1016/S0304-3959(03)00293-8

Fava A, Pirritano D, Consoli D, Plastino M, Casalinuovo F, Cristofaro S, et al. Chronic migraine in women is associated with insulin resistance: a cross-sectional study. *Eur J Neurol.* (2014) 21:267–72. doi: 10.1111/ene.12289

Ashina S, Serrano D, Lipton RB, Maizels M, Manack AN, Turkel CC, et al. Depression and risk of transformation of episodic to chronic migraine. *J Headache Pain.* (2012) 13:615–24. doi: 10.1007/s10194-012-0479-9

Robblee J, Starling AJ. SEEDS for success: Lifestyle management in migraine. *Cleve Clin J Med.* (2019) 86:741–9. doi: 10.3949/ccjm.86a.1 9009

Schwedt TJ. Preventive therapy of migraine: Contin lifelong. *Learn Neurol.* (2018) 24:1052–65. doi: 10.1212/CON.0000000000000635

Woldeamanuel YW, Cowan RP. The impact of regular lifestyle behavior in migraine: a prevalence case–referent study. *J Neurol.* (2016) 263:669– 76. doi: 10.1007/s00415-016-8031-5

Buse DC, Andrasik F. Behavioral medicine for migraine. *Neurol Clin.* (2009) 27:445–65. doi: 10.1016/j.ncl.2009.01.003

Andrasik F, Buse DC, Grazzi L. Behavioral medicine for migraine and medication overuse headache. *Curr Pain Headache Rep.* (2009) 13:241– 8. doi: 10.1007/s11916-009-0041-x

Adoukonou T, Agbetou M, Gahou A, Sossou CB, Houinato D. Migraine and obesity in parakou in 2017: case-control study. *Pain Stud Treat.* (2018) 6:15–23. doi: 10.4236/pst.2018.63003

Bigal ME, Lipton RB. Obesity is a risk factor for transformed migraine but not chronic tension- type headache. *Neurology.* (2006) 67:252– 7. doi: 10.1212/01.wnl.0000225052.35019.f9

Gelaye B, Sacco S, Brown WJ, Nitchie HL, Ornello R, Peterlin BL. Body composition status and the risk of migraine: a meta-analysis. *Neurology.* (2017) 88:1795–804. doi: 10.1212/WNL.0000000000003919

Ornello R, Ripa P, Pistoia F, Degan D, Tiseo C, Carolei A, et al. Migraine and body mass index categories: a systematic review and meta-analysis of observational studies. *J Headache Pain*. (2015) 16:27. doi: 10.1186/s10194-015-0510-z

Berilgen M, Bulut S, Gonen M, Tekatas A, Dag E, Mungen B. Comparison of the effects of amitriptyline and flunarizine on weight gain and serum leptin, c peptide and insulin levels when use das migraine preventive treatment. *Cephalalgia*. (2005) 25:1048–53. doi: 10.1111/j.1468-2982.2005.00956.x

Guldiken B, Guldiken S, Demir M, Turgut N, Tugrul A. Low leptin levels in migraine: a case control study. *Headache J Head Face Pain*. (2008) 48:1103– 7. doi: 10.1111/j.1526-4610.2008.01152.x

Biousse V, Bruce BB, Newman NJ. Update on the pathophysiology and management of idiopathic intracranial hypertension. *J Neurol Neurosurg Psychiatry*. (2012) 83:488–94. doi: 10.1136/jnnp-2011-302029

Tilg H, Moschen AR. Adipocytokines: mediators linking adipose tissue, inflammation and immunity. *Nat Rev Immunol*. (2006) 6:772–83. doi: 10.1038/nri1937

Recober A, Goadsby PJ. Calcitonin gene-related peptide: a molecular link between obesity and migraine? *Drug News Perspect*. (2010) 23:112. doi: 10.1358/dnp.2010.23.2.1475909

Bigal ME, Serrano D, Buse D, Scher A, Stewart WF, Lipton RB. Acute migraine medications and evolution from episodic to chronic migraine: a longitudinal population-based study. *Headache J Head Face Pain*. (2008) 48:1157–68. doi: 10.1111/j.1526-4610.2008.01217.x

Peterlin BL, Rapoport AM, Kurth T. Migraine and obesity: epidemiology, mechanisms, and implications. *Headache J Head Face Pain*. (2010) 50:631– 48. doi: 10.1111/j.1526-4610.2009.01554.x

Peterlin BL, Calhoun AH, Siegel S, Mathew NT. Rational combination therapy in refractory migraine. *Headache J Head Face Pain*. (2008) 48:805– 19. doi: 10.1111/j.1526-4610.2008.01142.x

Bond DS, Thomas JG, O'Leary KC, Lipton RB, Peterlin BL, Roth J, et al. Objectively measured physical activity in obese women with and without migraine. *Cephalalgia*. (2015) 35:886–93. doi: 10.1177/0333102414562970

Cervoni C, Bond DS, Seng EK. Behavioral weight loss treatments for individuals with migraine and obesity. *Curr Pain Headache Rep*. (2016) 20:13. doi: 10.1007/s11916-016-0540-5

Expert panel report: Guidelines (2013) for the management of overweight and obesity in adults: Guidelines (2013) for Managing Overweight and Obesity. *Obesity*. (2014) 22:S41–410. doi: 10.1002/oby.20660

U.S. Department of Health and Human Services. *Physical Activity Guidelines for Americans, 2nd Edn*. Washington, DC: U.S. Department of Health and Human Services (2018) Available online at: https://health.gov/sites/default/files/2019-09/Physical_Activity_Guidelines_2nd_edition.pdf

Varkey E, Cider Å, Carlsson J, Linde M. Exercise as migraine prophylaxis: a randomized study using relaxation and topiramate as controls. *Cephalalgia*. (2011) 31:1428–38. doi: 10.1177/0333102411419681

Irby MB, Bond DS, Lipton RB, Nicklas B, Houle TT, Penzien DB. Aerobic exercise for reducing migraine burden: mechanisms, markers, and models of change processes. *Headache J Head Face Pain*. (2016) 56:357– 69. doi: 10.1111/head.12738

Darabaneanu S, Overath CH, Rubin D, Lüthje S, Sye W, Niederberger U, et al. Aerobic exercise as a therapy option for migraine: a pilot study. *Int J Sports Med*. (2011) 32:455–60. doi: 10.1055/s-0030-1269928

Martin VT, Vij B. Diet and headache: part 1: headache. *Headache J Head Face Pain*. (2016) 56:1543–52. doi: 10.1111/head.12953

Zis P, Julian T, Hadjivassiliou M. Headache associated with coeliac disease: a systematic review and meta-analysis. *Nutrients*. (2018) 10:1445. doi: 10.3390/nu10101445

Mitchell N, Hewitt CE, Jayakody S, Islam M, Adamson J, Watt I, et al. Randomised controlled trial of food elimination diet based on IgG antibodies for the prevention of migraine like headaches. *Nutr J*. (2011) 10:85.doi:10.1186/1475-2891-10-85

Ferrara LA, Pacioni D, Di Fronzo V, Russo BF, Speranza E, Carlino V, et al. Low-lipid diet reduces frequency and severity of acute migraine attacks. *Nutr Metab Cardiovasc Dis*. (2015) 25:370–5. doi: 10.1016/j.numecd.2014.12.006

Gazerani P. Migraine and diet. *Nutrients*. (2020) 12:1658. doi: 10.3390/nu12061658

Evcili G. Early and long period follow-up results of low-glycemic index diet for migraine prophylaxis. *Agri - J Turk Soc Algol*. (2018) 30:8– 11. doi: 10.5505/agri.2017.62443

de Soares AA, Louçana PMC, Nasi EP, Sousa KM de H, Sá OM de S, Silva-Néto RP. A double- blind, randomized, and placebo-controlled clinical trial with omega-3 polyunsaturated fatty acids (OPFA ω-3) for the prevention of migraine in chronic migraine patients using amitriptyline. *Nutr Neurosci*. (2018) 21:219–23. doi: 10.1080/1028415X.2016.1266133

Razeghi Jahromi S, Ghorbani Z, Martelletti P, Lampl C, Togha M. Association of diet and headache. *J Headache Pain*. (2019) 20:106. doi: 10.1186/s10194-019-1057-1

Slavin M, Ailani J. A Clinical Approach to addressing diet with migraine patients. *Curr Neurol Neurosci Rep*. (2017) 17:17. doi: 10.1007/s11910-017-0721-6

Stanton AA. A comment on severe headache or migraine history is inversely correlated with dietary sodium intake: NHANES 1999–2004. *Headache J Head Face Pain*. (2016) 56:1214–5. doi: 10.1111/head.12861

Fila M, Chojnacki C, Chojnacki J, Blasiak J. Is an "Epigenetic Diet" for migraines justified? The case of folate and DNA methylation. *Nutrients*. (2019) 11:2763. doi: 10.3390/nu11112763

Nas A, Mirza N, Hägele F, Kahlhöfer J, Keller J, Rising R, et al. Impact of breakfast skipping compared with dinner skipping on regulation of energy balance and metabolic risk. *Am J Clin Nutr*. (2017) 105:1351– 61. doi: 10.3945/ajcn.116.151332

Abu-Salameh I, Plakht Y, Ifergane G. Migraine exacerbation during Ramadan fasting. *J Headache Pain*. (2010) 11:513–7. doi: 10.1007/s10194-010-0242-z

Dueland AN. Headache and alcohol. *Headache J Head Face Pain*. (2015) 55:1045–9. doi: 10.1111/head.12621

Panconesi A. Alcohol and migraine: trigger factor, consumption, mechanisms. A review. *J Headache Pain*. (2008) 9:19–27. doi: 10.1007/s10194-008-0006-1

Krymchantowski AV, da Cunha Jevoux C. Wine and headache. *Headache J Head Face Pain*. (2014) 54:967–75. doi: 10.1111/head.12365

Taylor FR. Tobacco, nicotine, and headache. *Headache J Head Face Pain*. (2015) 55:1028–44. doi: 10.1111/head.12620

Henry P, Auray JP, Gaudin AF, Dartigues JF, Duru G, Lantéri-Minet M, et al. Prevalence and clinical characteristics of migraine in France. *Neurology*. (2002) 59:232–7. doi: 10.1212/WNL.59.2.232

López-Mesonero L, Márquez S, Parra P, Gámez-Leyva G, Muñoz P, Pascual J. Smoking as a precipitating factor for migraine: a survey in medical students. *J Headache Pain*. (2009) 10:101–3. doi: 10.1007/s10194-009-0098-2

Blau JN. Water deprivation: a new migraine precipitant. *Headache J Head Face Pain*. (2005) 45:757–9. doi: 10.1111/j.1526-4610.2005.05143_3.x

Langdon R, DiSabella MT. Pediatric headache: an overview. *Curr Probl Pediatr Adolesc Health Care*. (2017) 47:44– 65. doi: 10.1016/j.cppeds.2017.01.002

Blau JN, Kell CA, Sperling JM. Water-deprivation headache: a new headache with two variants. *Headache J Head Face Pain*. (2004) 44:79– 83. doi: 10.1111/j.1526-4610.2004.04014.x

Spigt M, Weerkamp N, Troost J, van Schayck CP, Knottnerus JA. A randomized trial on the effects of regular water intake in patients with recurrent headaches. *Fam Pract*. (2012) 29:370– 5. doi: 10.1093/fampra/cmr112

Armstrong L, Johnson E. Water intake, water balance, and the elusive daily water requirement. *Nutrients*. (2018) 10:1928. doi: 10.3390/nu10121928

Panel on Dietary Reference Intakes for Electrolytes and Water Standing Committee on the Scientific Evaluation of Dietary Reference Intakes Food and Nutrition. *Board Dietary Reference Intakes for Water, Potassium, Sodium, Chloride, and Sulfate*. Washington, DC: National Academies Press (2005). 638. p.

Fried N, Elliott M, Oshinsky M. The Role of adenosine signaling in headache: a review. *Brain Sci*. (2017) 7:30. doi: 10.3390/brainsci7030030

Zaeem Z, Zhou L, Dilli E. Headaches: a review of the role of dietary factors. *Curr Neurol Neurosci Rep*. (2016) 16:101. doi: 10.1007/s11910-016-0702-1

Headache Classification Committee of the International Headache Society (IHS). *The International Classification of Headache Disorders, 3rd Edn*. Cephalalgia (2018) 38:1–211. doi: 10.1177/0333102417738202

Mollaoglu M. Trigger factors in migraine patients. *J Health Psychol*. (2013) 18:984–94. doi: 10.1177/1359105312446773

Fukui PT, Gonçalves TRT, Strabelli CG, Lucchino NMF, Matos FC, Santos JPM dos, et al. Trigger factors in migraine patients. *Arq Neuropsiquiatr*. (2008) 66:494–9. doi: 10.1590/S0004-282X2008000400011

Peres MFP, Mercante JPP, Tobo PR, Kamei H, Bigal ME. Anxiety and depression symptoms and migraine: a symptom-based approach research. *J Headache Pain*. (2017) 18:37. doi: 10.1186/s10194-017-0742-1

Breslau N, Lipton RB, Stewart WF, Schultz LR, Welch KMA. Comorbidity of migraine and depression: investigating potential etiology and prognosis. *Neurology*. (2003) 60:1308–12. doi: 10.1212/01.WNL.0000058907.41080.54

Sorbi MJ, Balk Y, Kleiboer AM, Couturier EG. Follow-up over 20 months confirms gains of online behavioural training in frequent episodic migraine. *Cephalalgia*. (2017) 37:236–50. doi: 10.1177/0333102416657145

Gu Q, Hou J-C, Fang X-M. Mindfulness meditation for primary headache pain: a meta-analysis. *Chin Med J*. (2018) 131:829– 38. doi: 10.4103/0366-6999.228242

Day MA, Thorn BE. The mediating role of pain acceptance during mindfulness-based cognitive therapy for headache. *Complement Ther Med*. (2016) 25:51–4. doi: 10.1016/j.ctim.2016.01.002

Williamson DA, Monguillot JE, Jarrell MP, Cohen RA, Pratt JM, Blouin DC. Relaxation for the treatment of headache: controlled evaluation of two group programs. *Behav Modif*. (1984) 8:407–24. doi: 10.1177/01454455840083007

Lund N, Westergaard ML, Barloese M, Glümer C, Jensen RH. Epidemiology of concurrent headache and sleep problems in Denmark. *Cephalalgia.* (2014) 34:833–45. doi: 10.1177/0333102414543332

Harnod T, Wang Y-C, Kao C-H. Association of migraine and sleep- related breathing disorder: a population-based cohort study. *Medicine.* (2015) 94:e1506. doi: 10.1097/MD.0000000000001506

Vgontzas A, Pavlović JM. Sleep disorders and migraine: review of literature and potential pathophysiology mechanisms. *Headache J Head Face Pain.* (2018) 58:1030–9. doi: 10.1111/head.13358

Kim J, Cho S-J, Kim W-J, Yang KI, Yun C-H, Chu MK. Insufficient sleep is prevalent among migraineurs: a population-based study. *J Headache Pain.* (2017) 18:50. doi: 10.1186/s10194-017-0756-8

Song T-J, Yun C-H, Cho S-J, Kim W-J, Yang KI, Chu MK. Short sleep duration and poor sleep quality among migraineurs: a population-based study. *Cephalalgia.* (2018) 38:855–64. doi: 10.1177/0333102417716936

Kim J, Cho S-J, Kim W-J, Yang KI, Yun C-H, Chu MK. Insomnia in probable migraine: a population-based study. *J Headache Pain.* (2016) 17:92. doi: 10.1186/s10194-016-0681-2

Calhoun AH, Ford S, Finkel AG, Kahn KA, Mann JD. The prevalence and spectrum of sleep problems in women with transformed migraine. *Headache J Head Face Pain.* (2006) 46:604–10. doi: 10.1111/j.1526-4610.2006.00410.x

Calhoun AH, Ford S. Behavioral sleep modification may revert transformed migraine to episodic migraine. *Headache J Head Face Pain.* (2007) 47:1178– 83. doi: 10.1111/j.1526-4610.2007.00780.x

Rains JC. Optimizing circadian cycles and behavioral insomnia treatment in migraine. *Curr Pain Headache Rep.* (2008) 12:213– 9. doi: 10.1007/s11916-008-0037-y

Smitherman TA, Walters AB, Davis RE, Ambrose CE, Roland M, Houle TT, et al. Randomized controlled pilot trial of behavioral insomnia treatment for chronic migraine with comorbid insomnia: randomized controlled pilot trial. *Headache J Head Face Pain.* (2016) 56:276–91. doi: 10.1111/head. 12760

Stone AA, Shiffman S, Schwartz JE, Broderick JE, Hufford MR. Patient compliance with paper and electronic diaries. *Control Clin Trials.* (2003) 24:182–99. doi: 10.1016/S0197-2456(02)00320-3

Park JYE, Li J, Howren A, Tsao NW, De Vera M. Mobile phone apps targeting medication adherence: quality assessment and content analysis of user reviews. *JMIR MHealth UHealth.* (2019) 7:e11919. doi: 10.2196/11919

Hundert AS, Huguet A, McGrath PJ, Stinson JN, Wheaton M. Commercially available mobile phone headache diary apps: a systematic review. *JMIR MHealth UHealth.* (2014) 2:e36. doi: 10.2196/mhealth.3452

Ramsey RR, Holbein CE, Powers SW, Hershey AD, Kabbouche MA, O'Brien HL, et al. A pilot investigation of a mobile phone application and progressive reminder system to improve adherence to daily prevention treatment in adolescents and young adults with migraine. *Cephalalgia.* (2018) 38:2035– 44. doi: 10.1177/0333102418756864

Minen MT, Jalloh A, Ortega E, Powers SW, Sevick MA, Lipton RB. User design and experience preferences in a novel smartphone application for migraine management: a think aloud study of the relaxahead application. *Pain Med.* (2019) 20:369–77. doi: 10.1093/pm/pny080

21

Type D Personality, Stress Level, Life Satisfaction and Alcohol Dependence in Older Men

Grzegorz Bejda[1], Agnieszka Kułak-Bejda[2*], Napoleon Waszkiewicz[2] and
Elzbieta Krajewska-Kułak[3]

[1] The School of Medical Science in Białystok, Białystok, Poland, [2] Department of Psychiatry, Medical University of Białystok,
Białystok, Poland, [3] Department of Integrated Medical Care, Medical University of Białystok, Białystok, Poland

*Correspondence:
Agnieszka Kułak-Bejda
agnieszka.kulak.bejda@gmail.com

Alcohol consumption among older adults is becoming an increasing public health problem due to the rapidly growing elderly population. There is a theory that Type D personality is positively correlated with alcohol dependence. The study aimed to assess the style of coping with stress, emotions and anxiety in elder men addicted to alcohol and the relationship between the above. The study included 170 men aged 60 years and older (mean age - 63 ± 3.1 years) addicted to alcohol staying in the Department of Alcohol Addiction Therapy for Men. They were tested with the questionnaire sheet and the following scales: Perceived Family Wealth (PFW), Family Affluence Scale (FAS), Cantril's Ladder of Life Scale, Satisfaction with Life Scale, Type D Personality Scale-14 (DS14), and the 10-item Perceived Stress Scale (PSS-10). The respondents' wealth on a scale of 1–5 points was assessed on avg. 3.1 ± 0.2. The above was confirmed by the results of the FAS scale study, where the respondents obtained an average of 3.9 ± 1.9 (min. 1, max. 8), which proves their average level of affluence. The evaluation of the satisfaction with life using Cantril's Ladder showed that the respondents were also satisfied with life on average (on average 5.5 ± 1.9). The assessment of life satisfaction using the Satisfaction with Life Scale (SWLS) scale allowed for the conclusion that the respondents were very dissatisfied with their lives (mean 17.2 ± 4.9). The evaluation of the measurement of perceived stress (PSS-10 scale) showed that the respondents obtained an average of 23.5 ± 3.7, and on the sten scale, a mean of 7.7 ± 0.98, which proves a high level of perceived stress. The study using the DS14 scale showed that the respondents were in the negative emotionality (NE) subscale - 17.4 ± 4.5 points, and in the HS scale - 16.2 ± 3.2, which proves that they can be classified as a Type D personality. The participants were very dissatisfied with their lives, with a high perceived stress and Type D personality.

Keywords: elderly, alcohol dependence, stress, life satisfaction, personality

INTRODUCTION

Alcoholism, as a multidimensional phenomenon, can be considered in interdisciplinary categories, i.e., on the physiological, medical, psychiatric, psychological and social levels, due to both its specific conditions and specific consequences.

It should be emphasized that alcohol addiction becomes a social and medical problem in the case of older adults (1). The risk of developing alcohol problems does not decrease with age. Unfortunately, there are cases of medical misdiagnosis that attribute the effects of alcohol to the aging process, e.g., cognitive impairment, malnutrition and unsteady gait (1).

Alcohol use disorder (AUD) has been associated with neurodegenerative diseases such as Alzheimer's and Parkinson's disease (2). Prolonged excessive alcohol intake contributes to increased production of reactive oxygen species that trigger neuroimmune response and cellular apoptosis and necrosis *via* lipid peroxidation, mitochondrial, protein and DNA damage. In addition, long-term binge alcohol consumption upregulates the glutamate receptors, glucocorticoids. It reduces the reuptake of glutamate in the central nervous system, resulting in glutamate excitotoxicity and eventually mitochondrial injury and cell death.

In this review, we delineate the following principles in alcohol-induced neurodegeneration: (1) alcohol-induced oxidative stress; (2) neuroimmune response toward increased oxidants and lipopolysaccharide; (3) glutamate excitotoxicity and cell injury; (4) interplay between oxidative stress, neuroimmune response and excitotoxicity leading to neurodegeneration; and (5) potential chronic alcohol intake-induced development of neurodegenerative diseases, including Alzheimer's and Parkinson's disease.

The literature on the subject emphasizes that alcohol is the drug most often chosen by older adults, although the frequency of its consumption decreases with age. It should be remembered that the consumption of alcoholic beverages among people of post-working age is hazardous due to the more severe health consequences of drinking in this group than in younger people. High alcohol levels in the body last longer because these individuals experience a decline in muscle mass and increased body fat. Drinking large amounts of alcohol contributes to osteoporosis, liver cirrhosis, atherosclerosis and heart attack, neurological disorders and breast cancer. Also, alcohol consumption is hazardous among people who take medications or suffer from chronic diseases. Unfortunately, chronic, progressive disease, common in seniors, and the inability to accept it, may be an additional cause of addiction (3–5).

Reasons for reaching for alcoholic beverages may also be problems resulting from the aging process, dependence on other people, low social and economic status and loss of a close family member. People with problems of old age start drinking alcohol most often after reaching the age of 65, and the symptoms of intoxication are masked by the environment (5).

Gerstenkorn and Suwała (6) report that half of the seniors had exposure to alcohol in the year prior to their research to varying degrees. Karakiewicz et al. (7) emphasizes that 25% of men over 65 with heart disease drink up to four glasses of vodka a day.

Dabrowska and Wieczorek (8), in the "Report on the implementation of the study: Analysis of risk factors and factors protecting the use of psychoactive substances among seniors," showed, for example, that the compulsion to drink the next day after drinking alcohol affected 7.5% of their respondents. The percentage of seniors who drank a lot (15%) was comparable to the results of American research. Lehmann and Fingerhood (9) found that 14.5% of Americans aged 65 and over consumed more alcohol than the local "safety" standards (a maximum of three drinks per day and a maximum of seven per week counted in standard alcohol portions).

There are many tools for measuring personality types. One example is the Structure of Temperament Questionnaire (STQ). It was developed by Rusalov within an experimental tradition for studying properties of nervous systems. Using human subjects, Rusalov measured multiple behavioral and psycho-physiological indices, including EEGs and evoked potentials. This resulted in the first activity-specific model of temperament separating physical-motor and social-verbal traits of temperament (10). The Functional Ensemble of Temperament (FET) model was created based on this researcher's tool. It contains links to many neurochemical systems (neurochemistry and neuropharmacology) and uses double-word names of the scales (motor-physical or social-verbal) (10). The concept of affective temperament was also created. This temperament style is characterized by one or more of five main affective dimensions: anxious, irritable, cyclothymic, hyperthymic and depressive (11).

Some authors suggest that one important predictor of treatment outcome, e.g., in depression, is affective experience, specifically the experience of positive affect (PA) and negative affect (NA). PA and NA are two distinct and relatively independent dimensions. They show a moderate correlation between them (12). On the other hand, the five-factor model of personality, created by Costa and McCrae, is a hierarchical organization of personality traits in terms of five basic dimensions: extraversion, agreeableness, conscientiousness, neuroticism and openness to experience (13).

The Temperament and Character Inventory is an objective questionnaire that assesses a seven-factor psychobiologic model of quantifiable personality traits. It has been validated based on various genetic and neurobiological data. Its four temperament dimensions—harm avoidance, novelty-seeking, reward dependence and persistence—are rooted primarily in various neurobiological data. Further, the three character dimensions—self-directedness, cooperativeness and self-transcendence—develop based on social learning (14).

Cox and Klinger believed that personality influences alcohol addiction through specific motives that prompt individuals to drink (15).

However, with regard to people with alcohol addiction, some researches have found the link between personality type D and addiction (16, 17). This stress-prone personality is characterized by negative affect and social inhibition. People with the personality type D experience negative emotions in various situations and inhibit their expression (16). Type D personality is stable across time and has a substantial underlying genetic component (18), and established cross-cultural measurement equivalence (19). The type D personality is a vulnerability factor for future episodes of emotional stress such as depressive episodes, anxiety and addiction to alcohol (16, 17, 20, 21).

In a cross-sectional study, 862 participants (mean age 26.1 years) completed the Type D Personality Scale, Drinking Motives Questionnaire and Severity of Alcohol Dependence Questionnaire; Type D personality was positively correlated with alcohol dependence. Furthermore, this relationship was mediated by coping and conformity drinking motives (16). Williams et al. (17) studied whether Type D personality was associated with higher levels of alcohol use in a group of 138 young participants (mean age 31.8 years). Their results report that Type D was associated with higher levels of alcohol use, stress and desire for alcohol at stressor and recovery.

The present study aimed to assess the style of coping with stress, emotions and anxiety in elder men addicted to alcohol and the relationship between the above. Furthermore, the correlation of Type D personality with alcohol dependence was assessed.

The following research questions were formulated:

- Are people addicted to alcohol satisfied with their lives?
- What level of stress do they feel?
- Do they present Type D personality? People with negative emotionality, social withdrawal, prone to experiencing strong emotions (fear, anger, hostility or irritation), tend to avoid social contact for fear of lack of approval, with a tendency not to manifest their emotions and behavior.
- Is there a statistically significant relationship between the age of the respondents and life satisfaction, having a Type D personality and the stress level presented?

MATERIALS AND METHODS

Study Group

One hundred seventy men aged 60–68 years (mean age - 63 ± 3.1 years), mostly from a rural environment (78%), participated in the study. Twenty-two percentage of respondents lived in the city. The respondents had primary education (23%), vocational (45%), secondary (22%), or higher (10%). The respondents' wealth on a scale of 1–5 points was 3.1 ± 0.2. The above was confirmed by the results of the FAS scale study, where the respondents obtained an average of 3.9 ± 1.9 (min. 1, max. 8), which proves their average level of affluence.

Study Design

A cross-sectional study was conducted from 2017 to 2020 in patients treated for alcohol addiction in the Alcohol Addiction Therapy Department for Men. Apart from age and 2 weeks abstinence from alcohol before admission to the Department, an additional inclusion criterion was the consent to participate in the study. Mental and physical condition at the admission to the department was assessed. It was satisfactory with no signs of active disease. The exclusion criteria were: (1) age under 60; (2) lack of literacy skills (a respondent who completed at least primary school could have participated in the survey); and (3) refusal to participate in the study. Each participant could withdraw from the study at any time. The completion rate was 100%, as the respondents completed the questionnaires during their stay in the Alcohol Addiction Therapy Department for Men.

The research was conducted with approval of the Local Ethical Committee of the Medical University of Bialystok.

Research Tools

The study was conducted using a self-questionnaire consisting of a part supplemented by the authors and a part supplemented by the respondent. In addition, Cantril's Ladder (self-anchoring scale) and standardized questionnaires: Family Affluence Scale (FAS), the Satisfaction with Life Scale (SWLS), Perceived Stress Scale (PSS10), and DS-14 scale were used to assess Type D personality.

FAS was used to assess the material resources of the respondent's family (22). Four questions form the basis of FAS: Does your family have a car or a multi-person car (van)? - response categories: no; yes one; yes, two or more; Do you have your room for your use? Response categories: no, yes. How many times in the last 12 months have you taken your family away from home for holidays or holidays? Response categories: I did not travel at all, once, two times, more than two times; and How many computers does your family have? Response categories: none, one, two, more. The FAS scale ranges from 0 to 7 points. For this study, it was divided into four ranges: 0–1 points (extremely poor families); 2–3 points (relatively poor); 4–5 points (average wealth); 6–7 points (wealthy families) (22).

The Satisfaction with Life Scale (SWLS) is five statements participants may agree or disagree with. Instructions are as follows: Using the 1–7 scale below, indicate your agreement with each item by placing the appropriate number on the line preceding that item. Please be open and honest in responding: 7—Strongly agree; 6—Agree; 5—Slightly agree; 4—Neither agree nor disagree; 3—Slightly disagree; 2—Disagree; 1—Strongly disagree (23). The scores obtained were summed up, and the overall result was the participant's degree of satisfaction with his own life. The range of results could be from 5 to 35 points; the higher the score, the greater the sense of satisfaction with life: 31–35 points—extremely satisfied; 26–30 points—satisfied; 21–25 points—slightly satisfied; 20 points—neutral; 15–19 points—slightly dissatisfied; 10–14 points—dissatisfied; 5–9 points—extremely dissatisfied. In the interpretation of the result, the properties characterizing the sten scale were also applied. Results in the ranges 1–4 of the sten were treated as low; 7–10 as high; and 5 and 6 as average. The reliability index (Cronbach's alpha) of SWLS is 0.81. The scale stability index, determined in the double study of 30 people with an interval of 6 weeks, was 0.86 (23).

Cantril's Ladder (self-anchoring scale) has a graphical form of a ladder, with steps marked with consecutive numbers from 0 to 10. Next to the ladder, a text explains that the top (10) is the best life there can be, and the bottom (0) is the worst life (24, 25). The respondent is to decide what his life is like at the moment and put an X in the appropriate place on the ladder. It is assumed that 0–5 points are obtained by people dissatisfied with their life; 6–8 points—average satisfaction; 9–10 points—very satisfied (24, 25).

The PSS10 contains 10 questions about various subjective feelings related to personal problems and events, behaviors and ways of coping (23). The respondents answered by entering the

TABLE 1 | Assessment of life satisfaction of the respondents assessed using the SWLS scale.

	Strongly agree	Agree	Slightly agree	Neither agree nor disagree	Slightly disagree	Disagree	Strongly disagree
In most ways, my life is close to my ideal			11.8%	11.8%	41.2%	11.8%	23.4%
The conditions of my life are excellent	17.6%	29.4%	17.6%	17.6%	11.9%	5.9%	
I am satisfied with my life	11.8%	29.4%	17.6%	17.6%	11.8%	11.8%	
So far I have gotten the important things I want in life	5.9%	17.6%	41.2%	29.4%	5.9%		
If I could live my life over. I would change almost nothing			17.6%	11.8%	17.6%	29.4%	23.6%

correct number (0—never, 1—rarely, 2—sometimes, 3—quite often, 4—very usually). The overall score is the sum of all points, with a theoretical distribution from 0 to 40. The higher the score, the greater the severity of the perceived stress. The overall index after conversion to standardized units is interpreted according to the properties characterizing the sten scale. Scores in the range 1–4 sten are treated as low, 7–10 sten as high and 5–6 sten as average (23).

The DS-14 scale to assess Type D personality - an adaptation by Ogińska-Bulik et al. (26) of the Type D Personality Scale (DS14) by Johan Denollet (27), was used for the measurement of distressed personality. The scale includes 14 statements; seven refer to negative emotionality (NE) and seven to social inhibition (HS). The examined person responds to the given statements using a five-point scale (0—false to 4—true). To qualify for Type D, the respondent must obtain at least 10 points in both dimensions. The opposite of Type D is non-D (both sizes result below 10 points).

Statistical Analysis

Statistical analysis of data was conducted using Statistica® version 13.3. We used descriptive statistics such as percentage calculation of results, arithmetic mean, standard deviation, tabular and graphical representation of data.

RESULTS

The study included 170 men treated in the Alcohol Addiction Therapy Department for Men. The longest duration of alcohol consumption was 35 years, the shortest-15 years (24.3 ± 14.2 years). The therapy lasted from 1 to 7 weeks (3.5 ± 2.1 weeks).

The subjects used Cantril's Ladder to decide what their life was like at the examination time. The respondents obtained an average of 5.5 ± 1.9 points. The respondents most often marked 5 points (47.1%) and least frequently marked 9.8, and 4 (5.6%). The results obtained indicate that the respondents were, on average satisfied with their lives.

According to the SWLS scale, the respondents were very dissatisfied with their lives (17.2 ± 4.9). Detailed results are presented in **Table 1**. In the group dissatisfied with their lives, 5.9%, very dissatisfied with their lives—17.6%, rather dissatisfied

with their lives—41.2%, neither satisfied nor dissatisfied with their lives—5.9% and somewhat satisfied with their lives—29.4%.

There was no significant correlation between the age of the respondents and life satisfaction ($p = 0.36339$), having a Type D personality, age ($p = 0.20274$) and wealth ($p = 1.000$). Significant correlations between age and stress level ($p = 0.00524$) and between affluence and life satisfaction ($p = 0.00077$) and level of stress ($p < 0.001$) were found. Detailed results are presented in **Tables 2**, **3**.

DISCUSSION

The study aimed to assess the style of coping with stress, emotions, and anxiety, Type D personality in elder men addicted to alcohol, and the relationship between the above.

The participants were very dissatisfied with their lives, with a high level of perceived stress and Type D personality. There was no significant relationship between the respondents' age and life satisfaction or respondents' age, having a Type D personality, and wealth. However, there was a correlation between age and level of stress and wealth, life satisfaction and stress level.

It is estimated that 2.3 billion people worldwide drink alcohol today. In terms of average consumption per capita, Europe is the leader, even though alcohol consumption has fallen by more than 10% since 2010. According to WHO, global alcohol consumption will increase in the next 10 years, especially in Southeast Asia, the Western Pacific and the Americas. Europeans and Americans drink the most alcohol, averaging 9.8 and 8 L of pure ethyl alcohol per day, respectively (28). In 2019, among men, respondents aged 45–54 used alcohol most often; in this group, it is practically common at 99%, and 83% in people over 65. Vodka was used by 22% of people aged 55–64 and 26% of people over 65. Seventy-three percentage of people over 65 used alcohol more often with their family than with friends (29).

It is worth emphasizing that alcohol abuse among seniors does not always have to refer to the stereotypical consumption of alcohol during loud feasts, and sometimes it may refer to drinking one's favorite beer before bedtime or a large glass of wine every evening (28, 29). The problem begins when alcohol becomes a habit, and a person cannot imagine a day without it. Unfortunately, in recent times, the context

TABLE 2 | Assessment of the perceived stress using the PSS-10 scale.

	Never	Almost never	Sometimes	Fairly often	Very often
In the last month, how often have you been upset because of something that happened unexpectedly?			58.8%	23.5%	17.7%
In the last month. how often have you felt that you were unable to control the important things in your life?		23.5%	17.6%	41.1%	17.8%
In the last month. how often have you felt nervous and "stressed"?		10.9%	17.1%	47.1%	24.9%
In the last month. how often have you felt confident about your ability to handle your personal problems?	33.5%	17.6%	24.7%	24.2%	
In the last month. how often have you felt that things were going your way?	16.8%	24.4%	23.5%	35.3%	
In the last month. how often have you found that you could not cope with all the things that you had to do?	5.9%	10.9%	24.4%	41.2%	17.6%
In the last month. how often have you been able to control irritations in your life?	5.9%	17.6%	35.3%	41.2%	
In the last month. how often have you felt that you were on top of things?	17.7%	17.6%	52.9%	5.9%	5.9%
In the last month. how often have you been angered because of things that were outside of your control?		11.8%	24.9%	46.2%	17.1%
In the last month. how often have you felt difficulties were piling up so high that you could not overcome them?	5.8%	5.9%	41.2%	35.3%	11.8%

TABLE 3 | Type D personality in the study group.

	False	Rather false	Neutral	Rather true	True
I make contact easily when I meet people		11.8%	23.5%	41.2%	23.5%
I often make a fuss about unimportant things		11.8%	23.5%	24.9%	39.8%
I often feel unhappy	5.9%	23.5%	17.6%	24.9%	28.1%
I am often irritated	5.9%	17.6%	23.5%	35.3%	17.7%
I often feel inhibited in social interactions		17.6%	23.5%	41.3%	17.6%
I take a gloomy view of things	5.9%	11.8%	23.5%	35.3%	23.5%
I find it hard to start a conversation	5.9%	24.9%	24.9%	24.9%	19.4%
I am often in a bad mood	5.9%	11.8%	24.9%	24.9%	32.5%
I am a closed kind of person	5.9%	35.3%	24.9%	17.6%	16.3%
I would rather keep other people at a distance	5.9%	17.6%	5.9%	58.8%	11.8%
I often find myself worrying about something	5.9%	23.5%	5.9%	41.2%	23.5%
I am often down in the dumps		35.3%	17.6%	24.9%	22.2%
When socializing. I don't find the right things to talk about above		35.3%	23.5%	20.4%	20.8%

of alcohol use and aging is a common phenomenon, both among men and women. Such alcohol consumption causes irreversible changes and damage to internal organs and consequently, reduces the life expectancy and condition of the senior's body drastically. Excessive alcohol consumption causes individuals to neglect daily duties, including, for example, missing regular visits to the doctor and not carrying out tests. Addicts often ignore the disease symptoms and do not care about their health until it is, unfortunately, too late to start treatment. Furthermore, hyperkatifeia is very interesting fenomenon. It is defined as the negative emotional state of drug withdrawal. It drives the negative reinforcement source of motivation for compulsive-like alcohol seeking and using. Moreover, hyperkatifeia can drive impulsivity like relapse in the preoccupation or anticipation stage and then a return to the binge or intoxication stage (30).

Data from the UK (31) summarizing hospital admissions related to alcohol abuse indicate that among the 337,110 people admitted, 56,240 were aged 64–75, and 43,910 were over 75 years of age. Thus, the cited data confirm a relatively large percentage of seniors in this group.

In a Polish study (5) that included 110 older adults living in Lubelskie Voivodeship, Poland, most seniors (83.6%) used alcohol occasionally. In this study, alcohol consumption was more common among older adults from rural rather than urban environments, and the majority of alcohol drinkers had primary education and were single. Indeed, the low level of education implies minor criticism of the older adults in relation to the advice given to them by other people. Also, in the present study, the majority of respondents came from the country.

In the study conducted by Wadd and Papadopoulos (32), older adults experienced high levels of alcohol-related harm but drink less than younger adults, and levels of alcohol-related harm in older adults are increasing. Similar findings were described in a US study (33), where single people (without support from family members, divorced, widowed) were more likely to seek consolation through drinking alcohol.

Researchers studying with alcohol addiction have long been looking for factors that may play an essential role in the genesis of addiction and the course of treatment (34). Only a small number articles have been published on the life satisfaction and quality of life of alcohol addicts.

In the analysis of life satisfaction of the elderly population in the example of Sweden, Austria and Germany, the author found that aging does not necessarily worsen one's perception of life. Based on the data shown here, there is no evidence from Austria and Spain that all people systematically, regardless of the year of birth, go through a stage of a lower level of life satisfaction. An important factor of life satisfaction is health self-assessment (35).

Data from the literature indicate the coexistence of anxiety, depressive disorders, somatization and phobias to a greater extent in women addicted to alcohol than in men. Also, the role of fear, optimism, self-efficacy and life satisfaction was studied (34). People also see alcohol as a way to cope with economic stress, stress at work and marital problems, often due to a lack of social support (36). Whether an individual will drink under stress depends on many factors, including genetics, the individual's drinking behavior, type of stressor, personal sense of control stress and the range of stress coping methods (36–39).

Some researchers believe that high levels of stress impact alcohol consumption when there are no alternative resources; when alcohol is available, the person believes alcohol will help reduce stress (36–39). This is confirmed by the current study, which shows that those respondents had a high level of perceived stress.

However, according to Pohorecky (36), whether people drink under stress beyond their control is not obvious. In his review of research on the relationship between alcohol consumption and stress, Pohorecky took into account several studies that examined people living in areas affected by a natural disaster. One study found a 30% increase in alcohol consumption in the 2 years following the Buffalo Creek floods in West Virginia. Similar increases were recorded in cities near Mount St. Helens after a volcanic eruption (35). However, after the Three Mile Island nuclear power plant disaster, alcohol was rarely used to deal with stress (39). Some studies show that drinking can occur when stress is anticipated or experienced (40).

It is also worth remembering that, in non-drinking people addicted to alcohol, personally threatening, severe and chronic life stressors can lead to alcohol relapse (37, 41). Brown (41) conducted a study on a group of men who discontinued inpatient therapy and then experienced acute and chronic psychosocial stress. The researchers found that patients who relapsed experienced acute and chronic stress twice as often before returning to drinking as those who continued abstinence.

The authors believe that while many factors contribute to the resumption of drinking, stress may have the most significant impact on the first alcohol consumption after a period of abstinence (42).

Research on the personality types of people addicted to alcohol and attempts to create a uniform personality profile has not yielded unequivocal results. Therefore, Cloninger et al. (43) investigated the inheritance of personality traits in susceptibility to alcohol addiction. In their prospective, longitudinal study, three dimensions of personality that could be a harbinger of a later addiction were distinguished: seeking novelty and impressions, avoiding unpleasantness and dependence of behavior on reward, but these features were not correlated with each other.

It is well-known that certain personality traits are associated with alcohol use (44). Because less is known about these traits, we wished to investigate whether changes in alcohol use were longitudinally associated with personality changes and in which direction the influence or causation might flow. Data came from the self-reported questionnaire answers of 5,125 young men at two time points during the Cohort Study on Substance Use Risk Factors (C-SURF). Their average ages were 20.0 and 25.4 years old at the first and second wave assessments, respectively. Four personality traits were measured: (a) aggression–hostility; (b) sociability; (c) neuroticism-anxiety; and (d) sensation-seeking. Alcohol use was measured by volume (drinks per week) and binge drinking (about 60+ g per occasion). Cross-lagged panel models and two-wave latent change score models were used. Aggression-hostility, sensation-seeking and sociability were significantly and positively cross-sectionally associated with both alcohol use variables. Drinking volume and these three personality traits bidirectionally predicted each other. Binge drinking was associated with sensation-seeking only, whereas aggression-hostility and sociability only predicted binge drinking, but not vice versa. Changes in alcohol use were significantly positively related to differences in aggression-hostility, sensation-seeking and sociability. Associations reached small Cohen's effect sizes for sociability and sensation-seeking, but not for aggression-hostility. Associations with neuroticism-anxiety were mainly not significant. The direction of effects confirmed findings from other studies, and the association between changes in personality and alcohol use supports the idea that prevention programs should simultaneously target both.

In the present study, we tried to assess whether the study participants addicted to alcohol belong to Type D personality, i.e., tend to feel negative emotions (negative emotionality), e.g., anger, fear, have a pessimistic approach to life, constantly feel tension, worry, feel insecure, are withdrawn in social relationships (social inhibition), and are reluctant to show negative emotions due to fear of rejection.

Our current study has some potential limitations. First, the study group was too small to generalize the results to Poland's entire population of drinking seniors. The study concerned only men, so it is worth verifying the results in other studies in an equally large group of women. It is known that alcohol consumption among women differs from that among men.

Women have different prognostic factors for alcohol abuse than men. Intoxication occurs in women after drinking less alcohol; chronic alcohol abuse causes more deaths in women; and alcohol has a more harmful effect on women's health than in men.

Despite these limitations, the results of this study may constitute a starting point for further research into the problems of older people addicted to alcohol. Optimally, these findings should be verified in a longitudinal examination and extended to a control group.

CONCLUSIONS

The men surveyed were very dissatisfied with their lives, had a high level of perceived stress and displayed personality traits of Type D. No significant relationships were found between the age of the respondents and life satisfaction and their wealth and having a Type D personality. Significant associations between age

and the level of stress and affluence and the level of stress and life satisfaction were found.

ETHICS STATEMENT

The studies involving human participants were reviewed and approved by the Local Ethical Committee of the Medical University of Bialystok. The patients/participants provided their written informed consent to participate in this study.

AUTHOR CONTRIBUTIONS

GB created the research concept. AK-B and GB were collecting materials to the study and prepared the initial version of the manuscript, which was corrected, supervised, and completed by NW and EK-K. EK-K conducted data analysis. All authors contributed to the article and approved the submitted version.

REFERENCES

Bronowski P, Sawicka M. Kluczyńska S. Prevalence of using alcohol among general hospitals patients at the age over 60. *Gerontologia Polska.* (2011) 19:47– 52.

Kamal H, Tan GC, Ibrahim SF, Shaikh MF, Mohamed IN, Mohamed R, et al. Alcohol use disorder, neurodegeneration, Alzheimer's and Parkinson's disease: interplay between oxidative stress, neuroimmune response and excitotoxicity. *Front Cell Neurosci.* (2020) 14:282. doi: 10.3389/fncel.2020.00282

Barret P, Vogel-Sprott M. Age, drinking habits and the effects of alcohol. *J Stud Alcohol Drugs.* (1984) 45:517–21. doi: 10.15288/jsa.1984.45.517

Ross S. Alcohol use disorders in the elderly. *Psychiatria po Dyplomie.* (2005) 4:17–28. doi: 10.5281/zenodo.55179

Bartoszek A, Kocka K, Zielonka E, Łuczyk M, Rzaca M, Deluga A, et al. The problem of the use of drugs among seniors living in the home environment. *J Educ Health Sport.* (2016) 6:235–44.

Gerstenkor A, Suwała M. Smoking and drinking alcohol in the metropolitan elderly population. *Psychogeriatria Polska.* (2006) 4:191–200.

Karakiewicz B, Kozielec T, Późniak J, Sałacka A. Selected health behaviors of elderly patients under the care of family doctors and cardiovascular diseases. *Polska Medycyna Rodzinna.* (2000) 2:159–61.

Dabrowska K, Wieczorek Ł. Report on the implementation of the study: analysis of risk factors and factors protecting the use of psychoactive substances among seniors. *Inst Psychiatr Neurol.* (2018).

Lehmann SW. Fingerhood M. Substance-use disorders in later life. *N Engl J Med.* (2018) 79:2351–60. doi: 10.1056/NEJMra1805981

Trofimova IN, Sulis W. A study of the coupling of FET temperament traits with major depression. *Front Psychol.* (2016) 7:1848. doi: 10.3389/fpsyg.2016.01848

Russo M, Mahon K, Shanahan M, Ramjas E, Solon C, Braga RJ, et al. Affective temperaments and neurocognitive functioning in bipolar disorder. *J Affect Disord.* (2014) 169:51–6. doi: 10.1016/j.jad.2014.07.038

Oren-Yagoda R, Björgvinsson T, Aderka IM. The relationship between positive affect and negative affect during treatment for major depressive disorder. *Psychother Res.* (2018) 28:958–68. doi: 10.1080/10503307.2017.1292066

McCrae RR, John OP. An introduction to the five-factor model and its applications. *J Pers.* (1992) 60:175–215. doi: 10.1111/j.1467-6494.1992.tb00970.x

Siddiqi SH, Chockalingam R, Cloninger CR, Lenze EJ, Cristancho P. Use of the temperament and character inventory to predict response to repetitive transcranial magnetic stimulation for major depression. *J Psychiatr Pract.* (2016) 22:193–202. doi: 10.1097/PRA.0000000000000150

Cox WM, Klinger E. A motivational model of alcohol use. *J Abnorm Psychol.* (1988) 97:168–80. doi: 10.1037/0021-843X.97.2.168

Bruce G, Curren C, Williams L. Type D personality, alcohol dependence, and drinking motives in the general population. *J Stud Alcohol Drugs.* (2013) 74:120–4. doi: 10.15288/jsad.2013.74.120

Williams L, Bruce G, Knapton C. Type D personality is associated with increased desire for alcohol in response to acute stress. *Stress Health.* (2018) 34:411–5. doi: 10.1002/smi.2800

Kupper N, Boomsma DI, de Geus EJ, Denollet J, Willemsen G. Nine-year stability

of type D personality: contributions of genes and environment. *Psychosom Med.* (2011) 73:75–82. doi: 10.1097/PSY.0b013e3181fdce54

Kupper N, Pedersen SS, Höfer S, Saner H, Oldridge N, Denollet J. Cross-cultural analysis of type D (distressed) personality in 6222 patients with ischemic heart disease: a study from the International HeartQoL Project. *Int J Cardiol.* (2013) 166:327–33. doi: 10.1016/j.ijcard.2011.10.084

Al-Qezweny MN, Utens EM, Dulfer K, Hazemeijer BA, van Geuns RJ, Daemen J, et al. The association between type D personality, depression anxiety ten years after PCI. *Neth Heart J.* (2016) 24:538–43. doi: 10.1007/s12471-016-0860-4

Doyle F, McGee H, Delaney M, Motterlini N, Conroy R. Depressive vulnerabilities predict depression status and trajectories of depression over 1 year in persons with acute coronary syndrome. *Gen Hosp Psychiatry.* (2011) 33:224–31. doi: 10.1016/j.genhosppsych.2011.03.008

Mazur J. Family affluence scale - validation study and suggested modification. *Hyg Public Health.* (2013) 48:211–7.

Juczyński Z, Ogińska-Bulik N. *Tools for Measuring Stress and Coping With Stress.* Warszawa: Pracownia Testów Psychologicznych (2009).

Cantril H. *The Patterns of Human Concerns.* New Brunswick, NJ: Rutgers University Press (1965).

Mazur J, Małkowska-Szkutnik A, Oblacińska A. Kołoło H. Cantril ladder in the studies on health and health inequalities among 11-18-year-old pupils. *Problem Hig Epidemiol.* (2009) 90:355–61.

Ogińska-Bulik N, Juczyński Z, Denollet J. D-type measurement scale. In: Juczyński Z. Ogińska-Bulik ZN, editors. *Tools for Measuring Stress Coping With Stress.* Warszawa: Pracownia Testów Psychologicznych Polskiego Towarzystwa Psychologicznego (2009). p. 71–85.

Denollet J. DS14: standard assessment of negative affectivity, social inhibition, and type D personality. *Psychosom Med.* (2005) 67:89–97. doi: 10.1097/01.psy.0000149256.81953.49

Poznyak V, Rekve D, Akselrod S, Saxena S, Fleischmann A, Gehring E, et al. *Global Status Report on Alcohol and Health 2018.* Geneva: World Health Organization (2018).

Bozewicz M. *Alcohol Consumption in Poland.* Warsaw: Komunikat CBOS 151 (2019).

Koob GF, Powell P, White A. Addiction as a coping response: hyperkatifeia, deaths of despair, and COVID-19. *Am J Psychiatry.* (2020) 177:1031–7. doi: 10.1176/appi.ajp.2020.20091375

Alcohol-Related Hospital Admissions - Statistical Tables for England. Available online at: https://fingertips.phe.org.uk/profile/local-alcohol- profiles/supporting-information/additional-data (accessed January 12, 2021).

Wadd S, Papadopoulos C. Drinking behaviour and alcohol-related harm amongst older adults: analysis of existing UK datasets. *BMC Res Notes.* (2014) 7:741. doi: 10.1186/1756-0500-7-741

Brennan P, Moos R, Schutte K. Predicting the development of late-life late- onset drinking problems: a 7-year prospective study. *Alcohol Clin Exp Res.* (1998) 6:1349–58. doi: 10.1111/j.1530-0277.1998.tb03918.x

Chodkiewicz J. The role of personal resources in maintaining abstinence by men dependent on alcohol. *Alkohol Narkomania*. (2015) 14:277–87.

Kutubaeva Rh. Analysis of life satisfaction of the elderly population on the example of Sweden, Austria and Germany. *Popul Econ*. (2019) 3:102–16. doi:10.3897/popecon.3.e47192

Pohorecky LA. Stress and alcohol interaction: an update of human research. *Alcohol Clin Exp Res*. (1991) 15:438–59. doi: 10.1111/j.1530-0277.1991.tb00543.x

Jennison KM. The impact of stressful life events and social support on drinking among older adults: a general population survey. *Int J Aging Hum Dev*. (1992) 35:99–123. doi: 10.2190/F6G4-XLV3-5KW6-VMBA

Sadava SW, Pak AW. Stress-related problem drinking and alcohol problems: a longitudinal study and extension of Marlatt's model. *Can J Behav Sci*. (1993) 25:446–64. doi: 10.1037/h0078841

Volpicelli JR. Uncontrollable events and alcohol drinking. *Br J Addict*. (1987) 82:381–92. doi: 10.1111/j.1360-0443.1987.tb01494.x

Kasl SV, Chisholm RF, Eskenazi B. The impact of the accident at the Three Mile Island on the behavior and well-being of nuclear workers. Part II: job tension, psychophysiological symptoms, and indices of distress. *Am J Public Health*. (1981) 71:484–95. doi: 10.2105/AJPH.71.5.484

Brown S. *Safe Passage*. Warszawa: IPZiT (1995).

Brown SA, Vik PW, McQuaid JR, Patterson TL, Irwin MR, Grant I. Severity of psychosocial stress and outcome of alcoholism treatment. *J Abnorm Psychol*. (1990) 99:344–8. doi: 10.1037/0021-843X.99.4.344

Cloninger CR, Sigvardsson S, Bohman M. Type I and type II alcoholism: an update. *Alcohol Health Res World*. (1996) 20:18–23.

Gmel G, Marmet S, Studer J, Wicki M. Are changes in personality traits and alcohol use associated? A cohort study among young Swiss men. *Front Psychiatry*. (2020) 23:591003 doi: 10.3389/fpsyt.2020. 591003

22

Moods in Clinical Depression are more Unstable than Severe Normal Sadness

Rudy Bowen[1]*, Evyn Peters[1], Steven Marwaha[2,3], Marilyn Baetz[1] and Lloyd Balbuena[1]

[1] University of Saskatchewan, Saskatoon, SK, Canada, [2] Division of Mental Health and Wellbeing, Warwick Medical School, Warwick University, Coventry, UK, [3] Affective Disorder Service (IPU 3-8), Caludon Centre, Coventry, UK

*Correspondence:
Rudy Bowen
r.bowen@usask.ca

Objective: Current descriptions in psychiatry and psychology suggest that depressed mood in clinical depression is similar to mild sadness experienced in everyday life, but more intense and persistent. We evaluated this concept using measures of average mood and mood instability (MI).

Method: We prospectively measured low and high moods using separate visual analog scales twice a day for seven consecutive days in 137 participants from four published studies. Participants were divided into a non-depressed group with a Beck Depression Inventory score of ≤ 10 ($n = 59$) and a depressed group with a Beck Depression Inventory score of ≥ 18 ($n = 78$). MI was determined by the mean square successive difference statistic.

Results: Mean low and high moods were not correlated in the non-depressed group but were strongly positively correlated in the depressed group. This difference between correlations was significant. Low MI and high MI were weakly positively correlated in the non-depressed group and strongly positively correlated in the depressed group. This difference in correlations was also significant.

Conclusion: The results show that low and high moods, and low and high MI, are highly correlated in people with depression compared with those who are not depressed. Current psychiatric practice does not assess or treat MI or brief high mood episodes in patients with depression. New models of mood that also focus on MI will need to be developed to address the pattern of mood disturbance in people with depression.

Keywords: depression, distress, low mood, high mood, mood instability

INTRODUCTION

The purpose of this paper is to distinguish between sadness and depression. Current descriptions suggest that depression is caused mainly by exposure to stress and the ups and downs of life (1, 2). If depression were simply extreme sadness, then patients would have more control over symptoms, and it would be less stigmatizing as a consequence (3, 4). Freud provided a clinical foundation for this idea by concluding that mourning and melancholia were comparable because the symptoms are similar, they are both precipitated by loss and improve with time (5). He noted that people with melancholia could become over-talkative and manic but did not adequately explain why this is so (5).

Other influential writers in psychiatry and psychology have endorsed similar notions. Bowlby compared negative emotions in adults to those that occur during separation from the attachment figure in infants (6). Beck attributed depression to dysfunctional negative thoughts of defeat, failure, and rejection (7). He dismissed mood-swings as a normal phenomenon (7). Although Watson paid more attention to mood instability (MI), he also dismissed negative mood variability as mundane and of little importance (8).

Kraepelin was a notable exception in that he emphasized brief moods swings and rapidly alternating mood symptoms in patients with manic–depressive illness (9). Consistent with his work, recent studies have shown that patients with mood disorders report increased affective lability and emotional instability; and this also occurs during euthymic periods in bipolar patients (10–12).

Depression could be understood as a consequence of loss or stress, but if high moods do occur during a depressive episode, they tend to be ignored (2, 6), dismissed (7, 8), or isolated to separate categories with low prevalences of about 1% such as bipolar mood disorder (13) and borderline personality disorder (14). Recently, DSM-5 has introduced the specifier "with mixed features" to acknowledge manic/hypomanic symptoms, but three out of seven symptoms are required (13). Any attempt to expand the bipolar spectrum to account for brief periods of high mood (15–17) has been vigorously criticized (18–21).

The reliance on retrospective methods for clinical and research interviewing (22) has made it easier to dismiss brief high moods because retrospective recall in depressed people is biased toward the negative. Recalling mood over the previous 2 weeks is more likely to result in smoothing away mood variation (23–25). If so, the raw data for clinically diagnosing major depression are systematically distorted (26). Ecological momentary assessment, which asks patients to record affect at a given moment over a specified duration, provides a fuller picture of mood by capturing variation in addition to severity. As early as 2006, the US Food and Drug Administration recommended that pharmaceutical companies make use of real-time data instead of patient recollection (26). Increasingly, smartphones are being used as a tool for ecological momentary assessment in psychological and clinical studies (27, 28).

Another way by which recalled moods are distorted is the "common-sense" view that low mood and high mood are mutually exclusive or negatively correlated (8, 29). Since negative affect predominates in depressed people, brief episodes of positive affect tend to be subsumed under overall gloom in patient recollections. There is evidence, however, that positive and negative affect are independent of each other (30) and that people can feel both happy and sad at the same time (31).

Among clinical samples, when low and high moods are measured prospectively on separate axes, the rapid cyclic recurrence of high moods with low moods becomes apparent, a phenomenon known as mood instability (11, 32–34). MI has been shown to exist in up to 13.9% of the adult population (34). MI seems to be the essential component of neuroticism (35, 36) and is an antecedent to major depression (37), psychotic symptoms (38), severity of distress (39), suicidal thoughts (35), and self-harm behavior

(40). In this study, we investigated how MI might characterize the experience of people who were depressed as compared with those who were not depressed.

Hypothesis

People who are depressed (distressed with negative mood and symptoms) are more likely to have more strongly correlated low and high unstable moods than people who are not depressed.

MATERIALS AND METHODS

Participants

We used data from participants in four controlled studies ($n = 168$) that we have published (32, 41–43). All patients had been referred by family physicians for treatment and were all under treatment at the time of the study. In three of the studies, males and females had been referred to general outpatient practices, in one study women had been referred for alcohol abuse, but all had been alcohol free for 3 weeks. All patients completed mood diaries (described in the next section) over a week. All of the studies received approval from the university ethics board. The patient group ($n = 104$) was assessed with the Mini-International Neuropsychiatric Interview (MINI English Version 5.0.0 for DSM-IV), and 49 met criteria for major depression (44). There was high comorbidity with anxiety disorders. Twenty-two of those with major depression (45%) reported hyperthymic symptoms in the past, which did not meet criteria for hypomania (45). The controls ($n = 64$) included health-care personnel and 17 graduate students.

Procedure

Participants completed the Beck Depression Inventory-IA (46, 47), which is a 21-item retrospective self-report questionnaire. Statements are presented in the first-person ("I feel sad"), and subjects select the item that best reflects their recent state from a choice of four items. It is reliable and correlates well with other measures of depression but may in part assess a general distress or neuroticism factor (48–50). In a study with undergraduate students, the BDI showed strong latent dimensional structure that is there was no evidence that a cut-score defined a latent class of depression (50).

Participants completed separate visual analog scales (VAS) (8) for low mood and high mood. They rated their moods in the morning after awakening and at night before bedtime, for 7 consecutive days (41, 51). The anchor points were "not at all" and "very much so."

For clarity, we define "low mood" as participant ratings for "sad/blue" or "depressed" over 1 week (twice daily ratings for a total of 14 ratings). Similarly, "high mood" is defined as participant ratings for "enthusiastic/interested" or "high mood." "Low MI" refers to the fluctuation of low mood, and "high MI" refers to the fluctuation of high mood over the same period. MI is operationalized as the mean square successive difference (MSSD) statistic across 14 ratings (52). One can think of MSSD as the SD of ratings, taking temporal sequence into account.

Analysis

We used the BDI scores to divide the participants into two distinct groups: those who were within a "normal" range of BDI scores (BDI ≤10) ($n = 59$) (47) and those with BDI scores ≥18 or who were likely clinically depressed ($n = 78$) (46, 47). The remaining participants ($n = 31$) fell outside of these two groups and were excluded from the sample. We used the conventional terms "non-depressed" (BDI ≤10) and "depressed" (≥18) to designate the two groups without assuming that the cut-score of BDI ≥18 defined a latent class of major depression or any particular form of depression. The mean BDI scores of the non-depressed and depressed groups were 4.51 (SD: 2.59) and 20.05 (SD: 13.89), respectively.

We used Pearson's correlation as a measure of association between low and high moods. We then tested whether the correlations between (a) mean low and high mood and (b) low and high MI were different between the non-depressed and depressed groups. This comparison of correlation magnitudes is, in principle, similar to Meehl's MAXCOV procedure in which the correlation of two variables is compared along successive cuts in a third variable (22).

RESULTS

In the original group of referred patient participants ($N = 104$), mean low mood was correlated with low MI; as were mean high mood and high MI ($p < 0.001$). In the original group of controls ($N = 64$), mean low mood was correlated with low MI ($p < 0.001$); as were mean high mood and high MI ($p < 0.01$).

Sample and Group Demographics

The participants ($n = 137$) ranged in age from 15 to 64 years (mean age = 30.0 years, SD = 10.9), and 104 (75.9%) were females. The "depressed" group ($n = 78$) (mean age = 30.62, SD = 11.60; 80.8% females) was composed of 51 patients, 24 volunteers as "controls" in the original studies, and 3 graduate students. The "non-depressed group" ($n = 59$) (mean age = 29.15 years, SD = 9.66; 69.5% females) included 40 people who volunteered as controls from the original studies, 14 graduate students, and 5 people referred as patients. There was no difference in age or sex distribution between the two groups.

Mean Mood

Table 1 shows mood scores for both groups. Compared to the non-depressed group, the depressed group experienced more severe low mood ($t = -4.73$, df = 129, $p < 0.001$) and less severe high mood ($t = 5.41$, df = 135, $p < 0.001$), consistent with the selection into non-depressed and depressed groups. **Table 2** shows mean low and mean high mood correlations for both groups. Notably, in the non-depressed group, the correlation between mean low and mean high moods was not significant ($r = -0.01$), but in the depressed group, mean low and high moods were positively correlated ($r = 0.38$). The Fisher r-to-z transformation indicated that the difference between these correlations was significant ($z = -2.30$, $p = 0.02$, two-tailed).

TABLE 1 | Mood and mood instability (MI) in depressed and non-depressed groups.

	Non-depressed			Depressed			t	df	Sig (two-tailed)
	N	Mean	SD	N	Mean	SD	–	–	–
Low mood	59	1.50	1.34	78	2.95	2.22	−4.73	129.22	<0.00
High mood	59	4.81	1.69	78	3.05	2.13	5.41	134.68	<0.00
Low MI	59	1.72	1.30	78	2.40	1.49	−2.81	135	<0.01
High MI	59	2.84	1.06	78	2.44	1.60	1.77	132.94	0.08

Low, high mood: mean visual analog scale mood ratings for low and high moods.
Low, high MI: mean square successive difference statistic for low mood and high mood.

Mood Instability

The depressed group experienced more severe low MI than the non-depressed group, as consistent with the findings of the original individual studies. The difference in high MI between the depressed and non-depressed groups was not significant. **Table 2** shows the important finding that low MI and high MI were correlated in both the depressed and the non-depressed groups, but the magnitude of correlation for the depressed group ($r = 0.61$) was almost twice that for the non-depressed group ($r = 0.31$). The difference between these correlations was significant ($z = -2.18$, $p = 0.03$, two-tailed).

DISCUSSION

On the VAS ratings, the depressed group experienced more severe low moods and less severe high moods than the non-depressed group, as would be expected given the selection criteria. This is consistent with reports of more severe negative emotions and variable positive emotions in ecological momentary assessment studies of patients with major depression (12, 33, 53).

In the non-depressed group, the overall means of low mood and high mood were uncorrelated. This supports the observation that in normal people low and high moods are not strongly related and easily distinguished (8). In the depressed group, however, mean low mood and mean high mood were moderately positively correlated. This indicates that the depressed group experienced high moods concurrent with low moods (54, 55). This is contrary to the common-sense view that low mood should not be associated with high moods.

Low MI and high MI were weakly correlated in the non-depressed group. In the depressed group, the correlation was moderate to large, and the difference between these correlations was significant. In other words, in the depressed group, the fluctuations of low moods and high moods are more closely related (**Table 2**).

Taken together, these results suggest that in people with depression, mood is a complex combination of rapidly fluctuating seemingly polar opposite emotions. This distinction is more easily understood if MI is considered along with stable low mood (56). Other studies have shown complex emotional patterns in anxiety

TABLE 2 | Correlations.[a]

	Non-depressed			Depressed				
	n	r^0	95% confidence limits	n	r	95% confidence limits	Z	Sig of the difference in r^0 and r (two-tailed)
Correlation mean low mood and high mood	59	−0.01	−0.27–0.25	78	0.38[b]	0.17–0.55	−2.3	0.02
Correlation mean square successive difference (MSSD) (mood instability) low mood and MSSD high mood	59	0.31[a]	0.06–0.53	78	0.61[a]	0.45–0.73	−2.18	0.03

[a]Correlations between mean low and mean high moods for the non-depressed and depressed groups and MSSD low and MSSD high moods for the non-depressed and depressed groups.
[b]Correlation is significant at the 0.05 level (two-tailed).

and mood disorders (12, 56–58). Two clinical applications are (a) that the usual semi-structured retrospective assessment might provide a limited appreciation of "nuanced" mood symptoms (12) and (b) that attention to mood stabilization might add an extra dimension to treatment (12, 59). In other words, since MI reflects neuroticism (36) that is an antecedent of depression (60), attention to the assessment and treatment of MI in addition to specific symptoms of depression (61, 62) might increase the treatment efficacy.

Our study had several methodological limitations. First, the number of participants was relatively small and from one center. Second, the wording of the questions for low mood and high mood varied slightly between studies, although the words were similar. This might be an advantage by reflecting real-world interviewing conditions. Third, paper and pencil diaries were used, raising the possibility of people retrospectively filling in data. Participants understood that they were to record momentary mood ratings, and the method of calculating MI was not intuitively apparent to the participant (52). Furthermore, all of the individual study results produced clear differences suggesting that the participants understood the instructions. Fourth, choosing graduate students as controls in one of the studies was a convenience sample, but we considered that graduate students would be generally more stable than undergraduates and that they would be older and closer in age to patients. Fifth, for simplicity we considered only low and high moods. Moods in broadly defined depression would likely appear even more complex and distressing if anxiety, irritability, and psychotic symptoms were included (63). Sixth, five people in the "non-depressed" group had been referred as patients. These people may have improved while waiting for treatment or may have had symptoms that were not detected by the way that they completed the BDI. Finally, during the diagnostic interview we did not probe sufficiently for hypomanic symptoms during the depressive episode, so we cannot say how many of the participants would have met criteria for the DSM-5 category of major depression with mixed features (13).

There are also limitations to the conclusions that can be drawn. The correlation between low and high MI might not be the best representation of complex emotions. The data do not address the question of the relative merits of continuous or categorical approaches to classification in psychiatry. Recent taxometric analyses indicate that in the mood and anxiety domains, dimensional distributions are much more likely (64, 65). We studied MI as a phenomenon, similar to instability in physical parameters such as blood pressure (66) and blood sugar (67) and without assumptions as to cause. MI is considered to be a simpler concept than "affective instability due to a marked reactivity of mood" (13) or emotional dysregulation (68). One question for further studies would be whether MI leads to unstable interpersonal relationships or *vice versa*. The relationship of MI to interpersonal and social–environmental events is a matter for further research. Instability of low moods is not entirely accounted for by reactivity to negative events (12). Finally, associating MI with neuroticism does not detract from evidence that certain kinds of stress can affect depression (69, 70). The main advantage to this study is the longitudinal collection of data, which is likely to give a more accurate depiction of moods than retrospective studies (23).

The results show that low and high moods, and low and high MI, are highly correlated in people with depression compared with those who are not depressed. Current psychiatric practice does not assess or treat MI or brief high mood episodes in patients with depression. New models of mood that also focus on MI will need to be developed to address the pattern of mood disturbance in people with depression.

ETHICS STATEMENT

This study was carried out in accordance with the recommendations of the Canadian Tri-Council Policy Statement for Ethical Conduct in research involving humans with written informed consent from all subjects. All subjects gave written informed consent in accordance with the Declaration of Helsinki. The protocol was approved by the University of Saskatchewan Behavioural Ethics Board.

AUTHOR CONTRIBUTIONS

RB: study conception, drafting the article, revised the article after peer review, and responded to reviewer comments. EP: contributing to the concepts as well as reading and adding to the final version. SM and MB: contributing to the concepts as well as reading and providing approval to the final version. LB: conception of the work, analysis of the data, and revised the article after peer review.

REFERENCES

Link BG, Phelan JC, Bresnahan M, Stueve A, Pescosolido BA. Public concep- tions of mental illness: labels, causes, dangerousness, and social distance. *Am J Public Health* (1999) 89(9):1328-33. doi:10.2105/AJPH.89.9.1328

Brown G, Harris T. *The Social Origins of Depression: A Study of Psychiatric Disorder in Women*. London, England: Tavistock Publications (1978).

Klerman GL. History and development of modern concepts of anxiety and panic. In: Ballenger JC, editor. *Clinical Aspects of Panic Disorder*. New York, NY: Wiley-Liss Inc. (1990). p. 67-82.

Speaker SL. From "happiness pills" to "national nightmare": changing cultural assessment of minor tranquilizers in America, 1955-1980. *J Hist Med Allied Sci* (1997) 52(3):338-76. doi:10.1093/jhmas/52.3.338

Freud S. Mourning and melancholia. In: Strachey J, editor. *On the History of the Psycho-Analytic Movement: Papers on Metapsychology and Other Works XIV*. London: The Hogarth Press and the Institute of Psycho-Analysis (1914- 1916). p. 243-58.

Bowlby J. *Attachment and Loss 2. Separation, Anxiety and Anger*. New York, NY: Basic Books (1973).

Beck AT. *Depression: Clinical, Experimental, and Theoretical Aspects*. New York, NY: Hoeber Medical Division, Harper & Row (1967).

Watson D. *Mood and Temperament*. New York, NY: Guilford Press (2000). 340 p.

Kraepelin E. Manic depressive insanity and paranoia. *J Nerv Ment Dis* (1921) 53(4):350. doi:10.1097/00005053-192104000-00057

Henry C, Van den Bulke D, Bellivier F, Roy I, Swendsen J, M'Bailara K, et al. Affective lability and affect intensity as core dimensions of bipolar disorders during euthymic period. *Psychiatry Res* (2008) 159(1-2):1-6. doi:10.1016/j.psychres.2005.11.016

Jahng S, Wood PK, Trull TJ. Analysis of affective instability in ecological momentary assessment: indices using successive difference and group comparison via multilevel modeling. *Psychol Methods* (2008) 13(4):354-75. doi:10.1037/a0014173

Thompson RJ, Mata J, Jaeggi SM, Buschkuehl M, Jonides J, Gotlib IH. The everyday emotional experience of adults with major depressive disorder: examining emotional instability, inertia, and reactivity. *J Abnorm Psychol* (2012) 121(4):819-29. doi:10.1037/a0027978

American Psychiatric Association. *Diagnostic and Statistical Manual of Mental Disorders (DSM-5*)*. Arlington, VA: American Psychiatric Association (2013).

Ten Have M, Verheul R, Kaasenbrood A, van Dorsselaer S, Tuithof M, Kleinjan M, et al. Prevalence rates of borderline personality disorder symptoms: a study based on the Netherlands mental health survey and incidence study-2. *BMC Psychiatry* (2016) 16:249. doi:10.1186/s12888-016-0939-x

Angst J, Gamma A, Benazzi F, Ajdacic V, Eich D, Rossler W. Toward a re-definition of subthreshold bipolarity: epidemiology and proposed criteria for bipolar-II, minor bipolar disorders and hypomania. *J Affect Disord* (2003) 73(1-2):133-46. doi:10.1016/S0165-0327(02)00322-1

Judd LL, Akiskal HS. The prevalence and disability of bipolar spectrum disor- ders in the US population: re-analysis of the ECA database taking into account subthreshold cases. *J Affect Disord* (2003) 73(1-2):123-31. doi:10.1016/ S0165-0327(02)00332-4

Akiskal HS, Benazzi F. Optimizing the detection of bipolar II disorder in outpatient private practice: toward a systematization of clinical diagnostic wisdom. *J Clin Psychiatry* (2005) 66(7):914-21. doi:10.4088/JCP.v66n0715

Baldessarini RJ. A plea for integrity of the bipolar disorder concept. *Bipolar Disord* (2000) 2(1):3-7. doi:10.1034/j.1399-5618.2000.020102.x

Patten SB, Paris J. The bipolar spectrum – a bridge too far? *Can J Psychiatry* (2008) 53(11):762-8. doi:10.1177/070674370805301108

Russell JJ, Moskowitz DS, Zuroff DC, Sookman D, Paris J. Stability and variability of affective experience and interpersonal behavior in bor- derline personality disorder. *J Abnorm Psychol* (2007) 116(3):578-88. doi:10.1037/0021-843x.116.3.578

Paris J. The bipolar spectrum: a critical perspective. *Harv Rev Psychiatry* (2009) 17(3):206-13. doi:10.1080/10673220902979888

Meehl PE, Yonce LJ. Taxometirc analysis: II. Detecting taxonicity using covariance of two quantitative indicators in successive intervals of a third indi- cator (MAXCOV procedure). *Psychol Rep* (1996) 78:1091-227. doi:10.2466/pr0.1996.78.3c.1091

Moffitt TE, Caspi A, Taylor A, Kokaua J, Milne BJ, Polanczyk G, et al. How common are common mental disorders? Evidence that lifetime prevalence rates are doubled by prospective versus retrospective ascertainment. *Psychol Med* (2010) 40(6):899-909. doi:10.1017/s0033291709991036

Ebner-Priemer UW, Kuo J, Welch SS, Thielgen T, Witte S, Bohus M, et al. A valence-dependent group-specific recall bias of retrospective self-reports: a study

of borderline personality disorder in everyday life. *J Nerv Ment Dis* (2006) 194(10):774-9. doi:10.1097/01.nmd.0000239900.46595.72

Solhan MB, Trull TJ, Jahng S, Wood PK. Clinical assessment of affective instability: comparing EMA indices, questionnaire reports, and retrospective recall. *Psychol Assess* (2009) 21(3):425-36. doi:10.1037/a0016869

Ebner-Priemer UW, Trull TJ. Ecological momentary assessment of mood disorders and mood dysregulation. *Psychol Assess* (2009) 21(4):463-75. doi:10.1037/a0017075

Hofmann W, Patel PV. SurveySignal: a convenient solution for experience sampling research using participants' own smartphones. *Soc Sci Comput Rev* (2015) 33(2):235-53. doi:10.1177/0894439314525117

Silk JS, Forbes EE, Whalen DJ, Jakubcak JL, Thompson WK, Ryan ND, et al. Daily emotional dynamics in depressed youth: a cell phone ecological momentary assessment study. *J Exp Child Psychol* (2011) 110(2):241-57. doi:10.1016/j.jecp.2010.10.007

Zautra AJ, Potter PT, Reich JW. The independence of affects is context-depen- dent: an integrative model of the relationship between positive and negative affect. *Annual Review of Gerontology and Geriatrics* (1997) 17:75-103.

Russell JA, Carroll JM. On the bipolarity of positive and negative affect. *Psychol Bull* (1999) 125(1):3-30. doi:10.1037/0033-2909.125.1.3

Larsen JT, McGraw AP, Cacioppo JT. Can people feel happy and sad at the same time? *J Pers Soc Psychol* (2001) 81(4):684-96. doi:10.1037/0022-3514.81. 4.684

Bowen R, Baetz M, Hawkes J, Bowen A. Mood variability in anxiety disorders. *J Affect Disord* (2006) 91(2-3):165-70. doi:10.1016/j.jad.2005.12.050

Santangelo P, Bohus M, Ebner-Priemer UW. Ecological momentary assess- ment in borderline personality disorder: a review of recent findings and methodological challenges. *J Pers Disord* (2014) 28(4):555-76. doi:10.1521/ pedi_2012_26_067

Marwaha S, Parsons N, Flanagan S, Broome M. The prevalence and clinical associations of mood instability in adults living in England: results from the adult psychiatric morbidity survey 2007. *Psychiatry Res* (2013) 205(3):262-8. doi:10.1016/j.psychres.2012.09.036

Bowen R, Baetz M, Leuschen C, Kalynchuk LE. Predictors of suicidal thoughts: mood instability versus neuroticism. *Pers Individ Dif* (2011) 51:1034-8. doi:10.1016/j.paid.2011.08.015

Bowen R, Balbuena L, Leuschen C, Baetz M. Mood instability is the distinctive feature of neuroticism. Results from the British Health and Lifestyle Study (HALS). *Pers Individ Dif* (2012) 53(7):896-900. doi:10.1016/j.paid.2012. 07.003

Marwaha S, Balbuena L, Winsper C, Bowen R. Mood instability as a precur- sor to depressive illness: a prospective and mediational analysis. *Aust N Z J Psychiatry* (2015) 49(6):557-65. doi:10.1177/0004867415579920

Marwaha S, He Z, Broome M, Singh SP, Scott J, Eyden J, et al. How is affective instability defined and measured? A systematic review. *Psychol Med* (2014) 44(9):1793-808. doi:10.1017/s0033291713002407

Bowen R, Wang Y, Balbuena L, Houmphan A, Baetz M. The relationship between mood instability and depression: implications for studying and treating depression. *Med Hypotheses* (2013) 81(3):459-62. doi:10.1016/j.mehy.2013.06.010

Peters EM, Balbuena L, Marwaha S, Baetz M, Bowen R. Mood instability and impulsivity as trait predictors of suicidal thoughts. *Psychol Psychother* (2016) 89(4):435-44. doi:10.1111/papt.12088

Bowen R, Clark M, Baetz M. Mood swings in patients with anxiety disor- ders compared with normal controls. *J Affect Disord* (2004) 78(3):185-92. doi:10.1016/s0165-0327(02)00304-x

Bowen R, Block G, Baetz M. Mood and attention variability in women with alcohol dependence: a preliminary investigation. *Am J Addict* (2008) 17(1):77-81. doi:10.1080/10550490701756013

Bowen R, Balbuena L, Baetz M. Lamotrigine reduces affective instability in depressed patients with mixed mood and anxiety disorders. *J Clin Psychopharmacol* (2014) 34(6):747-9. doi:10.1097/jcp.0000000000000164

Sheehan DV, Lecrubier Y, Sheehan KH, Amorim P, Janavs J, Weiller E, et al. The Mini-International Neuropsychiatric Interview (M.I.N.I.): the development and validation of a structured diagnostic psychiatric interview for DSM-IV and ICD-10. *J Clin Psychiatry* (1998) 59(Suppl 20):22-33.

Angst J, Cui L, Swendsen J, Rothen S, Cravchik A, Kessler RC, et al. Major depressive disorder with subthreshold bipolarity in the National Comorbidity Survey Replication. *Am J Psychiatry* (2010) 167(10):1194-201. doi:10.1176/appi.ajp.2010.09071011

Beck AT, Steer RA. Beck Depression Inventory (BDI). In: American Psychiatric Association, editor. *Handbook of Psychiatric Measures*. Washington, DC: American Psychiatric Association (2000). p. 519-23.

Beck AT, Steer RA, Garbin MG. Psychometric Properties of the Beck Depression

Inventory: twenty-five years of evaluation. *Clin Psychol Rev* (1988) 8:77–100. doi:10.1016/0272-7358(88)90050-5

Beck AT, Steer RA, Brown GK. *BDI-II: Beck Depression Inventory – Manual.* 2nd ed. San Antonio, TX: The Psychological Corporation. Harcourt Brace & Company (1996).

Enns MW, Cox BJ, Parker JD, Guertin JE. Confirmatory factor analysis of the Beck Anxiety and Depression Inventories in patients with major depression. *J Affect Disord* (1998) 47(1–3):195–200. doi:10.1016/S0165-0327(97)00103-1

Ruscio AM, Ruscio J. The latent structure of analogue depression: should the Beck Depression Inventory be used to classify groups? *Psychol Assess* (2002) 14(2):135–45. doi:10.1037/1040-3590.14.2.135

Tellegen A, Watson D, Clark LA. On the dimensional and hierarchical struc- ture of affect. *Psychol Sci* (1999) 10(4):297–303. doi:10.1111/1467-9280.00157

Ebner-Priemer UW, Eid M, Kleindienst N, Stabenow S, Trull TJ. Analytic strategies for understanding affective (in)stability and other dynamic processes in psychopathology. *J Abnorm Psychol* (2009) 118(1):195–202. doi:10.1037/a0014868

Ebner-Priemer UW, Kuo J, Kleindienst N, Welch SS, Reisch T, Reinhard I, et al. State affective instability in borderline personality disorder assessed by ambulatory monitoring. *Psychol Med* (2007) 37(7):961–70. doi:10.1017/s0033291706009706

Cassano GB, Rucci P, Frank E, Fagiolini A, Dell'Osso L, Shear MK, et al. The mood spectrum in unipolar and bipolar disorder: arguments for a unitary approach. *Am J Psychiatry* (2004) 161(7):1264–9. doi:10.1176/appi. ajp.161.7.1264

Akiskal HS. The prevalent clinical spectrum of bipolar disorders: beyond DSM-IV. *J Clin Psychopharmacol* (1996) 16(2 Suppl 1):4s–14s. doi:10.1097/00004714-199604001-00002

Ruscio J, Brown TA, Meron Ruscio A. A taxometric investigation of DSM-IV major depression in a large outpatient sample: interpretable structural results depend on the mode of assessment. *Assessment* (2009) 16(2):127–44. doi:10.1177/1073191108330065

Selby EA, Franklin J, Carson-Wong A, Rizvi SL. Emotional cascades and self-injury: investigating instability of rumination and negative emotion. *J Clin Psychol* (2013) 69(12):1213–27. doi:10.1002/jclp.21966

McGrath JJ, Saha S, Al-Hamzawi A, Andrade L, Benjet C, Bromet EJ, et al. The bidirectional associations between psychotic experiences and DSM-IV mental disorders. *Am J Psychiatry* (2016) 173(10):997–1006. doi:10.1176/appi.ajp.2016.15101293

ten Have M, Vollebergh W, Bijl R, Nolen WA. Bipolar disorder in the general population in The Netherlands (prevalence, consequences and care utilisa-tion): results from The Netherlands Mental Health Survey and Incidence Study (NEMESIS). *J Affect Disord* (2002) 68(2–3):203–13. doi:10.1016/ S0165-0327(00)00310-4

Cuijpers P, Smit F, Penninx BW, de Graaf R, ten Have M, Beekman AT. Economic costs of neuroticism: a population-based study. *Arch Gen Psychiatry* (2010) 67(10):1086–93. doi:10.1001/archgenpsychiatry.2010.130

Regeer EJ, Kupka RW, Have MT, Vollebergh W, Nolen WA. Low self-recogni- tion and awareness of past hypomanic and manic episodes in the general pop-ulation. *Int J Bipolar Disord* (2015) 3(1):22. doi:10.1186/s40345-015-0039-8

Holmes EA, Bonsall MB, Hales SA, Mitchell H, Renner F, Blackwell SE, et al. Applications of time-series analysis to mood fluctuations in bipolar disorder to promote treatment innovation: a case series. *Transl Psychiatry* (2016) 6:e720. doi:10.1038/tp.2015.207

Kendler KS. The phenomenology of major depression and the representa- tiveness and nature of DSM criteria. *Am J Psychiatry* (2016) 173(8):771–80. doi:10.1176/appi.ajp.2016.15121509

Haslam N, Holland E, Kuppens P. Categories versus dimensions in personality and psychopathology: a quantitative review of taxometric research. *Psychol Med* (2012) 42(5):903–20. doi:10.1017/s0033291711001966

Balbuena L, Baetz M, Bowen R. The dimensional structure of cycling mood disorders. *Psychiatry Res* (2015) 228(3):289–94. doi:10.1016/j. psychres.2015.06.031

Mehlum M, Liestol K, Julius S, Kjeldsen SE, Hua TA, Rothwell PM, et al. 3D.01: visit-to-visit blood pressure variability increases risk of stroke or cardiac events in patients given valsartan or amlodipine in the value trial. *J Hypertens* (2015) 33(Suppl 1):e40. doi:10.1097/01.hjh.0000467454.55397.ea

Hanefeld M, Sulk S, Helbig M, Thomas A, Kohler C. Differences in glycemic variability between normoglycemic and prediabetic subjects. *J Diabetes Sci Technol* (2014) 8(2):286–90. doi:10.1177/1932296814522739

Glenn CR, Klonsky ED. Emotion dysregulation as a core feature of bor-derline personality disorder. *J Pers Disord* (2009) 23(1):20–8. doi:10.1521/pedi.2009.23.1.20

Shalev I, Moffitt TE, Braithwaite AW, Danese A, Fleming NI, Goldman-Mellor S, et al. Internalizing disorders and leukocyte telomere erosion: a prospective study of depression, generalized anxiety disorder and post-traumatic stress disorder. *Mol Psychiatry* (2014) 19(11):1163–70. doi:10.1038/mp.2013.183

Fergusson DM, Horwood LJ, Boden JM, Mulder RT. Impact of a major disas- ter on the mental health of a well-studied cohort. *JAMA Psychiatry* (2014) 71(9):1025–31. doi:10.1001/jamapsychiatry.2014.652

23

Lifestyle Behaviors and Quality of Life among Older Adults after the First Wave of the COVID-19 Pandemic in Hubei China

Yanping Duan [1,2,3†], D. L. I. H. K. Peiris [1†], Min Yang [1†], Wei Liang [1,2], Julien Steven Baker [1,2], Chun Hu [4] and Borui Shang [5]*

[1] Department of Sport, Physical Education and Health, Faculty of Social Sciences, Hong Kong Baptist University, Kowloon Tong, Hong Kong SAR, China, [2] Centre for Health and Exercise Science Research, Hong Kong Baptist University, Kowloon Tong, Hong Kong SAR, China, [3] College of Health Sciences, Wuhan Institute of Physical Education, Wuhan, China, [4] Student Mental Health Education Center, Northwestern Polytechnical University, Xian, China, [5] Department of Social Science, Hebei Sport University, Shijiazhuang, China

Correspondence:
Yanping Duan
duanyp@hkbu.edu.hk

[†] *These authors share first authorship*

Background: Older adult quality of life (QoL) is facing huge challenges during the COVID-19 pandemic. New normal lifestyle behaviors, including getting adequate physical activity (PA), consuming sufficient fruits and vegetables (FV) and enacting individual preventive behaviors (frequent hand washing, facemask wearing, and social distancing), as a significant determinant for QoL, have not been adequately addressed in older adults during the pandemic. This study aimed to investigate the characteristics of QoL in Chinese older adults after the first wave of the COVID-19 pandemic in Hubei China. The objective of the study was to examine any associations of lifestyle behaviors with QoL, and to identify the moderating role of socioeconomic indicators in the associations identified.

Methods: A cross-sectional study was conducted in Hubei, China, from June 15, 2020, to July 10, 2020. Five hundred sixteen older adults completed an online survey (mean age $= 67.6 \pm 6.6$; 57.9% women). The questionnaire consisted of demographic information, covariates (chronic diseases and infected cases of acquaintances), lifestyle behaviors [PA stage, FV intake (FVI) stage and three preventive behaviors], and QoL. *T*-tests, ANOVA tests, multiple linear regression models with simple slope analyses were used to test the hypotheses.

Results: QoL significantly differed in relation to economic situation, chronic diseases, marital status, education, living situation, age group, and professional status. Participants' economic situation ($\beta_{\text{average vs. below average}} = 0.17$, $p < 0.01$; $\beta_{\text{above average vs. below average}} = 0.15$, $p < 0.01$), chronic diseases ($\beta_{\text{yes vs. no}} = 0.19$, $p < 0.001$), FVI stage ($\beta = 0.21$, $p < 0.001$), and preventive behaviors ($\beta = 0.10$, $p < 0.05$) indicated a significant association with QoL. Education level and economic situation significantly interacted with preventive behaviors on QoL, respectively ($\beta_{\text{preventive behaviors} \times \text{educational level}} = -1.3$, $p < 0.01$; $\beta_{\text{preventive behaviors} \times \text{economic situation}} = -0.97$, $p < 0.05$).

Conclusions: Findings emphasize the importance of enhancing FVI and preventive behaviors on QoL improvement in older adults during the COVID-19 pandemic. Older adults who are in a lower economic situation with lower education levels should be given priority when implementing interventions to improve preventive behaviors and QoL in older adults.

Keywords: physical activity, fruit and vegetable intake, preventive behaviors, quality of life, socioeconomic status, older adults, COVID-19 pandemic

BACKGROUND

The novel coronavirus disease (COVID-19), a global health emergency and worldwide threat, contributed to over 161 million confirmed cases and over 3 million deaths worldwide as of 20th July 2021, including 119,784 confirmed cases and 5,617 deaths in China (1). Considerable evidence demonstrates that the likelihood of suffering from severe illness and death related to COVID-19 increases with age (2). Older adults (60 years old and above) are one of the most susceptible and vulnerable populations for being infected with COVID-19 (3).

During the COVID-19 pandemic, healthy aging advocacy is facing a big challenge. Maintaining a relatively high quality of life (QoL) in the elderly is an important indicator of healthy aging. QoL is considered, in general, a broad-ranging concept affected in a complex way by physical health, psychological state, personal beliefs, individual social relationships, and their relationships with the environment (4). A recent systematic review indicated that individuals' quality of life worsened during the COVID-19 pandemic and was more serious for older adults (5). Thus, it is crucial to identify and understand the factors contributing to a good QoL among older adults during the pandemic.

Many studies have indicated that healthy lifestyle behaviors relevant to health promotion and disease prevention present a considerable contributor to improved quality of life and lower morbidity and mortality among older adults (6–9). Performing adequate physical activity and consuming sufficient fruit and vegetables have been identified as two important health promotion behaviors because of their effective roles in improving physical and mental health in older adults (10–14). However, self-isolation and restrictions during the pandemic dramatically reduced the opportunities for the public to be physically active (15). In addition, there has been a high prevalence of unhealthy diets (e.g., insufficient fruit and vegetable intake) during the pandemic (16). These behavior changes may lead to negative health consequences and a low level of QoL among older adults (17).

Also, during the COVID-19 pandemic, individual disease preventive behaviors, including frequent hand washing, facemask wearing, and social distancing in public areas, play an important role in reducing the transmission of COVID-19 in the community (18). Because there is still not enough vaccination

prevention for COVID-19 worldwide and in anticipation of rapidly mutating viruses which transitions may not be prevented by vaccinations, performing individual preventive behaviors in daily life, as a new healthy lifestyle behavior, will be paramount in preventing the spread of the virus. A recent study indicated that preventive behaviors could directly affect the QoL among the general population (19). As older adults are at a higher risk of infection of COVID-19, investigating the impact of preventive behaviors on QoL in older adults should be prioritized. To the best of our knowledge, few studies have examined the relationship between all three healthy lifestyle behaviors (two health promotion behaviors including physical activity, fruit and vegetable intake, as well as one disease preventive behavior) and QoL among old adults during the COVID-19 pandemic.

Socioeconomic status (SES), including educational level, professional status, and economic situation, have been demonstrated to be important predictors for physical activity, diet, preventive behaviors and QoL in the general population, respectively (20–23). For example, many studies have reported positive associations with adequate physical activity, healthy eating, and performing preventive behaviors with high economic status during the COVID-19 pandemic (16, 24–26). In addition, a recent systematic review indicated that low education levels, unemployment status, and low economic situation correlated with poorer QoL (26). However, the moderating effects of SES on the association between lifestyle behaviors and QoL among older adults are still unknown. This deserves further examination and can help to develop tailored strategies to enhance the efficacy of an intervention to improve QoL of the elderly. This can be achieved using PA, healthy diet, and preventive behaviors during the COVID-19 outbreak and future pandemics (26).

The current study aimed to (1) investigate the characteristics of QoL among Chinese older adults during the COVID-19 pandemic; (2) examine the associations of three lifestyle behaviors (physical activity, fruit and vegetable intake, and preventive behaviors) with older adults' QoL levels; (3) identify the moderating role of SES indicators (education level, professional status, and economic situation) in the associations between lifestyle behaviors and QoL levels among Chinese older adults. It was hypothesized that (1) older adults' QoL levels would differ significantly for several demographic characteristics; (2) taking up healthier lifestyle behaviors would be significantly associated with higher QoL levels among Chinese older adults; (3) specific SES indicators would significantly moderate the associations between lifestyle behaviors and QoL levels in Chinese older adults. The research may assist in understanding

Abbreviations: COVID-19, coronavirus disease 2019; PA, physical activity; FVI, fruit and vegetable intake; QoL, quality of life; SES, socioeconomic status; WHO, World Health Organization; BMI, Body Mass Index; SD, standard deviation; CI, confidence interval.

older adults' QoL and their potential contributors. Such information may provide useful information to inform public health and social policies focused on maintaining the overall well-being of older adults during the COVID-19 pandemic.

METHODS

Participants

A cross-sectional study design with a convenient sampling approach was used in this study. The sample size was calculated by using G*Power 3.1 software with Linear Multiple Regression Fixed Model (27). For achieving a medium effect size (Cohen's $f^2 = 0.15$) on the association between PA and QoL in previous studies in older adults (28, 29), with an alpha of 0.05, the statistical power of 80%, and a response rate of 60%, a total of 205 participants were required. Seven hundred and twenty-seven community-dwelling older adults aged 60 years and above were contacted from five cities in the Hubei province of China, including Wuhan, Xiaogan, Jingzhou, Shiyan, and Xiangyang. A total of 609 older adults (609/727, 83.8%) agreed to participate in this online survey. Participants met the eligibility criteria, including (1) aged 60 years and above; (2) not infected with COVID-19; (3) having no cognitive disorders or impairments; (4) having access to mobile phones or computers; and (5) having sufficient reading skills in Chinese. Finally, data of 516 eligible participants were included in the analysis, where 93 participants were excluded due to following reasons (1) no access to mobile phones or computer; (2) having reading disorders, and (3) repeated completion. For participants who had difficulties using mobile phones or computer operations, their family members and friends were invited to assist them in completing the online survey. The survey was conducted from 15th June 2020 to 10th July 2020, which were 3 months after the first wave of the COVID-19 pandemic in Hubei province with no lockdown restrictions in this region.

Procedure

The online questionnaire survey was administered using an online survey platform in China, namely SOJUMP (Changsha Ranxing Information Technology Co., Ltd., China). All recruitment posters and the survey hyperlink were disseminated through mobile Short Message Service (SMS) and popular social media platforms in China such as WeChat, Weibo, and QQ. There were three approaches used for recruiting participants: (1) Relying on the researchers' social networks in five cities of Hubei province, the eligible family members, friends, and relatives of researchers were also invited. These initial participants then encouraged their friends to join the survey. (2) Researchers contacted the directors of community neighborhood committees in Wuhan and Xiaogan and sought their collaboration and support. Upon receiving the directors' agreement, researchers were permitted to enter their community neighborhood WeChat groups to recruit eligible participants. (3) Researchers contacted officials who oversaw the retirement in two universities in Wuhan. With the support of officials, a recruitment poster and survey hyperlink were delivered to their internal WeChat group, especially for retirement colleagues.

The duration of the online survey was around 15 min. Participants who completed the online survey was offered a 30 RMB incentive by electronic transfer *via* WeChat or Alipay or by prepaid telephone recharge. Participants were asked to sign an informed consent form prior to completing the questionnaire. Ethical approval for the study was obtained from the Research Ethics Committee of Hong Kong Baptist University (REC/19-20/0490).

Measures

Demographic Information

Demographic characteristics included age, gender (male/female), marital status (single/married/divorced or widowed), living situation (alone/with others such as a spouse, partner or children), and three socioeconomic status (SES) related variables (26), which included educational level (primary school or below/middle or high school/college or above), professional status (unemployed/pensioner or retired/employed), and economic situation (below average/average/above average). Body weight and height were also collected for calculating the body mass index [BMI, body weight (kg)/body height squared (m^2)]. The BMI was categorized into four levels (underweight BMI < 18.5/ healthy weight $18.5 \leq BMI < 23$/overweight $23 \leq BMI < 26$/obese $BMI \geq 26$) based on previous studies for Chinese populations (30, 31).

Covariates

Having chronic diseases and infected cases of acquaintances were considered as health-related covariates (32, 33). Participants were asked if they had a chronic disease (e.g., heart diseases, diabetes, cancer, respiratory illnesses, liver, or kidney diseases) and if any acquaintances were (or had been) infected with COVID-19 (e.g., friends, family members, and neighbors). Answers were recorded as Yes/No.

Lifestyle Behaviors

Physical activity (PA) was measured using the algorithm of the stages of change for PA, adapted from a previous study (34). Participants were asked one question about PA; "Currently, do you perform at least 150 min of moderate-intensity (slightly sweating and some increase in respiration) physical activity (e.g., brisk walking, bicycling, or swimming) every week?" Answers were given on a five-point Likert-scale with "1 = No, I don't intend to start, 2 = No, but I'm considering it; 3 = No, but I seriously intend to start; 4 = Yes, but only during the outbreak of COVID-19; and 5 = Yes, this was true for a long time before the outbreak of COVID-19." A higher score indicated a higher PA level, at which participants performed more PA.

Fruit and vegetable intake (FVI) was measured using the algorithm of the stages of change for FVI, adapted from a previous study (34). Participants were asked one question about "Currently, do you eat at least five servings of fruit and vegetable every day?" Answers were given on a five-point Likert-scale with "1 = No, I don't intend to start, 2 = No, but I'm considering it; 3 = No, but I seriously intend to start; 4 = Yes, but only during the outbreak of COVID-19; and 5 = Yes, this was true for a long period before the outbreak of COVID-19." A higher score indicated a higher FVI level, at which participants eat more fruits and vegetables.

COVID-19 preventive behaviors include hand washing, facemask wearing, and social distancing in public areas according to the recommendations of WHO (35). A six-item structured scale was used to measure preventive behaviors, with two items for each of the three behaviors (36). In particular, the items for hand washing were "during the previous week, I adhered to washing my hands frequently with soap and water or alcohol-based hand rub (for at least 20 s, on all surfaces of the hands)" followed by two situations including "(a) in a daily life situation, e.g., before eating, and (b) in a disease-related situation, e.g., after caring for the sick." The items for facemask wearing were "during the previous week; I adhered to wearing a face mask properly", followed by two situations including "(a) when visiting public places, and (b) when caring for the sick." The items for social distancing were "during the previous week, I adhered to social distancing" followed by two situations including "(a) staying out of crowded places and avoiding mass gatherings when going outside of my home, and (b) keeping space (at least 1.5 m) between myself and other people who were coughing or sneezing." All responses were indicated on a four-point Likert scale ranging from "1 = strongly disagree" to "4 = strongly agree." A mean score of the total six items was then computed.

Quality of Life (QoL)

The self-reported scale of the World Health Organization Quality of Life (WHOQOL)-BREF (37) was used to assess QoL. Two items were used from general QoL in this study based on the parsimonious principle. One item assessed the overall rating of each participant's QoL using a 5-point Likert-scale with "1 = very bad; 2 = bad; 3 = ordinary; 4 = good; 5 = very good." The other one assessed how participants were satisfied with health using a 5-point Likert scale ranging from "1 = very dissatisfied" to "5 = very satisfied." A mean score of two items was then calculated. The Cronbach's alpha coefficient was 0.761. In addition, the QoL was classified into three categories, including low level (mean score <3), middle level (mean score = 3), and high level (mean score >3) (38).

Data Analysis

Data were analyzed using the IBM SPSS version 26.0. The diagnostic testing (e.g., outlier screening and distribution checking) was first conducted, and all data adhered to the normal distribution and the absolute values of skewness and kurtosis were <2. Descriptive statistics including means, standard deviation, and percentages were used to describe characteristics. T-tests and One-way analyses of variance (ANOVAs) tests were applied to assess the characteristics of QoL. To examine the association of PA stage, FVI stage and preventive behaviors with QoL, multiple linear regression models were used. First, the significant demographics were set as predictors entered into Model 1. Then, two covariates were added to Model 2. Subsequently, the PA stage, FVI stage, and preventive behaviors were included in Model 3.

The role of SES indicators in moderating the associations of PA stage, FVI stage, and preventive behaviors with QoL were examined using multiple linear regression analyses, respectively. Before the regression analysis, Pearson correlation analyses was used to assess the association between SES and QoL. Only SES showing significant correlation with QoL were included in the multiple linear regressions. For each multiple linear regression analysis, the significant SES were entered into Model 1. Then the significantly correlated behavior was entered into Model 2. Finally, the interaction terms between SES and significantly correlated behavior were entered into Model 3. Finally, to test the interaction terms, all the variables were mean-centered. For significant interaction terms, simple slope analyses were conducted to assess the association between QoL and behavior at low and high levels (+ 1 standard deviation) of SES. The 5% level (two-tailed) was taken as the statistical significance cutoff point.

RESULTS

Characteristics of the Participants

Five hundred and sixteen eligible participants aged 60–90 years old (Mean age = 67.6 ± 6.6 yrs.) participated in the study. As shown in **Table 1**, the sample includes 57.9% females, and 68.6% of the participants were aged between 60 and 69 years. Most of the elderly were married (83.7%) and reported living with their spouse, partner, or children (90.7%). Nearly half (46.5%) of the old adults received college or above education, and more than half (57.9%) reported an average household income level. A total of 92.6% were pensioners/retired. 52.1% of the elderly participants were identified as overweight or obese (BMI ≥ 26 kg/m^2). In terms of medical history, about half of the participants (50.8%) suffered from chronic diseases (e.g., heart diseases, diabetes, or cancer). A few participants reported that their acquaintances (e.g., family members, friends, or neighbors) had been confirmed with COVID-19 (9.7%). According to QoL levels, the majority of the participants (78.5%) reported high-level QoL, while 6.0% of the elderly reported low-level QoL and 15.5% of the elderly indicated middle-level QoL during the outbreak of COVID-19. The means of behaviors are shown in **Table 1** [mean PA stage = 3.83 (1.54); mean FVI stage = 3.77 (1.49); mean PB = 3.61 (0.40)].

Characteristics of Quality of Life

As shown in **Table 2**, older adults' QoL differed significantly for different characteristics. There were no significant differences in QoL across gender [$t_{(514)} = -0.26$, $p = 0.796$], BMI intervals [$F_{(3, 512)} = 1.96$, $p = 0.119$], and infected cases of acquaintances [$t_{(514)} = -1.61$, $p = 0.109$]. The QoL was significantly higher for participants who had better economic situations [$t_{(2, 513)} = 14.52$, $p < 0.001$] and reported no chronic diseases [$t_{(514)} = -5.43$, $p < 0.001$]. Old adults who were married [$F_{(2, 513)} = 5.18$, $p < 0.01$] with better education [$F_{(2, 513)} = 6.98$, $p < 0.01$] reported significantly better QoL. The poorer QoL was identified among those who lived alone [$t_{(514)} = -2.43$, $p < 0.05$] and were aged over 80 years old [$F_{(2, 513)} = 4.38$, $p < 0.05$]. The employed old adults reported better QoL compared with those who were unemployed, pensioners and those who retired elderly [$F_{(2, 513)} = 4.25$, $p < 0.05$).

Lifestyle Behaviors and Quality of Life among Older Adults after the First Wave of the COVID-19...

207

TABLE 1 | Descriptive characteristics of the study sample ($n = 516$).

Variable	N (%)
Gender, n (%)	
Male	217 (42.1%)
Female	299 (57.9%)
Living situation, n (%)	
Live alone	48 (9.3%)
Live with others	468 (90.7%)
Age group, n (%)	
60–69 years old	354 (68.6%)
70–79 years old	128 (24.8%)
80 years old and above	34 (6.6%)
Marital status, n (%)	
Single	14 (2.7%)
Married	432 (83.7%)
Divorced or widowed	70 (13.6%)
Educational level, n (%)	
Primary school or below	45 (8.7%)
Middle or high school	231 (44.8%)
College or above	240 (46.5%)
Professional status, n (%)	
Unemployed	22 (4.3%)
Pensioner or retired	478 (92.6%)
Employed	16 (3.1%)
Economic situation, n (%)	
Below average	113 (21.9%)
Average	299 (57.9%)
Above average	104 (20.2%)
Body mass index (BMI), n (%)	
BMI < 18.5 kg/m^2	19 (3.7%)
18.5 kg/m^2 ≤ BMI < 23 kg/m^2	228 (44.2%)
23 kg/m^2 ≤ BMI < 26 kg/m^2 ≤ BMI < 26 kg/m2	206 (39.9%)
BMI ≥ 26 kg/m^2	63 (12.2%)
Chronic diseases, n (%)	
Yes	262 (50.8%)
No	254 (49.2%)
Infected cases of acquaintances, n (%)	
Yes	50 (9.7%)
No	466 (90.3%)
QoL, mean (SD): 3.76 (0.61)	
Low	31 (6.0%)
Middle	80 (15.5%)
High	405 (78.5%
Lifestyle behaviors	
PA stage, mean (SD): 3.83 (1.54)	
FVI stage, mean (SD): 3.77 (1.49)	
Preventive behaviors, mean (SD): 3.61 (0.40)	

SD, standard deviation; PA, physical activity; FVI, fruit and vegetable intake.

TABLE 2 | Characteristics of quality of life ($n = 516$).

Variable	QoL mean (SD)	F/t	P
Gender, n (%)		$t_{(514)} = -0.26$	0.796
Male	3.75 (0.60)		
Female	3.77 (0.62)		
Living situation, n (%)		$t_{(514)} = -2.43$	**<0.05**
Live alone	3.51 (0.77)		
Live with others	3.78 (0.59)		
Age group, n (%)		$F_{(2, 513)} = 4.38$	**<0.05**
60–69 years old	3.80 (0.60)		
70–79 years old	3.70 (0.61)		
80 years old and above	3.51 (0.68)		
Marital status, n (%)		$F_{(2, 513)} = 5.18$	**<0.01**
Single	3.64 (0.82)		
Married	3.80 (0.57)		
Divorced or widowed	3.54 (0.74)		
Educational level, n (%)		$F_{(2, 513)} = 6.98$	**<0.01**
Primary school or below	3.44 (0.78)		
Middle or high school	3.77 (0.59)		
College or above	3.81 (0.58)		
Professional status, n (%)		$F_{(2, 513)} = 4.25$	**<0.05**
Unemployed	3.41 (0.68)		
Pensioner or retired	3.77 (0.60)		
Employed	3.90 (0.58)		
Economic situation, n (%)		$F_{(2, 513)} = 14.52$	**<0.001**
Below average	3.50 (0.68)		
Average	3.83 (0.57)		
Above average	3.86 (0.58)		
Body mass index (BMI)			
BMI < 18.5 kg/m^2	3.82 (0.630)	$F_{(3, 512)} = 1.96$	0.119
18.5 kg/m^2 ≤ BMI < 23 kg/m^2	3.72 (0.61)		
23 kg/m^2 ≤ BMI < 26 kg/m^2 ≤ BMI < 26 kg/m^2	3.84 (0.59)		
BMI ≥ 26 kg/m^2	3.67 (0.61)		
Chronic diseases, n (%)		$t_{(514)} = -5.43$	**<0.001**
Yes	3.62 (0.61)		
No	3.90 (0.58)		
Infected cases of acquaintances			
Yes	3.63 (0.67)	$t_{(514)} = -1.61$	0.109
No	3.78 (0.60)		

SD, standard deviation. Bold values denote statistical significance p-value < 0.05.

Association of PA Stage, FVI Stage, and Preventive Behaviors With QoL

Based on the characteristics of QoL, 6 significant demographic variables (living situation, age group, marital status, educational level, professional status, and economic situation) were entered as predictors in Model 1. Dummy variables were applied for all categorical predictors. Model 1 explained 9% of the variance in QoL ($p < 0.001$). Medical history of chronic diseases and infected cases of acquaintances were entered as covariates into Model 2 contributing to the additional explanation of 5% of the variance in QoL ($\Delta R^2 = 0.05, p < 0.001$). After controlling demographics and covariates, PA stage, FVI stage and preventive behaviors the lifestyle behaviors were entered to Model 3, contributing to a significant improvement in the variance explanation ($\Delta R^2 = 0.06, p < 0.001$). Model 3 accounted for 20% explanation

TABLE 3 | Multiple linear regression analysis of demographics, covariate, and lifestyle behaviors with QoL (n = 516).

Variable	Model 1			Model 2			Model 3		
	B (SE)	95%CI	β	B (SE)	95%CI	β	B (SE)	95%CI	β
BLOCK 1: DEMOGRAPHICS									
Living situation									
Live alone	Reference	N/A	N/A	Reference	N/A	N/A	Reference	N/A	N/A
Live with others	0.12 (0.10)	(−0.08, 0.33)	0.06	0.13 (0.10)	(−0.07, 0.32)	0.06	0.90 (0.10)	(−0.10, 0.28)	0.04
Age group									
60–69 years old	Reference	N/A	N/A	Reference	N/A	N/A	Reference	N/A	N/A
70–79 years old	−0.04 (0.06)	(−0.16, 0.09)	−0.03	0.01 (0.06)	(−0.11, 0.13)	0.01	0.02 (0.06)	(−0.09, 0.14)	0.02
80 years old and above	−0.25 (0.11)	(−0.47, −0.04)	−0.10*	−0.20 (0.11)	(−0.41, 0.01)	−0.08	−0.13 (0.11)	(−0.34, 0.07)	−0.05
Marital status									
Single	Reference	N/A	N/A	Reference	N/A	N/A	Reference	N/A	N/A
Married	0.13 (0.16)	(−0.19, 0.45)	0.08	0.11 (0.16)	(−0.20, 0.42)	0.07	0.09 (0.15)	(−0.22, 0.39)	0.05
Divorced or widowed	0.06 (0.18)	(−0.29, 0.40)	0.03	0.06 (0.17)	(−0.28, 0.39)	0.03	0.04 (0.17)	(−0.29, 0.36)	0.02
Educational level									
Primary school or below	Reference	N/A	N/A	Reference	N/A	N/A	Reference	N/A	N/A
Middle or High school	0.16 (0.11)	(−0.05, 0.37)	0.13	0.21 (0.11)	(0.00, 0.42)	0.17*	0.14 (0.10)	(−0.06, 0.34)	0.12
College or above	0.13 (0.11)	(−0.09, 0.35)	0.11	0.19 (0.11)	(−0.02, 0.41)	0.16	0.11 (0.11)	(−0.10, 0.32)	0.09
Professional status									
Unemployed	Reference	N/A	N/A	Reference	N/A	N/A	Reference	N/A	N/A
Pensioner or retired	0.16 (0.14)	(−0.11, 0.44)	0.07	0.21 (0.14)	(−0.06, 0.48)	0.09	0.17 (0.13)	(−0.09, 0.43)	0.07
Employed	0.24 (0.21)	(−0.16, 0.65)	0.07	0.26 (0.20)	(−0.13, 0.65)	0.07	0.29 (0.19)	(−0.09, 0.67)	0.08
Economic situation									
Below average	Reference	N/A	N/A	Reference	N/A	N/A	Reference	N/A	N/A
Average	0.30 (0.07)	(0.16, 0.43)	0.24***	0.26 (0.07)	(0.13, 0.39)	0.21***	0.21 (0.07)	(0.08, 0.33)	0.17**
Above average	0.32 (0.09)	(0.16, 0.49)	0.21***	0.29 (0.08)	(0.12, 0.45)	0.19***	0.23 (0.08)	(0.07, 0.39)	0.15**
BLOCK 2: COVARIATES									
Chronic diseases									
Yes	–	–	–	Reference	N/A	N/A	Reference	N/A	N/A
No	–	–	–	0.26 (0.05)	(0.16, 0.36)	0.21***	0.24 (0.05)	(0.14 0.34)	0.19***
Infected cases of acquaintances									
Yes	–	–	–	Reference	N/A	N/A	Reference	N/A	N/A
No	–	–	–	0.12 (0.09)	(−0.05, 0.29)	0.06	0.10 (0.09)	(−0.07, 0.27)	0.05
BLOCK 3: LIFESTYLE BEHAVIORS									
PA stage	–	–	–	–	–	–	0.01 (0.02)	(−0.03, 0.04)	0.02
FVI stage	–	–	–	–	–	–	0.08 (0.02)	(0.05 0.12)	0.21***
Preventive behaviors	–	–	–	–	–	–	0.16 (0.07)	(0.03 0.29)	0.10*

* Coefficient is significant at the 0.01 level; ** Coefficient is significant at the 0.05 level, *** Coefficient is significant at the 0.0001 level.

power of the variance in QoL. The economic situation ($\beta_{\text{average vs. below average}}$ = 0.17, $p < 0.01$, 95%CI = 0.08–0.33; $\beta_{\text{above average vs. below average}}$ = 0.15, $p < 0.01$, 95%CI = 0.07–0.39), chronic diseases ($\beta = 0.19$, $p < 0.001$, 95%CI = 0.14–0.34), FVI stage ($\beta = 0.21$, $p < 0.001$, 95%CI = 0.05–0.12) and preventive behaviors ($\beta = 0.10, p < 0.05$, 95%CI = 0.03–0.29) can significantly predict the QoL of old adults. Details of regression analysis is shown in **Table 3**.

Moderating Effect of Socioeconomic Status

Correlation analyses revealed that educational level ($r = 0.13$, $p < 0.01$), professional status ($r = 0.12$, $p < 0.01$), and economic situation ($r = 0.20$, $p < 0.001$) were significantly associated with

QoL. In addition, except PA stage ($r = 0.02, p = 0.449$), FVI stage ($r = 0.21$, $p < 0.001$), and preventive behaviors ($r = 0.10$, $p < 0.05$) were significantly related to QoL.

In terms of the moderating effects of socioeconomic status between FVI and QoL, **Table 4** shows that educational level, professional status, and economic situation significantly predicted old adults' QoL in model 1 ($R^2 = 0.22$, $p < 0.001$), FVI stage significantly contributed to model 2 ($\Delta R^2 = 0.14$, $p < 0.001$), the interactions of SES with FVI stage did not significantly contribute to model 3 ($\Delta R^2 = 0.00$, $p = 0.510$). In terms of moderating effects of socioeconomic status between preventive behaviors and QoL, **Table 5** shows that economic situation significantly predicted old adults' QoL in model 1 ($R^2 = 0.22$, $p < 0.001$), preventive behaviors significantly contributed

TABLE 4 | Multiple linear regression examining main and interaction effects of socioeconomic status and FVI measures on QoL (n = 516).

Variable	Model 1			Model 2			Model 3		
	B (SE)	95%CI	β	B (SE)	95%CI	β	B (SE)	95%CI	β
Educational level	0.05 (0.04)	(−0.03, 0.14)	0.06	0.03 (0.04)	(−0.05, 0.11)	0.03	0.14 (0.11)	(−0.08, 0.36)	0.15
Professional status	0.17 (0.10)	(−0.03, 0.37)	0.08	0.17 (0.10)	(−0.02, 0.36)	0.08	0.28 (0.22)	(−0.15, 0.7)	0.12
Economic situation	0.16 (0.04)	(0.07, 0.24)	0.17***	0.14 (0.04)	(0.05, 0.22)	0.14***	0.07 (0.11)	(−0.14, 0.29)	0.08
FVI stage	–	–	–	0.12 (0.02)	(0.08, 0.15)	0.28***	0.23 (0.11)	(0.01, 0.45)	0.56*
FVI stage × Educational level	–	–	–	–	–	–	−0.03 (0.03)	(−0.09, 0.02)	−0.23
FVI stage × Professional status	–	–	–	–	–	–	−0.04 (0.06)	(−0.15, 0.08)	−0.18
FVI stage × Economic situation	–	–	–	–	–	–	0.02 (0.03)	(−0.04, 0.07)	0.11

FVI, fruit and vegetable intake; B, unstandardized coefficient; SE, standard error; β, standardized coefficient; –, data do not include in this model. *p < 0.05; ***p < 0.001, 2 tailed. Model 1 R² = 0.22; Model 2 R² = 0.36; Model 3 R² = 0.36.

TABLE 5 | Multiple linear regression examining main and interaction effects of socioeconomic status and preventive behaviors on QoL (n = 516).

Variable	Model 1			Model 2			Model 3		
	B (SE)	95%CI	β	B (SE)	95%CI	β	B (SE)	95%CI	β
Educational level	0.05 (0.04)	(−0.03, 0.14)	0.06	0.03 (0.04)	(−0.06, 0.11)	0.03	1.11 (0.39)	(0.34, 1.87)	1.16**
Professional status	0.17 (0.10)	(−0.03, 0.37)	0.08	0.17 (0.10)	(−0.02, 0.37)	0.08	−0.41 (0.76)	(−1.91, 1.08)	−0.18
Economic situation	0.16 (0.04)	(0.07, 0.24)	0.17***	0.13 (0.04)	(0.05, 0.22)	0.14**	0.95 (0.37)	(0.24, 1.67)	1.01**
Preventive behaviors	–	–	–	0.28 (0.07)	(0.15, 0.41)	0.18***	1.09 (0.43)	(0.24, 1.93)	0.71*
Preventive behaviors × Educational level	–	–	–	–	–	–	−0.30 (0.11)	(−0.51, −0.09)	−1.30**
Preventive behaviors × Professional status	–	–	–	–	–	–	0.16 (0.22)	(−0.27, 0.58)	0.32
Preventive behaviors × Economic situation	–	–	–	–	–	–	−0.23 (0.10)	(−0.43, −0.03)	−0.97*

B, unstandardized coefficient; SE, standard error; β, standardized coefficient; –, data do not include in this model. *p < 0.05; ***p < 0.001, 2 tailed. Model 1 R² = 0.22; Model 2 R² = 0.28; Model 3 R² = 0.33.

to model 2 ($\Delta R^2 = 0.06$, $p < 0.001$), the interactions of SES with preventive behaviors significantly contributed to model 3 ($\Delta R^2 = 0.05$, $p < 0.01$). In particular, 2 out of 3 interaction terms (preventive behaviors * educational level, $\beta = -1.3$, $p < 0.01$, 95%CI $= -0.51$ to -0.09; preventive behaviors * economic situation, $\beta = -0.97$, $p < 0.05$, 95%CI $= -0.43$ to -0.03) were significantly associated with QoL among old adults.

To further analyze the significant interaction effects, simple slopes analyses was conducted. In terms of the moderating effects of education level on the relationship between preventive behaviors and QoL, **Figure 1** shows that preventive behaviors were significantly associated with QoL at primary school or below of educational level [$\beta = 0.78$, $t_{(510)} = 3.86$, 95%CI $= 0.38$–1.18, $p < 0.001$] and at the middle or high school educational level [$\beta = 0.34$, $t_{(510)} = 3.79$, 95%CI $= 0.16$–0.52, $p < 0.001$], while the association was not significant at college or above for educational level [$\beta = 0.09$, $t_{(510)} = 0.82$, 95%CI $= -0.13$ to 0.32, $p = 0.411$]. In terms of the moderating effects of economic situation on the relationship between preventive behaviors and QoL, **Figure 2** shows that preventive behaviors were significantly associated with QoL at the below average level for economic situation [$\beta = 0.58$, $t_{(510)} = 4.46$, 95%CI $= 0.33$–0.84, $p < 0.001$] and at the average economic situation [$\beta = 0.18$, $t_{(510)} = 2.06$, 95%CI $= 0.01$–0.36, $p = 0.040$], while the association was not significant at the above average level for economic situation [$\beta = 0.11$, $t_{(510)} = 0.73$, 95%CI $= -0.18$ to 0.41, $p = 0.464$].

DISCUSSION

To the best of our knowledge, this is the first online cross-sectional study to explore the characteristics of QoL, to examine the association between lifestyle behaviors and QoL, and to identify the moderating role of SES on the association between lifestyle behaviors and QoL among Chinese older adults during the COVID-19 pandemic. The findings from the study have fully supported the proposed hypotheses. Specifically, during the outbreak of COVID-19, older adults' QoL differed significantly for demographic characteristics; healthy lifestyle behaviors significantly associated with higher QoL and SES indicators such as economic situation and educational level moderated the association between lifestyle behaviors and QoL levels in Chinese older adults.

In terms of the characteristics of QoL, as suggested in previous studies, older adults with better economic situations showed higher levels of QoL than those with lower economic conditions (39, 40). In line with previous evidence, the findings revealed that the elderly with higher levels of education showed higher QoL levels (41, 42). Employed participants and the elderly below 69 years of age showed higher QoL, confirming previous research results (42). As suggested in previous studies (41), the elderly with lesser family associations demonstrated significantly poorer QoL than those with sufficient socialization. Therefore, it is not surprising that older adults who were married and lived

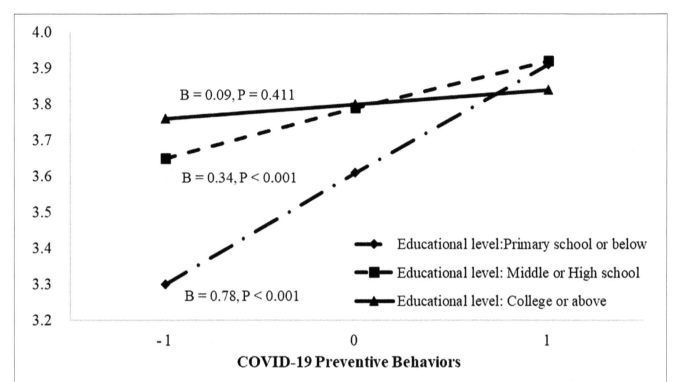

FIGURE 1 | The association between COVID-19 preventive behavior and quality of life (QoL) at different categories of educational level. The plot shows the predicted values of QoL at mean and ±1 SD of preventive behavior and educational level.

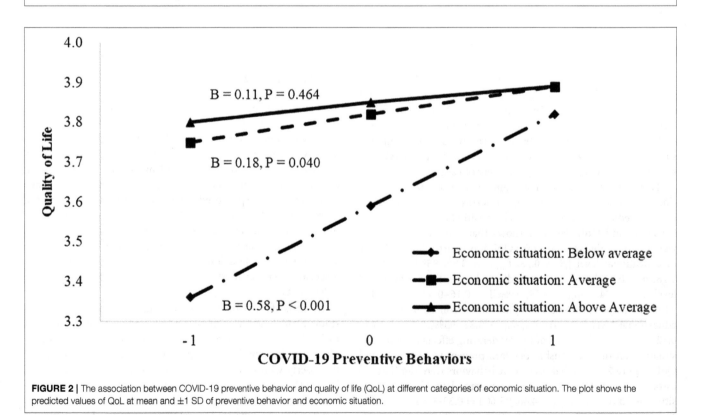

FIGURE 2 | The association between COVID-19 preventive behavior and quality of life (QoL) at different categories of economic situation. The plot shows the predicted values of QoL at mean and ±1 SD of preventive behavior and economic situation.

with others (e.g., spouse, partner, or children) indicated higher QoL. Also, the older adults with chronic diseases showed a significantly poorer QoL. This finding is consistent with a recent study in Moroccan populations, which observed that the impact of COVID-19 on QoL was more marked in people with chronic health problems (43). Consistent with previous evidence, the current study did not indicate significant differences in gender and BMI (44, 45). A discrepancy with previous evidence occurred in the infected cases of acquaintances (39) where no significant differences were found in this study. This may be attributed to the reason that most of our participants reported no infected cases of acquaintances (90.3%).

In terms of the association of lifestyle behaviors with QoL, our findings were consistent with a recent cross-sectional study among polish adults (46). Older adults who were at a higher FVI stage (eating more fruits and vegetables) and adopted more individual preventive behaviors (e.g., hand washing, facemask wearing, and social distancing) were more likely to show higher QoL during the COVID-19 pandemic. Notably, the lifestyle behaviors during the COVID-19 pandemic accounted for 6% of the variance in QoL, while economic situation, SES and chronic diseases as covariates also played an important role in predicting older adults' QoL status. These findings emphasize the significance of promoting FVI and preventive behaviors during the COVID-19 pandemic among older adults. The findings also highlight the importance of considering economic and health conditions when making relevant policies and designing interventions to enhance QoL among older adults.

In terms of the moderating effects of SES indicators in the association between lifestyle behaviors and QoL, educational level, and economic situation were found to be significant moderators in preventive behaviors and QoL association. To the best of our knowledge, there are no previous studies revealing such findings. Our recent study found that economic situations could modify the relationship between COVID-19 preventive behaviors and depression among Chinese older adults (36). As depression is significantly associated with QoL in older adults (47) we infer that the moderating role of economic situation might also occur between preventive behaviors and QoL. However, more empirical research using similar study designs among older adults from other regions and countries are needed in the future. The findings of the SES moderating role in the current study revealed that when authorities motivate older adults to enact COVID-19 preventive behaviors to improve their QoL status, they need to especially focus on older adults who are at a lower economic status with lower education levels. From a social policy aspect, the findings indicate the importance and necessity of public welfare targeting socioeconomic-specific population during the pandemic prevention. For example, local government can provide relief funding and epidemic prevention appliances (e.g., face masks, disinfection alcohol, and hand sanitizer) for low-income households to facilitate their preventive behaviors (48). In addition, community administrators can organize workshops and campaigns for older adults who are at lower education levels to increase their health literacy about preventive behaviors. All these policies and measures are useful for those older adults with socio-economic disadvantages to enact more preventive behaviors, which in turn can improve their level of health-related QoL during the pandemic.

Limitations of the current study should be acknowledged. Firstly, older adults who were at low socioeconomic status may have no access to mobile phones or computers to participate in this online survey. In addition, we applied snowball sampling approach to recruit older adults from Hubei province in China. Such investigation mode and sampling method may weaken the representativeness of samples and findings. Future studies should enlarge sample size, employ randomized sampling approaches, and administrate both online and offline surveys to enhance the generalization. Secondly, all the variables were measured using self-reported subjective scales, which might lead to recall bias and social desirability effects. In addition, due to the consideration on the parsimonious mode of online survey among older adults, only two general items of QoL were addressed in this study. We acknowledge that these items were not representative enough to capture the specific domains of QoL. For PA and FVI, only the simple algorithms were used to measure the stages of change of behaviors although the validity and reliability of the questionnaire were approved in previous studies (34). Therefore, applying comprehensive questionnaires to measure QoL, PA, and FVI should be warranted in future studies. Thirdly, the socio-demographic and behavioral factors identified in the present study only explained 20% of the variance of QoL. Hence, more socio-demographics such as the number of children an older adult has, how much financial support older adults receive from their children (49) and other healthy behaviors such as restful sleep (6) should be investigated in future studies among older adults. Notwithstanding the limitations, this study provides important information on the association between lifestyle behaviors and QoL during the COVID-19 pandemic. The study also provides detail relating to the role of SES indicators in moderating lifestyle behaviors and QoL among Chinese older adults. The research findings from this study inform interventions and policy makers to improve the health and QoL of older adults by means of enhancing their lifestyle behaviors (FVI and preventive behaviors) during the COVID-19 outbreak and future pandemics.

CONCLUSION

The current study investigated how Chinese older adults' demographic characteristics differ in QoL during the COVID-19 pandemic. The study also examined the association of lifestyle behaviors and QoL and identified the role of SES indicators in moderating the behavior–QoL relationship. All the study hypotheses were supported. The QoL of older adults differed significantly for living situations, age group, marital status, educational level, professional status, economic situation, and chronic diseases. The positive association of FVI and preventive behaviors with QoL was also identified in the current study. For SES indicators, only education level and economic situation significantly moderated the relationships between preventive behaviors and QoL. The research findings highlight the need for enacting preventive behaviors and FVI on enhancing QoL among older adults during the COVID-19 pandemic. The findings also revealed the importance of considering socioeconomic disparities such as economic status and education level when promoting preventive behaviors and QoL among the elderly during the pandemic. The findings presented here could be informative in implementing public health and social policies to maintain the overall well-being of older adults during the COVID-19 pandemic.

ETHICS STATEMENT

The studies involving human participants were reviewed and approved by REC/19-20/0490 Hong Kong Baptist University. The patients/participants provided their written informed consent to participate in this study.

AUTHOR CONTRIBUTIONS

YD and WL conceived and designed the study. YD, WL, CH, and BS contributed to the preparation of study materials. YD, WL, MY, CH, and BS collected the data. MY, WL, and YD screened and analyzed the data. MY, DP, and YD drafted the manuscript. YD, JB, and WL revised and polished the manuscript. All authors have read and agreed to the published version of the manuscript.

FUNDING

This research was supported by the Start-Up Grant of Hong Kong Baptist University. The funding organization had no role in the study design, study implementation, data collection, data analysis, manuscript preparation, or publication decision. This work was responsibility of the authors.

ACKNOWLEDGMENTS

We acknowledge support from the Hong Kong PhD Fellowship Scheme 2020.

REFERENCES

World Health Organization. *China: WHO Coronavirus Disease (COVID-19) Dashboard With Vaccination Data*. WHO (COVID-19) (2021). Available online at: https://covid19.who.int/region/wpro/country/cn (accessed July 20, 2021).

Bidzan-Bluma I, Bidzan M, Jurek P, Bidzan L, Knietzsch J, Stueck M, et al. A polish and german population study of quality of life, well-being, and life satisfaction in older adults during the COVID-19 pandemic. *Front Psychiatry*. (2020) 11:585813. doi: 10.3389/fpsyt.2020.5 85813

Chen X, Wang S Bin, Li XL, Huang ZH, Tan WY, Lin HC, et al. Relationship between sleep duration and sociodemographic characteristics, mental health and chronic diseases in individuals aged from 18 to 85 years old in Guangdong province in China: A population-based cross-sectional study. *BMC Psychiatry*. (2020) 20:455. doi: 10.1186/s12888-020-02866-9

World Health Organization. *WHOQOL Measuring Quality of Life*. Geneva (1997). Available online at: https://www.who.int/mental_health/media/en/68. pdf (accessed May 16, 2021).

Oliveira AKBD, Araújo MSD, Alves SFL, Rocha LDB, Da Silva ML, Rocha RSB, et al. Quality of life and social distancing: systematic review of literature. *Res Soc Dev*. (2020) 9:e318985885. doi: 10.33448/rsd-v9i8.5885

Tan SL, Storm V, Reinwand DA, Wienert J, de Vries H, Lippke S. Understanding the positive associations of sleep, physical activity, fruit and vegetable intake as predictors of quality of life and subjective health across age groups: a theory based, cross-sectional web-based study. *Front Psychol*. (2018) 9:977. doi: 10.3389/fpsyg.2018.00977

Schweitzer SO, Atchison KA, Lubben JE, Mayer-Oakes SA, De Jong FJ, Matthias RE. Health promotion and disease prevention for older adults: opportunity for change or preaching to the converted? *Am J Prev Med*. (1994) 10:223–9. doi: 10.1016/S0749-3797(18)30595-6

Akosile CO, Igwemmadu CK, Okoye EC, Odole AC, Mgbeojedo UG, Fabunmi AA, et al. Physical activity level, fear of falling and quality of life: a comparison between community-dwelling and assisted-living older adults. *BMC Geriatr*. (2021) 21:12. doi: 10.1186/s12877-020-01982-1

Kwon SC, Wyatt LC, Kranick JA, Islam NS, Devia C, Horowitz C, et al. Physical activity, fruit and vegetable intake, and health-related quality of life among older Chinese, Hispanics, and Blacks in New York City. *Am J Public Health*. (2015) 105:S544–52. doi: 10.2105/AJPH.2015.302653

Langhammer B, Bergland A, Rydwik E. The importance of physical activity exercise among older people. *Biomed Res Int*. (2018) 2018:7856823. doi: 10.1155/2018/7856823

Baugreet S, Hamill RM, Kerry JP, McCarthy SN. Mitigating nutrition and health deficiencies in older adults: a role for food innovation? *J Food Sci*. (2017) 82:848–55. doi: 10.1111/1750-3841.13674

Robinson SM. Improving nutrition to support healthy ageing: what are the opportunities for intervention? *Proc Nutr Soc*. (2018) 77:257–64. doi: 10.1017/S0029665117004037

Wang X, Ouyang Y, Liu J, Zhu M, Zhao G, Bao W, et al. Fruit and vegetable consumption and mortality from all causes, cardiovascular disease, and cancer: systematic review and dose-response meta-analysis of prospective cohort studies. *BMJ*. (2014) 349:g4490. doi: 10.1136/bmj.g4490

Catalan-Matamoros D, Gomez-Conesa A, Stubbs B, Vancampfort D. Exercise improves depressive symptoms in older adults: an umbrella review of systematic reviews and meta-analyses. *Psychiatry Res*. (2016) 244:202–9. doi: 10.1016/j. psychres.2016.07.028

Pinto AJ, Dunstan DW, Owen N, Bonfá E, Gualano B. Combating physical inactivity during the COVID-19 pandemic. *Nat Rev Rheumatol*. (2020) 16:347–8. doi: 10.1038/s41584-020-0427-z

Butler MJ, Barrientos RM. The impact of nutrition on COVID-19 susceptibility and long-term consequences. *Brain Behav Immun*. (2020) 87:53–4. doi: 10.1016/j. bbi.2020.04.040

Barber SJ, Kim H. COVID-19 worries and behavior changes in older and younger men and women. *Journals Gerontol Ser B*. (2021) 76:e17–23. doi: 10.1093/geronb/gbaa068

Doung-Ngern P, Suphanchaimat R, Panjangampatthana A, Janekrongtham C, Ruampoom D, Daochaeng N, et al. Associations between mask-wearing, hand washing, and social distancing practices and risk of COVID-19 infection in public: a case-control study in Thailand. *medRxiv*. (2020). 26. doi: 10.1101/2020.06.11.20128900

Armbruster S, Klotzbücher V. *Lost in Lockdown? COVID-19, Social Distancing, and Mental Health in Germany*. Freiburg im Breisgau: Albert-Ludwigs-Universität Freiburg, Wilfried-Guth-Stiftungsprofessur für Ordnungs- und Wettbewerbspolitik (2020).

Pieh C, O Rourke T, Budimir S, Probst T. Relationship quality and mental health during COVID-19 lockdown. *PLoS ONE*. (2020) 15:e0257118. doi: 10.1371/journal.pone.0238906

Jehn A. COVID-19 health precautions: identifying demographic and socioeconomic disparities and changes over time. *Can Public Policy*. (2021) 47:252–64. doi: 10.3138/cpp.2020-138

Petrovic D, de Mestral C, Bochud M, Bartley M, Kivimäki M, Vineis P, et al. The contribution of health behaviors to socioeconomic inequalities in health: a systematic review. *Prevent Med*. (2018) 113:15–31. doi: 10.1016/j. ypmed.2018.05.003

Zhu Y, Duan MJ, Dijk HH, Freriks RD, Dekker LH, Mierau JO. Association between socioeconomic status and self-reported, tested and diagnosed COVID-19 status during the first wave in the Northern Netherlands: a general population-based cohort from 49 474 adults. *BMJ Open*. (2021) 11:e048020. doi: 10.1136/bmjopen-2020-048020

Niu Z, Wang T, Hu P, Mei J, Tang Z. Chinese Public's engagement in preventive and intervening health behaviors during the early breakout of COVID-19: Cross-sectional study. *J Med Internet Res*. (2020) 22:e19995. doi: 10.2196/19995

Fearnbach SN, Flanagan EW, Höchsmann C, Beyl RA, Altazan AD, Martin CK, et al. Factors protecting against a decline in physical activity during the COVID-19 pandemic. *Med Sci Sports Exerc*. (2021) 53:1391–9. doi: 10.1249/MSS.0000000000002602

Knorst JK, Sfreddo CS, Meira FG, Zanatta FB, Vettore MV, Ardenghi TM. Socioeconomic status and oral health-related quality of life: a systematic review and meta-analysis. *Commun Dent Oral Epidemiol.* (2021) 49:95–102. doi: 10.1111/cdoe.12616

Faul F, Erdfelder E, Lang A, Buchner A. G*Power 3: a flexible statistical power analysis program for the social, behavioral, and biomedical sciences. *Behav Res Methods.* (2007) 39:175–91. doi: 10.3758/BF03193146

McAuley E, Konopack J, Motl R, Morris K, Doerksen S, Rosengren K. Physical activity and quality of life in older adults: influence of health status and self-efficacy. *Ann Behav Med.* (2006) 31:99–103. doi: 10.1207/s15324796abm3101_14

Kang H, Park M, Wallace Hernandez J. The impact of perceived social support, loneliness, and physical activity on quality of life in South Korean older adults. *J Sport Heal Sci.* (2018) 7:237–44. doi: 10.1016/j.jshs.2016.05.003

Ko GTC, Tang J, Chan JCN, Sung R, Wu MMF, Wai HPS, et al. Lower BMI cut-off value to define obesity in Hong Kong Chinese: an analysis based on body fat assessment by bioelectrical impedance. *Br J Nutr.* (2001) 85:239–42. doi: 10.1079/BJN2000251

Liang W, Duan YP, Shang BR, Wang YP, Hu C, Lippke S. A web-based lifestyle intervention program for Chinese college students: study protocol and baseline characteristics of a randomized placebo-controlled trial. *BMC Public Health.* (2019) 19:1097. doi: 10.1186/s12889-019-7438-1

Mazza C, Ricci E, Biondi S, Colasanti M, Ferracuti S, Napoli C, et al. A nationwide survey of psychological distress among italian people during the COVID-19 pandemic: immediate psychological responses and associated factors. *Int J Environ Res Public Health.* (2020) 17:3165. doi: 10.3390/ijerph17093165

Maertl T, De Bock F, Huebl L, Oberhauser C, Coenen M, Jung-Sievers C. Physical activity during COVID-19 in German adults: analyses in the COVID- 19 snapshot monitoring study (COSMO). *Int J Environ Res Public Health.* (2021) 18:507. doi: 10.3390/ijerph18020507

Duan YP, Wienert J, Hu C, Si GY, Lippke S. Web-based intervention for physical activity and fruit and vegetable intake among Chinese university students: a randomized controlled trial. *J Med Internet Res.* (2017) 19:e106. doi: 10.2196/jmir.7152

Culp WC. Coronavirus disease 2019: in-home isolation room construction. *AA Pract.* (2020) 14:e01218. doi: 10.1213/XAA.0000000000001218

Liang W, Duan Y, Shang B, Hu C, Baker JS, Lin Z, et al. Precautionary behavior and depression in older adults during the covid-19 pandemic: an online cross-sectional study in Hubei, China. *Int J Environ Res Public Health.* (2021) 18:1853. doi: 10.3390/ijerph18041853

World Health Organization. *The World Health Organization Quality of Life (WHOQOL)-BREF.* (2004). Available online at: https://www.who.int/ substance_abuse/research_tools/en/english_whoqol.pdf (accessed May 16, 2021).

Duan YP, Liang W, Guo L, Wienert J, Si GY, Lippke S. Evaluation of a web-based intervention for multiple health behavior changes in patients with coronary heart disease in home-based rehabilitation: pilot randomized controlled trial. *J Med Internet Res.* (2018) 20:e12052. doi: 10.2196/12052

Algahtani FD, Hassan SUN, Alsaif B, Zrieq R. Assessment of the quality of life during covid-19 pandemic: a cross-sectional survey from the Kingdom of Saudi Arabia. *Int J Environ Res Public Health.* (2021) 18:847. doi: 10.3390/ijerph18030847

Netuveli G, Wiggins RD, Hildon Z, Montgomery SM, Blane D. Quality of life at older ages: evidence from the English longitudinal study of aging (wave 1). *J Epidemiol Commun Health.* (2006) 60:357–63. doi: 10.1136/jech.2005.040071

Zaninotto P, Falaschetti E, Sacker A. Age trajectories of quality of life among older adults: results from the English longitudinal study of ageing. *Qual Life Res.* (2009) 18:1301–9. doi: 10.1007/s11136-009-9543-6

Grassi L, Caruso R, Da Ronch C, Härter M, Schulz H, Volkert J, et al. Quality of life, level of functioning, and its relationship with mental and physical disorders in the elderly: results from the MentDis_ICF65+ study. *Health Qual Life Outcomes.* (2020) 18:61. doi: 10.1186/s12955-020-01310-6

Samlani Z, Lemfadli Y, Ait Errami A, Oubaha S, Krati K. The impact of the COVID-19 pandemic on quality of life and well-being in Morocco. *Arch Commun Med Public Health.* (2020) 6:130–4. doi: 10.17352/2455-5479.000091

Somrongthong R, Hongthong D, Wongchalee S, Wongtongkam N. The influence of chronic illness and lifestyle behaviors on quality of life among older thais. *Biomed Res Int.* (2016) 2016:2525941. doi: 10.1155/2016/2525941

Siette J, Dodds L, Seaman K, Wuthrich V, Johnco C, Earl J, et al. The impact of COVID-19 on the quality of life of older adults receiving community-based aged care. *Australas J Ageing.* (2021) 40:84–9. doi: 10.1111/ajag.12924

Górnicka M, Drywien´ ME, Zielinska MA, Hamułka J. Dietary and lifestyle changes during covid-19 and the subsequent lockdowns among polish adults: a cross-sectional online survey plifecovid-19 study. *Nutrients.* (2020) 12:2324. doi: 10.3390/nu12082324

Levkovich I, Shinan-Altman S, Essar Schvartz N, Alperin M. Depression and health-related quality of life among elderly patients during the COVID-19 pandemic in Israel: a cross-sectional study. *J Prim Care Commun Health.* (2021) 12:2150132721995448. doi: 10.1177/21501327219 95448

Lu Q, Cai Z, Chen B, Liu T. Social policy responses to the covid-19 crisis in China in 2020. *Int J Environ Res Public Health.* (2020) 17:5896. doi: 10.3390/ijerph17165896

van Leeuwen KM, van Loon MS, van Nes FA, Bosmans JE, de Vet HCW, Ket JCF, et al. What does quality of life mean to older adults? A thematic synthesis. *PLoS ONE.* (2019) 14:e0213263. doi: 10.1371/journal.pone.02 13263

24

Experiment *in vivo*: How COVID-19 Lifestyle Modifications Affect Migraine

Vesselina Grozeva[1]*, Ane Mínguez-Olaondo[2] and Marta Vila-Pueyo[3]

[1] *Neurology Practice Polyclinic, Sofia, Bulgaria,* [2] *Department of Neurology, Hospital Universitario Donostia, San Sebastián, Spain,* [3] *Headache Group, Wolfson Centre for Age Related Diseases, Institute of Psychiatry, Psychology and Neuroscience, King's College London, London, United Kingdom*

*Correspondence:
Vesselina Grozeva
v.grozeva@yahoo.com

Introduction: The coronavirus disease 2019 (COVID-19) pandemic represents a unified lifestyle modification model, which was developed by the globally applied measures. The lockdowns designed the perfect study settings for observing the interaction between migraine and the adopted changes in lifestyle. An experiment *in vivo* took place unexpectedly to determine how the lockdown lifestyle modifications can influence migraine.

Subsection 1: Overall lifestyle modifications during the pandemic: People stay home, and outdoor activities and public contacts are restricted. Sleep is disturbed. Media exposure and prolonged screen use are increased. Working conditions change. In-person consultations and therapies are canceled. The beneficial effects of short-term stress, together with the harmful effects of chronic stress, were observed during the pandemic.

Subsection 2: Short-term effects: Substantial lifestyle changes happened, and knowing how vulnerable migraine patients are, one could hypothesize that this would have resulted in severe worsening of headache. Surprisingly, even though the impacts of changing social conditions were significant, some patients (including children) experienced a reduction in their migraine during the first lockdown.

Subsection 3: Long-term effects: Unfortunately, headache frequency returned to the basal state during the second pandemic wave. The risk factors that could have led to this worsening are the long-term disruption of sleep and dietary habits, stress, anxiety, depression, non-compliance to treatment, and working during the pandemic.

Discussion: Sudden short-term lifestyle changes taking migraine patients out of their usual routine may be beneficial for headache management. It is not necessary to have a natural disaster in place for a drastic lifestyle modification with 6–8-week duration, if we know that this will improve migraine.

Keywords: COVID-19, pandemic, migraine, lifestyle, modifications

INTRODUCTION

Migraine is an invisible disabling and undertreated disease (1). It is among the most prevalent disorders and one of the main causes of disability worldwide (2). A relationship between migraine and some environmental factors exists (3). However, the exact pathophysiology and how such factors affect the course of migraine remain unclear (4). Among the described triggers and aggravating factors (5) are emotional stress (6), sleep disturbances (7), nutrition, physical exercise, and others (8, 9). Avoidance of these triggers/factors through lifestyle changes is recommended because there is evidence that certain modifications of lifestyle can be beneficial for a better management of migraine (5, 6, 8). Despite the lack of well-designed studies to prove this link, the coronavirus disease 2019 (COVID-19) pandemic represents a unified lifestyle modification model that was followed in several countries because the preventative measures were globally applied. The COVID-19 lockdown designed the perfect study settings for observing the interaction between migraine sufferers and the adopted changes in lifestyle. This exceptional *in vivo* experiment took place unexpectedly and allowed us to determine how the lockdown lifestyle modifications can influence migraine.

SUBSECTION 1: OVERALL LIFESTYLE MODIFICATIONS DURING THE PANDEMIC

Substantial lifestyle changes happen during pandemic lockdowns, especially when global restrictions are applied. Social isolation is required to prevent spreading of the disease. People stay home, and outdoor activities and public contacts are restricted (9). Working conditions and some jobs change, while others disappear completely (10). Home-based working combined with homeschooling children under one and the same shelter carries additional burden. Parent–child relationships become challenging when all family members are required to stay close together under one shelter for a long time. Caregiving fatigue can add on (11, 12). Maintaining regular eating habits during an outbreak can become a real challenge as well (11). Shopping food restrictions and related food insecurity have been linked to risk of weight gain and obesity (13). Weight gain is very likely to happen during lockdown. Closed restaurants and limited physical exercise and outdoor activities could facilitate it (14). Of note, obesity is negatively associated with increased migraine frequency and disability (15). Both weight gain and obesity can be accompanied by sedentary life features such as prolonged sitting and poor posture, which are also very common in lockdowns and can be triggers of migraine attacks (16, 17). On the same line, the reduction in physical activity as a direct effect of lockdowns can only be a negative factor for migraine frequency, intensity, and duration (11). Sleep is another factor that could be possibly disturbed when having to cope with the pandemic emergency, increased stress, and fear of the unknown. Such disturbances can affect mood and quality of life (18), and this is essential for all aspects of health (11). Poor sleep has been linked to headache severity and disability, especially in the youth (19, 20). Media exposure, constant influx

of news, and prolonged screen use can lead to shorter and poorer quality of sleep (21); during the pandemic, a higher social media exposure was associated with severe psychological distress among migraineurs (22, 23) and also with an increased risk of migraine in adolescents and young adults (24). Besides the increased use of screens, brightness of computer screens is also considered a trigger for migraine attack exacerbation (25). Furthermore, it is important to mention that usual healthcare is modified during a pandemic, and in-person consultations and migraine therapies are canceled or substituted (10). It is well-known that pandemics increase stress, anxiety, and negative emotional reactions such as anger, fear, and risk perception (26). Social isolation, in turn, produces depressive symptoms, uncertainty about the future, and concerns for the health of family members (27).

The COVID-19 pandemic is a stressor, and its effects on migraine patients can be divided into short and long term. Short-term stress is known to activate multiple physiological systems as a response to enable survival (28) and may improve adaptive mechanisms. However, a transition can be observed from adaptive short-term stress to harmful chronic stress (28). Chronic stress results in stress-related biological changes that can last for months and even years (28). It may be hypothesized that under certain conditions, chronic prolonged stress could worsen a disease (28). The COVID-19 pandemic can be considered as an ideal experiment to observe the beneficial effects of short-term stress (during the beginning of the pandemic and the first lockdown), together with the harmful effects of the chronic stress observed during the ongoing pandemic. The COVID-19 pandemic has modified daily life in a negative way, and knowing how vulnerable migraine patients are, it could be suggested that this natural disaster would have resulted in severe worsening of the disease. Surprisingly, the study data show different results, especially for the first lockdown that could be possibly related to the short-term effects of the changes that occurred in the beginning of the pandemic.

SUBSECTION 2: SHORT-TERM EFFECTS

The COVID-19 pandemic entirely changed the daily living of migraine patients. Contrary to the expectations, several studies have shown that the lockdown has been beneficial for different groups of migraine patients. A study conducted in Italy showed that the lockdown led to a reduction in reported headache intensity and frequency in Italian children and adolescents (29). Another study investigated the impact of COVID-19 on young migraine patients. The results of the survey of the study showed a reduction in reported headache intensity and frequency as well (10, 29). A subsequent Dutch study also proved that the change in lifestyle caused by the pandemic has been beneficial for individuals with migraine (14). The number of migraine days and the acute medication intake days decreased along the first lockdown (14). During that period, an increase in general well-being was noted, compared with the month before the lockdown. Furthermore, for those patients who provided extended electronic diary data, this change was maintained even during the 2nd month of lockdown (10, 14). A Japanese group initially hypothesized that increased stress during the COVID-19 pandemic would affect the migraine population in a negative way (30). In line with this, a significant number of patients reported increased stress, and a negative impact of the first wave of the COVID-19 pandemic on their daily lives, together with concerns about COVID-19 and changes in mood and sleep. However, headache-related disability, the number of headache days and headache intensity did not change during the first wave of the COVID-19 pandemic. Thus, the results did not support the hypothesis for a negative impact on migraine course during the first lockdown (30). This study, though, highlighted the development of a new-onset headache in younger age individuals with worsened mood, sleep, and increased stress due to the pandemic (30).

SUBSECTION 3: LONG-TERM EFFECTS

The COVID-19 lockdowns have led to multiple lifestyle changes, which turned out to be time and quantity dependent in terms of effects on migraine. Long-lasting insecurity and stress related to the pandemic could potentially have led to an increased migraine disability (14). In contrast with the evidence presented in the previous section, a Spanish study found out that the overall long-term effects of COVID-19 lockdowns on migraine are negative (9). Approximately half of the studied patients shared a negative lockdown-related impact on their headache (9). The worsening was represented by higher intensity of attacks, and it was associated with higher levels of post-traumatic stress, anxiety, and depression (9). Increased intensity and frequency of migraine during lockdown were both related to new, but long-term triggers, such as changes in life habits or insomnia, and the negative emotional impact of COVID-19 (9). This phenomenon was explained with moderate-to-severe symptoms of post-traumatic-stress (9). Psychological distress among migraine patients is considered as one of the most important factors for worsening and poor management of migraine (31). Another study conducted in July 2020 during lockdown showed increased migraine frequency and severity among the majority of patients with migraine in Kuwait. Migraineurs were overusing analgesics, and around 10% transformed to chronic migraine during lockdown (31). Sixty percent reported worsening of their headaches, and 80 percent reported anxiety and depression. The risk factors that led to this worsening were sleep disturbances and bad dietary habits, associated with anxiety and depression, lack of communication with their treating neurologist, non-compliance to treatment, and working during the pandemic (31). Chinese patients with migraine also reported increased levels of insomnia, anxiety, and depressive symptoms during the COVID-19 pandemic (32). Perceived stress was more strongly associated with brooding and COVID-related rumination among patients with migraine than healthy controls (33). Perceived stress is known to be more common in chronic migraine, depression, and anxiety (34) and it might have been one of the risk factors that contributed to the worsening of migraine during the pandemic. The positive effects on migraine from the first lockdown in Italy

reverted to negative during the second lockdown, especially for the patients with episodic migraine (26). This resulted from more pronounced emotional reactions (anger, disgust, fear) toward the pandemic in the second wave that were correlated to higher headache intensity and frequency (26). Negative psychological effects and stressors included longer quarantine duration, factors associated with infection, economic crisis, and uncertainty of government measures (35). Frequency of migraine came back to its basal condition, and even worsened in episodic patients, with a potential transformation into chronic form (26). Thus, the long-lasting effects of the pandemic were found to have a negative impact on migraine evolution (33).

DISCUSSION

The COVID-19 pandemic lockdowns entirely changed the daily living of migraine patients. Multiple lifestyle changes modified the susceptibility to a migraine attack (14). Professionals initially suggested that migraine patients should stick to their previous routine to avoid worsening of their headache during the pandemic (31). However, our clinical practice and studies showed that the sudden and abrupt change in their routine was initially favorable for migraine patients. Stressful, challenging, and emotionally overwhelming experiences in the school environment may cause overreaction of the central nervous system to environmental requests that are perceived as too intense by the individual. Thus, the risk of headache and migraine is increased (36). This is also valid for the adult population, although the environment is different, and this population is considered to have more resilience to deal with such stressors. Lifestyle modifications during lockdown seem to have led to a reduction in the intensity and frequency of migraine in children and adolescents (29). These effects were explained mainly with the lower level of school-related stress during lockdown (29). We agree with the speculation that these unexpected improvements in migraine symptoms could be related to a reduction in external or internal demands for high performance in daily social settings, such as school/or work and sport or leisure activities (37, 38). Psychological stressors are potential migraine triggers. In the beginning of this unknown natural disaster, it was difficult to determine which were the bigger stressors: the usual daily demands that might had exceeded the capability of migraine patients or the fear of the unknown virus that took over the whole world, but there was still little information about it. A logical explanation for the improvement of migraine during the first pandemic wave could be the reduction of all known stressors in daily life. Since the actual hazard and harm of COVID-19 disease could not have been estimated in the beginning of the pandemic, the elimination of the old and usual stressors seems to have been very beneficial. The Dutch group proposed that working flexibility, reduction in social demands, and freedom to choose how to organize one's time might have led to a reduction in migraine frequency, intensity, and disability (14). This speculative conclusion was made for both children and adults with migraine (14, 29). The appropriate modification of the impact of school, work, and social demands on migraine patients could be beneficial for their migraine symptoms, and actually, the results indicate that short-term changes in some elements of their lifestyle can have a positive influence on the course of migraine (10).

In the first pandemic wave, the limited impact of the emotional behavior on migraine may be explained by the occurrence of a phenomenon called resilience (26). Unfortunately, during the second wave, negative psychological effects due to the prolonged stress and health emergency state prevailed (35). Negative emotional reactions against the pandemic, such as anger, anxiety, fear, and risk perception, linked to headache intensity, were absent during the first lockdown (26). The second wave of the pandemic led to an extension of the restrictive measures (35) and the emotional impact of the quarantine was enhanced by the uncertainty about the pandemic outcome, restrictive measures, and continuous viral diffusion (35). In the long term, factors like insecurity and stress may have worsened migraine disability (14). This COVID-19 experiment *in vivo* taught us that sudden short-term lifestyle changes that take migraine patients out of their usual routines may be beneficial for headache management. It is not necessary to have a natural disaster in place for a drastic lifestyle modification with 6–8-week duration, if we know that this will improve migraine. Short-lasting abrupt changes of lifestyle under less stressful circumstances can have even larger benefits than those observed in the first COVID-19 lockdown (14).

LIMITATIONS

This review provides a narrative approach by using all the current evidence to show the positive impact of the first COVID-19 wave on migraine patients. We acknowledge that using this approach, and not a systematic review, could be considered a limitation of the study.

We did not compare the effects of COVID-19 pandemic in migraine patients with previous pandemics because of several reasons. First, previous pandemics, such as the one in 1918, happened in a different historical moments where lifestyle was completely different from the current one, making the comparison irrelevant. Another point is the global effect that the COVID-19 pandemic has had, which is a unique characteristic of this pandemic. Future research could investigate further what is common between the pandemic eras and what is clearly distinct in terms of lifestyle, technology, and medicine evolution.

It would be interesting to understand if the pandemic has also modified other diseases or if it is a unique feature of migraine. Although there are some studies that support the changes induced by the pandemic in patients with Parkinson's disease or multiple sclerosis (39, 40), it is difficult to establish a comparison with migraine as those studies do not make a distinction between the two pandemic waves.

AUTHOR CONTRIBUTIONS

VG created the perspective idea and drafted the first manuscript. AM-O, VG, and MV-P reviewed the literature, processed and analyzed the data, interpreted the results, and edited and reviewed the language. MV-P conceptualized and designed the article and critically revised the manuscript. All authors contributed to the article and approved the submitted version.

FUNDING

MV-P received support from the Wellcome Trust (Grant number 104033). There were no funders involved in the study design, collection, analysis, interpretation of data, the writing of this article, or the decision to submit it for publication.

ACKNOWLEDGMENTS

We thank our families, our mentors, and clinical staff who participated in our professional pathway.

REFERENCES

Angus-Leppan H, Guiloff AE, Benson K, Guiloff RJ. Navigating migraine care through the COVID-19 pandemic: an update. *J Neurol.* (2021) 17:1–8. doi: 10.1007/s00415-021-10610-w

Stovner LJ, Nichols E, Steiner TJ, Abd-Allah F, Abdelalim A, Al- Raddadi RM, et al. Global, regional, and national burden of migraine and tension-type headache, 1990-2016: a systematic analysis for the Global Burden of Disease Study (2016). *Lancet Neurol.* (2018) 17:954–76. doi: 10.1016/S1474-4422(18)30322-3

Lipton RB, Pavlovic JM, Haut SR, Grosberg BM, Buse DC. Methodological issues in studying trigger factors and premonitory features of migraine. *Headache.* (2014) 54:1661–9. doi: 10.1111/head.12464

Szperka CL, Ailani J, Barmherzig R, Klein BC, MinenMT, Halker Singh RB, et al. Migraine care in the era of COVID-19: clinical pearls and plea to insurers. *Headache.* (2020) 60:833–42. doi: 10.1111/head.13810

Finocchi C, Sivori G. Food as trigger and aggravating factor of migraine. *Neurol Sci.* (2012) 33:S77–80. doi: 10.1007/s10072-012-1046-5

Radat F. Stress and migraine. *Rev Neurol.* (2013) 169:406–12. doi: 10.1016/j.neurol.2012.11.008

Mollao_glu M. Trigger factors in migraine patients. *J Health Psychol.* (2013) 18:984–94. doi: 10.1177/1359105312446773

Amin FM, Aristeidou S, Baraldi C, Czapinska-Ciepiela EK, Ariadni DD, et al. The association between migraine and physical exercise. *J Headache Pain.* (2018) 19:83. doi: 10.1186/s10194-018-0902-y

Gonzalez-Martinez A, Planchuelo-Gómez Á, Guerrero ÁL, García-Azorín D, Santos-Lasaosa S, Navarro-Pérez MP, et al. Evaluation of the Impact of the COVID-19 Lockdown in the Clinical Course of Migraine. *Pain Med.* (2021) 28:pnaa449. doi: 10.1093/pm/pnaa449

Grazzi L, Rizzoli P. Lessons from lockdown - behavioural interventions in migraine. *Nat Rev Neurol.* (2021) 17:195–196. doi: 10.1038/s41582-021-00475-y

Karvounides D, Marzouk M, Ross AC, VanderPluym JH, Pettet C, Ladak A, et al. The intersection of COVID-19, school, and headaches: problems and solutions. *Headache.* (2021) 61:190–201. doi: 10.1111/head. 14038

Prime H, Wade M, Browne DT. Risk and resilience in family well- being during the COVID-19 pandemic. *Am Psychol.* (2020) 75:631–43. doi: 10.1037/amp0000660

Metallinos-Katsaras E, Must A, Gorman K. A longitudinal study of food insecurity on obesity in preschool children. *J Acad Nutr Diet.* (2012) 112:1949–58. doi: 10.1016/j.jand.2012.08.031

Verhagen IE, van Casteren DS, de Vries Lentsch S, Terwindt GM. Effect of lockdown during COVID-19 on migraine: a longitudinal cohort study. *Cephalalgia.* (2021) 41:865–70. doi: 10.1177/0333102420981739

Oakley CB, Scher AI, Recober A, Peterlin BL. Headache and obesity in the pediatric population. *Curr Pain Headache Rep.* (2014) 18:416. doi: 10.1007/s11916-014-0416-5

Park S-Y, Yoo W-G. Effects of the sustained computer work on upper cervical flexion motion. *J Phys Ther Sci.* (2014) 26:441–42. doi: 10.1589/jpts.26.441

Smith L, Louw Q, Crous L, Grimmer-Somers K. Prevalence of neck pain and headaches: impact of computer use and other associative factors. *Cephalalgia*. (2009) 29:250–7. doi: 10.1111/j.1468-2982.2008.01714.x

Zeitlhofer J, Schmeiser-Rieder A, Tribl G, Rosenberger A, Bolitschek J, Kapfhammer G, et al. Sleep and quality of life in the Austrian population. *Acta Neurol Scand*. (2000) 102:249–57. doi: 10.1034/j.1600-0404.2000.102004249.x

Clementi MA, Chang YH, Gambhir R, Lebel A, Logan DE. The impact of sleep on disability and school functioning: results from a Tertiary Pediatric Headache Center. *J Child Neurol*. (2020) 35:221–7. doi: 10.1177/0883073819887597

Gilman DK, Palermo TM, Kabbouche MA, Hershey AD, Powers SW. Primary headache and sleep disturbances in adolescents. *Headache*. (2007) 47:1189–94. doi: 10.1111/j.1526-4610.2007.00885.x

Kenney EL, Gortmaker SL. United States adolescents' television, computer, videogame, smartphone, and tablet use: associations with sugary drinks, sleep, physical activity, and obesity. *J Pediatr*. (2017) 182:144–9. doi: 10.1016/j.jpeds.2016.11.015

Gao J, Zheng P, Jia Y, Chen H, Mao Y, Chen S, et al. Mental health problems and social media exposure during COVID-19 outbreak. *PLoS ONE*. (2020) 15:e0231924. doi: 10.1371/journal.pone.0231924

Chao M, Xue D, Liu T, Yang H, Hall BJ. Media use and acute psychological outcomes during COVID-19 outbreak in China. *J Anxiety Disord*. (2020) 74:102248. doi: 10.1016/j.janxdis.2020.102248

Montagni I, Guichard E, Carpenet C, Tzourio C, Kurth T. Screen time exposure and reporting of headaches in young adults: a cross-sectional study. *Cephalalgia*. (2016) 36:1020–7. doi: 10.1177/0333102415620286

Hysing M, Pallesen S, Stormark KM, Jakobsen R, Lundervold AJ, Sivertsen B. Sleep and use of electronic devices in adolescence: results from a large population-based study. *BMJ Open*. (2015) 5:e006748. doi: 10.1136/bmjopen-2014-006748

Delussi M, Gentile E, Coppola G, Prudenzano AMP, Rainero I, Sances G, et al. Investigating the effects of COVID-19 quarantine in migraine: an observational cross-sectional study from the Italian National Headache Registry (RICe). *Front Neurol*. (2020) 11:597881. doi: 10.3389/fneur.2020.597881

Fegert JM, Vitiello B, Plener PL, Clemens V. Challenges and burden of the coronavirus 2019 (COVID-19) pandemic for child and adolescent mental health: a narrative review to highlight clinical and research needs in the acute phase and the long return to normality. *Child Adolesc Psychiatr Ment Health*. (2020) 14:1–11. doi: 10.1186/s13034-020-00329-3

Dhabhar FS. The short-term stress response - Mother nature's mechanism for enhancing protection and performance under conditions of threat, challenge, and opportunity. *Front Neuroendocrinol*. (2018) 49:175–92. doi: 10.1016/j.yfrne.2018.03.004

Papetti L, Loro PAD, Tarantino S, Grazzi L, Guidetti V, Parisi P, et al. I stay at home with headache. A survey to investigate how the lockdown for COVID-19 impacted on headache in Italian children. *Cephalalgia*. (2020) 40:459–73. doi: 10.1177/0333102420965139

Suzuki K, Takeshima T, Igarashi H, Imai N, Danno D, Yamamoto T, et al. Impact of the COVID-19 pandemic on migraine in Japan: a multicentre cross-sectional study. *J Headache Pain*. (2021) 7:53. doi: 10.1186/s10194-021-01263-1

Al-Hashel JY, Ismail II. Impact of coronavirus disease 2019 (COVID-19) pandemic on patients with migraine: a web-based survey study. *J Headache Pain*. (2020) 24:115. doi: 10.1186/s10194-020-01183-6

Li Y, Qin Q, Sun Q, Sanford LD, Vgontzas AN, Tang X. Insomnia and psychological reactions during the COVID-19 outbreak in China. *J Clin Sleep Med*. (2020) 16:1417–8. doi: 10.5664/jcsm.8524

Kovacs LN, Baksa D, Dobos D, Eszlari N, Gecse K, Kocsel N, et al. Perceived stress in the time of COVID-19: the association with brooding and COVID-related rumination in adults with and without migraine. *BMC Psychol*. (2021) 9:68. doi: 10.1186/s40359-021-00549-y

Moon HJ, Seo JG, Park SP. Perceived stress in patients with migraine: a case-control study. *J Headache Pain*. (2017) 18:73. doi: 10.1186/s10194-017-0780-8

Brooks SK, Webster RK, Smith LE, Woodland L, Wessely S, Greenberg N, et al. The psychological impact of quarantine and how to reduce it: rapid review of the evidence. *SSRN Electron J*. (2020) 395:912–20. doi: 10.1016/S0140-6736(20)30460-8

Ashina S, Bendtsen L, Ashina M. Pathophysiology of tension-type headache. *Curr Pain Headache Rep*. (2005) 9:415–22. doi: 10.1007/s11916-005-0021-8

Balottin U, Chiappedi M, Rossi M, Termine C, Nappi G. Childhood and adolescent migraine: a neuropsychiatric disorder? *Med Hypotheses*. (2011) 76:778–81. doi: 10.1016/j.mehy.2011.02.016

Dallavalle G, Pezzotti E, Provenzi L, Toni F, Carpani A, Borgatti R. Migraine symptoms improvement during the COVID-19 lockdown in a cohort of children and adolescents. *Front Neurol*. (2020) 8:579047. doi: 10.3389/fneur.2020.579047

Prasad S, Holla VV, Neeraja K, Surisetti BK, Kamble N, Yadav R, et al. Impact of prolonged lockdown due to COVID-19 in patients with Parkinson's disease. *Neurol India*. (2020) 68:792–5. doi: 10.4103/0028-3886.293472

Morris-Bankole H, Ho, A.K. The COVID-19 pandemic experience in multiple sclerosis: the good, the bad and the neutral. *Neurol Ther*. (2021) 10:279–91. doi: 10.1007/s40120-021-00241-8

Mental Disorders, Cognitive Impairment and the Risk of Suicide in Older Adults

Agnieszka Kułak-Bejda¹*, Grzegorz Bejda² and Napoleon Waszkiewicz¹

¹ *Department of Psychiatry, Medical University of Bialystok, Bialystok, Poland,* ² *The School of Medical Science in Bialystok, Bialystok, Poland*

Correspondence:
Agnieszka Kułak-Bejda
agnieszka.kulak.bejda@gmail.com

More than 600 million people are aged 60 years and over are living in the world. The World Health Organization estimates that this number will double by 2025 to 2 billion older people. Suicide among people over the age of 60 is one of the most acute problems. The factors strongly associated with suicide are mentioned: physical illnesses, such as cancer, neurologic disorder, pain, liver disease, genital disorders, or rheumatoid disorders. Moreover, neurologic conditions, especially stroke, may affect decision-making processes, cognitive capacity, and language deficit. In addition to dementia, the most common mental disorders are mood and anxiety disorders. A common symptom of these disorders in the elderly is cognitive impairment. This study aimed to present the relationship between cognitive impairment due to dementia, mood disorders and anxiety, and an increased risk of suicide among older people. Dementia is a disease where the risk of suicide is significant. Many studies demonstrated that older adults with dementia had an increased risk of suicide death than those without dementia. Similar conclusions apply to prodromal dementia Depression is also a disease with a high risk of suicide. Many researchers found that a higher level of depression was associated with suicide attempts and suicide ideation. Bipolar disorder is the second entity in mood disorders with an increased risk of suicide among the elderly. Apart from suicidal thoughts, bipolar disorder is characterized by high mortality. In the group of anxiety disorders, the most significant risk of suicide occurs when depression is present. In turn, suicide thoughts are more common in social phobia than in other anxiety disorders. Suicide among the elderly is a serious public health problem. There is a positive correlation between mental disorders such as dementia, depression, bipolar disorder, or anxiety and the prevalence of suicide in the elderly. Therefore, the elderly should be comprehensively provided with psychiatric and psychological support.

Keywords: suicide, elderly, cognitive impairment, dementia, depression, bipolar disorder, anxiety

INTRODUCTION

The World Health Organization (WHO) reported that more than 600 million people age 60 years and older worldwide. The WHO further estimated that, by 2025, this number would double to two billion older people (1). It is well-known that older people are at greater risk for diseases and body injuries, poverty, social isolation, loneliness, and loss of independence, all of which contribute to deterioration in mental health (2, 3). The prevalence rate of suicide ranges from 8.54 to 33% (3–5). In older adults, the most frequently diagnosed mental disorders are anxiety disorders (10.9%) and mood disorders such as depression (7.4%) (3, 6). Moreover, suicide is a global concern. Almost 78% of all completed suicides occur in low- and middle-income countries, and in general, suicides account for 1.4% of premature deaths worldwide (7).

The rate of suicide has been shown to increase with advancing age, and one of the most acute problems is suicide among people over the age of 60. Older men and women have been identified as having the highest suicide rate in almost every country, reaching 48.7/100,000 in the US for white men (more than four times that nation's age-adjusted rate of 11.1/100,000) and 140/100,000 in rural China for men (6, 8).

Among the factors strongly associated with suicide are physical illnesses, such as cancer, neurologic disorder, pain, liver disease, genital disorders, and rheumatoid disorders. Moreover, neurologic conditions, especially stroke, may affect decision-making processes, cognitive capacity, and language (9, 10). These risk factors, combined with a lack of social connection and a sense of meaninglessness, contribute to the occurrence of suicidal behavior (9–11).

In older adults, suicide is often a consequence of mental disorders such as depression, anxiety disorder, insomnia, Alzheimer's disease, and vascular dementia (12). All these disease entities are also strongly associated with cognitive impairment.

Cognitive appraisal theory is a theory of emotions. It states that a person's evaluative judgment (or appraisal) of a situation, event, or object determines or contributes to their emotional response to it. Cognitive appraisal theory is based on the James-Lange theory of emotions and considers that a given physiological response can give rise to various emotional responses. The theory was initially proposed by American psychologist Stanley Schachter in 1964 and has later been developed further by other researchers. In an experiment carried out by Schachter and Singer, participants were injected with adrenaline and not told that this would cause a heightened level of physiological arousal. When placed in situations designed to elicit either anger or euphoria, these subjects would attribute their state of arousal to their problem (13).

Cognitive impairment plays a role in attempted suicide among older people. The literature mentions the following risk factors: dysfunctional cognitive control, executive function, and problem-solving. The loss of these abilities makes it difficult to cope with life problems functionally and, thus, increases the risk of suicide (14).

Older people newly diagnosed with dementia are significantly more at risk for suicide than their peers without dementia. Individuals diagnosed with dementia had a 54% increased risk for suicide within the 1st year after diagnosis. The risk was exceptionally high among those aged 74 years and younger (12).

Several studies have considered cognitive impairment in late-life depression both qualitatively and quantitatively. Studies that included a clinical diagnosis of major depression, a comprehensive assessment of cognition, and a healthy comparison group have documented deficits in episodic memory, speed of information processing, executive functioning, and visual-spatial ability (15).

Deficits in the speed of information processing and executive functioning might be particularly pertinent. Three recent studies reported that slowed rate of information processing or working memory deficits appears to mediate the cognitive impairment associated with depression predominantly. Mechanisms that might increase the risk depression poses for developing Alzheimer's disease (16). Late-life depression is associated with both chronic elevations of adrenal glucocorticoid production and cerebrovascular disease. Together, these factors may lead to hippocampal atrophy and generalized ischemia (17).

Generalized ischemia often has a preference for frontostriatal regions, leading to abnormalities that could also serve to maintain or cause subsequent depressive episodes. These factors can also lower brain or cognitive reserve. When other pre-existing Alzheimer's disease casual risk factors are present, this can hasten the progression of underlying Alzheimer's disease pathology to clinical manifestation of this disease entity (17).

Some reports show depressive symptoms are linked to suicide in patients with cognitive impairment (12, 18–21). Little is yet known about the relationship between cognitive impairment itself and suicide.

Worse cognitive functioning is associated with more frequent suicidal ideas in those individuals with depression even when depression severity was taken into account (22).

This study aimed to present the relationship between cognitive impairment due to dementia, mood disorders and anxiety, and an increased risk of suicide among older adults. The authors provide an overview of the literature from the main databases (Medline, Web of Science, EMBASE, and the Cochrane Database of Systematic Reviews) from the latest years.

DEMENTIA

Dementia is a disease entity characterized by progressive cognitive impairment and behavioral changes. Dementia is a general term used to refer to diseases including Alzheimer's disease, vascular dementia, Lewy body dementia, frontotemporal dementia, and mixed dementia (23, 24). Data have shown that about 50% of all dementia is related to Alzheimer's disease (24, 25). Generally, patients with dementia present the following symptoms: progressive impairments in memory, thinking, and behavior, which have a strong negative influence on everyday activities. Other common symptoms include difficulties with language, decreased motivation, and emotional problems, such as depression, psychotic hallucinations, delusions, apathy, anxiety, or aggression (26).

Tu et al. analyzed data from the Taiwan National Health Insurance Research Database and compared 1,189 patients age ≥ 65 who attempted suicide and 4,756 age- and sex-matched control subjects. The methods used by suicide attempters included drug overdose (13.5%), hanging or drowning (4.1%), physical injury (44.2%), and poison (38.5%). The researchers also found that the elderly who attempted suicide had a significantly ($p < 0.001$) higher likelihood of developing dementia than controls. Another conclusion they reached is that demographic geriatric suicide attempts were significantly associated with an elevated risk of developing dementia (hazard ratio [HR]: 7.40, 95% CI: 6.11–8.97, $p < 0.001$) in later life (27).

Annor et al. analyzed data from 2013 to 2016 from the Georgia Alzheimer's Disease and Related Dementia registry that were linked with data from the Georgia Vital Records and Georgia Violent Death Reporting System. They identified 91 residents with dementia who died by suicide. The suicide rate among persons with dementia was 9.3 per 100,000 person-years overall and higher among those diagnosed in the past 12 months (424.5/100,000 person-years). They concluded that male gender, the onset of dementia before age 65, and a recent diagnosis of dementia are predictive factors of suicide (28).

Zucca et al. determined the prevalence of suicidal ideation and attempts in patients with behavioral frontotemporal dementia (bvFTD) by assessing possible risk factors for suicide. They found that patients with bvFTD who attempted suicide showed a higher global Scale for Suicide Ideation (SSI) score in comparison to those who presented suicidal ideation alone ($P < 0.001$). Patients with bvFTD were found to have significantly higher functional and cognitive impairment levels and were more apathetic and impulsive. However, no differences in neuropsychological characteristics were identified when comparing patients with bvFTD at risk for suicide and patients with bvFTD with no suicide risk (29).

Lai et al. analyzed data from two databases, the US Department of Veterans Affairs (VA) National Patient Care Database and the Department of Veterans Affairs (VA) National Suicide Prevention Applications Network (SPAN), and estimated the 2-year prevalence of mental health disorders across five dementia subtypes during fiscal years 2012 and 2013. They found that patients with FTD had the highest 2-year prevalence of psychiatric disorders and suicidal behavior (nearly 4% having suicidal ideation and 0.5% having a suicidal plan or having attempted suicide). Likewise, patients with VD showed a high 2-year prevalence of suicidal behavior (3%) and other psychiatric disorders such as anxiety (14%) and substance use (17%) (30).

Choi et al. used the National Health Insurance Service Senior Cohort data. They included 36,541 older adults with newly diagnosed dementia such as Alzheimer's disease, vascular dementia, and other/unspecified dementia from 2004 to 2012. They attempted to estimate suicide risk within 1 year of dementia diagnosis. They verified 46 deaths by suicide during the 1st year after a dementia diagnosis. Older adults with dementia had an increased risk of death by suicide than those without dementia (31).

Koyama et al. examined 634 patients with dementia and observed suicidal ideation in 10%. These results correlated with the severity of behavioral and psychological dementia symptoms (32).

Richard-Devantoy et al. suggested that poor cognitive control may contribute to high suicide rates in old age. They also demonstrated that cognitive control deficits in older patients with any high-lethality suicide attempt might undermine their ability to solve real-life problems, precipitating a catastrophic accumulation of stressors (33).

By contrast, a link has been identified between suicide and prodromal dementia. Gujral et al. compared 67 non-suicidal depressed older adults, 63 depressed suicide ideators, 44 late-onset and 48 early-onset suicide attempters, and 56 non-psychiatric comparison groups. They found that both attempter groups presented worse executive functioning than the non-suicidal depressed group. Moreover, poorer global cognition and processing speed were demonstrated by late-onset attempters compared to non-suicidal depressed older adults. They also showed more flawed memory than early-onset attempters (34).

MOOD DISORDERS

Depressive disorders are described in the Diagnostic and Statistical Manual for Mental Disorders (5th edition; DSM-5). Among the group of mood disorders, the DSM-5 includes major depressive disorder (MDD), persistent depressive disorder (dysthymia), bipolar I and II disorder (BD), cyclothymic disorder, and premenstrual dysphoric disorder (35).

The prevalence of the major depressive disorder in adults age 65 and older ranges from 1–5% in the community. Furthermore, significant depressive symptoms are present in approximately 15% of older adults (36).

Lee and Atteraya analyzed data from the Survey of Living Conditions and Welfare Needs of Korean Older Persons, which included 10,279 persons. They found that people between 65 and 69 years old have suicide ideation more often than those 80 years and older. A higher level of depression (OR = 1.19) was strong associated with suicide ideation. In addition, poverty (OR = 1.59) and exposure to abuse (OR = 2.37) were associated with suicide ideation (37).

Nakamura et al. analyzed data from 63,026 men and 72,268 women age 65 years and older. They showed that the male suicide standardized mortality ratio (SMR) was positively correlated with depressive symptoms ($p = 0.002$). The female suicide SMR was positively correlated with the rate of depressive symptoms ($\rho = 0.258$) (38).

Choi et al. focused on a specific group of patients. They assessed suicide risk in the elderly within 1 year after stroke and attempted to correlate it with depression. Patients with depression had an increased risk of suicide after stroke (AHR = 2.9; 95% CI, 1.8–4.8), and this applied to post-stroke depression as well (AHR = 4.1; 95% CI, 1.8–9.5) (31). However, compared to stroke patients without depression, both pre-and post-stroke depression suicidality was higher (AHR = 4.8; 95% CI, 2.1–11.1) (39).

For their study, Kiosses et al. recruited 74 older participants (65–95 years old) with MDD and cognitive impairment. They found that the Montgomery–Aasberg Depression Rating Scale's negative emotions scores were significantly associated with suicidal ideation during treatment ($F_{[1,165]} = 12.73$, $p = 0.0005$) (40).

Yeh et al. analyzed data from national health insurance databases in Taiwan. They showed that the risk of suicide was higher in those who had depression (OR = 3.49, 95% CI = 2.2–5.4) and bipolar disorder (OR = 1.98, 95% CI = 1.1–3.6) (41).

Tan et al. attempted to identify the differences between two age groups, middle-aged (45–64 years) and older-aged people (65+ years), who had self-harmed. They found that the 65+ age group had a history of depression ($p < 0.0001$) and had been diagnosed with depression at the time of their attempt ($p < 0.0001$). Moreover, suicidal intent was more common among older-aged people who had self-harmed ($p = 0.004$), and this group had lower survival rates in the 12 months following their self-harm attempt (risk ratio = 7.5; 95% CI = 3.1–18.1) (42).

Woo et al. characterized the high-intent suicide attempters admitted to emergency departments. They demonstrated that the number of older than 66 years increased as the strength of suicidal intent increased ($P = 0.04$). They also had higher Hamilton Depression Rating Scale (HDRS) scores, higher premeditation rates, and sustained suicidal ideation (43).

Park et al. analyzed the data from the Survey of Living Conditions and Welfare Needs of Korean Older Persons. The prevalences of depression and suicidal ideation were 30.3 and 11.2%, respectively. Moreover, they found that 60.5% of suicidal ideation could be prevented or reduced if depression was eliminated (44).

The 220 older adults with bipolar disorder (BD) recruited to the study conducted by O'Rourke et al. found that older adults with BD who reported low satisfaction with life and current depressive symptoms and misused alcohol also reported having significantly higher levels of suicidal ideation (45). The same authors attempted to describe predictors of suicidal ideation among older adults with BD. They confirmed that depressive symptoms and cognitive failures could be predictors of suicidal ideation (46).

Almeida et al. analyzed data from 37,768 men ages 65–85 years with bipolar disorder. They showed that BD was also associated with increased mortality (HR = 1.51, 95% CI 1.28–1.77). Suicide was one of the most common causes of death in this group of patients (47).

Belvederi Murri et al. drew interesting conclusions from their study. They found that cognitive impairments linked with BD were associated with an increased likelihood of disability and recent aggressive behavior but not suicidal thoughts (48).

ANXIETY DISORDERS

Generalized anxiety disorder (GAD) is a state of chronic, uncontrolled anxiety. This anxiety disrupts daily functioning and causes sleep disturbance. In turn, panic disorder is characterized by a recurrent, unexpected attack of intense anxiety. It causes physical and cognitive dysfunctions and impairs everyday functioning. By contrast, a specific phobia is an exaggerated fear of a particular object or situation (49, 50).

According to Pary et al., fear of falling occurs in about 50% of older persons who have fallen recently (49).

Bendixen et al. included 218 older adults in their study. They measured the severity of anxiety symptoms using the Geriatric Anxiety Inventory (GAI) and the Montgomery–Aasberg Depression Rating Scale (MADRS) to assess the severity of depression. They showed that higher GAI scores were significantly associated with suicidality ($\beta = 0.206$, $p = 0.006$). Moreover, higher GAI scores were related to scores on the MADRS ($\beta = 0.233$, $p = 0.002$) (51).

Petkus et al. examined age differences in death and suicidal ideation in patients with anxiety disorders. Interestingly, the authors showed that older participants with social anxiety disorder were significantly more likely to report thoughts of death and suicidal thoughts than older adults with other anxiety disorders (52).

DISCUSSION

Suicide is problem that affects older adults. In the USA, suicide rates are high among older men, with men ages 85 and older having the highest rate of any other group. Moreover, suicide attempts by the elderly are much more likely to end in death than among young people. The following factors influence this fact: older adults use more deadly methods, are less often found and saved, and they are less likely to recover from complications due to age and comorbidities (9, 11, 53).

In many studies, the relationship between disability, pain, physical illnesses (like cancer), and suicidal behavior in older adults has been demonstrated (9, 10, 54, 55).

Moreover, the systematic review conducted by Fässberg et al. showed that completed suicide specifically had been associated with psychiatric disorders (e.g., major depressive disorder), addictions, and sleep disturbances (54). Among other risk factors, the researchers mentioned marital status (widowed or divorced), family conflicts, material problems, and previous suicide attempts (55, 56).

Among the prisoners' specific study group, suicide rates are higher than those in the same age group in the general population. The authors associate these findings with the lack of proper diagnosis of mental disorders and their specific treatment (56).

Szanto et al. found three pathways to suicidal behavior in older adults, and the authors distinguished: very high levels of cognitive and dispositional risk factors, dysfunctional personality traits, and impulsive decision-making, and cognitive deficits (57).

Interestingly, Jung et al. showed that depression and suicidal ideation levels in the religiously affiliated group were not significantly different from that of the religiously non-affiliated group. Moreover, there were no significant differences between Christians and Buddhists (58).

Kiosses et al. presented psychosocial intervention to reduce suicide risk in older adults who have been hospitalized after a suicide attempt or with suicidal ideation. Cognitive Reappraisal Intervention for Suicide Prevention (CRISP) assumed: an emotional crisis precedes hospitalization for suicidality and patients have had difficulty dealing with this emotional crisis; this emotional crisis is related to personalized triggers; identifying these personalized triggers and the associated negative emotions and providing strategies for adaptive response and improvement of suicide prevention. The authors expect that CRISP may reduce suicide risk at the post-discharge period, where the patients are particularly vulnerable to suicide (40).

In turn, Kim et al. analyzed the effectiveness of a community-based program for suicide prevention among elders with early-stage dementia. They found that the developed suicide prevention program significantly affected the perceived health status, social support, depression, and suicidal ideation of elders with early-stage dementia (59).

Sakashita and Oyama concluded that community interventions are essential in reducing suicide in older adults. Furthermore, integrating universal, selective, and indicated prevention strategies might be necessary for this process. Perhaps the most important relationship is between selective and indicated preventive interventions (60).

The International Research Group for Suicide Among the Elderly proposes that multifaceted strategies should improve resilience and positive aging and involve family and community guardians. Also, telecommunications should be expanded to reach vulnerable older people and assess the impact of resource constraints. Moreover, physicians of all specialties should be educated on suicide by older people and actively participate in preventive programs (61).

Older people are most vulnerable to health problems due to various factors: depression, anxiety, dementia, neurocognitive disorders, social isolation, loss of relatives, pain, and chronic physical diseases. These mentioned factors increase the risk for suicidal behavior. So, these risk factors should be taken into account in suicide prevention strategies (9).

Our results have several medical implications. Family doctors should be involved in the prevention of suicidal behavior in older people. They are the first to have contact with older suicidal people. Older adults have a higher prevalence of physical disorders and more often visit their doctors (62).

Furthermore, older adults had more frequent contact with the family doctor than with the psychiatric services before suicide. Additionally, anxiety disorder and depression are associated with suicide, and the treatment of these psychiatric conditions should be enhanced in older adults (63).

The loss of a spouse, grief, hopelessness increase the risk of suicidal thoughts or behaviors. Older adults who have been widowed, socially isolated, and who have cognitive problems should increase our attention in health consultations (64).

STRENGTHS AND LIMITATIONS

This literature review presents the most recent findings on dementia, mood disorders, anxiety, and suicidal behaviors in older adults. However, some limitations should be highlighted. First, the most significant part of the studies has been performed on small population samples with clinical heterogeneity according to age and the disease stage. Second, very few studies explored the link between suicide and the different types of dementia. Third, we included the literature from recent years.

CONCLUSIONS

Suicide among people over the age of 60 is a frequent problem. Older men and women have been identified as having the highest suicide rate in almost every country. Dementia is a disease where the risk of suicide is significant. Older adults with dementia had an increased risk of suicide death compared to those without dementia. Also, prodromal dementia, depression, and bipolar disorder are diseases with a high risk of suicide.

Furthermore, bipolar disorder is characterized by high mortality. Families, social support systems, and health care providers should learn about suicide in older people. And they should discuss suicide warning signs and how to provide support. It is essential to make physicians who have contact with seniors aware of the possible occurrence of suicidal thoughts, especially if mental disorders accompany them. We suggest that family doctors should be able to perform suicide risk tests among seniors.

AUTHOR CONTRIBUTIONS

AK-B contributed to the conception and design of the study and wrote the first draft of the manuscript. AK-B and GB analyzed the database. NW supervised the preparation of the final version of the manuscript. All authors contributed to the revision of the manuscript and read and approved the presented version.

REFERENCES

World Health Organization. *Towards Age-Friendly Primary Health Care*. (2004). Available online at: http://www.who.int/ageing/publications/phc/en/ (accessed January 15, 2021).

World Federation for Mental Health. *Mental Health and Older People*. (2013). Available online at: http://lmentala.net/admin/archivosboletin/WMHDay_2013_v3_small_file.pdf (accessed January 15, 2021).

Kenbubpha K, Higgins I, Chan SW, Wilson A. Promoting active ageing in older people with mental disorders living in the community: an integrative review. *Int J Nurs Pract*. (2018) 24:e12624. doi: 10.1111/ijn.12624

Gum AM, King-Kallimanis B, Kohn R. Prevalence of mood, anxiety, and substance-abuse disorders for older Americans in the national comorbidity survey-replication. *Am J Geriatr Psychiatry*. (2009) 17:769–81. doi: 10.1097/JGP.0b013e3181a d4f5a

Ritchie K, Artero S, Beluche I, Ancelin M-L, Mann A, Dupuy A-M, et al. Prevalence of DSM-IV psychiatric disorder in the French elderly population. *Br J Psychiatry*.
(2004) 184:147–52. doi: 10.1192/bjp.184.2.147

Baladón L, Fernández A, Rubio-Valera M, Cuevas-Esteban J, Palao DJ, Bellon JA, et al. Prevalence of mental disorders in non- demented elderly people in primary care. *Int Psychogeriatr*. (2015) 27:757–68. doi: 10.1017/S1041610214002841

Bachmann S. Epidemiology of suicide and the psychiatric perspective. *Int J Environ Res Public Health*. (2018) 15:1425. doi: 10.3390/ijerph15071425

Conwell Y, Thompson C. Suicidal behavior in elders. *Psychiatr Clin North Am*. (2008) 31:333–56. doi: 10.1016/j.psc.2008.01.004

Conejero I, Olié E, Courtet P, Calati R. Suicide in older adults: current perspectives. *Clin Intervent Aging*. (2018) 13:691–9. doi: 10.2147/CIA.S130670

Finestone HM, Blackmer J. Refusal to eat, capacity, and ethics in stroke patients: a report of 3 cases. *Arch Phys Med Rehabil*. (2007) 88:1474–7. doi: 10.1016/j.apmr.2007.07.018

Wand A, Peisah C, Draper B, Brodaty H. Understanding self-harm in older people: a systematic review of qualitative studies. *Aging Ment Health*. (2018) 22:289–98.

doi: 10.1080/13607863.2017.1304522

An JH, Lee KE, Jeon HJ, Son SJ, Kim SY, Hong JP. Risk of suicide and accidental deaths among elderly patients with cognitive impairment. *Alzheimers Res Ther.* (2019) 11:32. doi: 10.1186/s13195-019-0488-x

Schachter S, Singer JE. Cognitive, social, and physiological determinants of emotional state. *Psychol Rev.* 69:379–99. doi: 10.1037/h0046234

Bermejo-Pareja F, Antequera D, Vargas T, Molina JA, Carro E. Saliva levels of Abeta1-42 as potential biomarker of Alzheimer's disease: a pilot study. *BMC Neurol.* (2010) 10:108. doi: 10.1186/1471-2377-10-108

Herrmann LL, Goodwin GM, Ebmeier KP. The cognitive neuropsychology of depression in the elderly. *Psychol Med.* (2007) 37:1693–702. doi: 10.1017/S0033291707001134

Butters MA, Whyte EM, Nebes RD, Begley AE, Dew MA, Mulsant BH, et al. The nature and determinants of neuropsychological functioning in late-life depression. *Arch Gen Psychiatry.* (2004) 61:587–95. doi: 10.1001/archpsyc.61.6.587

Sheline YI, Barch DM, Garcia K, Gersing K, Pieper C, Welsh-Bohmer K, et al. Cognitive function in late life depression: relationships to depression severity, cerebrovascular risk factors and processing speed. *Biol Psychiatry.* (2006) 60:58–65. doi: 10.1016/j.biopsych.2005.09.019

Andreescu C, Ajilore O, Aizenstein HJ, Albert K, Butters MA, Landman BA, et al. Disruption of neural homeostasis as a model of relapse and recurrence in late-life depression. *Am J Geriatr Psychiatry.* (2019) 27:1316–30. doi: 10.1016/j.jagp.2019.07.016

Lim WS, Rubin EH, Coats M, Morris JC. Early-stage Alzheimer disease represents increased suicidal risk in relation to later stages. *Alzheimer Dis Assoc Disord.* (2005) 19:214–9. doi: 10.1097/01.wad.0000189051.48688.ed

Vega U, Kishikawa Y, Ricanati E, Friedland R, Suicide P, Alzheimer disease. *Am J Geriatr Psychiatry.* (2002) 10:484–5. doi: 10.1097/00019442-200207000-00021

Seyfried LS, Kales HC, Ignacio RV, Conwell Y, Valenstein M. Predictors of suicide in patients with dementia. *Alzheimers Demen.* (2011) 7:567–73. doi: 10.1016/j.jalz.2011.01.006

Lara E, Olaya B, Garin N, Ayuso-Mateos JL, Miret M, Moneta V, et al. Is cognitive impairment associated with suicidality? A population-based study. *Eur Neuropsychopharmacol.* (2015) 25:203–13. doi: 10.1016/j.euroneuro.2014.08.010

Figueira J, Jonsson P, Nordin Adolfsson A, Adolfsson R, Nyberg L, Öhman A. NMR analysis of the human saliva metabolome distinguishes dementia patients from matched controls. *Mol bioSystems.* (2016) 12:2562–71. doi: 10.1039/C6MB00233A

Ship JA, DeCarli C, Friedland RP, Baum BJ. Diminished submandibular salivary flow in dementia of the Alzheimer type. *J Gerontol.* (1990) 45:M61–6. doi: 10.1093/geronj/45.2.M61

Kołodziej U, Maciejczyk M, Miasko A, Matczuk J, Kna´s M, Zukowski P, et al. Oxidative modification in the salivary glands of high fat-diet induced insulin resistant rats. *Front Physiol.* (2017) 8:20. doi: 10.3389/fphys.2017.00020

Burns A, Iliffe S. Dementia. *BMJ.* (2009) 338:b75. doi: 10.1136/bmj.b75

Tu YA, Chen MH, Tsai CF, Su TP, Bai YM, Li CT, et al. Geriatric suicide attempt and risk of subsequent dementia: a nationwide longitudinal follow-up study in Taiwan. *Am J Geriatr Psychiatry.* (2016) 24:1211–8. doi: 10.1016/j.jagp.2016.08.016

Annor FB, Bayakly RA, Morrison RA, Bryan MJ, Gilbert LK, Ivey-Stephenson AZ, et al. Suicide among persons with Dementia, Georgia, 2013 to 2016. *J Geriatr Psychiatry Neurol.* (2019) 32:31–9. doi: 10.1177/0891988718814363

Zucca M, Rubino E, Vacca A, Govone F, Gai A, De Martino P, et al. High risk of suicide in behavioral variant frontotemporal dementia. *Am J Alzheimers Dis Other Demen.* (2019) 34:265–71. doi: 10.1177/1533317518817609

Lai AX, Kaup AR, Yaffe K, Byers AL. High occurrence of psychiatric disorders and suicidal behavior across dementia subtypes. *Am J Geriatr Psychiatry.* (2018) 26:1191–201. doi: 10.1016/j.jagp.2018.08.012

Choi JW, Lee KS, Han E. Suicide risk within 1 year of dementia diagnosis in older adults: a nationwide retrospective cohort study. *J Psychiatry Neurosci.* (2021) 46:E119–27. doi: 10.1503/jpn.190219

Koyama A, Fujise N, Matsushita M, Ishikawa T, Hashimoto M, Ikeda M. Suicidal ideation and related factors among dementia patients. *J Affect Disord.* (2015) 178:66–70. doi: 10.1016/j.jad.2015.02.019

Richard-Devantoy S, Szanto K, Butters MA, Kalkus J, Dombrovski AY. Cognitive inhibition in older high-lethality suicide attempters. *Int J Geriatr Psychiatry.* (2015) 30:274–83. doi: 10.1002/gps.4138

Gujral S, Butters MA, Dombrovski AY, Szanto K. Late-Onset suicide: a dementia prodrome? *Am J Geriatr Psychiatry.* (2021) 29:709–13. doi: 10.1016/j.jagp.2020.12.004

Vandeleur CL, Fassassi S, Castelao E, Glaus J, Strippoli MF, Lasserre AM, et al. Prevalence and correlates of DSM-5 major depressive and related disorders in the community. *Psychiatry Res.* (2017) 250:50–8. doi: 10.1016/j.psychres.2017.01.060

Fiske A, Wetherell JL, Gatz M. Depression in older adults. *Annu Rev Clin Psychol.* (2009) 5:363–89. doi: 10.1146/annurev.clinpsy.032408.153621

Lee SY, Atteraya MS. Depression, poverty, and abuse experience in suicide ideation among older Koreans. *Int J Aging Hum Dev.* (2019) 88:46–59. doi: 10.1177/0091415018768256

Nakamura T, Tsuji T, Nagamine Y, Ide K, Jeong S, Miyaguni Y, et al. Suicide rates, social capital, and depressive symptoms among older adults in japan: an ecological study. *Int J Environ Res Public Health.* (2019) 16:4942. doi: 10.3390/ijerph16244942

Choi JW, Lee SG, Kim TH, Han E. Poststroke suicide risk among older adults in South Korea: a retrospective longitudinal cohort study. *Int J Geriatr Psychiatry.* (2020) 35:282–9. doi: 10.1002/gps.5245

Kiosses DN, Gross JJ, Banerjee S, Duberstein PR, Putrino D, Alexopoulos GS. Negative emotions and suicidal ideation during psychosocial treatments in older adults with major depression and cognitive impairment. *Am J Geriatr Psychiatry.* (2017) 25:620–9. doi: 10.1016/j.jagp.2017.01.011

Yeh ST, Ng YY, Wu SC. Risk of suicide according to the level of psychiatric contact in the older people: analysis of national health insurance databases in Taiwan. *Compr Psychiatry.* (2017) 74:189–95. doi: 10.1016/j.comppsych.2017.01.016

Tan YM, Cheung G. Self-harm in adults: a comparison between the middle-aged and the elderly. *N Z Med J.* (2019) 132:15–29.

Woo S, Lee SW, Lee K, Seo WS, Lee J, Kim HC, et al. Characteristics of high-intent suicide attempters admitted to emergency departments. *J Korean Med Sci.* (2018) 33:e259. doi: 10.3346/jkms.2018.33.e259

Park JI, Yang JC, Han C, Park TW, Chung SK. Suicidal ideation among korean elderly: risk factors and population attributable fractions. *Psychiatry.* (2016) 79:262–81. doi: 10.1080/00332747.2016.1175837

O'Rourke N, Heisel MJ, Canham SL, Sixsmith A, Yaghoubi-Shahir H, King DB, et al. Psychometric validation of the Geriatric Suicide Ideation Scale (GSIS) among older adults with bipolar disorder. *Aging Ment Health.* (2018) 22:794–801. doi: 10.1080/13607863.2017.1317333

O'Rourke N, Heisel MJ, Canham SL, Sixsmith A, BADAS Study Team. Predictors of suicide ideation among older adults with bipolar disorder. *PLoS ONE.* (2017) 12:e0187632. doi: 10.1371/journal.pone.0187632

Almeida OP, McCaul K, Hankey GJ, Yeap BB, Golledge J, Flicker L. Risk of dementia and death in community-dwelling older men with bipolar disorder. *Br J Psychiatry.* (2016) 209:121–6. doi: 10.1192/bjp.bp.115.180059

Belvederi Murri M, Respino M, Proietti L, Bugliani M, Pereira B, D'Amico E, et al. Cognitive impairment in late life bipolar disorder: risk factors and clinical outcomes. *J Affect Disord.* (2019) 257:166–72. doi: 10.1016/j.jad.2019.07.052

Pary R, Sarai SK, Micchelli A, Lippmann S. Anxiety disorders in older patients. *Prim Care Companion CNS Disord.* (2019) 21:18nr02335. doi: 10.4088/PCC.18nr02335

Moye J. Anxiety, physical functioning, and integrated care in older adults. *Clin Gerontol.* (2018) 41:269–70. doi: 10.1080/07317115.2018.1463484

Bakkane Bendixen A, Engedal K, Selbæk G, Hartberg CB. Anxiety symptoms in older adults with depression are associated with suicidality. *Dement Geriatr Cogn Disord.* (2018) 45:180–9. doi: 10.1159/000488480

Petkus AJ, Wetherell JL, Stein MB, Chavira DA, Craske MG, Sherbourne C, et al. Age differences in death and suicidal ideation in anxious primary care patients. *Clin Gerontol.* (2018) 41:271–81. doi: 10.1080/07317115.2017.1356893

Sinyor M, Tan LP, Schaffer A, Gallagher D, Shulman K. Suicide in the oldest old: an observational study and cluster analysis. *Int J Geriatr Psychiatry.* (2016) 31:33–40. doi: 10.1002/gps.4286

Fässberg MM, Cheung G, Canetto SS, Erlangsen A, Lapierre S, Lindner R, et al. A systematic review of physical illness, functional disability, and suicidal behaviour among older adults. *Aging Ment Health.* (2016) 20:166–94. doi: 10.1080/13607863.2015.1083945

Cao R, Jia C, Ma Z, Niu L, Zhou L. Disability in daily living activities, family dysfunction, and late-life suicide in rural China: a case-control psychological autopsy study. *Front Psychiatry.* (2019) 10:827. doi: 10.3389/fpsyt.2019.00827

Opitz-Welke A, Konrad N, Welke J, Bennefeld-Kersten K, Gauger U, Voulgaris A. Suicide in older prisoners in Germany. *Front Psychiatry.* (2019) 10:154. doi: 10.3389/fpsyt.2019.00154

Szanto K, Galfalvy H, Vanyukov PM, Keilp JG, Dombrovski AY. Pathways to late-life suicidal behavior: cluster analysis and predictive validation of suicidal behavior in a sample of older adults with major depression. *J Clin Psychiatry.* (2018) 79:17m11611. doi: 10.4088/JCP.17m11611

Jung J, Roh D, Moon YS, Kim DH. The moderating effect of religion on the relationship between depression and suicidal ideation in the elderly. *J Nerv Ment Dis.* (2017) 205:605–10. doi: 10.1097/NMD.0000000000000637

Kim JP, Yang J. Effectiveness of a community-based program for suicide prevention among elders with early-stage dementia: a controlled observational study. *Geriatr Nurs.* (2017) 38:97– 105. doi: 10.1016/j.gerinurse.2016.08.002

Sakashita T, Oyama H. Developing a hypothetical model for suicide progression in older adults with universal, selective, and indicated prevention strategies. *Front Psychiatry.* (2019) 10:161. doi: 10.3389/fpsyt.2019.00161

Lapierre S, Erlangsen A, Waern M, De Leo D, Oyama H, Scocco P, et al. A systematic review of elderly suicide prevention programs. *Crisis.* (2011) 32:88–98. doi: 10.1027/0227-5910/a000076

Cheung G, Merry S, Sundram F. Medical examiner and coroner reports: uses and limitations in the epidemiology and prevention of late-life suicide. *Int J Geriatr Psychiatry.* (2015) 30:781–92. doi: 10.1002/gp s.4294

Voshaar RC, van der Veen DC, Kapur N, Hunt I, Williams A, Pachana NA. Suicide in patients suffering from late-life anxiety disorders; a comparison with younger patients. *Int Psychogeriatr.* (2015) 27:1197– 205. doi: 10.1017/S1041610215000125

Koo YW, Kõlves K, De Leo D. Suicide in older adults: differences between the young-old, middle-old, and oldest old. *Int Psychogeriatr.* (2017) 29:1297– 306. doi: 10.1017/S1041610217000618

Permissions

List of Contributors

Jialin Fan
School of Psychology, Shenzhen University, Shenzhen, China
Centre for Occupational and Health Psychology, School of Psychology, Cardiff University, Cardiff, United Kingdom

Andrew P. Smith
Centre for Occupational and Health Psychology, School of Psychology, Cardiff University, Cardiff, United Kingdom

Nitin Shivappa and James R. Hebert
Cancer Prevention and Control Program, University of South Carolina, Columbia, SC, United States
Department of Epidemiology and Biostatistics, Arnold School of Public Health, University of South Carolina, Columbia, SC, United States

Asal Neshatbini Tehrani, Bita Bayzai and Bahram Rashidkhani
Department of Community Nutrition, Faculty of Nutrition Sciences and Food Technology, National Nutrition and Food Technology Research Institute (WHO Collaborating Center), Shahid Beheshti University of Medical Sciences, Tehran, Iran

Farah Naja
Nutrition and Food Sciences Department, American University of Beirut, Beirut, Lebanon

David Marchant and Kelly Marrin
Psychology of Sport, Exercise and Movement Research Group, Department of Sport and Physical Activity, Edge Hill University, Ormskirk, United Kingdom

Sophie Hampson
Manchester University NHS Foundation Trust, Manchester, United Kingdom

Lucy Finnigan
School of Sport and Exercise Sciences, Liverpool John Moores University, Liverpool, United Kingdom

Craig Thorley
Department of Psychology, James Cook University, Townsville, QLD, Australia

Wiepke Cahn
Department of Psychiatry, Rudolf Magnus Institute for Neuroscience, University Medical Center Utrecht, Utrecht, Netherlands

Thomas W. Scheewe
Department of Human Movement and Education, Windesheim University of Applied Sciences, Zwolle, Netherlands
Department of Psychiatry, Rudolf Magnus Institute for Neuroscience, University Medical Center Utrecht, Utrecht, Netherlands

Frederike Jörg
Rob Giel Research Center, University Center of Psychiatry, University Medical Center Groningen, University of Groningen, Groningen, Netherlands
Research Department, GGZ Friesland (Friesland Mental Health Services), Leeuwarden, Netherlands

Tim Takken
Child Development and Exercise Center, Wilhelmina Children's Hospital, University Medical Center Utrecht, Utrecht, Netherlands

Jeroen Deenik
GGz Centraal, Amersfoort, Netherlands

Davy Vancampfort
University Psychiatric Center KU Leuven, Leuven, Belgium
Department of Rehabilitation Sciences, KU Leuven, Leuven, Belgium

Frank J. G. Backx
Department of Rehabilitation, Physical Therapy Science and Sports, Rudolf Magnus Institute for Neuroscience, University Medical Center Utrecht, Utrecht, Netherlands

Min Hu and Ming-Qiang Xiang
Department of Sports and Health, Guangzhou Sport University, Guangzhou, China

Zebo Xu
Department of Sports and Health, Guangzhou Sport University, Guangzhou, China
Department of Linguistics and Modern Languages, The Chinese University of Hong Kong, Hong Kong, China

Zi-Rong Wang and Jin Li
Department of Graduation, Guangzhou Sport University, Guangzhou, China

Aura Shoval and Hilary F. Armstrong
Department of Rehabilitation and Regenerative Medicine, Columbia University, New York, NY, United States

Julia Vakhrusheva
Department of Psychiatry, Columbia University, New York, NY, United States

Jacob S. Ballon
Department of Psychiatry and Behavioral Science, Stanford University, Stanford, CA, United States

Matthew N. Bartels
Department of Rehabilitation Medicine, Albert Einstein College of Medicine, Bronx, NY, United States

David Kimhy
Department of Psychiatry, Icahn School of Medicine at Mount Sinai, New York, NY, United States

Anis Ben Chikha
Ksar-Saïd, Manouba University, ECOTIDI UR16ES10, Tunis, Tunisia

Aïmen Khacharem
LIRTES (EA 7313), UFR SESS-STAPS, Paris-East Créteil University, Créteil, France

Khaled Trabelsi
Research Laboratory: Education, Motricité, Sport et Santé, EM2S, LR19JS01, High Institute of Sport and Physical Education of Sfax, University of Sfax, Sfax, Tunisia

Nicola Luigi Bragazzi
Laboratory for Industrial and Applied Mathematics, Department of Mathematics and Statistics, York University, Toronto, ON, Canada

Scott B. Teasdale and Jackie Curtis
Keeping the Body in Mind Program, South Eastern Sydney Local Health District, Sydney, NSW, Australia
School of Psychiatry, UNSW Sydney, Sydney, NSW, Australia

Julia Lappin
School of Psychiatry, UNSW Sydney, Sydney, NSW, Australia

Rebecca Jarman, Tammy Wade and Elisa Rossimel
Keeping the Body in Mind Program, South Eastern Sydney Local Health District, Sydney, NSW, Australia

Philip B. Ward
School of Psychiatry, UNSW Sydney, Sydney, NSW, Australia
Schizophrenia Research Unit, South Western Sydney Local Health District, Ingham Institute for Applied Medical Research, Liverpool, NSW, Australia

Andrew Watkins
Keeping the Body in Mind Program, South Eastern Sydney Local Health District, Sydney, NSW, Australia
Faculty of Health, University of Technology Sydney, Ultimo, NSW, Australia

Katherine Samaras
Department of Endocrinology, St Vincent's Hospital, Sydney, NSW, Australia
Diabetes and Metabolism Division, Garvan Institute of Medical Research, Sydney, NSW, Australia
St Vincent's Clinical School, UNSW Sydney, Sydney, NSW, Australia

Xin Qi and Zhonghui He
Department of Physical Education and Research, Peking University, Beijing, China

Jiajin Tong and Xiangyi Zhu
Beijing Key Laboratory of Behavior and Mental Health, School of Psychological and Cognitive Sciences, Peking University, Beijing, China

Senlin Chen
School of Kinesiology, Louisiana State University, Baton Rouge, LA, United states

John A. Engh, Gry Bang-Kittilsen, Therese T. Bigseth, Tom L. Holmen and Jon Mordal
Division of Mental Health and Addiction, Vestfold Hospital Trust, Tønsberg, Norway

Jens Egeland
Division of Mental Health and Addiction, Vestfold Hospital Trust, Tønsberg, Norway
Department of Psychology, University of Oslo, Oslo, Norway

Ole A. Andreassen
NORMENT, KG Jebsen Centre for Psychosis Research, Oslo, Norway
Division of Mental Health and Addiction, Institute of Clinical Medicine, University of Oslo, Oslo, Norway

Egil W. Martinsen
Division of Mental Health and Addiction, Institute of Clinical Medicine, University of Oslo, Oslo, Norway

Eivind Andersen
Faculty of Humanities, Sports and Educational Science, University of South-Eastern Norway, Horten, Norway

Yingmin Zou, Ping Li and Xinghua Liu
Beijing Key Laboratory of Behavior and Mental Health, School of Psychological and Cognitive Sciences, Peking University, Beijing, China

Stefan G. Hofmann
Department of Psychological and Brain Sciences, Boston University, Boston, MA, United States

Michael de Manincor and Fiona Hargraves
NICM Health Research Institute, Western Sydney University, Westmead, NSW, Australia

Jerome Sarris
NICM Health Research Institute, Western Sydney University, Westmead, NSW, Australia
Professorial Unit, The Melbourne Clinic, Department of Psychiatry, Melbourne University, Melbourne, VIC, Australia

Jack Tsonis
NICM Health Research Institute, Western Sydney University, Westmead, NSW, Australia
THRI, Western Sydney University, Campbelltown, NSW, Australia

Lin Zhu and Long Li
School of Physical Education, Soochow University, Suzhou, China

Lin Wang and Xiaohu Jin
Department of Physical Education, Wuhan University of Technology, Wuhan, China

Huajiang Zhang
College of Physical Education, Hubei University of Arts and Science, Xiangyang, China

Astrid Roeh, Sophie K. Kirchner, Isabel Maurus, Peter Falkai and Alkomiet Hasan
Department of Psychiatry and Psychotherapy, University Hospital, Ludwig-Maximilians University Munich, Munich, Germany

Berend Malchow
Department of Psychiatry and Psychotherapy, Universitätsklinikum Jena, Jena, Germany

Andrea Schmitt
Department of Psychiatry and Psychotherapy, University Hospital, Ludwig-Maximilians University Munich, Munich, Germany
Laboratory of Neuroscience (LIM27), Institute of Psychiatry, University of São Paulo, São Paulo, Brazil

Luca Oppici
Psychology of Learning and Instruction, Department of Psychology, School of Science, Technische Universität Dresden, Dresden, Germany
Centre for Tactile Internet with Human-in-the-Loop (CeTI), Technische Universität Dresden, Dresden, Germany

Emily Frith
Cognitive Neuroscience of Creativity Laboratory, Department of Psychology, Penn State University, State College, PA, United States

James Rudd
Research Institute for Sport and Exercise Sciences, Liverpool John Moores University, Liverpool, United Kingdom

Patrick A. Ho
Department of Psychiatry, Geisel School of Medicine Dartmouth, Hanover, NH, United States

Danielle N. Dahle
Harvard Medical School, Division of Psychotic Disorders, McLean Hospital, Belmont, MA, United States

Douglas L. Noordsy
Department of Psychiatry and Behavioral Sciences, Stanford University School of Medicine, Stanford University, Stanford, CA, United States

Zhuxuan Zhan and Lin Li
Key Laboratory of Adolescent Health Assessment and Exercise Intervention of Ministry of Education, East China Normal University, Shanghai, China
College of Physical Education and Health, East China Normal University, Shanghai, China

Jingyi Ai and Chien-Heng Chu
Department of Physical Education, National Taiwan Normal University, Taipei, Taiwan

Feifei Ren
Graduate Institute of Athletics and Coaching Science, National Taiwan Sport University, Taoyuan, Taiwan
Department of Physical Education, Beijing Language and Culture University, Beijing, China

Yu-Kai Chang
Department of Physical Education, National Taiwan Normal University, Taipei, Taiwan
Institute for Research Excellence in Learning Science, National Taiwan Normal University, Taipei, Taiwan

Eleanor Chadwick and Sarah Reeve
Department of Psychiatry, University of Oxford, Oxford, United Kingdom

Felicity Waite, Jonathan Bradley and Daniel Freeman
Department of Psychiatry, University of Oxford, Oxford, United Kingdom
Sleep and Circadian Neuroscience Institute, University of Oxford, Oxford, United Kingdom
Oxford Health NHS Foundation Trust, Oxford, United Kingdom

Jessica C. Bird
Department of Psychiatry, University of Oxford, Oxford, United Kingdom
Oxford Health NHS Foundation Trust, Oxford, United Kingdom

Mojtaba Abbas-Zadeh
School of Cognitive Sciences, Institute for Research in Fundamental Sciences (IPM), Tehran, Iran

Gholam-Ali Hossein-Zadeh
School of Cognitive Sciences, Institute for Research in Fundamental Sciences (IPM), Tehran, Iran
School of Electrical and Computer Engineering, College of Engineering, University of Tehran, Tehran, Iran

Maryam Vaziri-Pashkam
Laboratory of Brain and Cognition, National Institute of Mental Health, Bethesda, MD, United States

Mendinatou Agbetou
Department of Neurology, University of Parakou, Parakou, Benin
Clinic of Neurology, Teaching Hospital of Parakou, Parakou, Benin

Thierry Adoukonou
Department of Neurology, University of Parakou, Parakou, Benin
Clinic of Neurology, Teaching Hospital of Parakou, Parakou, Benin
Inserm U1094, IRD U270, Univ. Limoges, CHU Limoges, EpiMaCT - Epidemiology of Chronic Diseases in Tropical Zone, Institute of Epidemiology and Tropical Neurology, OmegaHealth, Limoges, France

Grzegorz Bejda
The School of Medical Science in Białystok, Białystok, Poland

Elzbieta Krajewska-Kułak
Department of Integrated Medical Care, Medical University of Białystok, Białystok, Poland

Rudy Bowen, Evyn Peters, Marilyn Baetz and Lloyd Balbuena
University of Saskatchewan, Saskatoon, SK, Canada

Steven Marwaha
Division of Mental Health and Wellbeing, Warwick Medical School, Warwick University, Coventry, UK
Affective Disorder Service (IPU 3-8), Caludon Centre, Coventry, UK

D. L. I. H. K. Peiris and Min Yang
Department of Sport, Physical Education and Health, Faculty of Social Sciences, Hong Kong Baptist University, Kowloon Tong, Hong Kong SAR, China

Wei Liang and Julien Steven Baker
Department of Sport, Physical Education and Health, Faculty of Social Sciences, Hong Kong Baptist University, Kowloon Tong, Hong Kong SAR, China
Centre for Health and Exercise Science Research, Hong Kong Baptist University, Kowloon Tong, Hong Kong SAR, China

Yanping Duan
Department of Sport, Physical Education and Health, Faculty of Social Sciences, Hong Kong Baptist University, Kowloon Tong, Hong Kong SAR, China
Centre for Health and Exercise Science Research, Hong Kong Baptist University, Kowloon Tong, Hong Kong SAR, China
College of Health Sciences, Wuhan Institute of Physical Education, Wuhan, China

Chun Hu
Student Mental Health Education Center, Northwestern Polytechnical University, Xian, China

Borui Shang
Department of Social Science, Hebei Sport University, Shijiazhuang, China

Vesselina Grozeva
Neurology Practice Polyclinic, Sofia, Bulgaria

Ane Mínguez-Olaondo
Department of Neurology, Hospital Universitario Donostia, San Sebastián, Spain

Marta Vila-Pueyo
Headache Group, Wolfson Centre for Age Related Diseases, Institute of Psychiatry, Psychology and Neuroscience, King's College London, London, United Kingdom

Agnieszka Kułak-Bejda and Napoleon Waszkiewicz
Department of Psychiatry, Medical University of Białystok, Białystok, Poland

Index